Intrapartum Management Modules

A Perinatal Education Program

Intrapartum Management Modules

A Perinatal Education Program

Editor

E. JEAN MARTIN, RN, MS, MSN, CNM

Professor Emeritus
College of Nursing, Graduate Nurse-Midwifery
Medical University of South Carolina
Charleston, South Carolina

3RD
EDITION

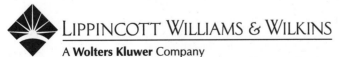

LIPPINCOTT WILLIAMS & WILKINS
A **Wolters Kluwer** Company

Philadelphia · Baltimore · New York · London
Buenos Aires · Hong Kong · Sydney · Tokyo

Acquisitions Editor: Jennifer Brogan
Managing Editor: Barclay Cunningham
Designer: Carolyn O'Brien

Third Edition

9 8 7 6 5

ISBN: 0-7817-3237-9
Library of Congress Cataloging-in-Publication Data is available upon request.

Care has been taken to confirm the accuracy of the information presented and to describe generally accepted practices. However, the authors, editors, and publisher are not responsible for errors or omissions or for any consequences from application of the information in this book and make no warranty, express or implied, with respect to the content of the publication.

The authors, editors, and publisher have exerted every effort to ensure that drug selection and dosage set forth in this text are in accordance with the current recommendations and practice at the time of publication. However, in view of ongoing research, changes in government regulations, and the constant flow of information relating to drug therapy and drug reactions, the reader is urged to check the package insert for each drug for any change in indications and dosage and for added warnings and precautions. This is particularly important when the recommended agent is a new or infrequently employed drug.

Some drugs and medical devices presented in this publication have Food and Drug Administration (FDA) clearance for limited use in restricted research settings. It is the responsibility of the health care provider to ascertain the FDA status of each drug or device planned for use in his or her clinical practice.

99 00
4 5 6 7 8 9 10

This edition is dedicated to you, the reader, who in rendering care touches not only the body but perhaps the soul. On behalf of the mothers and babies you care for in a knowledgeable, safe, and sensitive manner—"thank you."

P R E F A C E

There is no substitute for clinical competency in the provision of direct patient care—and no easy way to achieve and maintain competency. It presumes, among many efforts, the continual acquisition of new knowledge and a consummate ability to apply that information in a highly individualized, safe, and therapeutic manner.

This third edition continues to focus on aspects of perinatal care that are of interest to health care providers and primary care providers such as nurse-midwives, nurse-practitioners, family practice physicians, physician assistants, and students in medical and nursing programs. It is, however, dedicated to staff nurses who work in the intrapartal setting, because this special group of caregivers is thought to be our primary readership.

The key to sound perinatal care practice is prevention of potential problems and early recognition of existing problems. Deliveries occur in community hospitals far more frequently than in regional centers. However, funding and staffing constraints can result in limited continuing education opportunities for staff nurses in regional and community hospitals. The goal of this book is to provide the staff nurse or in-service educator with a self-paced, essentially self-instructional syllabus that addresses clinical practice knowledge, issues, and skills essential to the care of the laboring woman and the fetus. All learning activities may take place in the hospital. Written for busy professionals, this book is intended to educate, update, and motivate.

Standards, guidelines, and priorities for care are drawn from current literature and the collective wisdom of professional organizations such as AWHONN, ACNM, ACOG, AAP, and CDC, as well as consensus panels and research publications under NIH. Evidence-based practice issues are considered. The reader is referred to excellent resources under both References and Suggested Readings in the expectation that further study will be pursued. A keen curiosity, an open mind, and reflection are needed to recognize and optimize sound information as it evolves. Ensuring that a "best practice" approach is integrated into the perinatal care setting takes considerable team building between nurses and physicians. A reasoned, planned consensus on important aspects of care sustains the clinical application of the best information available.

This book is not intended to replace standard texts. Topics are pertinent to the assessment of the pregnant woman and fetus, as well as the newly delivered mother and her newborn. Most modules have undergone extensive revision. New topics have been added, such as perinatal issues of the intrauterine growth–restricted fetus, alternative therapies for intrapartum pain management, perinatal consequences of hepatitis C infection, CDC guidelines for hepatitis A immunization, and an overview of STDs and adverse pregnancy outcomes. The module on diabetes has been greatly expanded to include antepartum and postpartum management issues.

Care has been taken to ensure that the drugs and treatment regimens outlined are correct and compatible with the standards generally accepted at the time of publication. Clinical topics not addressed in this text are covered in other available resources. Your feedback will guide us in determining content to be included in future editions.

The program is organized into 17 modules of self-instructional material. Although you should progress through each module at your own pace, an effort should be made to complete the course in 12 weeks. The material reads more like a succinct study guide than a textbook. It requires thoughtful perusal. New content may need a reread and study. Do not become discouraged when reading. Knowledge and technology are evolving at a rapid pace. In keeping with this, the content of this book has become increasingly sophisticated. Some of the content involves very complex subject matter. A detailed description of each of the skills essential to intrapartal nursing care accompanies the appropriate module. If this program is being implemented by your institution or an outside agency, clinical preceptors will be appointed to assist you in the development or refinement of the skills you are learning. If you are studying this program independently, you will need to negotiate a contract with a clinician (nurse or primary care provider such as a physician or nurse-midwife) for supervision and, finally, validation of your skill achievement.

Practice/Review sections provide an opportunity for recall of what you have learned. If you need to review the information, you can do so immediately. The *Posttests* and *Posttest Answer Keys,* which follow the appendices, will enable you to validate your comprehension of material from the modules and find the correct answer for any questions missed.

"Guidelines for Implementing a Perinatal Education Program" are provided in Appendix D for hospital institutions or health department agencies who wish to offer the program on a large scale. These guidelines include overall protocols for implementing the program, a sample introductory letter, sample workshop agenda, participant checklist, and evaluation. The surveys will assist the sponsoring institution in making revisions for program offerings in the future.

Believe that the care you give has the ability to have a profound effect on the woman and her family. However, the dynamics of such interactions work both ways. And gratitude is ours for being allowed to participate in one of life's most incredible events!

E. Jean Martin, RN, MS, MSN, CNM

A C K N O W L E D G E M E N T S

As this text is readied for a third edition, I am reminded of its history and am very grateful to key individuals instrumental in its origins.

Special appreciation is owed to Henry C. Heins, Jr., MD, MPH, for his contributions, foresight, and leadership. Dr. Heins initiated the original perinatal outreach program for South Carolina under the auspices of the Department of Obstetrics and Gynecology and the Nurse-Midwifery Program and the Medical University of South Carolina with the support of the Robert Wood Johnson Foundation and the Improved Pregnancy Outcome Project of South Carolina.

I also thank members of the Department of Pediatrics, University of Virginia Health Sciences Center, Charlottesville, Virginia, who pioneered one of the first self-instructional perinatal outreach programs in the United States. They have generously granted permission for the use of their highly successful text format and program plan on which this book is based. Their program on maternal, fetal, and newborn evaluation and care continues to be updated and available. Components of the program and an address are cited at the end of Module 15 under a "resource of note."

Donna M. Childs-Vincent, RN, BSN, MA, formerly Nursing Consultant and Perinatal Outreach Clinical Specialist, Huntington Beach and Los Angeles, California, authored the Guidelines for Implementation for the first and second editions. Their relevance continues for this third edition.

Our thanks to the following staff members who assisted in the retrieval of fetal monitoring strips used in Module 6: from Overland Park Regional Medical Center, Overland Park, Kansas: Bob Davis, Surgical OBT; Becky Jackson, RNC, BSN; Cher Macek, RNC, BSN; Sharon Millberger, RNC; and Leslie Porch, RN, BSN. Thanks also to Mary Jane Dexter, BSN, and Christy Mazur, BSN, of St. Luke's South Hospital, Overland Park, Kansas.

Many hardworking, gifted people contributed to this present edition. It is a pleasure to thank them and acknowledge their expertise. To the following individuals for their review of selected manuscripts and helpful advice:

☐ Susan F. Bellebaum, RNC, Instructor, AWHONN Fetal Heart Monitoring Principles and Practices (FHMPP), Summerville Medical Center Summerville, South Carolina. Manuscript reviewer for the intrapartum fetal monitoring content in Module 6.

☐ Roberta A. Kimsey, MSN, CNM, in private practice with Carolina Nurse-Midwives, Charlotte, North Carolina. Manuscript reviewer for the intrapartum content and skills in Module 5.

☐ Jill Mauldin, MD, Assistant Professor, Medical University of South Carolina, College of Medicine, Department of Obstetrics and Gynecology, Division of Maternal-Fetal Medicine, Charleston, South Carolina. Consultant and manuscript reviewer for the content related to care of the HIV-infected laboring woman in Module 11 and care of the intrapartum patient with diabetes in Module 13.

☐ Stephen T. Vermillion, MD, Assistant Professor, Medical University of South Carolina, College of Medicine, Department of Obstetrics and Gynecology, Division of Maternal-Fetal Medicine, Charleston, South Carolina. Consultant and manuscript reviewer for the content related to care of the HIV-infected laboring woman in Module 11.

I am indebted to Francine R. Margolius, EdD, MSN, RN, FAAN, Associate Professor, Medical University of South Carolina, College of Nursing, for authorship of *Comfort Care for the Dying Newborn* in Appendix C. Throughout much of her academic career, pain management in the very young patient has been a key research and clinical focus. Despite extraordinarily difficult circumstances at the time of writing, she has been able to provide our readers with the key elements about effective pain management for the dying newborn. It is hoped that these elements will be used by health professionals in developing standards and policies to consistently prevent and relieve unnecessary discomfort and pain.

My thanks to Ida A. Desrosiers, who has devoted many after-work hours to assisting with literature searches and document retrieval.

One has only to scan the pages of this book to know that preparing an electronic manuscript or hardcopy would be exacting, requiring considerable computer skills and creativity. Stephanie Joy Lindsey has stayed with me every step of the way! I'm especially grateful that she thinks critically as she types. God bless!

This has not been a lonely effort. The College of Nursing administrative and departmental faculty agreed to let me retain my office and other coveted spaces. My work ethic centers here. Colleagues' queries and encouragement lent a quality to my life and this writing effort that could never have been achieved elsewhere.

William & Wilkins, publishers of the first and second editions of *Intrapartum Management Modules,* is now merged with Lippincott. I gratefully acknowledge the encouragement, patience, and editorial support given by Jennifer E. Brogan, Director of Nursing Practice; Susan Barta Rainey, Assistant Editor, Nursing Publishing; and Barclay Cunningham, Managing Editor. Special thanks to Barclay, who has guided, problem solved, and reassured throughout this effort.

Suzanne Kastner of Graphic World Publishing Services has seen this book through many phases of production. I appreciate the impact her expertise has made on the final product.

And finally, the contributors to this book are special people in my world. All are either faculty or graduates of the Nurse-Midwifery Education Program at the Medical University of South Carolina. They are expert clinicians, self-actualized individuals, who are sensitive and generous but exacting in setting professional standards for themselves and others through their clinical practice, teaching, and writing. My heartfelt thanks to each one for her unique assistance in producing this third edition.

CONTRIBUTORS

Joan G. Andres, RN, MSN, CNM
Nurse Midwife, Private Practice
Southside OB/GYN, P.C.
Richmond Hill, Georgia

Marcella T. Hickey, RN, MSN, CNM
Assistant Professor
Acting Director, Graduate Nurse-Midwifery
Education Program
College of Nursing
Medical University of South Carolina
Charleston, South Carolina

E. Jean Martin, RN, MS, MSN, CNM
Professor Emeritus
College of Nursing, Graduate Nurse-
Midwifery
Medical University of South Carolina
Charleston, South Carolina

Mary Copeland Myers, RN, BSN, MSN,
CNM, CDE
Instructor
Division of Maternal-Fetal Medicine
College of Medicine, Department of
Obstetrics and Gynecology
Medical University of South Carolina
Charleston, South Carolina

Meegan D. Page, RN, MS, MSN, CNM
Nurse-Midwife, Private Practice
For Women Only
Overland Park, Kansas

Patricia Ann Payne, RN, CNM, MPH
Adjunct Clinical Professor
Department of Family Medicine
Research Fellow, Cecil G. Sheps Center for
Health Services Research
University of North Carolina at Chapel Hill
Chapel Hill, North Carolina

Nancy Webster Smith, RN, MSN, CNM
Nurse Midwife, Private Practice
Lowcountry Obstetrics and Gynecology
Mt. Pleasant, South Carolina

Ann Mogabgab Weathersby, RN, MSN,
CNM
Assistant Manager of Obstetrics and
Gynecology
Piedmont Practice Service Director
Kaiser Permanente
Atlanta, Georgia

CONTENTS

M O D U L E   3
Admission Assessment of the Laboring Woman   61
E. JEAN MARTIN

M O D U L E   4
Admission Assessment of the Fetus   97
E. JEAN MARTIN

MODULE 7
Induction and Augmentation of Labor   293
MARCELLA T. HICKEY

MODULE 8
Caring for the Woman at Risk for Preterm Labor or With Premature Rupture of Membranes   321
NANCY WEBSTER SMITH

MODULE 9
Caring for the Laboring Woman With Hypertensive Disorders Complicating Pregnancy 349
E. JEAN MARTIN

M O D U L E   1 0
Intrauterine Growth Restriction: Perinatal Issues and Management   399

JOAN G. ANDRES

M O D U L E   1 1
Caring for the Laboring Woman With HIV Infection or AIDS   437

MARY COPELAND MYERS

M O D U L E   1 2
Hepatitis B Infection: Maternal–Newborn Management (Hepatitis A and C addressed) 473

E. JEAN MARTIN

M O D U L E   1 6
Informed Consent and Documentation   601

MARCELLA T. HICKEY

PART 1

PART 2

M O D U L E   1 7
Maternal Transport   617

E. JEAN MARTIN

Glossary   633

A P P E N D I X   A
Sexually Transmitted Diseases: Overview, Perinatal Issues, and Management   641

A P P E N D I X   B

M O D U L E   1

Overview of Labor

E. JEAN MARTIN

As you complete this module, you will learn:

1. Current theories and concepts on labor physiology and initiation
2. The stages of labor
3. The anatomic divisions of the uterus undergoing labor
4. Characteristics and terms used to describe uterine contractions
5. Characteristics of normal uterine contractions
6. Appropriate timing of vaginal examination to evaluate cervical dilatation
7. Techniques for evaluating uterine contractions
8. Effective ways to support the laboring woman
9. A definition of cultural competence and characteristics of a culturally competent practitioner.

When you have completed this module, you should be able to recall the meaning of the following terms. You should also be able to use the terms when consulting with other health professionals. The terms are defined in this module or in the glossary at the end of this book.

cervix
contraction
corticotropin-releasing factor (CRF)
cytokines
decidua
endogenous

gap junctions
macrophages
parturition
placenta
progesterone
prostaglandins

Labor and Birth: A Medical View

Identifying Features of Labor

■ What is labor?

Labor can be defined medically as regular, progressively intense uterine contractions that, over time, produce cervical effacement and dilatation, leading to the development of expulsive forces adequate to move the fetus through the birth canal against the resistance of soft tissue, muscle, and the bony structure of the pelvis.

A number of biochemical, physiologic, and pharmacologic pathways are thought to exist; it is through these pathways that labor is initiated and maintained. The exact mechanism for labor initiation and progression has not yet been fully revealed. Improved experimental laboratory techniques and increasingly sophisticated research approaches *in humans* are leading to better understanding of the numerous hormonal interactions in human labor and birth.[1]

There is no doubt that under hormonal influences, the uterus is maintained in a quiescent state throughout most of pregnancy. One investigative goal is to identify the stimulus that triggers the biochemical cascade leading to labor.[2] Certainly, a dramatic physiologic change is involved in taking a pregnancy from the state of relatively low-level antepartum uterine contractility to the coordinated, intense uterine contractility of labor.

Labor Initiation and Maintenance

- All parts of the uterus undergo preparation for labor and delivery *(parturition)*.[3]
- Hormonal mediators from the placenta and maternal and fetal endocrine glands are believed to affect the regulation of the uterine musculature (myometrium).
- In pregnancy the lining of the uterus (the endometrium) is referred to as the *decidua*. Experiencing marked change in thickness and vascularity, the decidua has the capacity to alter hormonal proportions (e.g., estrogen increases over progesterone content) and enzymes and to nourish the embryo. Special decidual cells called *macrophages* synthesize prostaglandins and another group of compounds called cytokines.[4]
- Direct tissue-to-tissue communication occurs among uterine musculature, the decidua, and fetal membranes.[4]
- The uterine myometrium consists of thick and thin contractile fibers grouped in bundles. Few intracellular contacts between them exist until late in pregnancy. At that time, areas between muscle fiber cells develop pathways for communication (cell to cell). These pathways are called *gap junctions*. They are clearly present in great numbers as parturition nears. These efficient cell-to-cell gap junctions serve as channels for the transfer of chemical and electrical signals from one muscle fiber cell to another. Simultaneous contractions of a majority of cells are needed to make an effective contraction. This synchronization of the uterine muscle fibers leads to efficient, coordinated *contractions,* which soften, thin, and dilate the cervix.[3]
- A placental hormone called *corticotropin-releasing factor* (CRF) is released into maternal circulation early in the second trimester, with concentrations rising significantly as pregnancy advances. CRF production increases the strength of contractions and stimulates production of oxytocin and prostaglandins.[2]
- *Prostaglandins* are chemicals derived from the fetus, amniotic membranes, decidua, and other sources. They cause smooth muscle contraction and vasoconstriction, soften ("ripen") cervical tissue, and modulate hormonal activity.[4,5] Not all clinical researchers are convinced that prostaglandins initiate labor, but all do postulate a key role for these hormones, particularly PGF and PGE_2.[4]
- *Cytokines* are an important group of compounds. These compounds have numerous functions in labor physiology, which act either synergistically or antagonistically.
- Calcium (the calcium ion) is vital for the contractile process in myometrial cells, which depends on the influx of extracellular free calcium. The calcium ion also plays a critical role in transmitting signals of excitation from the myometrial cell membranes to the contractile complex inside the cell.[3]

✳*NOTE: Agents that block this movement of calcium, called calcium channel blockers (e.g., nifedipine), are in fact used as tocolytic agents for the purpose of suppressing uterine contractility.*

- The initiation of labor depends on both maternal and fetal signals, both using oxytocin as a signal.[3]
- The nonpregnant or very early gravid uterus is not sensitive to oxytocin. However, oxytocin is secreted in pulses of low frequency throughout pregnancy.[3]
- As the uterus gradually approaches term, it is thought that the myometrium becomes increasingly responsive to oxytocic hormones, mainly PGE_2 and PGF. Toward the end of pregnancy, the number of oxytocin receptors increases, peaking in the myometrium and decidua in early labor.
- Secretion of oxytocin seems to be in a pulsatile fashion, even in labor.[3] See Figures 1.1 and 1.2.

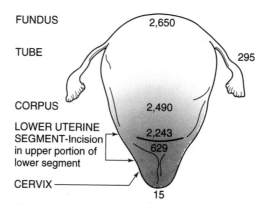

FIGURE 1.1 Distribution of oxytocin receptors in a pregnant human uterus, removed in preterm labor at 34 weeks. Numbers denote oxytocin receptors (OTRs) per unit measurement (fmol/mg DNA). (Reprinted with permission from Fuchs, A. R., & Fuchs, R. [1996]. Physiology and endocrinology of parturition. In S. G. Gabbe, J. R. Niebyl, & J. L. Simpson [Eds.] *Obstetrics: Normal and problem pregnancies* [3rd ed., p. 123]. New York: Churchill Livingstone.)

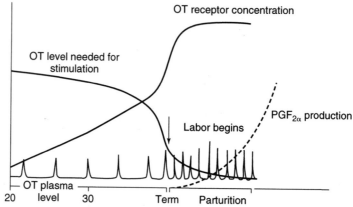

FIGURE 1.2 Diagrammatic representation of the concentration of myometrial oxytocin, the level of oxytocin needed to elicit contractions, and maternal plasma oxytocin levels at the end of gestation and during labor. Oxytocin is secreted in pulses of low frequency. During labor, pulse frequency increases. Fetal secretion of oxytocin can be considerable and may contribute to the oxytocin level reaching the myometrium. PGF production does not increase significantly until labor is in progress and then increases progressively throughout the third stage of labor. OT, oxytocin. (Reprinted with permission from Fuchs, A. R., & Fuchs, R. [1996]. Physiology and endocrinology of parturition. In S. G. Gabbe, J. R. Niebyl, & J. L. Simpson [Eds.]. *Obstetrics: Normal and problem pregnancies* [3rd ed., p. 124]. New York: Churchill Livingstone.)

- Maternal plasma concentrations of endogenous oxytocin are equivalent to a range of 4 to 6 mU/min during the first stage of labor.[6]

Identifying Stages and Phases of Labor

■ How are the parts of the labor process described?[3,7]

For the sake of description, labor is divided into the following four stages:

Stage I Stage I begins with the onset of regular uterine contractions and lasts until full dilatation of the cervix is achieved. Dilatation is the *gradual opening of the cervical entrance* to the uterus. Stage I can be divided further into *two phases*, which are predictable in normal labor.

Latent phase—begins with fairly regular contractions until rapid cervical dilatation begins. It usually lasts several hours.

Active phase—begins with rapid cervical dilatation and lasts until full dilatation of the cervix occurs.

Stage II Stage II begins with full cervical dilatation and lasts until the baby is born.

Stage III Stage III is that part of the process after the birth of the baby in which the placenta is delivered.

Stage IV Stage IV is that part of the process after the delivery of the placenta in which the uterus effectively contracts, preventing excessive bleeding. This is a period of adjustment as the mother's body functions begin to stabilize.

> Careful assessment of the laboring woman's progress through this predictable pattern can be helpful in early detection of problems.

Evaluating Contractions

■ How is the uterus suited to accomplish labor and birth?

The uterus is composed of *three* layers of tissue. These layers are arranged as shown in Figure 1.3.

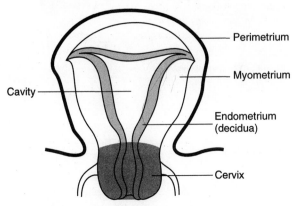

FIGURE 1.3 The three major tissue layers of the uterus.

NOTE: The endometrium is altered through hormonal influences during pregnancy to become what is called the decidua, which functions to maintain the pregnancy.

1. **Perimetrium**—a thick outer membrane covering the uterus.
2. **Myometrium**—the middle layer that contains special muscle cells called *myometrial cells.*
3. **Endometrium**—the innermost layer containing glands and nutrient tissue.

Figure 1.4 illustrates the changes in the uterus and cervix as normal labor progresses.

Under the influence of myometrial contractions, labor progresses with the uterus becoming separated into *two distinct parts*. The upper portion becomes *thicker* and more powerful because of shortening and thickening of the myometrial fibers. This prepares the uterus to exert the effort necessary to push the baby out at birth. The lower portion of the uterus becomes *thinner, softer,* and *more relaxed* as the myometrial fibers relax and become longer. As a result, the baby can more easily be pushed out at birth.

Downward pressure caused by the contraction of the fundal segment is gradually transmitted to the passive lower segment or cervical portion, causing effacement (thinning of the cervix)

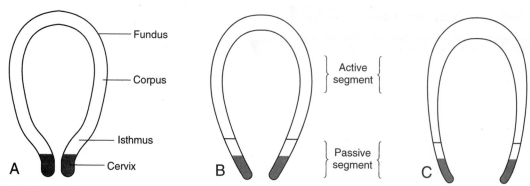

FIGURE 1.4 Changes in the uterus and cervix as normal labor progresses. **A.** Uterus and cervix at term. **B.** Uterus and cervix early in Stage I. **C.** Uterus and cervix in Stage II.

and dilatation. The cervix is drawn upward and over the baby, allowing it to descend into the passageway. The cervix is made up of an inner part called the internal os and an outer part called the external os. Figure 1.5 demonstrates how the internal and external os change position as effacement occurs.

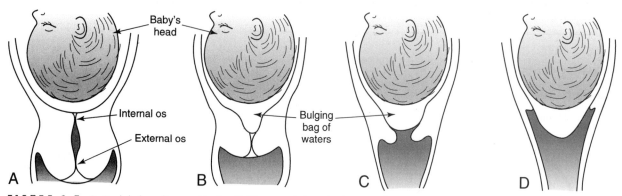

FIGURE 1.5 A. Cervix before effacement begins. **B.** Effacement in its early phase. **C.** Effacement with some dilatation. **D.** Complete effacement and dilatation.

■ How are uterine contractions described?

Contractions have a wavelike pattern that can be divided into segments (Fig. 1.6).

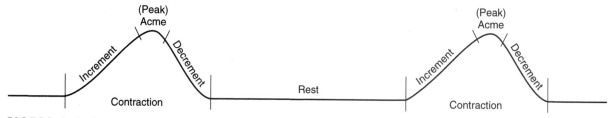

FIGURE 1.6 The segments of a contraction.

- Increment—usually makes up the *longest* part of the contraction.
- Acme—the *shortest,* but most intense, part of the contraction.
- Decrement—a fairly rapid diminishing of the contraction.

Four characteristics of a contraction have been identified:

1. **Frequency**—This is how often the contractions are occurring. Contractions can begin 10 to 15 minutes apart but get closer together as labor progresses. They can occur as frequently as 2 to 3 minutes apart late in the labor process.

2. **Regularity**—As labor becomes well established, contractions occur with a rhythmic pattern.
3. **Duration**—The length of contractions increases as labor progresses. Contractions in early labor can be as short as 30 seconds and gradually increase to 90 seconds.
4. **Intensity**—This characteristic can be assessed as mild, moderate, or strong. The strength of contractions increases as labor intensifies. To obtain an estimate of the intensity, you can palpate the mother's abdomen with your hand. A true assessment of the contraction's intensity can be obtained only by using an internal uterine monitor, which is described in detail in Module 6.

NOTE: In normal labor *the intensity (or amplitude) of the contraction varies from 30 to 55 mm Hg and the frequency is 2 to 5 contractions every 10 minutes.* In prolonged labor *the intensity of the contractions is less than 25 mm Hg and the frequency is fewer than 2 contractions every 10 minutes.* No labor is occurring if the intensity is less than 15 mm Hg.

The duration and frequency of a contraction can be diagrammed as in Figure 1.7.

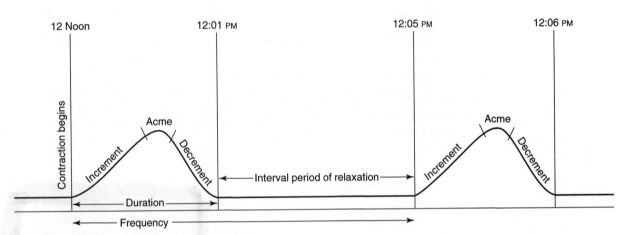

FIGURE 1.7 Frequency and duration of contractions.

Notice that the duration of a contraction is timed from the beginning of the increment to the end of the decrement. The frequency of a contraction is timed from the beginning of one contraction to the beginning of the next.

Although the interval between contractions is referred to as a period of relaxation, in fact, the uterus never entirely relaxes between contractions. It maintains what is called a resting tone, a result of increased tension and thickening of muscle fibers in the upper portion of the uterus.

Contractions are assessed in three basic ways:

1. **Subjectively**—This is a description given by the patient. She will respond to questions such as "When did they start?" "How often are they coming?" "How long do they last?" and "Are they getting stronger?"
2. **Palpation**—This is an efficient method of assessment using the palmar surface of the fingertips. Fingertips should be kept moving throughout the contraction to continually palpate the changing uterus through the abdominal wall.

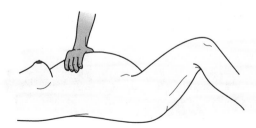

FIGURE 1.8 Palm or surface of the fingers palpates for intensity and duration of a contraction.

The intensity of the uterine contraction can be described as follows:

- Mild—The uterus can be indented with gentle pressure.
- Moderate—The uterus will indent only with firm pressure at the peak of a contraction.
- Strong—The uterus feels firm or hard and cannot be indented at the peak of a contraction.

> Your moving fingertips pick up the changes within a contraction as it gains in intensity and then recedes. Do this carefully so that you do not cause discomfort to the laboring woman.

3. **Electronic fetal monitoring**—This type of fetal monitoring can be used as an external or internal monitoring method. The external method involves the use of electronic equipment that measures and records the frequency and duration of contractions. The intensity of contractions can be truly measured only with the internal method. True representation of heart rate variability is obtained only with the internal method (fetal spiral electrode).

If you are assessing contractions, it is suggested that you sit at the bedside for 20 to 40 minutes (depending on the general frequency of contraction), with your fingertips lightly placed over the fundal portion of the mother's abdomen. This will enable you to detect accurately the beginning and end of the contraction. You cannot depend on signals from the mother—such as restlessness or a statement that the contraction is beginning—because she is often unaware of the initial changes in the uterine muscle.

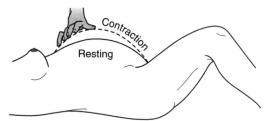

FIGURE 1.9 The palpating fingers are placed near the top of the uterus.

> When feeling for the general intensity and duration of a contraction, the best area of the mother's abdomen on which to place your fingertips is near the top of the uterus.

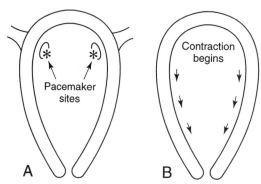

FIGURE 1.10 A. Sites where the uterine contraction begins (pacemaker sites). **B.** Contraction pathway.

The reason for placing your fingertips near the top of the uterus is that the uterus has pacemakers located there. These pacemakers are a group of highly excitable myometrial cells that are responsible for starting contractions. They are located on either side of the uterus near the oviducts or fallopian tubes: *The contraction begins at the top of the uterus and sweeps down over the main body of the uterus.*

Each contraction wave has three components:

1. **Propagation** of the wave starts at the pacemaker site. The wave starts above and moves downward toward the lower part of the uterus.
2. **Duration** of the contraction lessens progressively as the wave moves away from the pacemaker. Throughout any contraction the upper portion of the uterus is in action for a longer period than the lower portion.
3. **Intensity** of the contraction decreases from the top to the bottom of the uterus; that is, the upper segment of the uterus contracts more strongly than the lower.

NOTE: Analysis of wave properties of the uterine contraction indicates that the full impact of the contraction is not felt at the cervix until the last half of the contraction.

Vaginal examination to determine cervical dilatation should be performed throughout a contraction and not between contractions. The woman should be prepared for this and helped to understand why the examination is done during a contraction. It is imperative that the examiner also understand the rationale. Vaginal examinations between contractions in actively laboring women will not always provide a true picture of what is happening to the cervix. Vaginal examinations during labor are discussed in Module 5.

To obtain a true assessment of contraction length and frequency, carefully palpate the abdomen for at least 30 minutes.

NOTE: When using electronic uterine and fetal monitoring, always palpate uterine contractions and auscultate maternal and fetal heart rates in the first few minutes of using the equipment. This validates that the equipment is working properly.

Labor and Birth: Reflections From a Different View

"Birth is not only about making babies. Birth is also about making mothers—strong, competent, capable mothers who trust themselves and know their inner strength."[7]

The experience of pregnancy and childbirth, although shared with husbands or partners, is uniquely female. It is life-altering, one of nature's most powerful events. The manner in which a woman experiences birth has profound implications, possibly affecting the quality of her immediate infant interaction and subsequent parenting. Research shows that childbirth affects a woman's self-esteem and can also affect her emotional availability to her infant.[8]

McKay maintains that the birth setting and its participants powerfully influence the childbirth experience, shaping roles and the amount of control held by the woman herself, those who support her, and her caregivers.[9] McKay goes on to state, "The outcome can be an environment of support, enabling the woman to experience her power and control or, at the opposite end of the spectrum, [the result is] managed birth where the principal actors are the caregivers, their procedures, and technology" (p. 283).

Supporting the Laboring Woman

Effective labor support involves the following:

- A thorough understanding of the physiologic and anatomic adaptations involved in labor and birth
- Compassion for the enormous but individualized adaptive responses required on the part of the woman and her family in the birth process
- Knowledge of the woman's (and her support person's) preparation, understanding, and goals for the birth experience
- Commitment to provide continuous support for the woman and her family and to work at facilitating this philosophy of care on the birth unit.

> The continuous presence of a support person reduces the likelihood of medication for pain relief, operative vaginal delivery, cesarean delivery, and a 5-minute Apgar score of less than 7.[10]

Current efforts are directed at making birthing units in hospitals more family-centered, home-like, and baby-friendly. The World Health Organization has promoted the Baby-Friendly Hospital Initiative, urging hospitals worldwide to be baby-friendly by giving support to breastfeeding. However, much more current research and understanding of babies, their intimate relationship with their mothers, and their developmental life in the womb (i.e., in cognitive, sensory, and emotional dimensions) need to be embraced and applied to 21st century obstetric practices.[11]

"Babies are not what we thought they were in the 19th century or even what we thought they were twenty-five years ago. . . . The finding's of psychology are so revolutionary that virtually everything we believed a quarter of a century ago has been discredited and a new encyclopedia of knowledge has been written" (p. 127).[12]

Chamberlain has conducted extensive research and written about prenatal and newborn clinical findings for years.[12,13] He believes that a new paradigm for a new view of babies, both the newborn and unborn, is in order, stating, "babies of whatever age are aware, expressive, and affected by their interactions with us"[12] (p. 130). This is important information for everyone who has a role in birthing and caring for babies: nurses, physicians, midwives, practitioners, childbirth educators, and parents.

> "It is something to be able to paint a particular picture, or to carve a statue, and so to make a few objects beautiful; but it is far more glorious to carve and paint the very atmosphere and medium through which we look, which morally we can do. To affect the quality of the day, that is the highest of the arts."
>
> —Henry David Thoreau, *Walden*

Practices that will provide support for the laboring woman, her unborn baby, and her coach include the following:

1. *Make the mother and her unborn baby the central focus in the situation* and include her coach through all phases of labor and birth.
   - Introduce yourself and others who might be providing care.
   - Inform the mother and her coach of her progress.
   - Include the mother and her coach in conversations with others.
   - Offer choices when possible.
   - Actively support the coach in his or her efforts to help the mother.
   - Think of the unborn baby as a sensing, responsive, and social being as you give care. Use touch, sound, and light as soothing, even therapeutic, elements.
2. Ensure the mother's privacy.
   - Try to provide a private labor room.
   - Orient the mother to her surroundings.
   - Keep the mother draped adequately.
   - Request the mother's permission for procedures and examinations and keep her coach updated and involved.
   - Control the environment according to the mother's wishes (e.g., a darkened or bright room, open or closed door, quiet atmosphere).
3. Promote preparedness.
   - Assess the mother's knowledge level and preparedness. Give information about labor and birth that addresses where she is in labor. Use simple, direct terminology appropriate to her level of understanding and ability to take it in at the time. Orient the mother and coach to the expected time frame for labor. Update this as necessary.
   - Instruct the mother and coach in relaxation, breathing, and pushing techniques. For mothers who have attended classes, these techniques might need to be reviewed. Give brief, practical instructions to the unprepared mother.
4. Instill confidence.
   - Praise the efforts of the mother and her coach.
   - Speak positively about labor and delivery events. For example, when giving a sedative, tell the mother that the medication will help her relax.

- Stay with the mother if she is without a coach. If you must leave her for a brief time, tell her why and when you will return.
- Provide a call light or buzzer when you are out of the room.
- Inform the mother and coach in advance of special procedures or examinations.
- Use vocabulary that is suited to the needs of the mother and coach and ensure that they understand.
- Encourage a family member to remain with the mother throughout labor and include this person in your explanations and care. Remember, coaches need reassurance too.

5. Apply culturally competent care to each woman and family.

The perinatal nurse's care is often directed to women and families from diverse cultures. Major cultural groups in the United States include African Americans/Blacks, American Indians/Alaska Natives, Asian Americans/Pacific Islanders, Hispanics/Latinos, and Whites/Caucasians. These women and their families approach childbirth within their cultural context, that is, a set of core values, cultural beliefs, and practices.[14]

Cultural competence is defined by Rorie, Paine, and Barger as a set of behaviors, attitudes, and policies that enable a system, agency, and/or individual to function effectively with culturally diverse patients and communities.[15] Groups might also include the homeless, migrants, and refugees. Providing care in a cultural-competent manner is a progressive and developmental, but conscious, process that should be a focus for the clinically competent nurse. These authors go on to outline traits that identify the culturally competent practitioner (Display 1.1).

DISPLAY 1.1	Characteristics of the Culturally Competent Practioner

Moves from cultural unawareness to an awareness of and sensitivity to own cultural heritage

Recognizes own values and biases and is aware of how he or she may affect patients from other cultures

Demonstrates comfort with cultural differences that exist between self and patients

Knows specifics about the particular cultural group(s) with which he or she works

Understands the historical events that may have caused harm to particular cultural groups

Respects and is aware of the unique needs of patients from diverse communities

Understands the importance of diversity within as well as between cultures

Endeavors to learn more about cultural communities through patient interactions, participation in cultural diversity workshops and community events, readings on cultural dynamics, and consultations with community experts

Makes a continuous effort to understand the other's point of view

Demonstrates flexibility and tolerance of ambiguity; is nonjudgmental

Maintains a sense of humor and an open mind

Demonstrates a willingness to relinquish control in clinical encounters; to risk failure; and to look within for the source of frustration, anger, and resistance

Acknowledges that the process is as important as the product

Adapted with permission from Rorie, J. L, Paine, L. L., & Barger, M. K. (1996). Cultural competence in primary care services. *Journal of Nurse Midwifery, 41*(2), 99.

The care of the laboring woman is addressed further in Module 5.

PRACTICE/REVIEW QUESTIONS

After reviewing this module, answer the following questions.

1. Define *labor* in your own words. Compare your definition with that presented in the text.

Labor is a natural progression in pregnancy that causes dilation of the cervix and birth of the baby. There are 3 stages of labor. Rhythmic contractions of the uterus dilate the cervix.

2. There is probably one predominant factor that results in rhythmic contractions leading to labor initiation and birth.

   A. True

   B. False (circled)

3. Current evidence shows that the functions of the uterus during labor are controlled by hormonal mediators from the placenta and the maternal and fetal glands.

   A. (True)

   B. False

4. Match the actions listed in Column B with the description of probable hormones, chemicals, or functions in labor listed in Column A.

   Column A

   1. _f_ Calcium ions

   2. _a_ Decidua

   3. _c_ Increased number of oxytocin receptor sites in the myometrium

   4. _d_ Prostaglandins

   5. _b_ Oxytocin

   6. _e_ Both maternal and fetal signals

   Column B

   a. Part of the endometrium; in pregnancy plays an important role in increasing estrogen content and synthesizing prostaglandins

   b. Secretion is pulsatile even during labor

   c. Results in increasing uterine sensitivity to oxytocin

   d. Derived from the fetus, decidua, and amniotic membranes

   e. Initiation of labor

   f. Vital for the contractile process in myometrial cells

5. When does Stage I begin and end? _Begins c̄ the onset of regular Contractions and ends c̄ full dilation of the cervix_

6. Describe each of the two phases of Stage I.

   Latent phase: _Begins c̄ fairly Regular Contractions until rapid dilati_

   Active phase: _Begins c̄ Rapid dilation; ends c̄ full dilation_ Begin

7. When does Stage II begin and end? _Begins c̄ full dilation; ends c̄ birth of baby._

8. Describe what occurs in Stage III. _Placenta delivery_

9. Describe what occurs in Stage IV. _Stabilization; Contracting of uterus_

10. Briefly describe why it is important to assess what stage of labor a woman is in.

    helps c̄ early detection of any problems

11. What are the three layers of tissue that make up the uterus?

    a. _Endometrium_

    b. _Myometrium_

    c. _Perimetrium_

12. Which layer of the uterus contains special muscle cells that aid in expulsion of the baby at birth? _Myometrium_

13. What does *effacement* mean when referring to the labor process?

    the thinning of the Cervix

14. Describe the changes that take place in the uterus as labor progresses.

    Upper portion: _becomes thicker and more powerful_

    Lower portion: _becomes thinner, softer, and more relaxed_

15. Label the following diagram of the uterus.

Active Fundae Segment

c. ← *Fundus*

Passive b. { Segment

d. ← *Isthmus*
e. ← *Cervix*

16. Which group of women is likely to experience effacement before labor actually begins?

_____

17. The longest part of a contraction is the *Increment* segment.

18. The shortest and most intense part of a contraction is the *Acme* segment.

19. The contraction diminishes in the *decrement* segment.

20. List the four characteristics of a contraction.

a. *frequency – how often contractions are occurring*
b. *Regularity – Rhythmic Pattern*
c. *Duration – Length*
d. *Intensity – ex. mild, moderate, strong*

21. For each of the following statements, identify the characteristic of a contraction that is described.

a. Contractions last for 15 seconds: *Duration*

b. An internal electronic monitor is needed to assess this characteristic: *Intensity*

c. Contractions are 6 minutes apart: *frequency*

d. There is an established, predictable pattern: *Regularity*

22. Match the appropriate labor description in Column A with the contraction intensity described in Column B.

Column A

1. *C* Normal labor

2. *a* No labor

3. *b* Prolonged labor

Column B

a. The intensity of the contraction is less than 15 mm Hg.

b. The intensity of the contraction is less than 25 mm Hg (and the frequency is fewer than 2 contractions every 10 minutes).

c. The intensity of contractions varies from 30 to 55 mm Hg (and the frequency is 2 to 5 contractions every 10 minutes).

577-5100
577-5100 *Dr. Studer*
Paperwork

23. Refer to the following diagram to answer questions a through d.

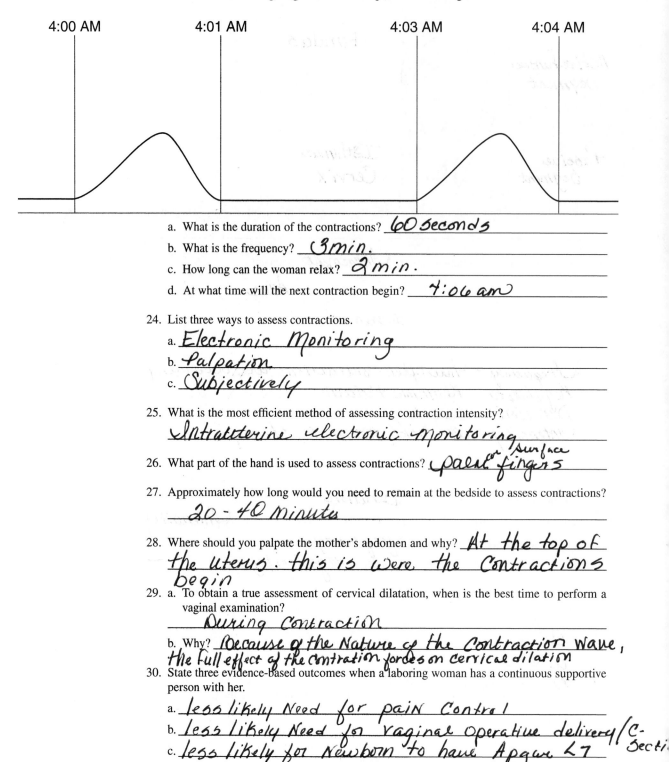

4:00 AM   4:01 AM   4:03 AM   4:04 AM

a. What is the duration of the contractions? _60 seconds_
b. What is the frequency? _3 min._
c. How long can the woman relax? _2 min._
d. At what time will the next contraction begin? _4:06 am_

24. List three ways to assess contractions.
a. _Electronic Monitoring_
b. _Palpation_
c. _Subjectively_

25. What is the most efficient method of assessing contraction intensity?
Intrauterine electronic monitoring

26. What part of the hand is used to assess contractions? _palm or surface fingers_

27. Approximately how long would you need to remain at the bedside to assess contractions?
20 - 40 minutes

28. Where should you palpate the mother's abdomen and why? _At the top of the uterus. this is were the Contractions begin_

29. a. To obtain a true assessment of cervical dilatation, when is the best time to perform a vaginal examination?
During Contraction
b. Why? _Because of the Nature of the Contraction wave, the full effect of the contration forces on cervical dilation_

30. State three evidence-based outcomes when a laboring woman has a continuous supportive person with her.
a. _less likely Need for pain Control_
b. _less likely Need for vaginal operative delivery/C-Secti_
c. _less likely for Newborn to have Apgar <7_

31. Which is *not necessarily* effective in providing support for the laboring woman?

    A. Telling her in advance about special procedures even though the procedure might be uncomfortable for her

    B. Protecting her privacy

    C. Keeping the visit of family members limited

    D. Including her in conversations when speaking with others in the room about her progress

32. In general, effective support during labor depends on which of the following?

    A. The health professional's interest and compassion

    B. The health professional's understanding of the physiologic and anatomic aspects of the birth process

    C. The health professional's appreciation of the psychological aspects of the birth process

    D. Knowledge of the level of preparation and the goals of the couple

    E. All of these

33. One of the first steps in becoming culturally competent is to increase awareness and sensitivity to one's own cultural heritage.

    A. True

    B. False

34. Relinquishing control in clinical situations does not play any role in culturally competent care.

    A. True

    B. False

PRACTICE/REVIEW ANSWER KEY

1. *Labor* is a process involving a series of integrated uterine contractions occurring over time, leading to the development of expulsive forces adequate to propel the fetus through the birth canal against the resistance of soft tissue, muscle, and the bony structure of the pelvis.

2. B

3. A

4. 1. f
   2. a
   3. c
   4. d
   5. b
   6. e

5. Stage I begins with true labor and ends with full dilatation of the cervix.

6. The *latent phase* begins with regular contractions and *lasts until* rapid cervical *dilatation begins.*
   The *active phase* begins with rapid cervical dilatation and lasts until *full dilatation* of the cervix occurs.

7. Stage II begins with full dilatation of the cervix and lasts until the baby is born.

8. In Stage III the placenta is delivered.

9. In Stage IV the uterus contracts and the mother's body functions begin to stabilize.

10. Assessment of a woman's progress through the stages of labor is helpful in detecting problems.

11. a. Perimetrium
    b. Myometrium
    c. Endometrium

12. Myometrium

13. In labor, *effacement* refers to the thinning of the cervix.

14. The upper portion of uterus becomes thicker because of shortening and thickening of the myometrial fibers.
    The lower portion of uterus becomes thinner, softer, and more relaxed as myometrial fibers become longer.

15. a. Active fundal segment
    b. Passive segment
    c. Fundus
    d. Isthmus
    e. Cervix

16. Mothers experiencing their first labor

17. Increment

18. Acme

19. Decrement

20. a. Frequency
    b. Regularity
    c. Duration
    e. Intensity

21. a. Duration
    b. Intensity
    c. Frequency
    d. Regularity

22. 1. c
    2. a
    3. b

23. a. 1 minute
    b. every 3 minutes
    c. 2 minutes
    d. 4:06 AM

24. a. Subjectively
    b. By palpation
    c. With use of electronic fetal monitoring

25. Internal electronic monitoring

26. Palmar surface of fingertips

27. At least 30 minutes

28. Fingertips should be placed lightly over the fundal portion of the abdomen, which is near the top of the uterus. This is an appropriate area because this is where contractions begin and end.

29. a. Throughout the entire contraction
    b. Because of the nature of the contraction wave, the full effects of the contraction forces on cervical dilatation will be appreciated only at the peak and toward the end of the contraction.

30. a. Less likelihood of medication need for pain relief
    b. Less likelihood of need for vaginal operative delivery
    c. Less likelihood of need for cesarean delivery
    d. Less likelihood of Apgar score less than 7 at 5 minutes

31. C

32. E

33. A

34. B

REFERENCES

1. Chaim, W., & Mazor, M. (1998). The relationship between hormones and human parturition. *Archives of Obstetrics and Gynecology, 62*(2), 43–51.
2. Farrington, P. F. & Ward, K. (1999). Normal labor, delivery and puerperium. In J. R. Scott, P. J. DiSaia, C. Hammond, & W. N. Spellacy (Eds.), *Danforth's obstetrics & gynecology* (8th ed.). Philadelphia: Lippincott Williams & Wilkins.
3. Fuchs, A. R., & Fuchs, F. (1996). Physiology and endocrinology of parturition. In S. G. Gabbe, J. R. Niebyl, & J. L. Simpson (Eds.), *Obstetrics: normal and problem pregnancies* (3rd ed.). New York: Churchill Livingstone.
4. Cunningham, F. G., Gant, N. F., Leveno, K. J., Gilstrap, L. C., III, Hauth, J. C., & Wenstrom, K. D. (Eds.) (2001). *Williams obstetrics* (21st ed.). New York: McGraw-Hill.
5. Pozaic, S. (1999). Induction and augmentation of labor. In L. K Mandeville, & N. H. Troiano (Eds.), *AWHONN's high-risk and critical care intrapartum nursing* (2nd ed., pp. 142–145). Philadelphia: Lippincott Williams & Wilkins.
6. Simpson, K. R., & Poole, J. H. (1998). *Cervical ripening and induction and augmentation of labor* (p. 27). Washington, DC: Association of Women's Health, Obstetric and Neonatal Nurses.
7. Rothman, B. K. (1996). Women providers and control. *Journal of Obstetric, Gynecologic, and Neonatal Nursing, 25*(3), 254.
8. Peterson, G. (1996). Childbirth: the ordinary miracle—Effects of childbirth on women's self-esteem and family relationships. *Pre- and Perinatal Psychology Journal, 11*(2), 101–109.
9. McKay, S. (1991). Shared power: The essence of humanized childbirth. *Pre- and Perinatal Psychology, 54*(4), 283–296.
10. Hodnett, E. D. (2000). Caregiver support for women during childbirth. *Cochrane Database System Review,* (2), CD000199.
11. Chamberlain, D. B., & Arms, S. (Fall/Winter, 1999). Obstetrics and the prenatal psyche. *Journal of Prenatal and Perinatal Psychology and Health, 14*(1–2), 97–118.
12. Chamberlain, D. B. (Winter/Fall, 1999). Babies are not what we thought: Call for a new paradigm. *Journal of Prenatal and Perinatal Psychology and Health, 14*(1–2), 127–144.
13. Chamberlain, D. B. (1994). The sentient prenate: What every parent should know. *Pre- and Perinatal Psychology Journal, 9*(1), 9–31.
14. Callister, L. C. (2001). Integrating cultural beliefs and practices into the care of childbearing women. In K. R. Simpson, & P. A. Creehan (Eds.), *Perinatal nursing* (2nd ed., pp. 73–80). Philadelphia: Lippincott Williams & Wilkins.
15. Rorie, J. L., Paine, L. L., & Barger, M. K. (1996). Cultural competence in primary care service. *Journal of Nurse Midwifery, 4*(2), 99.

SUGGESTED READINGS

Brach, C., & Fraser, I. (2000). *Can cultural competency reduce racial and ethnic health disparities? A review and conceptual model.* Agency for Healthcare Research and Quality. Rockville, MD: U.S. Department of Health and Human Services.

Enkin, M., Keirse, M. J. N. C., Neilson, J., Crowther, C., Duley, L., Hodnett, E., & Hofmeyer, J. (2000). *A guide to effective care in pregnancy and childbirth* (3rd ed.). New York: Oxford University Press.

Goer, H. (1999). *The thinking woman's guide to a better birth.* New York: Berkley Publishing Group.

Lowdermilk, D. L, Perry, S. E., & Bobak, I. M. (Eds.). (2000). *Maternity & women's health care* (7th ed.). St. Louis: Mosby.

Mandeville, L. K., & Troiano, N. H. (1999). *High-risk & critical care intrapartum nursing* (2nd ed.). Philadelphia: Lippincott Williams & Wilkins.

Pillitteri, A. (1999). *Maternal & child health nursing* (3rd ed.). Philadelphia: Lippincott.

Simkin, P., & Ancheta, R. (2000). *The labor progress handbook.* Malden, MA: Blackwell Science.

Simpson, K. R., & Creehan, P. A. (2001). *Perinatal nursing* (2nd ed.). Philadelphia: Lippincott Williams & Wilkins.

Willis, W. O. (1999). Culturally competent nursing care during the perinatal period. *Journal of Perinatal Nursing, 13*(3), 45–59.

MODULE 2

Maternal and Fetal Response to Labor

E. JEAN MARTIN

Identifying Features of the Pelvis That Make It Adequate for Labor

As you complete Part 1 of this module, you will learn:
1. Critical factors involved in labor
2. The significance of each type of pelvis to the birth process
3. Features of the pelvis that affect labor
4. Limitations of pelvic evaluation methods

When you have completed Part 1 of this module, you should be able to recall the meaning of the following terms. You should also be able to use the terms when consulting with other health professionals. The terms are defined in this module or in the glossary at the end of this book.

fetal attitude	fetal presentation
fetal lie	molding
fetal position	pelvic planes

Features of the Pelvis That Make It Adequate for Labor

There are four factors, often referred to as the "four P's," that affect the progress of labor.

1. *Passage* involves	–the size of the pelvis
	–the shape of the pelvis
	–the ability of the cervix to dilate and the vagina to stretch
2. *Passenger* involves	–fetal head size
	–fetal *attitude* describes the relation of the fetal head, shoulder, and legs to one another
	–fetal *lie* refers to the relationship of the long axis ($\updownarrow$) of the fetus to the long axis ($\updownarrow$) of the the mother
	–fetal *presentation* describes that part of the fetus entering the pelvis first
	–fetal *position* refers to the direction toward which the presenting part is pointing—front, side, or back of the maternal pelvis
3. *Powers* involves	–the frequency, duration, and intensity of uterine contractions
	–abdominal pressures resulting from pushing, which occur in Stage II of labor
4. *Psyche* involves	–the mother's physical, emotional, and intellectual preparation
	–her previous childbirth experiences
	–her cultural attitude
	–support from significant people in the mother's life

For labor to progress smoothly, there must be adaptations of both the fetal and maternal factors. Abnormalities of any of these critical factors can mean risk for baby, mother, or both.

■ What makes a pelvis adequate for labor?

The size and the shape of the pelvis make it adequate for labor. The female pelvis is uniquely suited to the demands of childbearing. However, not all women possess the same type of pelvis. The following four classic types of pelves are based on differences in shapes, diameters, and angles[1,2] (Display 2.1).

DISPLAY 2.1 Classic Types of Pelves[1,2]

TYPE	FEATURES
A. Gynecoid pelvis	–Typical female pelvis –Adequate for labor and birth –Found in 50% of women

TYPE	FEATURES
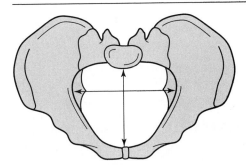 B. Android pelvis	–Typical male pelvis –Narrow dimensions –Slow descent of fetal head –Associated with the halting of labor –Forceps delivery often required –Found in 20% of women
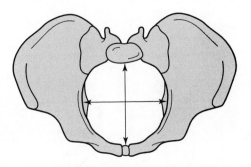 C. Arthropoid pelvis	–Apelike pelvis –Adequate for labor and birth –Found in 25% of women
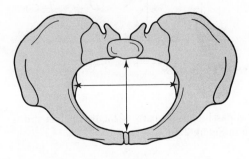 D. Platypelloid pelvis	–Unfavorable for labor –Frequent delay in descent –Found in 5% of women

A woman can have a pelvis that has a combination of characteristics from these classic types.

In obstetrics, the pelvis is divided into the following parts:

1. *False pelvis*—where there is ample room
2. *True pelvis*—which contains important narrow dimensions through which the fetus must pass

There is a ridge that provides an imaginary dividing line between the two areas. This ridge is the boundary for the inlet to the true pelvis.

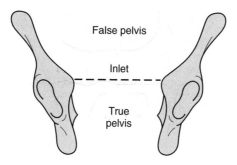

FIGURE 2.1 False pelvis and true pelvis.

The *true pelvis* can be divided into three key areas:

1. Inlet
2. Pelvic cavity, which extends from the inlet to the outlet
3. Outlet

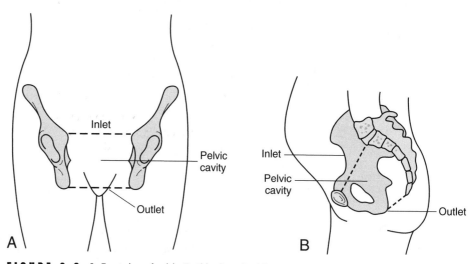

FIGURE 2.2 **A.** Front view of pelvis. **B.** Side view of pelvis.

The *pelvic planes* are imaginary flat surfaces passing across parts of the true pelvis at different levels. Three important planes are shown in Figure 2.3.

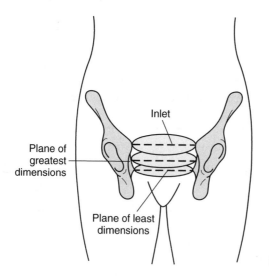

The plane of least dimensions is the narrowest section of the pelvis. Occasionally, labor will stop because the fetus cannot descend past this area.

FIGURE 2.3 Pelvic planes.

■ How is the adequacy of the pelvis evaluated?

The relationship of the fetal size to the pelvis must be evaluated. This relationship probably changes depending on the forces and stages of labor. Positioning of the mother can bring about subtle changes in one or two pelvic dimensions (e.g., McRoberts maneuver; see Module 14). Dynamic changes in the fetal head, thorax, and abdomen are believed to occur as the pelvic passageway is negotiated during descent.

Efforts to predict fetal–pelvic disproportion have included the following[1]:

- Clinical pelvimetry
- X-ray pelvimetry
- Ultrasonography
- Computed tomographic (CT) pelvimetry (CT scanning)
- Magnetic resonance imaging (MRI)

1. Clinical pelvimetry	–Estimation of pelvic shapes and dimensions by the examiner –Wide margin of error depending on the examiner's skill
2. X-ray pelvimetry	–Potential fetal exposure to low-dose radiation –Can provide critical pelvic diameters not otherwise obtainable –Sometimes used in breech presentations –Has been replaced by other pelvic imaging methods
3. Ultrasonography	–Uses sound waves, not ionizing energy –Not useful for evaluating maternal pelvic measurement –Useful for precisely measuring fetal biparietal diameters and fetal head circumference
4. CT scanning	–Has replaced x-ray pelvimetry at many institutions –Accuracy is improved over conventional x-ray pelvimetry –Involves a lower fetal radiation exposure than x-ray –Maternal movement during procedure needs to be minimal to prevent distortion –Expense is comparable to that of conventional x-ray
5. MRI	–Offers accurate pelvic measurements and complete fetal imaging –Has the potential to aid in diagnosing soft tissue dystocia and obstructed labor –Use is limited by expense, length of time needed to obtain the study, and availability of equipment

Additional considerations include the following:

Except for some relaxation of the pelvic joints because of hormonal influences, the bones of the pelvis cannot expand.

The relationship of the fetal head size to the pelvis is important.

The fetal head has the ability to change shape to fit through the pelvis. This ability of the head to change shape is called *molding*.

Because of the tilt of the pelvis, the fetus descends through this pathway during labor and birth, as shown in Figure 2.4.

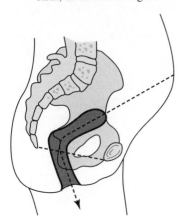

FIGURE 2.4 Pathway of fetal descent.

PRACTICE/REVIEW QUESTIONS
After reviewing Part 1, answer the following questions.

1. List four critical factors involved in the labor process.
   a. *Passage*
   b. *Pasanger*
   c. *Powers*
   d. *Psyche*

2. Match the definition in Column B with the correct term in Column A.
   Column A   Column B

   1. *a* Lie   a. Relationship of the long axis of the fetus to the long axis of the mother
   2. *c* Attitude
   3. *d* Position   b. That part of the fetal body that is entering the pelvis
   4. *b* Presentation   c. The relationship of fetal parts to one another
                               d. The direction toward which the presenting part is pointing with respect to the front, side, or back of the mother's pelvis

3. List the four main types of pelves.
   a. *Gynecoid*
   b. *Android*
   c. *Platypelloid*
   d. *Anthropoid*

4. The pelvis best suited for labor and birth is the *Gynecoid* pelvis. This type of pelvis is found in *50* % of women.

5. The pelvis that has narrow dimensions and is likely to result in labor stopping or a forceps delivery is the *Android* pelvis. This type of pelvis is found in *20* % of women.

6. Match the areas of the pelvis with the correct numbers in the diagram.
   1 a. Inlet
   2 b. False pelvis
   5 c. True pelvis
   3 d. Outlet
   4 e. Plane of least dimensions

7. The true pelvis is made up of three key planes called:
   a. *least dimensions*
   b. *greatest dimensions*
   c. *pelvic inlet*

8. The planes of the true pelvis are critical because *Contains important narrow dimensions in which the fetus must pass through*

9. Name two ways in which the female pelvis is evaluated for adequacy.
   a. *Clinical (pelvimeters)*
   b. *MRI*

10. Explain how it is possible for the fetal head to fit through the rigid, bony pelvis. *Molding - the fetal head has the ability to change shape*

PRACTICE/REVIEW ANSWER KEY

1. a. Passage
   b. Passenger
   c. Power
   d. Psyche

2. 1. a
   2. c
   3. d
   4. b

3. a. Gynecoid
   b. Android
   c. Platypelloid
   d. Anthropoid

4. Gynecoid; 50

5. Android; 20

6. a. 1
   b. 2
   c. 5
   d. 3
   e. 4

7. a. Least dimensions
   b. Greatest dimensions
   c. Pelvic inlet

8. The fetus must pass through these areas, some of which are narrow.

9. a. X-ray
   b. Pelvic examination

10. The head flexes and the bones of the scalp mold somewhat.

Identifying Relationships Between the Fetus and Pelvis

As you complete Part 2 of this module, you will learn:

1. Relationships of the fetal position and presenting part to the outcome of labor
2. Landmarks used to identify the position of the fetus
3. Features of the pelvis that affect labor
4. How to determine and describe fetal lie, presentation, attitude, and position

When you have completed Part 2 of this module, you should be able to recall the meaning of the following terms. You should also be able to use the terms when consulting with other health professionals. The terms are defined in this module or in the glossary at the end of this book.

biparietal diameter	mentum
denominator	occiput
fetal anencephaly	placenta previa
fetal hydrocephaly	prematurity
fontanelle	sinciput
grandmultiparity	suture
hydramnios	vertex

Relationships Between the Fetus and Pelvis

■ **How does the fetal passenger accommodate to the pelvis during labor?**

The position of the fetus as the mother is ready to go into labor largely determines how smoothly the labor and delivery will progress.

The fetal head is the largest part of the baby and is composed of both fixed and flexible parts. You must become familiar with the parts of the fetal skull because the identification of certain landmarks will assist you when performing vaginal examinations to determine the mother's labor progress.

The skull consists of three major divisions:

1. Face
2. Back of the skull
3. Cranium, or top of the skull

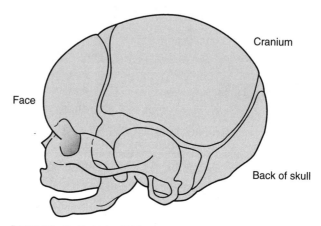

FIGURE 2.5 Major divisions of the fetal skull.

The bones of the face and the back of the skull are fused and fixed, but the cranium consists of several large bones that are not fused together at the time of birth. This permits the shape of the head to change somewhat as the fetus passes through the narrow, rigid pelvis.

The force of uterine contractions on the fetal head can cause overlapping of the cranial bones; this is called *molding* and can be felt during a vaginal examination.

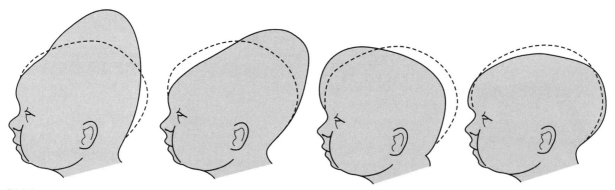

FIGURE 2.6 Molding of the fetal head in different cephalic presentations.

■ **What other landmarks of the fetal skull are used in describing the fetal head?**

There are four landmarks that are important in describing the general areas of the fetal head.

1. *Sinciput*—brow area
2. *Vertex*—area between the anterior and posterior fontanelles
3. *Occiput*—area beneath the posterior fontanelle where the occipital bone is located
4. *Mentum*—fetal chin

NOTE: *Learn these terms now because later in this module they will be used to denote which part of the fetal head is leading as the fetus descends.*

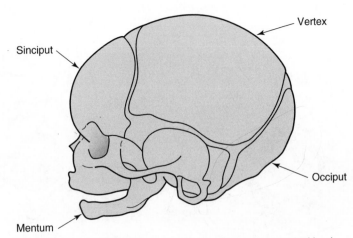

FIGURE 2.7 Bony landmarks used in describing areas of the fetal head.

If looking down at the fetal cranium, you would see the divisions between the bones of the head, as depicted in Figure 2.8.

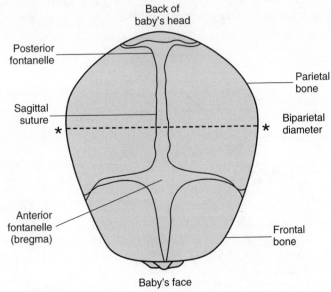

FIGURE 2.8 Suture, fontanelle, and bony landmarks used in describing the position of the fetal head.

A *suture* is a space between the cranial bones that is covered by a membrane. A *fontanelle*, or *fontanel*, is a space covered by a membrane where the cranial sutures meet.

> Feeling the suture lines and fontanelles during a vaginal examination helps in identifying the position of the fetal head.

There are two important *landmarks* formed by the sutures that are useful in identifying the position of the fetal head in the pelvis.

1. *Anterior fontanelle*—is *diamond-shaped* and measures 2 × 3 cm. This is sometimes referred to as the *bregma*. When the head is *moderately* flexed or hyperextended, this fontanelle can be palpated. It remains open approximately 18 months after birth to allow for brain growth.

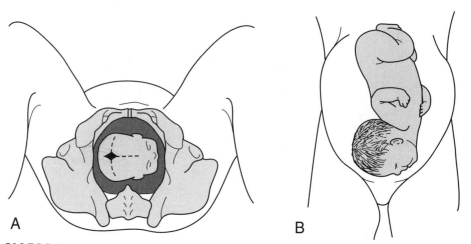

FIGURE 2.9 **A.** Vaginal view (hyperextended head). **B.** Abdominal view (hyperextended head).

2. *Posterior fontanelle*—is *smaller* and *triangular* in shape. When the head is well flexed, this fontanelle can be felt. The posterior fontanelle closes approximately 12 weeks after birth.

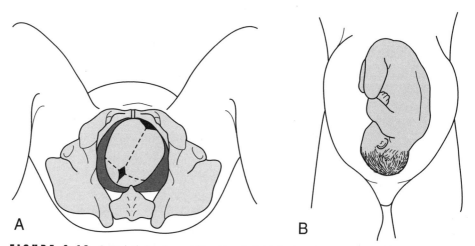

FIGURE 2.10 **A.** Vaginal view (normal flexed head). **B.** Abdominal view (normal flexed head).

■ **How is the position of the fetus in the mother's abdominal cavity and pelvis described?**

You must understand the relationship of the fetus to the mother's abdominal and pelvic cavities because careful observation of these relationships can alert you to potential problems.

To review, four aspects of this relationship are as follows:
1. *Lie*—the relationship of the long axis of the fetus to that of the mother
2. *Presentation*—that part of the fetus entering the pelvic inlet first
3. *Attitude*—the relationship of the fetal parts (e.g., chest, chin, arms) to each other
4. *Position*—the relationship of the presenting part to a specific area of the mother's pelvis

Types of Fetal Lie

Display 2.2 illustrates longitudinal and transverse lies.

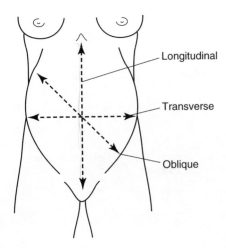

NOTE: Only a longitudinal lie is normal.

FIGURE 2.11 Types of fetal lie.

| DISPLAY 2.2 | Illustrations of Fetal Lie |

A longitudinal lie, occurring in 99.5% of pregnancies, is when the long axis of the fetal body is parallel to the mother's spine.[2]
  A longitudinal lie can be either *cephalic* or *breech*.

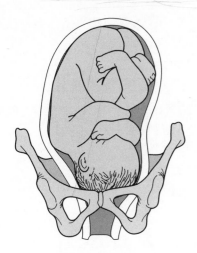

When the head is leading, it is called a *cephalic lie.*

A. Cephalic lie

display continues on page 34

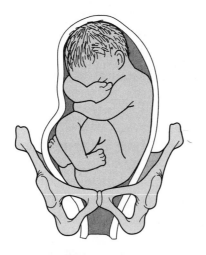

If the buttocks are coming first, it is called a *breech lie.*

B. Breech lie

The fetus can assume a *transverse lie,* in which the long axis of the fetus lies directly across the mother's spine. It occurs in approximately 0.3% of pregnancies.[1]

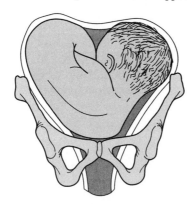

C. Transverse lie

Transverse lie is often associated with the following:

1. Grandmultiparity (having five or more pregnancies)
2. A small (contracted) pelvis
3. A placenta previa

Vaginal delivery is not possible with a transverse lie.

Types of Fetal Attitude

Attitude refers to the relationship of the fetal parts to each other. Normally, the attitude is one of *flexion* or *extension* (Display 2.3).

DISPLAY 2.3 | Illustrations of Fetal Attitude

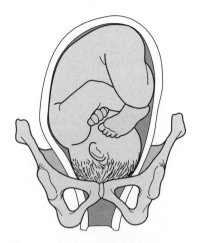

Flexion is when the chin is near the chest, the arms and legs are folded in front of the body, and the back is curved.

This position of the fetus presents the smallest possible fetal head measurements in relation to the pelvic passageway and is the only normal attitude.

A. Attitude of flexion

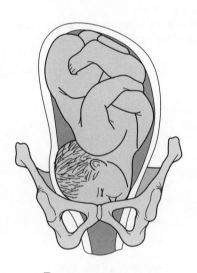

Extension occurs when the head is bent back and the chest and abdomen are slightly curved.

In the extreme of this position, the fetal face is the leading part as it descends through the pelvis. It is traumatic for the baby, who is often not deliverable vaginally because a larger diameter of the fetal head presents, unlike when the head is well flexed.

B. Attitude of extension

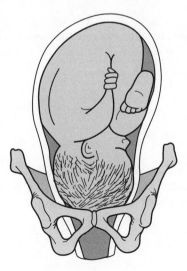

Military attitude occurs when the fetal position is not one of flexion or extension.

C. Military attitude (neither flexed nor extended)

display continues on page 36

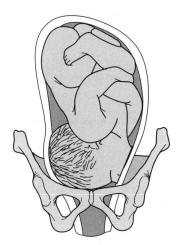

Partial extension occurs when there is moderate extension of the head.

D. Attitude of partial extension

The *cephalic prominence* describes that part of the fetal head that can be felt by placing both hands on the sides of the uterus and feeling down toward the pelvis.

When the head is in normal flexion, the cephalic prominence is felt on the opposite side of the fetal back; in Figure 2.12 it is found in the lower left of the mother's abdomen.

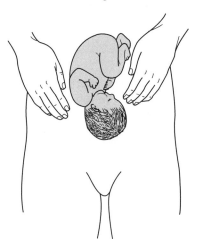

FIGURE 2.12 Position of the cephalic prominence in normal flexion.

Hyperextension of the head results in the face presenting for birth. The cephalic prominence is felt on the same side as the fetal back; in Figure 2.13 it is found in the lower right of the mother's abdomen.

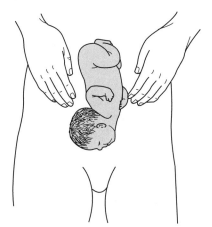

> The location of the cephalic prominence can aid in diagnosing the attitude of the fetus and any malpositions (discussed further in Module 4).

FIGURE 2.13 Position of the cephalic prominence in hyperextension.

Types of Fetal Presentation

Presentation refers to that part of the fetus entering the pelvic inlet first. The main presentations are as follows:

- Shoulder
- Breech
- Cephalic

DISPLAY 2.4	Types of Fetal Presentation	
Shoulder	Either shoulder leads	Fortunately, shoulder presentation rarely occurs.
Breech	Buttocks lead	Breech presentation occurs in 3% to 4% of pregnancies and is more common in preterm pregnancies.[1]
Cephalic	Head leads	Cephalic presentation occurs in 96% to 97% of term pregnancies.[1]

Shoulder Presentation

The shoulder is entering the pelvis first (↓) (Fig. 2.14). This presentation occurs infrequently.

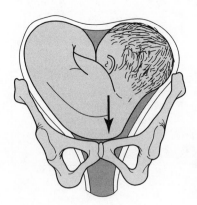

FIGURE 2.14 Shoulder presentation.

Breech Presentation

The buttocks or breech enters the pelvis first (Figs. 2.15, 2.16, and 2.17). Breech presentation can be complete, frank, or footling breech.

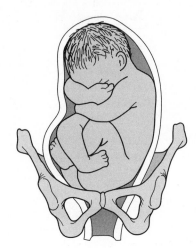

FIGURE 2.15 Complete breech presentation.

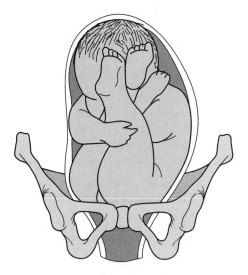

FIGURE 2.16 Frank breech presentation.

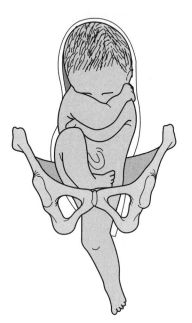

Breech presentations can occur when the following conditions exist:

Placenta previa	Grandmultiparity
Hydramnios	Fetal hydrocephaly
Twin pregnancies	Fetal anencephaly
Preterm labor/birth	

FIGURE 2.17 Footling breech presentation.

Cephalic Presentation

Cephalic presentation (96% to 97% of term pregnancies) can occur[1]:

When the head is *well flexed* and the vertex presents first, as in Figure 2.18

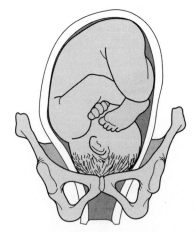

> This is the only normal presentation.

FIGURE 2.18 Vertex presents in cephalic presentation.

When the head is *poorly flexed* and the brow presents first, as in Figure 2.19

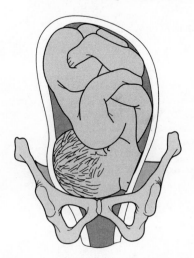

FIGURE 2.19 Brow presents in cephalic presentation.

When the head is *poorly flexed* and the face presents first, as in Figure 2.20

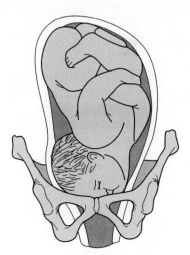

FIGURE 2.20 Face presents in cephalic presentation.

Types of Fetal Position

■ How are the fetal positions described?

Position refers to the relationship of the presenting part to a specific area on the woman's pelvis. In describing fetal position, certain landmarks on the fetus, called *denominators,* are used.

In *vertex* presentations, the *occiput* is the denominator (Fig. 2.21).

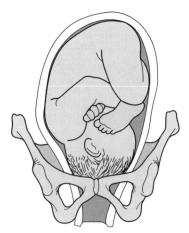

FIGURE 2.21 Vertex presentation with occiput as the denominator.

In *face* presentations, the *mentum* (chin) is the denominator (Fig. 2.22).

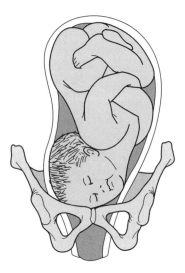

FIGURE 2.22 Face presentation with chin as the denominator.

In *breech* presentations, the *sacrum* is the denominator (Fig. 2.23).

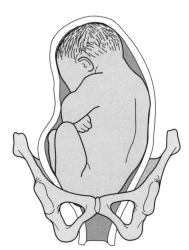

FIGURE 2.23 Breech presentation with sacrum as the denominator

In *shoulder* presentations, the *scapula,* or the *acromial process,* is the denominator (Fig. 2.24).

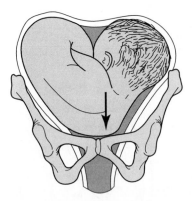

FIGURE 2.24 Shoulder presentation with the scapula (acromial process) as the denominator.

Having determined which denominator is the leading part of the fetus, its *position* can be described further. Note whether the denominator is pointing to the left (**L**) or right (**R**) side of the mother's pelvis. For example:

The *occiput* of the fetus leads and points to the mother's *right* (Fig. 2.25).

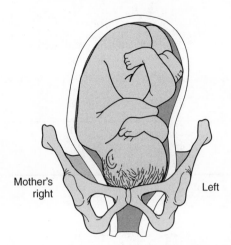

Mother's right

Left

FIGURE 2.25 Occiput leading and pointing to mother's right.

The *sacrum* of the fetus leads and points to the mother's *left* (Fig. 2.26).

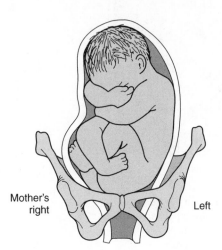

Mother's right

Left

FIGURE 2.26 Sacrum leading and pointing to mother's left.

Finally, in describing position, note whether the denominator is in the front (anterior), directly to the side (transverse), or in the back (posterior) of the *mother's* pelvis (Display 2.5).

DISPLAY 2.5	Examples of Denominator Positions in Cephalic Presentation

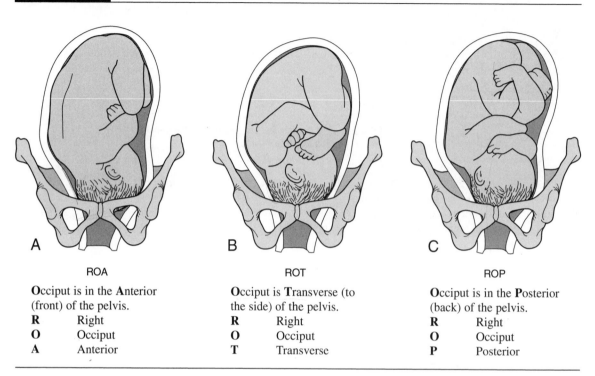

A	B	C
ROA	ROT	ROP

Occiput is in the **A**nterior (front) of the pelvis.		**O**cciput is **T**ransverse (to the side) of the pelvis.		**O**cciput is in the **P**osterior (back) of the pelvis.	
R	Right	**R**	Right	**R**	Right
O	Occiput	**O**	Occiput	**O**	Occiput
A	Anterior	**T**	Transverse	**P**	Posterior

Display 2.6 shows breech positions.

DISPLAY 2.6	Examples of Denominator Positions in Breech Presentation

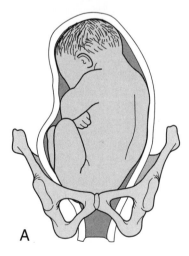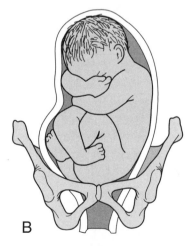

A	B
LSA	LSP

Sacrum is in the **A**nterior (front) of the pelvis.		**S**acrum is in the **P**osterior (back) of the pelvis.	
L	Left	**L**	Left
S	Sacrum	**S**	Sacrum
A	Anterior	**P**	Posterior

Display 2.7 shows a face presentation with the *mentum* (chin) leading.

DISPLAY 2.7	Example of Denominaor Position in Cephalic Presentation with Face Presenting

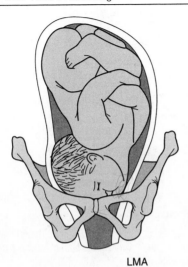

LMA

The **Mentum** (chin) is in the **Left**
Anterior of the pelvis.
L   Left
M   Mentum
A   Anterior

Figures 2.27 and 2.28 illustrate how various positions for vertex and breech presentations can be described.

Vertex Positions

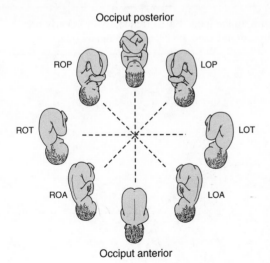

Occiput posterior

ROP   LOP

ROT   LOT

ROA   LOA

Occiput anterior

NOTE: The occiput is the denominator.

FIGURE 2.27 Variety of fetal positions with vertex presentations. (Adapted with permission from Oxorn, H. [1986]. *Oxorn-Foote human labor & birth* [5th ed., p. 59]. New York: Appleton-Century-Crofts.)

Breech Positions

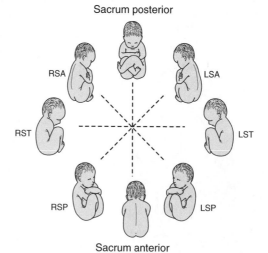

NOTE: *The sacrum is the denominator.*

FIGURE 2.28 Variety of fetal positions with breech presentations. (Adapted with permission from Oxorn, H. [1986]. *Oxorn-Foote human labor & birth* [5th ed., p. 59]. New York: Appleton-Century-Crofts.)

■ **How can fetal position and presentation be determined?**

It is important to determine fetal position and presentation to predict the course of labor. Several methods are available:

- Combined abdominal inspection and palpation (Leopold's maneuvers)
- Vaginal examination
- Sonography
- CT scanning
- X-ray examination

> Because x-rays are known to be harmful to the fetus if used frequently or in early pregnancy, they are used only when fetal position cannot be determined in any other way.

PRACTICE/REVIEW QUESTIONS

After reviewing Part 2, answer the following questions.

1. Label the following diagrams.

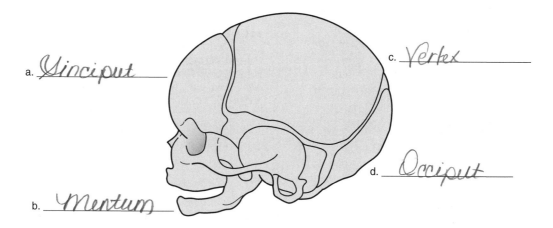

a. *Sinciput*

b. *Mentum*

c. *Vertex*

d. *Occiput*

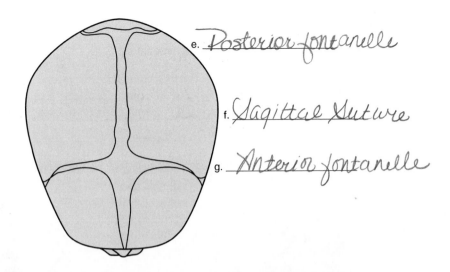

e. ~~Posterior fontanelle~~

f. *Sagittal Suture*

g. *Anterior fontanelle*

2. The posterior fontanelle closes approximately _____ *3* _____ months after birth. It is ~~triangular~~-shaped and can be felt when the head is *Well* flexed.

3. The anterior fontanelle closes approximately _____ *18* _____ months after birth. It is *diamond*-shaped and can be felt when the head is *Moderately* flexed.

4. The only normal lie is *a logitudinal lie*

5. A longitudinal lie can be *Cephalic* when the head leads, or *Breech* when the buttocks come first.

6. Why is vaginal delivery impossible with a transverse lie? *Because the long Axis of the fetus lies across the long axis of the Mother.*

7. The only normal attitude is one of . *flexion*

8. Why is a fetus positioned in extreme extension often not deliverable vaginally? *Because it can be traumatizing to the infant, a larger part of the head tries to go through the pelvis*

9. Locating the cephalic prominence is helpful in diagnosing fetal *Attitude* and malpositions.

10. The three primary types of presentations are:
    a. *Cephalic* (approximately 96%)
    b. *Breech* (3% to 4% of pregnancies)
    c. *Shoulder* (infrequent)

11. The only normal presentation is *Cephalic*, when the *Vertex* presents first.

12. Prematurity, placenta previa, and/or grandmultiparity can be associated with a *Breech* presentation.

13. State the denominator used to describe the fetal position in each of the following presentations:

Fetal Position	Denominator
a. Vertex	Occiput
b. Face	Mentum
c. Breech	Sacrum
d. Shoulder	Scapula

14. Fully describe each of the following according to fetal lie, presentation, and position.

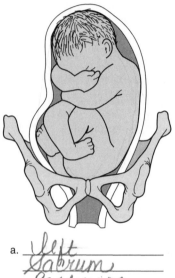

a. 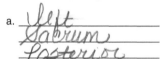 Left Sacrum Posterior

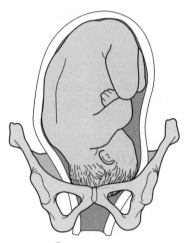

b. 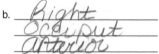 Right Occiput Anterior

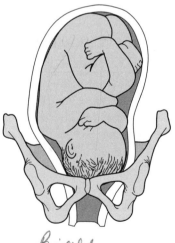

c. Right Occiput Posterior

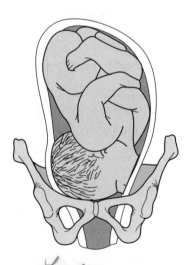

d. 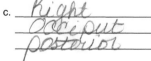 Left Mentum Anterior

15. State five ways in which fetal position and presentation can be determined.

    a. _Leopolds Maneuver_

    b. _Vaginal Examination_

    c. _Sonography_

    d. _CT Scanning_

    e. _X-ray examination_

16. The term *position* refers to which of the following?

    A. The relationship of the long axis of the fetus to that of the mother

    B. The part of the fetus that first enters the inlet of the pelvis

    C. The degree of descent of the fetus through the maternal pelvis

    D. The relationship of a specific point of the fetus to one of the four quadrants of the mother's pelvis

17. Which statement accurately describes the fetal attitude, lie, presentation, and position in the following illustration?

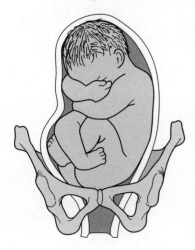

    A. Attitude is one of extension, longitudinal lie, breech presentation, and position is LSP.

    B. Attitude is one of flexion, longitudinal lie, breech presentation, and position is LSA.

    C. Attitude is one of flexion, longitudinal lie, breech presentation, and position is LSP.

    D. Attitude is one of extension, longitudinal lie, cephalic presentation, and position is RSP.

PRACTICE/REVIEW ANSWER KEY

1. a. Sinciput
   b. Mentum
   c. Vertex
   d. Occiput
   e. Posterior fontanelle
   f. Sagittal suture
   g. Anterior fontanelle (bregma)

2. 3; triangular; well

3. 18; diamond; moderately

4. longitudinal

5. cephalic; breech

6. Vaginal delivery is not possible with a transverse lie because the long axis of the fetus lies across the mother's spine.

7. Flexion

8. In extreme extension, the face is often the leading part as the fetus descends through the pelvis. This is traumatic for the baby. A larger diameter is presented to the vaginal passageway than when the head is well flexed.

9. Attitude

10. a. Cephalic
    b. Breech
    c. Shoulder

11. Cephalic; vertex

12. Breech

13. a. Occiput
    b. Mentum
    c. Sacrum
    d. Scapula or acromial process

14. a. Longitudinal (breech) lie
       Breech presentation
       LSP
    b. Longitudinal (cephalic) lie
       Cephalic presentation
       ROA
    c. Longitudinal (cephalic) lie
       Cephalic presentation
       ROP
    d. Longitudinal (cephalic) lie
       Cephalic presentation
       LMT (You may interpret the diagram to be LMA.)

15. a. Abdominal inspection and palpation
    b. Vaginal examination
    c. Sonography
    d. CT scanning
    e. X-ray examination

16. D

17. C

Describing Fetal Descent During Labor

As you complete Part 3 of this module, you will learn:

1. How to describe the descent of the fetus
2. The significance of engagement and pelvic adequacy
3. How fetal descent through the pelvis is evaluated
4. How molding of the fetal head can affect the evaluation of descent

When you have completed Part 3 of the module, you should be able to recall the meaning of the following terms. You should also be able to use the terms when consulting with other health professionals. The terms are defined in this module or in the glossary at the end of this book.

caput succedaneum   multipara
dipping   primigravida
engagement   station
floating

Fetal Descent During Labor

■ How is the descent of the fetus described and assessed?

The degree of descent of the fetus through the pelvis is assessed by abdominal, vaginal, and rectal examination. The relationship of the presenting part of the fetus to an imaginary line drawn between the ischial spines of the pelvis is called *station* (Fig. 2.29A).

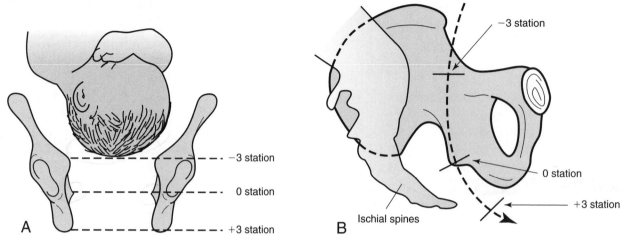

FIGURE 2.29 A. Descent of the presenting fetal part to station −3. Front view using a scale of −3 to +3. **B.** Descent pathway, side view.

The ischial spines are approximately halfway between the pelvic inlet and the pelvic outlet. When the presenting fetal part (e.g., the head) is at the level of the ischial spines, it is said to be at *station 0*.

The long axis of the birth canal above and below the ischial spines is divided into thirds (Fig. 2.29B). If the presenting part is above the spines and at the level of the pelvic inlet, it is said to be at −3 station. If it has descended one third the distance past the inlet, it is at −1 station. A similar division is assigned to the distances between the ischial spines and the pelvic outlet. If the level of the presenting part is one third or two thirds the distance between the spines and the outlet, is it said to be +1 or +2 station, respectively. When the presenting fetal part descends to the bony outlet, it is resting on the muscles of the vaginal opening and is at +3 station.

To measure station, sometimes a scale of −5 to +5 (Fig. 2.30) is used instead of the −3 to +3 scale described here. In this case, the numbers represent the position of the presenting part if 1, 2, 3, 4, or 5 cm above or below the level of the ischial spines.

The same scale should be understood and used consistently by all staff within the labor and delivery unit.

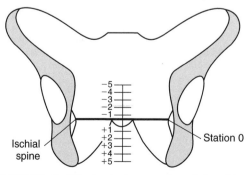

FIGURE 2.30 Levels of progress through the pelvis using a scale of −5 to +5.

■ **When is the pelvis considered adequate?**

When the presenting part of the fetal head is at station 0, the widest part of the head usually has passed through the inlet and the pelvis is then thought to be adequate. This is called *engagement* (Fig. 2.31).

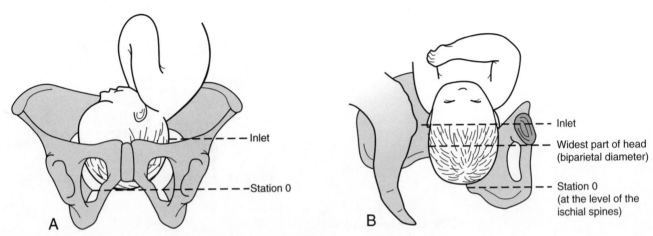

FIGURE 2.31 Engaged presenting fetal head. **A.** Front view. **B.** Side view.

Vaginal examinatio*n will assist you in determining the amount of descent.*

CAUTION: • In women with deep pelves, this relationship might not be exact, and even though engagement has occurred, the presenting part can be slightly above the spines.
• Sometimes the fetal scalp becomes edematous with the pressure of labor exerted on it. This can be felt as a soft, swollen layer over the hard bony surface of the skull and is called *caput succedaneum*. Also, it is possible for molding of the fetal skull to occur, which can distort the examiner's evaluation of the fetal head descent.

If the fetal head is severely molded, there is considerable caput succedaneum, or both, engagement might not have taken place *even though the tip of the presenting part is at station 0.*

Progressive cervical dilatation without fetal descent can suggest fetal–pelvic disproportion.

For women pregnant for the first time (primigravidas), engagement occurs approximately 2 to 3 weeks before labor begins.

For women who have had more than one pregnancy (multiparas), engagement occurs any time before or during labor.

Other terms used to describe the relationship of the fetal presenting part to the pelvic passageway are as follows:

Floating—when the presenting part is entirely out of the pelvis and can be moved by the examiner abdominally just above the symphysis pubis bone (Fig. 2.32)

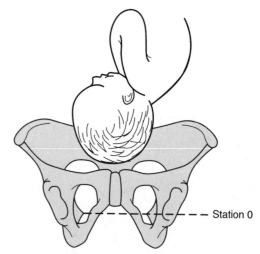

FIGURE 2.32 Floating. Fetal head is entirely out of the pelvis.

Dipping—when the presenting part has descended into the false pelvis but is not through the inlet. The examiner has to feel more deeply abdominally, and the presenting part is not easily moved.

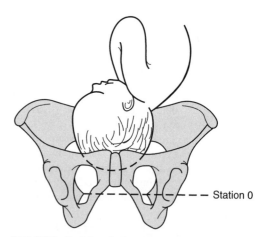

FIGURE 2.33 Dipping. Fetal head is approaching but not through the pelvic inlet.

■ What else can station tell you?

You should recognize some situations that can predict problems[2]:

- An unengaged presenting part in a primigravida can indicate fetal–pelvic disproportion and bears careful watching. However, this actually happens frequently, and women often make good progress in labor.
- The occurrence of disproportion is more likely when the presenting part is high (e.g., station +3, as labor begins).
- Women who begin labor with high presenting parts tend to have achieved less cervical dilatation during early labor. Women with presenting parts at lower stations (station 0 or +2) tend to have cervices that are more effaced and dilated at the beginning of labor.
- The higher the station, the longer labor tends to be.
- Dysfunctional (nonprogressive) labor is more common when the presenting part is at a high station.
- The high presenting part that descends rapidly is usually not related to abnormal labor.

PRACTICE/REVIEW QUESTIONS

After reviewing Part 3, answer the following questions.

1. When the presenting fetal part is at the pelvic inlet, it is said to be at ___−3___ station.

2. When the presenting fetal part is at the level of the ischial spines, it is said to be at ___0___ station.

3. When the presenting fetal part is halfway between the ischial spines and the pelvic outlet, it is at ___+2___ station.

4. When the widest part of the fetal head has passed through the pelvic inlet, _Engagement_ has occurred.

5. When engagement has taken place, the pelvis is thought to be _Adequate_.

6. What effect does molding have on assessment for the amount of descent? _It can distort the examiners Assessment of descent; engagement May not have occured_

7. Why is it important to assess the degree of descent? _helps determine normal/abnormal progress in labor over time._

PRACTICE/REVIEW ANSWER KEY

1. −3 (or −5, depending on the scale used)

2. 0

3. Close to +2 station using the −3 to +3 scale; at +3 station using the −5 to +5 station

4. Engagement

5. Adequate

6. Sometimes, if severe molding of the fetal head has occurred, the examiner's assessment of the amount of descent can be distorted. That is, engagement might not have occurred even though the leading edge of the presenting part is at 0 station.

7. Assessment of the degree of descent is necessary to determine normal/abnormal progress in labor over time.

Evaluating for Fetal Malpresentation

As you complete Part 4 of this module, you will learn:

1. What is meant by *fetal malpresentation*
2. To identify maternal and fetal conditions that can lead to fetal malpresentation
3. What to do if you suspect a fetal malpresentation
4. Steps to take when a prolapse of the cord is suspected or detected

When you have completed Part 4 of the module, you should be able to recall the meaning of the following terms. You should also be able to use the terms when consulting with other health professionals. The terms are defined in this module or in the glossary at the end of this book.

anoxia
dystocia
prolapsed cord

Fetal Malpresentation

■ What is fetal malpresentation?

Malpresentation means that some other part of the fetus, such as buttocks, shoulder, or face, is presenting at or near the pelvic inlet.

Maternal and Fetal Conditions That Can Lead to Fetal Malpresentation

Maternal factors leading to malpresentation include the following:

- Contracted (small) pelvis (the most commonly occurring factor)
- Lax abdominal muscles so that the uterus and fetus fall forward, preventing good fetal descent
- Uterine tumors (fibroids), which can block the entry to the pelvic passageway
- Uterine malformations, which can prevent efficient labor
- Abnormalities of placental size or location that lead to the fetus assuming a position unfavorable to labor and/or descent

Fetal factors leading to malpresentation include the following:

- Breech presentation or transverse lie
- Abnormal fetal attitude (e.g., hyperextension)
- Multiple pregnancy
- Fetal abnormalities (e.g., hydrocephalus)
- Hydramnios (excessive amounts of fluid permit greater freedom for fetal movement and, therefore, abnormal positions)

Effects of Malpresentation on Labor

- Weak and irregular contractions that are inefficient
- Prolonged labor
- Slow and incomplete cervical dilatation
- Failure of presenting part to descend
- Increased need for operative delivery
- Increased risk of uterine rupture

Effects of Malpresentation on the Mother

- Maternal exhaustion because of prolonged labor
- Greater chance of lacerations along the birth canal because of wider presenting parts
- Heavier bleeding because of lacerations and/or an exhausted uterus, which fails to contract after delivery
- Increased risk of infection caused by the following:
  –Early rupture of membranes
  –Increased blood loss
  –Tissue damage because of lacerations and bruising
  –Prolonged labor
- Decreased peristalsis of the bowel and bladder

Effects of Malpresentation on the Fetus

- Difficult fit through the pelvis, which leads to edema of the presenting part and excessive molding
- Long labor, which can be hard on the fetus, increasing the possibility of anoxia and intrauterine death
- Increased incidence of forceps and cesarean birth
- More frequently occurring prolapsed cord

When a prolapsed cord occurs, a delay of more than 30 minutes in delivering the baby increases fetal mortality fourfold.[2]

■ What should you do if you suspect fetal malpresentation?

The nurse is often the first person to recognize a malpresentation such as breech presentation.

Fetal malpresentation is detected through careful abdominal palpation and vaginal examination. If you suspect malpresentation during your nursing assessment, take the following steps:

1. Alert the primary care provider immediately.
2. Monitor the baby closely until the primary care provider arrives.
3. Closely assess the mother's status and progress in labor. Do not leave her alone.

In all patients who have a breech presentation or any presentation that does not fit the pelvis well or is not settled well into the pelvis, it is essential to inspect the perineum, to listen to fetal heart tones, and to conduct a vaginal examination as soon as the membranes rupture.

> When the presenting part fails to fit the pelvic inlet closely, the danger of a prolapsed cord exists.

A vaginal examination should be performed in the following situations:

- There is unexplained fetal distress (this is especially true when the presenting part is high).
- The membranes rupture with a high presenting part.
- The membranes rupture in a woman presenting with a malpresentation.
- The baby is premature.
- There is a twin gestation.

■ Why is it necessary to be able to recognize a breech presentation?

A prolapsed cord can occur in a breech presentation because the pelvic cavity is not well filled when the feet or buttocks are coming first.

Once the cord is out of the uterus or vagina, the fetal blood and oxygen supply can be blocked because of (a) a drop in temperature, (b) spasm of the blood vessels, or (c) compression between the pelvic brim and the presenting part.

> A prolapsed cord means that the umbilical cord lies beside or below the presenting part of the fetus. This occurs in 0.3% to 0.6% of all pregnancies.[2]

A prolapsed cord can:

- Extend through the vaginal opening

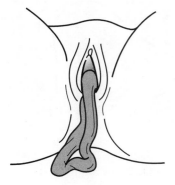

> If the cord extends through the vagina, cover it with a sterile gauze pad moistened with saline solution to keep it from drying out.

FIGURE 2.34 Prolapse of cord through the vaginal opening.

• Be palpable at the cervix

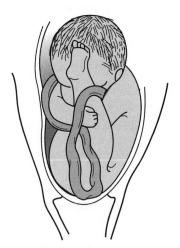

In breech presentations, if membranes rupture spontaneously, a vaginal examination should be performed immediately to feel for the presence of a prolapsed cord.

FIGURE 2.35 Prolapsed cord can be felt at the cervical opening.

• Be hidden and unable to be palpated

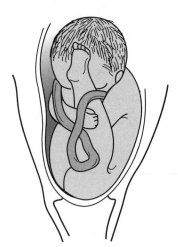

With a prolapsed cord, if no remedies are effected within approximately 40 minutes, fetal death is likely to occur.

FIGURE 2.36 Hidden prolapsed cord.

■ What should you do after detecting or suspecting a prolapsed cord?

1. Place the mother in a position that reduces compression of the cord by the presenting part.

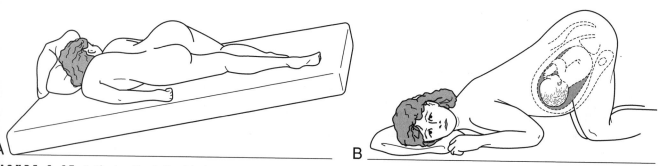

FIGURE 2.37 A. Sims' position in Trendelenburg. **B.** Knee–chest position.

2. DO NOT HANDLE THE CORD because it can cause the cord to spasm, shutting off the fetal blood supply.
3. Perform a vaginal examination. Place two gloved fingers on either side of the cord or both fingers on one side of the cord to avoid compressing the cord and exert upward pressure against the presenting part to relieve pressure on the cord.
4. The primary care provider must be called at the slightest suspicion of a prolapsed cord.
5. If the cord extends through the vagina, cover it with a sterile gauze pad moistened with saline solution to keep it from drying out.

A prolapsed cord in a viable fetus requires prompt delivery, which usually means a cesarean section. Preparation for this should begin immediately.

PRACTICE/REVIEW QUESTIONS

After reviewing Part 4, answer the following questions.

1. Define *malpresentation*. _Is presentation of buttocks, Mentum, shoulder or leg at the pelvis outlet_

2. State at least four maternal or fetal factors that can lead to malpresentation.
   a. _Small pelvis_
   b. _lax abdominal muscles_
   c. _Breech presentation or transverse lie_
   d. _multiple pregnancy_

3. Why is it critical that you be able to recognize a breech presentation? _It could cause fetal death_

4. Explain the first step that you would take when a prolapsed cord is detected.
   1) Place the mother in a position that reduce compression of the cord

5. If you suspect a prolapsed cord and the membranes rupture spontaneously, what should you do? _SVE, hold cord so it does not get compressed_

6. If the cord extends through the vagina, what should you do? _Cover c gauze + sterile water do not handle it because it could spasm_

7. Why is it not advisable to handle a prolapsed cord? _Because it can spasm + shut of fetal blood supply_

8. State five situations in which the danger of a prolapsed cord exists, necessitating a vaginal examination.
   a. _Unexplained fetal distress, especially when fetal presentation is_
   b. _When membranes rupture + presenting part is high (high)_
   c. _When membranes rupture + the fetus has malpresentation_
   d. _When the baby is premature_
   e. _When there is more than 1 gestation_

PRACTICE/REVIEW ANSWER KEY

1. *Malpresentation* means that a part other than the vertex, such as buttocks, shoulder, or face, is presenting at or near the pelvic inlet.

2. Maternal factors are a contracted pelvis, lax abdominal muscles, uterine tumors blocking entry to the pelvic passageway, uterine malformations preventing efficient labor, and abnormalities of placental size or locations. Fetal factors are breech or transverse lie, abnormal fetal attitude, multiple pregnancy, fetal abnormalities, and hydramnios.

3. A prolapsed cord can occur in a breech presentation. The prolapsed cord can result in blockage of blood supply to the fetus, which could result in fetal death.

4. Place the mother in a position that reduces compression of the cord by the presenting part. Use the extreme Trendelenburg or modified Sims' position.

5. Perform a vaginal examination. If you encounter a prolapsed cord, leave your hand in the vagina, holding up the presenting part to alleviate compression on the cord.

6. Do not touch it. Cover the cord with a sterile gauze pad moistened with saline solution. Place the mother in the knee–chest or Sims' position and call the primary care provider.

7. Handling the cord can cause it to go into spasms, shutting off the fetal blood supply.

8. a. When there is unexplained fetal distress (especially when the presenting part is high)
   b. When membranes rupture with a high presenting part
   c. When membranes rupture in a woman with a malpresentation
   d. When the baby is very premature
   e. In a twin gestation

REFERENCES

1. Cunningham, F. G., Gant, N. F., Leveno, K. J., Gilstrap, L. C., III, Hauth, J. C., & Wenstrom, K. D. (Eds.) (2001). *Williams obstetrics* (21st ed., pp. 291–307). New York: McGraw-Hill.
2. Oxorn, H. (1986). *Oxorn-Foote human labor & birth* (5th ed.). New York: Appleton-Century-Crofts.

SUGGESTED READINGS

Lowdermilk, D. L., Perry, S. E., & Bobak, I. M. (Eds.). (2000). *Maternity & women's health care* (7th ed.). St. Louis: Mosby.

MODULE 3

Admission Assessment of the Laboring Woman

E. JEAN MARTIN

As you complete this module, you will learn:

1. Key questions to ask the woman being admitted to the labor unit
2. To identify factors that make the laboring woman a high-risk patient
3. To recognize those characteristics that help distinguish between true labor and false labor
4. Physical assessment measures for admitting the laboring woman
5. How to use the fern test, the Nitrazine paper test, and a sterile speculum examination to determine whether membranes have ruptured
6. To evaluate cervical effacement, dilatation, fetal presentation, and station during labor
7. The importance of preparing for and informing the expectant mother of examination and test procedures

KEY TERMS

When you have completed Part 1 of this module, you should be able to recall the meaning of the following terms. You should also be able to use the terms when consulting with other health professionals. The terms are defined in this module or in the glossary at the end of this book.

ABO incompatibility
abruptio placentae
amniotic fluid index (AFI)
arborization
bradycardia
chancroid
chorioamnionitis
cleft palate
clonus
Down's syndrome
eclampsia
esophageal atresia
group B streptococcus (GBS)
herpes simplex virus (HSV) type 1, type 2
hydramnios (polyhydramnios)
macrosomia
meconium

meconium aspiration syndrome (MAS)
microcephaly
multipara
nullipara
oligohydramnios
perinatal
perinatal morbidity
perinatal mortality
postterm infant
pyloric stenosis
Rh incompatibility
spina bifida
tachycardia
term infant
thrombophlebitis
vertical transmission

Identifying Critical Information

■ **What critical information must be identified for the woman being admitted to the labor unit?**

Certain information is needed immediately to evaluate the following:

- The extent of the woman's labor
- Her general physical condition
- Her risk status
- Her preparation for labor and delivery

This assessment must be carried out quickly to determine how active the labor is and to become alert to the woman with a history of rapid deliveries or with problems denoting risk.

Questions	Information Needed
What made you come to the hospital?	Presenting complaint
When were you told the baby was due?	Expected date of delivery/confinement (EDD/EDC) –by dates –by size –by ultrasound
How many babies have you had?	Projection about possible rapid labor due to multiparity
When did your labor begin? How far apart are the contractions? Have they changed in intensity? Have you had any bleeding?	Stage of labor she is in: –frequency, duration, and intensity of contractions –amount and character of bloody show –identification of abnormal bleeding versus bloody show
Has the bag of water (membranes) broken, and when did it occur? What color was the fluid?	Whether or not membranes have ruptured Risk of chorioamnionitis due to prolonged rupture of membranes Presence or absence of meconium-stained amniotic fluid
How has your pregnancy been? Did you have any problems that required special treatment? Have you had any bleeding?	Any abnormalities in her pregnancy—specifically ask about problems with blood pressure, bleeding, or infections
When did you last have anything to eat or drink? What were these foods?	Extent of gastric fullness
Are you allergic to any foods or drugs that you know of?	Any known allergies to drugs
Who has come with you? Will they be staying with you during labor? Have you had any preparation for this labor and delivery?	Presence of a support system Knowledge level of birth experience
Is there anything special about your pregnancy that I should know?	Important unelicited information that could affect her labor/delivery or the newborn

Guidelines for History-taking

- Keep eye contact.
- **Introduce yourself** and confirm the name by which the woman wishes to be called.
- Inform the woman that you need to ask several questions and that you will stop whenever a contraction begins.
- Ask open-ended questions when possible. For example, "Can you tell me about any infections (or problems) you have had during this pregnancy?" instead of "Have you had an infection (or problem) during this pregnancy?" and "What preparation have you had for your labor and delivery?" instead of "Have you attended childbirth preparation classes?"

> You might need to ask specific questions to follow up on her answers to your open-ended questions.

Identifying the High-Risk Mother and Fetus

■ **How can you identify a mother and fetus who are at risk?**

Mothers with high-risk pregnancies tend to have high-risk babies. These patients need to be identified as early as possible on admittance to the labor unit.

> Taking a good history and reviewing the prenatal record of the woman when she is admitted to the labor unit is necessary for identifying the high-risk intrapartal patient.

Perinatal mortality is a greater cause of death than all other causes combined until age 65. Every year 700 American women die of pregnancy-related complications during their pregnancy or within 1 year of delivery. Leading causes are hemorrhage, preeclampsia and eclampsia, emboli, and infection.[1] The risk of a pregnancy-related death is four times greater among Black women and two times greater among Hispanic women than among white women.[1]

High-Risk Factors for Laboring Women

Age 16 years or younger
Nulliparous at age 35 or older
Multiparous at age 40 or older
Fifth or more pregnancy
Height 60 inches or less and prepregnant weight of 20% less than or 20% more than standard for height and age
Little or no weight gain during pregnancy
Heavy cigarette smoking
Rh incompatibility or ABO incompatibility problems
Two or more previous premature deliveries
Previous birth to a large infant (more than 4,000 g/9 lb—*macrosomia*)
Previous perinatal loss
Less than a high school education or in the poverty-level income group
Single marital status or is an unplanned pregnancy
Little or no antenatal care
History of a congenital anomaly or medical disorder, such as anemia, diabetes, renal disease, cardiac problems, malignant tumors, or psychiatric disorders

> There is nearly a twofold differential in infant birth weights between mothers who smoke and nonsmokers.[2]

> Mothers with limited education are more likely to have low-birth-weight infants. Infants born to mothers with less than a high school education are less likely to survive.[3]

Symptoms of oral (type 1) or genital (type 2) *herpes simplex virus (HSV)* or a current positive herpes culture; current symptoms especially significant if the genital herpes infection present is the woman's first infection (primary infection) experienced during pregnancy

Lesions appear as blisterlike vesicles, which progress to a crusted or ulcer-type appearance. HSV of either type 1 or 2 can be shed at the cervix in symptomatic and asymptomatic women. Women with prior HSV type 2 infections who are asymptomatic have a low risk of shedding the virus during delivery.

Universal viral culturing is not recommended at the time of delivery for asymptomatic women with a history of recurrent infection or whose partner has had a herpetic lesion.

> **NOTE:** *Ulcerative genital complaints are symptomatic of many kinds of infections (e.g., chancroid, secondary infected syphilis, contact dermatitis).*

Primary HSV is a first infection with the virus and can be symptomatic or asymptomatic. It has a 33% to 50% neonatal vertical transmission rate.[4]

Nonprimary first episode HSV is a recurrent infection but is first clinically recognized. It has a 2% to 5% transmission rate.[4] *Recurrent HSV and genital lesions at the time of delivery* have a 0% to 3% transmission rate.[5]

> Viral cultures are costly and imprecise. A negative culture does not rule out the possibility of neonatal infection because the culture sensitivity is well below 100%.[5]

Partner currently has or has a history of herpes

Active herpes in a partner can expose the sexually active mother and can unwittingly infect a newborn after birth. Parents should be educated on the possible risks that HSV imposes on the newborn. Sources of risk include children, grandparents, etc., who have oral lesions as well. Contact with the newborn should be avoided by anyone with a current infection.

At risk for hepatitis B carrier status and no documentation of a negative screen

Approximately 1,500 to 2,000 newborns contract neonatal herpes each year.[5]

Newborns born vaginally or by cesarean delivery to a mother with active HSV lesions should be physically separated from other babies and managed with precautions while remaining in the nursery. An isolation room is not necessary.[4]

See Appendix A for further discussion.

> The hepatitis B virus can be transmitted to the fetus during delivery and, perhaps, in rare cases, transplacentally. See Module 12.

At risk for HIV infection or AIDS

History of previous obstetric complications, such as preeclampsia, multiple pregnancy, or hydramnios

Abnormal presentation (breech presentation or transverse lie)

> Without ZDV therapy, the risk of mother to infant transmission of HIV is 25%. With ZDV therapy, the risk is reduced to 5% to 8%.[6] See Module 11.

Fetus has failed to grow normally or fetus does not reach the expected size for dates

> A preterm birth is one that occurs before 37 completed weeks of gestation. *Gestational age is more important than weight in determining perinatal morbidity or mortality.* See Module 8.

> ■ **Can women who are clearly at risk for problems during labor be identified ahead of time?**

The following factors have a high association of problems developing for either the mother or the baby during or after labor.

Factors From the Mother's History

- Diabetes
- Preeclampsia or eclampsia
- Rh sensitization
- Sickle cell disease
- Heart disease

> Women who are partners of intravenous drug abusers or bisexual males or those who have multiple partners demonstrate high-risk sexual behavior for sexually transmitted diseases, some of which could be life-threatening to both the mother and the fetus. Screening for syphilis, hepatitis B, and HIV infection is strongly recommended.[4]

- Chronic hypertension
- Previous perinatal loss
- Anemia
- Renal disease
- Carrier state for bloodborne infectious disease (e.g., hepatitis B, syphilis, or HIV)

> Maternal syphilis is associated with drug abuse (especially crack cocaine) and lack of prenatal care. Syphilis during pregnancy can cause preterm labor, fetal abnormalities, fetal death, and neonatal infections. In 1999, 556 cases of congenital syphilis were reported.[7,8]

- Group B streptococcus carrier status

> *Group B streptococcus (GBS)* sepsis occurs annually at a rate of 1.8 per live births in the United States. It results in 300 deaths annually among infants less than 90 days of age. *Primary prevention is intrapartum antibiotic chemoprophylaxis for pregnant women with clinical risk factors or a positive GBS culture between 35 and 37 weeks' gestation.*[4] See Appendix A for further discussion.

Factors Developing During This Pregnancy

- Preeclampsia
- Postterm pregnancy (more than 42 weeks' gestation)
- Hydramnios or oligo-hydramnios
- Third trimester bleeding of undetermined origin
- Abruptio placentae or placenta previa

> One in four women will be physically abused during her lifetime, and pregnancy is a risk factor for abuse.[4]

Factors Related to the Fetus

- Irregularity in fetal heart rate (FHR)
- Intrauterine growth restriction
- Prematurity
- Malpresentation, such as breech
- Significant increase or decrease in current fetal activity
- Meconium staining
- Bradycardia or tachycardia

Factors Developing During Early Labor

- Amnionitis
- Premature labor
- Premature rupture of membranes

- Fresh meconium-stained fluid
- Abnormal fetal heart tones
- Suspected cephalopelvic disproportion

> The presence of any one of these factors requires that the mother and fetus be continually evaluated throughout labor. Electronic fetal monitoring is recommended.

Determining True Labor

■ Is the woman in true labor?

The uterus undergoes intermittent contractions once pregnancy is established. These contractions are called Braxton Hicks contractions, and they are often associated with false labor. After the twenty-eighth week of pregnancy, these contractions become definite and more noticeable by the woman.

As the thirty-seventh week of pregnancy approaches, contractions can be strong and are sometimes perceived by the expectant mother as a sign of true labor. Braxton Hicks contractions usually stop or become highly irregular with a change of activity.

True Labor

Show—is often present. Show is blood-tinged mucus released from the cervical canal as labor nears or begins. It is pink, red, or brownish.
NOTE: Bloody show without contractions indicates that the body is preparing for labor but labor is not present without regular contractions lasting approximately 1 minute.
Contractions—tend to occur at regular intervals. They start at the back and sweep around to the abdomen, increasing in intensity and duration over several hours. They often intensify with walking.
NOTE: Regular and intensifying contractions are the single most important indication that labor might have begun.
Fetal movement—no significant change is noted.
Cervix—becomes effaced and dilated.
NOTE: Progressive cervical dilatation is the hallmark of progress in labor.

Walking—increases the intensity of contractions.

Sedation—does not stop true labor.

In addition, for some women:
Bowel status—can have loose stools 1 or 2 days before the onset of labor.
Nesting—women tend to experience a flurry of activity in housecleaning 1 or 2 days before the onset of labor.

False Labor

Show—is absent or can be related to intercourse or to a recent vaginal examination. It is brownish when the bleeding occurs hours before discovery.

Contractions—are irregular. They can be felt only in the back or in the lower abdomen. They do not intensify with walking and gradually diminish over several hours.

Fetal movement—can increase for a short time or remain the same.
Cervix—no change is noted or very small changes in thinning out (Braxton Hicks) occur. Contractions help bring about effacement.

Walking—does not change the intensity of contractions.

Sedation—tends to stop false labor or prodromal labor.

Bowel status—is usually unchanged.

Nesting—none is present.

If uncertainty exists regarding the status of labor, the mother might need to walk for 2 to 3 hours, taking frequent rests. Walking often assists in establishing a good contraction pattern.

> When the mother is asked to walk, tell her to return if the following occur:
> - Bag of water breaks
> - Contractions become more frequent than 3 to 4 minutes apart
> - Bloody show increases
> - Nausea and vomiting occur
> - Urge to push occurs
> - Contractions become so strong that she is having difficulty coping

Evaluating the Status of Membranes

■ What is meant by "membranes"?

While developing inside the uterus, the fetus lives in a sac. The sac has two layers: the inner layer, called the *amnion,* and the outer covering, called the *chorion.* This sac is filled with fluid that is made up of water, various chemicals (e.g., salts), and particles that come from the fetus itself (e.g., body cells and hair).

■ What is normal amniotic fluid like?

By the end of pregnancy, the uterus contains approximately 1 L of amniotic fluid. The fluid is clear or straw-colored and has a characteristic (not foul) odor. When tested for its acid-base content, it ranges from neutral to slightly alkaline. A close relationship exists between the status of the fluid and the health of the fetus. By studying various components of amniotic fluid, one can learn much about the sex, health, and maturity of the baby.

■ Does the fluid serve a special purpose?

The fetus derives many benefits from amniotic fluid, which does the following:

- Protects it from a direct blow that the mother might receive. Pressure from a blow spreads in all directions within the fluid-filled sac, so the fetus does not receive the full impact of the blow.
- Provides a fluid environment in which the fetus moves. This fluid continually changes in amount and consistency, promoting the growth and development of the fetus.
- Prevents loss of heat and permits the fetus to maintain a constant body temperature.
- Provides a source of oral intake. The fetus swallows amniotic fluid from approximately the fourth month until delivery.
- Acts as a collection system for the waste products of the fetus. The fetus urinates into the amniotic fluid from the fourth month until delivery.

■ What can happen to the amniotic fluid and membranes that indicates something is wrong?

A. Premature Rupture of Membranes (PROM) Before Labor Begins With a Term Fetus at 37 Completed Weeks' or More Gestational Age

Membranes ("bag of waters") can rupture before labor begins. The break in the membranes can be complete, with a large gushing of fluid from the birth canal or a small tear with a slow leak.

> Most women go into labor spontaneously within a few hours after membranes rupture.

B. Preterm Premature Rupture of Membranes (pPROM) Before Labor Begins With a Preterm Fetus 36 Weeks' or Less Gestational Age

When rupture occurs before the fetus has reached the thirty-seventh completed week of gestation, perinatal morbidity and mortality increase.

> BE PREPARED FOR THE BIRTH OF A HIGH-RISK INFANT.

C. Meconium-Stained Amniotic Fluid

Fetal stool is referred to as *meconium.* It is largely made up of water but also contains proteins, cholesterol, lipids, vernix, and other substances. Large concentrations of bile pigments give meconium its green color. Meconium present for more than 24 hours begins to turn yellow-green. Bacteria are not present in fresh meconium.[9]

Meconium at delivery in a term fetus is present in 7% to 22% (some say 30%) but approaches an incidence of 40% to 50% in postterm infants.[9,10]

Fetal physiologic mechanisms that result in relaxation of the sphincter required for meconium passage are not well understood.

- May be associated with a hypoxic event
- May simply be the result of a mature fetal vagal response[11]

The significance of meconium-stained amniotic fluid as a predictor of fetal compromise depends on the following factors[10]:

- Concentration (grading) (Table 3.1)
- Gestational age
- Stage of labor when the meconium is passed (often not known)
- The presence of other fetal compromise markers such as FHR abnormalities or oligohydraminios

TABLE 3.1	Grading of Meconium Staining
Grade 1 (mild)	Yellow-green staining
Grade 2 (moderate)	Green color with moderate thickness
Grade 3 (severe)	Thick green meconium of pea soup consistency

Meconium aspiration syndrome (MAS) is thought to be caused by an initial hypoxic event resulting in the release of meconium into amniotic fluid. The normal fetal response to hypoxemia is to gasp, and thus in this instance, the meconium is aspirated (can be seen below the cords on examination).

The pathophysiologic process set up in meconium aspiration syndrome often leads to a poor perinatal outcome.

*NOTE: Babies who aspirate meconium **but are not hypoxemic during labor** are not likely to experience any serious consequences, and 90% will be asymptomatic.[10]*

Related Facts

Meconium is rarely passed before the thirty-fourth gestational week.

Clinical studies indicate an association of meconium passage with maternal high-risk situations, such as the following:

- Acute chorioamnionitis
- PROM
- Abruptio placentae
- Cocaine use
- Postterm pregnancy

Meconium alone is not an indicator of fetal hypoxia. Look at other fetal assessment parameters.

FRESH MECONIUM STAINING IN THE **ABSENCE** OF POOR FETAL HEART PATTERNS CAN INDICATE THAT THE FETUS IS NOT IN DISTRESS.

FRESH MECONIUM STAINING IN THE **PRESENCE** OF POOR FETAL HEART PATTERNS INDICATES **SEVERE** FETAL DISTRESS.

Signs of chronic intrauterine stress and meconium passage are often seen in postterm pregnancies.

> Postterm pregnancies are defined as lasting beyond 42 weeks' gestation. See Module 4.

In postterm laboring women, you should look for the following:

- The presence of meconium-stained fluid
- The absence of any amniotic fluid (This should alert you to the almost certain presence of meconium even though you cannot see it!)
- Placental dysfunction
  –Watch for late decelerations.
- Umbilical cord compression
  –This often presents with decreased amniotic fluid.
- Variable decelerations
- Macrosomia

> Many pregnancies thought to be at term can actually be postterm. Primigravidas are more likely to have prolonged pregnancies.

> **BE PREPARED FOR A HIGH-RISK BABY.**

The relationship of intrapartum meconium to low Apgar scores and acidosis remains controversial. However, heavy meconium does appear to increase the risk of low Apgar scores, MAS, and death.[9,10]

A policy of elective labor induction at term to reduce the incidence of meconium staining of amniotic fluid has consistently failed to reduce the incidence of meconium aspiration.[10]

Electronic internal monitoring is recommended when meconium is noted.

Suctioning should be anticipated and the neonatal specialist alerted (Display 3.1).

DISPLAY 3.1 Selective Suctioning

The American Academy of Pediatrics[4] recommends the following:

1. Oropharyngeal suctioning of the infant upon delivery of the head and before delivery of the shoulders of all infants (cephalic presentation) who have meconium-stained amniotic fluid

2. Suctioning after delivery of the head in a breech presentation with meconium-stained amniotic fluid

3. That in presence of thick meconium, visualization of the larynx and removal of any meconium present

4. That if meconium is present and the infant is depressed, intubation of the trachea and suctioning to remove meconium or other aspirated material from beneath the glottis

5. That in a vigorous and spontaneously breathing infant who may have aspirated meconium, there is less cause for aggressive suctioning because it could result in vocal cord injury

> When suctioning with a mechanical apparatus, set the suction pressure so that when the suction tubing is occluded, negative pressure never exceeds 100 mm Hg.

> The presence of meconium-stained amniotic fluid, no matter what the color, should alert you to the potential for fetal aspiration of meconium at birth. Prompt suctioning of the mouth and nose of the infant with a DeLee suction apparatus before delivery of the baby's shoulders and trunk is important to reduce the occurrence of meconium aspiration syndrome (a form of aspiration pneumonia that occurs most often in term or postterm infants who have passed meconium in utero). Even when DeLee suctioning is done, meconium aspiration can be present because aspiration can occur in utero.

D. Infection

Amniotic membranes and fluid can become infected, especially after 24 hours of ruptured membranes. Infection can be detected by the presence of a foul odor and an elevated temperature in the mother.

> In all instances of *premature rupture of membranes,* the woman's temperature should be taken and recorded every 2 hours. An elevated temperature (99.6°F) can indicate the presence of an infection and should be reported immediately to the primary care provider.

E. Port Wine–Colored Amniotic Fluid—AN EMERGENCY

Port wine–colored amniotic fluid is an indicator of a premature separation of the placenta from the uterine wall, called *abruptio placentae* (Display 3.2).

DISPLAY 3.2   Signs of Abrutio Placentae

The following signs indicate that the placenta has partially or totally separated from the uterine wall:

- Tender abdomen
- Hard or rigid tone to abdomen
- Absence of fetal heart tones
- Mother has had a few sharp piercing pains in her abdomen in the past 1 or 2 hours
- Mother *might* or *might not* have vaginal bleeding

Abruptio placentae occurs in approximately 1 of 200 pregnancies.[12] It is often found in women who have the following:

- Hypertension
- Hydramnios
- Multiple pregnancy
- Trauma
- History of heavy smoking
- Cocaine use (especially intravenous use)

F. Hydramnios/Oligohydramnios

There can be too much or too little fluid within the amniotic sac. Normally, the fluid volume is about 1 L toward the end of pregnancy. The presence of 2 L of amniotic fluid is considered excessive and called *polyhydramnios* or *hydramnios.* This condition occurs in about 1% of all pregnancies.[13] The mother's abdomen can look unusually large, tight, and glistening. When there is less than 500 mL of fluid, the condition is called *oligohydramnios.*

Ultrasonic techniques are used to measure amounts of amniotic fluid. The measurement is reported as a number (e.g., 24 cm), which is compared with standardized values for normal pregnancies at expressed gestational weeks. The calculation involves adding the vertical depths of the largest packets of fluid in each of four equal uterine quadrants. The numerical value is called the *amniotic fluid index (AFI).*[13]

> Amniotic fluid volume normally peaks at approximately 800 mL by the thirty-fourth week and then slowly decreases until 40 weeks. It can decrease quickly after 40 weeks.[14]

Clinical studies indicate that the AFI tends to be reliable in determining normal and increased fluid but is not accurate in diagnosing oligohydramnios. Factors such as maternal hydration/dehydration and altitude may affect the AFI.[13]

Hydramnios, an AFI of greater than 20 to 25 cm, is commonly associated with fetal malformations and chromosomal abnormalities. The infant should be carefully screened for the following:

- Hydrocephaly
- Microcephaly
- Anencephaly
- Spina bifida
- Cleft palate
- Esophageal atresia
- Pyloric stenosis
- Down's syndrome
- Congenital heart disease
- Prematurity

Oligohydramnios, an AFI of 5 cm or less, is not common in early pregnancy but is associated with poor outcomes. When pregnancies continue beyond term, diminished fluid volume is often found (12% in one study cited in Cunningham and others[13]). Electronic fetal monitoring is recommended.

Oligohydramnios is primarily associated with the following:

- Congenital defects of the fetal urinary tract
- Intrauterine growth restriction
- Postterm pregnancies

> Common maternal antepartal complications with which hydramnios is associated are as follows:
>
> - Diabetes
> - Multifetal pregnancies

> Be alert for maternal intrapartal complications such as the following:
>
> - Placental abruption
> - Uterine dysfunction
> - Postpartum hemorrhage

> Cord compression during labor is common with oligohydramnios. Whenever women are diagnosed as having oligohydramnios or when there is no amniotic fluid on rupture of membranes, electronic fetal monitoring is recommended.

> It is not enough to screen the infant in the delivery room for congenital problems associated with hydramnios. The infant must be screened for respiratory and feeding difficulties during the first 48 hours of life.

PRACTICE/REVIEW QUESTIONS

After reviewing this part, answer the following questions. ONE OR MORE THAN ONE of the choices may be correct.

1. List at least five types of information you need to elicit from a woman being admitted to the labor unit.

a. *Do you have labor coach, who is c you, did you take childbirth preparation class*
b. *How far apart are your contractions*
c. *Have your membranes ruptured*
d. *have you had a bloody show*
e. *Do the contraction get stronger when you walk; Do they continue when you rest*
f. *Have you had any infections*
g. *What is your EDC*

2. Which of the following are considered high-risk categories for a laboring woman?

   (A.) Age of 37 years

   (B.) Unmarried

   C. High school graduate

   D. Fourth pregnancy

   (E.) Previous perinatal loss

   F. First pregnancy

   (G.) Current history of an active herpes lesion

3. Which of the following factors predict a strong possibility of problems developing for the mother or baby during or after labor and delivery?

   (A.) Maternal history of heavy smoking

   → (B.) Fresh meconium-stained fluid

   C. Induction of labor

   → (D.) Fetal tachycardia

   → (E.) Multiple pregnancy

   (F.) Mild anemia

   → (G.) Prematurity

4. A birth occurring before ___*37*___ completed weeks' gestation is identified as preterm birth.

5. A fetus of more than ___*42*___ completed weeks' gestation (postterm) is considered high risk.

6. Which one of the following is an indication of *true* labor?

   A. Pinkish mucus present

   B. Regular and intensifying contractions

   C. Loose stools 1 to 2 days before labor

   D. Effaced cervix

   E. Increase in fetal movement

7. Define *primary HSV infection:* *it is the first injection c the virus + can by symptomatic or asymptomatic. It has a 33% to 50% neonatal vertical transmission rate.*

8. Define *nonprimary first episode HSV:* *recurring injection but is 1st clinically recognized*

9. Amniotic fluid generally peaks in volume by the ___*34*___ gestational week and then slowly ___*↓*___ until the ___*40th*___ week. It can ___*↓*___ quickly after 40 weeks.

   AFI after 41 wks <5 needs delivered

10. Which of the following descriptions are characteristic of normal amniotic fluid?

    A. Clear or straw-colored

    B. Neutral to slightly acid

    C. Composed of water, salts, and other particles from the fetus

    D. Alkaline

11. Which of the following situations indicates that you should prepare for the birth of a high-risk infant?

    A. Rupture of membranes before labor begins with a 38-week gestational age fetus

    B. Rupture of membranes before labor begins with a fetus less than 37 weeks' gestational age

    C. A laboring woman at a documented 43 weeks' gestation

    D. Rupture of membranes with little fluid at 41 weeks' gestation

12. Which of the following can indicate that the fetus is in distress?

    A. Greenish brown meconium staining with a cephalic presentation

    B. Mother's temperature of 99°F

    C. Tender abdomen

    D. Excessive amniotic fluid

    E. Port wine–colored amniotic fluid

    F. Absence of amniotic fluid

13. State the difference between PROM (premature rupture of membranes) and pPROM (preterm premature rupture of membranes). *PROM - rupture before labor begins c̄ a term fetus 37 or > completed weeks pPROM - rupture before 37 completed weeks*

14. Meconium passage at delivery in a term fetus is present in approximately *7-22* % of women. Two situations that increase the chances of this happening are *hypoxic event* and *mature vagal response*.

15. Heavy meconium-stained amniotic fluid does not appear to increase the risk of a low Apgar score.

    A. True

    B. False

16. The American Academy of Pediatrics recommends that in a vigorous and spontaneously breathing infant who may have aspirated meconium aggressive suctioning may not be warranted.

    A. True

    B. False

17. When pregnancy is prolonged beyond 42 completed weeks of gestation, one should be prepared for a high-risk baby that is *Postmature / Dysmature*

18. In prolonged pregnancies, one should watch for placental dysfunction that can be reflected in an electronic fetal monitoring strip depicting *late decelration*.

19. DeLee (endotracheal) suctioning done on infants with moderate or thick meconium-stained amniotic fluid ensures that meconium aspiration will not occur.

    A. True

    B. False

20. The amniotic fluid index (AFI) is defined as *an US technique used to determine the amount amniotic fluid.*

21. The AFI tends to be less reliable in diagnosing *Oligohydramnios*.

Calculations taken by measuring 4 quadrants (pockets of fluid)

22. If a woman is diagnosed as having oligohydramnios, electronic fetal monitoring is recommended.
     A) True
     B. False

PRACTICE/REVIEW ANSWER KEY

1. Presenting complaint and symptoms, EDC, stage of labor, abnormalities in pregnancy, time of last snack or meal, known allergies to drugs, support system, review of patient's history (family and past history, current laboratory data, present obstetric status)

2. A, B, E, G

3. B, D, E, G

4. 37

5. 42

6. A, B, D, E, G

7. *Primary HSV* is a first infection with the virus; it can be symptomatic or asymptomatic.

8. *Nonprimary first episode HSV* is actually a recurrent infection but at the time is first clinically diagnosed as such.

9. Thirty-fourth, decreases, fortieth, decreases

10. A, C, D

11. B, C, D

12. A, C, E, F

13. PROM pertains to rupture of membranes after the thirty-seventh completed gestational week, whereas pPROM signifies rupture of membranes before the thirty-seventh completed gestational week.

14. 7% to 22% (some say 30%); any two of the following: acute chorioamnionitis, premature rupture of membranes, abruptio placentae, cocaine use, postterm pregnancy

15. B

16. A

17. Postmature/Dysmature (see glossary)

18. Late decelerations

19. B

20. A numerical value expressing calculations of amniotic fluid volume found during ultrasonography as compared with standardized values for normal pregnancies at expressed gestational weeks.

21. Oligohydramnios

22. A

Physical Examination of the Laboring Woman
SKILL UNIT 1

This section details how to perform a modified physical examination to screen for problems in the woman being admitted to labor and delivery. Study this section and then attend a skill practice and demonstration session scheduled with your preceptor. You will need to demonstrate the examination and correctly interpret the results. The steps of the examination are summarized at the end of this unit.

ACTIONS	REMARKS

What Are the Techniques to Be Used in Performing the Physical Examination?

1. *Inspection*–observing the general health and outstanding characteristics of the patient in a thorough, unhurried manner	
2. *Palpation*–feeling or touching parts to be evaluated	The physical examination of the laboring woman is not as extensive as that given at her first prenatal visit.
3. *Auscultation*–listening, usually with a stethoscope, for the sounds produced by the body	

What Steps Should You Take to Prepare for the Examination?

1. Ask the woman to empty her bladder.	A full bladder can make examination of the abdomen or bladder uncomfortable.
2. Follow a logical order of assessment. Use all of your senses as the assessment is carried out.	In general, it is suggested that you begin at the head of the patient and work toward the toes. You are not likely to miss anything this way.
3. Explain to the woman what you are doing.	
4. Warm your hands by rubbing them together or holding them under warm water.	
5. Chart your findings in a logical order.	Unless you have a checklist, chart your findings in the same order in which you conduct the examination.

When Is the Best Time to Perform the Physical Examination?

The initial assessment is carried out immediately to evaluate the labor and any signs of problems.	The examination is conducted as quickly as possible. The woman can then assume a side-lying or upright sitting position. Cardiac output is better for the mother, and uteroplacental circulation for the fetus is optimized in these positions.

Assess the following:
   General appearance
      –Look for edema in face, hands, and feet
	Early and careful assessment of the patient's physical status will provide clues to problems.

Vital signs
   Abdominal
      –Determine frequency, duration, intensity of contractions
   Fetal position
   Fetal heart tones
   Height of the fundus (top of uterus)
	For example, if the blood pressure is elevated, evaluate for the following:
	   –Edema in hands and feet
	   –Protein in the urine
	   –Presence of headache and blurred vision
	   –Elevated preeclampsia laboratory indices

Perform a vaginal examination to determine the following:

    Cervical effacement
    Cervical dilatation and station
    Amount of bloody show
    Whether membranes have ruptured
    Amount of amniotic fluid

NOTE: *Women with preterm or term pregnancies who are not in labor and who present with ruptured membranes and no signs of fetal distress should not have a vaginal examination on arrival. Wait for the primary care provider to arrive.*

Vaginal examination should not be done on a nonlaboring woman who presents with ruptured membranes. A sterile speculum examination using strict aseptic techniques will tell you whether she is dilated. A single vaginal examination can compromise both mother and fetus by leading to chorioamnionitis. Management of the expectant woman will depend on whether membranes have ruptured, not on dilatation.

> If the fetus is in a transverse position and labor is active, you will need to alert the primary care provider immediately. If the membranes are ruptured and there are signs of fetal distress, you will need to perform a sterile vaginal examination to determine that there is not a prolapsed cord.

What Position Is Best for the Examination?

Ask the patient to lie on her back as you begin the examination.

Elevate the head of the bed or the examining table enough to make the patient comfortable.

Completing a General Assessment

Give *thoughtful attention* to the general appearance of the patient.

Note the following:
    Signs of distress
    Skin color
    Movements
    Personal hygiene
    Odor
    Facial expression
    Speech
    Manner
    Mood
    State of awareness

The woman who comes to the labor unit in active labor might appear stressed because contractions are strong and frequent. Note how she is coping with them—whether she is using a breathing technique or tensing up. You can reinforce her technique or teach her an effective one.

If she has come with a support person, find out whether she wishes the support person to remain with her during as much of the admission as possible. If she has no partner, you may need to assume a supporting role.

Vital Signs

1. Blood pressure (BP)
    a. The cuff must fit snugly on the arm and be of appropriate size. The cuff should be approximately 20% wider than the width of the arm.

    b. Take BP measurements with the woman in a sitting position or left lateral (side-lying) position.

    c. Taking BP measurements using the Korotkoff IV (muffled) sound or the V (disappearing) sound has been an issue. A recent consensus states

A cuff too small or too large can result in BP readings that are inaccurately high or low, respectively.

BP in the arteries is affected by position. When sitting, the pressure in the brachial artery is highest; when lying on the right or left side, it is lowest.

BP taken while the woman is flat on her back (supine) can be inaccurate, especially toward the end of pregnancy.

that the Korotkoff V sound should be used for reading the diastolic pressure.[16]

The method for taking BP readings (e.g., patient position and which Korotkoff sound to use) should be consistently used by all caretakers on the unit.

> An elevated systolic but normal diastolic blood pressure can indicate anxiety.

Compare the reading you obtain with the mother's prenatal BP readings.

The patient has a hypertensive disorder if the BP is:

- 140/90 mm Hg or higher (mild hypertension)
- 160/110 mm Hg or higher (severe hypertension)

To determine hypertension in the mother, *her baseline BP must be known.*

A woman with either of these BP changes can have pregnancy-induced hypertension, chronic hypertension, or transient hypertension.

You also need to do the following:

–Determine whether the mother's urine has protein in it

–Check for facial, fingertip, and pretibial edema

–Test for hyperreflexia

–Ask the mother if she is having headaches or blurred vision or is seeing spots before her eyes

–Notify the primary care provider immediately of proteinuria (other than trace), BP elevations approaching 140/90 mm Hg, hyperreflexia, marked edema (>2+), and complaints of headaches or blurred vision or spots before the eyes.

A multiparous woman presenting before term (30 to 36 weeks) with flulike symptoms, nausea, vomiting, or gastrointestinal upset should be immediately assigned a differential diagnosis of HELLP syndrome. Elevated BP *might not* be present. These women are very ill and need immediate evaluation and intervention (see Module 9).

2. Pulse (normal range is 60 to 90 bpm)

Increased pulse rate can result from excitement, anxiety, dehydration, and in rare cases, cardiac problems.

3. Respirations

Avoid counting respirations during a uterine contraction because they can be abnormally high or low as a result of stress or because of the use of a breathing technique.

4. Temperature (normal range is 97.6° to 99.6°F [36.2° to 37.6°C])

Look for signs of infection or dehydration if the temperature is above 99.6°F.

NOTE: *In the past, an increase of 30 mm Hg systole or 15 mm Hg diastole above a baseline BP on at least two occasions 6 hours apart was diagnostic for pregnancy-induced hypertension. This is no longer considered a reliable diagnostic marker. However, rising systolic and/or diastolic BP readings are always cause for increased surveillance of the pregnant woman. See Module 9 for a detailed discussion of this topic.*

Abdomen

1. Inspect for scars, striae (stretch marks), rashes, and symmetry of the abdomen.

Striae are shiny, reddish lines that appear on the breasts, abdomen, thighs, and buttocks of approximately half of pregnant women as a result of stretching of the skin and underlying tissue.

2. If you detect a scar that the woman tells you is the result of surgery done on the uterus and the woman is in active labor, notify the primary care provider immediately.

Vertical scars from previous classic cesarean births are much more likely to rupture than horizontal scars down low on the abdomen. Maternal morbidity from rupture of vertical scars is close to 5%, but the perinatal mortality rate is near 50%

3. Assess the following:
   - Fundal height
   - Fetal position
   - Fetal heart tones

An abnormal shape of the abdomen should alert you to fetal malposition (such as a transverse lie)

See Skill Unit "Measuring Fundal Height" in Module 4.

Bladder

Gently palpate the lower abdominal area just above the symphysis pubis bone to determine bladder fullness or tenderness.

Suprapubic tenderness might suggest a bladder infection. Signs and symptoms of elevated temperature, burning on urination, and frequency of urination should be discussed.

Lower Extremities

1. Inspect for the presence of *varicosities.* If present, feel for warmth.

Warmth over a varicosity can indicate a *thrombophlebitis* (inflammation of a vein associated with a blood clot). The primary care provider should be alerted.

Using both hands, palpate for *tenderness,* beginning behind the knee and working your way down the leg to the ankle (Fig. 3.1)

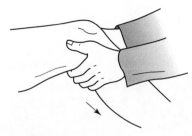

FIGURE 3.1

If the woman experiences tenderness to your touch, dorsiflex the foot (i.e., bend it back toward the knee) and ask her whether this causes any calf pain (Fig. 3.2). Calf pain with dorsiflexion of the foot indicates possible thrombophlebitis. This is called Homans' sign.

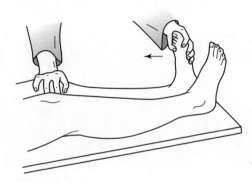

FIGURE 3.2

2. Press firmly with the thumb approximately 5 seconds over the pretibial (shin) area to test for *edema* in both legs (Fig. 3.3).

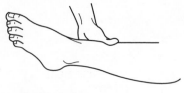

FIGURE 3.3

Edema of the legs measuring 3+ and 4+ is often accompanied by facial and hand edema. BP and proteinuria should be evaluated, as well as the presence of headaches and blurred vision, to diagnose preeclampsia.

Pretibial edema is assessed as follows:

1+ = small suggestion of fullness felt
2+ = sense of fullness
3+ = blanching of the skin and depression seen as finger presses down

3. To elicit a deep tendon reflex (DTR), the patient must be relaxed. Position the leg by supporting the knee in a somewhat flexed position with one hand or arm while asking the patient to relax that leg completely (Fig. 3.4). Briskly tap the patellar tendon just below the kneecap. This can also be done with the patient in a sitting position (Fig. 3.5). Watch for some degree of a brisk jerk.

NOTE: *Many women, including adolescents, will have brisk reflexes. Do not use this as a major indication of a pathologic condition.*

4+ = indentation made by finger pressure (pitting), which remains for several seconds and gradually declines

> Edema is not considered a reliable diagnostic criterion for preeclampsia.

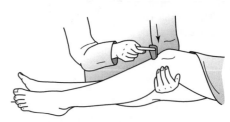

FIGURE 3.4

Reflexes are graded on a 0 to 4+ scale.
4+ = extremely brisk (called hyperactive); often indicates a disease state of the central nervous system
3+ = brisker than average
2+ = average, normal
1+ = somewhat diminished, low normal
 0 = flat, no response

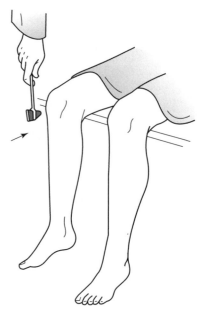

FIGURE 3.5

Test for clonus if reflexes are 4+ (hyperactive). Support the knee in a partially flexed position. With your other hand, sharply dorsiflex the foot and maintain it in dorsiflexion (see Fig. 3.2). If clonus is present, you will see the foot moving back and forth in small rhythmic movements.

The presence of clonus indicates that the central nervous system is highly irritated, although in some patients it can simply be the result of anxiety. Clonus is often associated with moderate to severe preeclampsia.

You will need to attend a skill session(s) to practice these skills with the help of your preceptor. Mastery of the skill is achieved when you can demonstrate techniques of physical assessment, including the following:

- Preparatory steps
- Logical order
- Appropriate positions for examining various areas of the body
- Accurate assessment of vital signs
- Abdomen (fundal height, fetal position, and fetal heart tones are demonstrated
  in Module 4)
- Bladder
- Lower extremities, including checking for edema, reflexes, and tenderness

Testing for Ruptured Membranes
–Sterile Speculum Examination
–Nitrazine Paper Test
SKILL UNIT 2

This section details the only accurate way to test for the rupture of amniotic membranes. Study this section and then attend a skill practice and demonstration scheduled with your preceptor. You will need to demonstrate that you can perform and interpret the steps of this procedure. These steps are summarized at the end of this unit.

ACTIONS	REMARKS

Selecting the Speculum

1. The speculum is composed of two blades and a handle. A thumb piece attaches to the top blade; the bottom blade is fixed (Fig. 3.6).

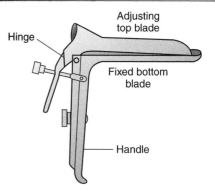

FIGURE 3.6

The top blade is hinged, and the thumb piece controls its motions (Fig. 3.7).

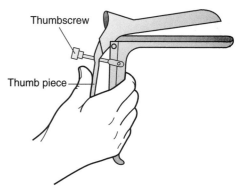

FIGURE 3.7

The thumbscrew, when turned, tightens and fixes the top blade in position (Fig. 3.8).

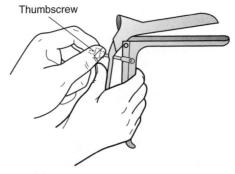

Thumbscrew

FIGURE 3.8

When the speculum is opened by using the thumb piece, a space is created between the blades, which, if placed in the vagina, permits a clear view of the vaginal walls and cervix (Fig 3.9).

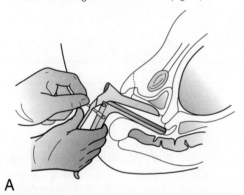

A

FIGURE 3.9

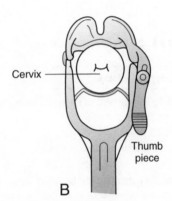

Cervix

Thumb piece

B

2. Two basic types of specula are as follows:
   a. The Graves speculum (Fig. 3.10)
      • Is the most common
      • Is used in the examination of the adult female
      • Comes in two sizes, standard and large, which vary in length from 3.5 to 5 inches and in width from 0.75 to 1.5 inches

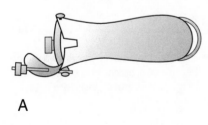

A

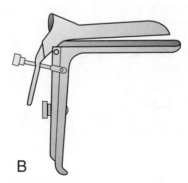

B

FIGURE 3.10 Graves speculum.

b. The Pedersen speculum (Fig. 3.11)
- Is as long as the Graves speculum but narrower and flatter
- Is used more in women who have not had intercourse, women who have never had a baby, or women who are so tense that insertion of the Graves speculum is difficult

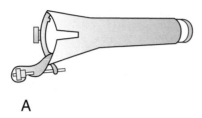

A

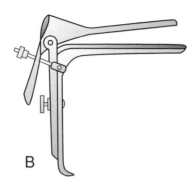

B

FIGURE 3.11 Pedersen speculum.

Preparing the Woman

3. Tell the woman what you are going to be doing in terms she can understand.

An informed woman is more relaxed. She is more likely to cooperate with you throughout the examination.

4. Ask the woman to empty her bladder.

A full bladder can make the examination uncomfortable for the woman and more difficult to perform.

5. Have the woman remove her underclothing and lie on the examining table. Assist her to relax with her legs bent, feet resting flat on the table or in the stirrups. Place a pillow under her head and ask that she rest her hands across her abdomen or at her sides.

This increases her comfort and relaxation. Sometimes women put their hands above their heads during a vaginal examination, which tightens abdominal muscles and makes the examination more difficult and uncomfortable.

What Should You Do Before Beginning the Examination?

6. Drape the mother's legs so that you cover her up to her knees. Make sure that you can see her face when you are sitting down.

7. Position a gooseneck lamp so that the perineum is well lit.

Position the stool on which you will sit for the examination so that you will not need to move it again.

If the perineum appears wet and glistening, there is a good chance that the membranes have ruptured.

8. Select the appropriate speculum. The speculum must be *sterile*.

9. Wash your hands.

10. Put on sterile gloves.

The appropriate speculum is the one that will cause the least amount of discomfort to the woman while providing a good view of the vagina and cervix.

11. If you are alone, open the package containing the sterile speculum in such a way that you can grasp the handle for removal after you have put on a sterile glove.

It is a good idea to have someone assist you and support the woman throughout the examination.

Take care! Maintaining strict aseptic technique throughout the sterile speculum examination can reduce the risk of chorioamnionitis if membranes are ruptured.

What Is the Best Way to Begin the Examination?

12. Sit down on the stool and ask the woman to separate or spread her legs. *Do not try to use force or even gently separate her legs.*

13. Tell the woman *how to relax.* If she knows a relaxation and breathing technique learned previously, have her use it. If not, have her do slow, deep, relaxed breathing. Ask her to let herself go limp, to think of herself as a rag doll.

14. If the woman becomes upset or tense during the examination, *stop whatever you are doing.* Do not remove your fingers; simply hold your hand still. Find out what is bothering her. Try to distinguish among discomfort as a result of pressure, fear, or actual pain. Wait until she has regained control, helping her to relax.

15. Hold the speculum near the gooseneck lamp to warm it.

    Often, additional lubricant is not needed because the vagina is moist from bloody show when the mother goes into labor. If a lubricant is needed, only *sterile* water should be used.

16. Tell the woman what you are doing as you touch her inner thigh with the back of the gloved hand that is not holding the speculum.

17. Using this same hand, place two fingers just inside the introitus and gently press down on the base of the vagina.

18. With your other hand, introduce the *closed* speculum past your fingers at approximately a 45-degree angle downward (Fig. 3.12). Keep a moderate downward pressure on the blades to avoid upward pressure on the sensitive bladder and top vaginal wall.

Because this examination is an intrusive procedure, it should be carried out when the woman is ready for it.

If you use running tap water or a lubricant, you will lose the sterility of the speculum. This could introduce an infectious organism to the mother and to the fetus if membranes are ruptured.

This accustoms her to your touch and prepares her for the more intrusive part of the examination.

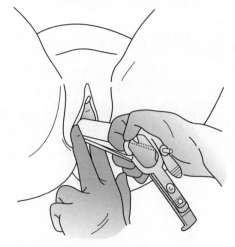

FIGURE 3.12

19. After the speculum is in the vagina, remove your fingers from the base of the vaginal opening. Turn the blades of the speculum into a horizontal position, all the while keeping a moderate downward pressure (Fig. 3.13).

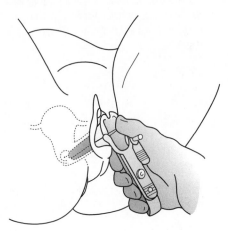

FIGURE 3.13

20. Tell the woman she might feel pressure. Move your thumb to the thumb piece and press to open the blades so that the cervix is in view (Fig. 3.14).
21. Sweep the blades slowly upward by gently pressing on the handle. If this does not bring the cervix into view, close the blades and withdraw the speculum a little. Warn the mother of the extra pressure she might feel. Then, while pressing down firmly, move the blades toward the back of the vagina again. Sometimes the tip of the blades needs to be directed more anteriorly or posteriorly, depending on the position of the cervix.
22. When the cervix is in view, tighten the thumbscrew to keep the blades open.

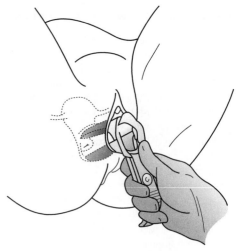

FIGURE 3.14

What Will You See If the Membranes Are Ruptured?

---

23. Fluid will be seen leaking from the cervical opening.

> Viewing leaking fluid from the cervical opening is the best method for determining that the membranes have ruptured.

Note the color and odor.

- *Deep yellow color* indicates the release of meconium approximately 1 to 2 days previously.
- *Greenish brown color* indicates *fresh* meconium staining of amniotic fluid.

Use this opportunity to screen for any signs of abnormalities, such as bleeding. Heavy bloody show can alert you to an advanced state of labor.

Amniotic fluid is clear or straw-colored. It does not have an unpleasant odor.

The presence of meconium is an indication of a potentially poor outcome for the fetus and requires further evaluation. It is not necessarily a predictor of poor fetal outcome, but it must be evaluated in light of other assessment and findings (e.g., fetal heart rate tracings). The release of meconium during labor means that the fetus is in distress (however, this might not be true if the fetus is in a breech position).

24. Obtain a specimen of the suspected leaking fluid by placing a *sterile* cotton-tipped applicator into the pool of fluid accumulating in the lower blade (Fig. 3.15).

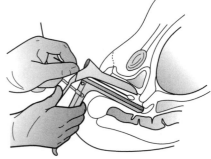

FIGURE 3.15

25. Touch the cotton-tipped applicator or cotton ball on a fresh strip of Nitrazine paper, moistening it well.

Nitrazine paper contains a dye that changes color when alkaline substances such as amniotic fluid moisten it.

How Do You Interpret the Color Change?

26. Compare the color that appears on the moistened paper against the standard color chart.

Findings on Nitrazine Paper		
Color	**pH**	**Interpretation**
Yellow	5.0	Probably membranes are *not* ruptured
Olive	5.5	
Olive-green	6.0	
Blue-green	6.5	Probably membranes are ruptured
Blue-gray	7.0	
Deep blue	7.5	May be caused by blood or cervical mucus

Be aware of the possibility of false readings.

A standard color chart can be found on the box of Nitrazine paper, with a range of colors used to interpret the alkaline nature of substances. Because amniotic fluid is neutral (pH 7.0) or slightly alkaline (pH 7.25), it will change the yellow color of Nitrazine paper. The pH values of blood, vaginal mucus, and certain secretions from vaginal infections are also alkaline. If the amount of amniotic fluid is small or absent but the above substances are present in large amounts, a false-positive test could result.

The Nitrazine test is not considered a definitive test for diagnosing ruptured membranes. See the fern test for this.

How Do You Remove the Speculum?

27. Release the thumbscrew on the thumb piece. Hold the blades apart by pressing on the thumb piece and begin withdrawing the speculum until the cervix is released from between the blades.

28. Release your pressure on the thumb piece and allow the blades to close. Avoid pinching the vaginal tissue or pubic hair when the blades close. Rotate the blades to a sideways position and exert downward pressure. As the blades are eased out, hook your index finger over the top blade to control it.

This avoids pressure to the sensitive urethra and top vaginal wall.

29. Note the odor of any vaginal discharge pooled in the bottom blade.

Foul-smelling discharge might indicate amniotic fluid infection.

30. Deposit the speculum in the proper container.

31. Wipe any moisture or discharge from the perineal area.

You will need to attend a skill session(s) to practice this skill with the help of your preceptor. Mastery of the skill is achieved when you can demonstrate the following:

- Selection and operation of an appropriately sized speculum for a variety of women
- Positioning and preparation of the woman for speculum examination
- The procedure for a sterile speculum examination
- How to obtain a specimen for Nitrazine paper testing
- Interpretation of color changes indicating that membranes have ruptured

Fern Testing for Ruptured Membranes
SKILL UNIT 3

This section details how to do the fern test to determine whether membranes have ruptured. Study this section and then attend a skill practice and demonstration section scheduled with your preceptor. You will need to demonstrate that you can perform the procedure and correctly interpret the results. These steps are summarized at the end of this unit.

ACTIONS	REMARKS
Preparing to Conduct the Test	
1. Who might need this test?	
• Any pregnant woman suspected of having ruptured membranes	Amniotic fluid contains a high amount of a salt called sodium chloride. If drops of the fluid are spread on a glass slide, allowed to dry, and examined through a microscope, a characteristic palm leaf pattern can be seen. This is why it is called *arborization* or the fern test.
2. What equipment is needed?	No bacteria or other foreign material should be introduced into the vagina if ruptured membranes are suspected.
• Sterile gloves	
• Sterile speculum	
• Two clean microscope slides	
• Two small, sterile cotton-tipped applicators	
Performing the Test	
1. Assemble all the necessary equipment.	
2. Explain to the woman exactly what you will be doing.	Many people use no lubricant. If a lubricant is needed for the speculum examination, use only sterile water. There is some concern that water dilutes the amniotic fluid specimen and interferes with the arborization process.
3. Help her assume the position for a speculum examination.	
4. Put on sterile gloves.	
5. Insert the sterile speculum.	
6. Locate the cervix.	
7. Insert a sterile cotton-tipped applicator and place it in the fluid accumulating in the lower blade. Be certain to use pooled fluid in the lower blade. Avoid touching the cervical opening.	If the membranes are ruptured, fluid can leak from the cervix if the woman is asked to cough or bear down.
8. Roll the cotton-tipped applicator on the first slide,	

spreading the specimen *thinly* over at least two thirds of the slide (Fig. 3.16).

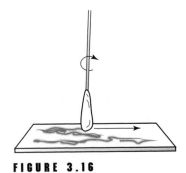

FIGURE 3.16

9. Repeat the procedure but place the second cotton-tipped applicator in the back of the vagina below the cervix.

10. Roll the cotton-tipped applicator on the second slide.

Testing from two different areas offers a better chance of obtaining leaking fluid, which might otherwise be overlooked.

Some people remove the speculum and dip the cotton-tipped applicator in the fluid that has pooled in the lower blade.

11. Allow the slide to dry for 5 to 7 minutes.

Drying permits the sodium chloride in the amniotic fluid to "arborize," or develop the typical "ferning" pattern (Fig. 3.17).

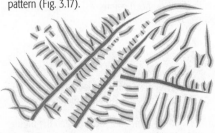

FIGURE 3.17

12. Put the microscope on *low* power and examine all areas of each slide for the ferning pattern. If you have any doubt about the ferning pattern you see under low power, check again under high power.

The presence of the ferning pattern is a positive test result for ruptured membranes. Cervical and vaginal fluids per se will not fern. If you see ferning on the first slide, it is not necessary to check the second slide. However, you should always check the second slide if you do not see ferning on the first slide.

You will need to attend a skill session(s) to practice this skill with the help of your preceptor. Mastery of the skill is achieved when you can demonstrate the following:

- Collection of a specimen for testing
- Preparation of the slides for microscope viewing
- Use of low and high power on the microscope
- Interpretation of the ferning pattern seen under the microscope

Vaginal Examination
SKILL UNIT 4

This section details how to do a vaginal examination to determine cervical effacement, dilatation, the status of membranes, and fetal presenting part and station. Study this section and then attend a skill practice and demonstration session scheduled with your preceptor. You will need to demonstrate that you can perform the procedure and correctly interpret the results. These steps are summarized at the end of this unit.

ACTIONS	REMARKS

Preparing the Woman for a Vaginal Examination

Information you need before performing a vaginal examination:

- Gravidity
- Parity
- Gestational age
- History of any bleeding/spotting
- History of possible ruptured membranes

Caution: If membranes are ruptured and the mother is not in active labor, do not perform a vaginal examination.

1. Ask the woman to empty her bladder before the examination.
2. Tell the woman, in terms she can understand, what you will be doing and share your findings with her throughout the examination using her name.
3. Warn the woman in advance if you are going to be exerting extra pressure or doing something that might be particularly uncomfortable.
4. Help her to lie down on the examining table with legs bent so that her feet are resting on the table or in the stirrups. Place a pillow under her head and ask that she rest her hands across her abdomen or at her sides.
5. Drape the woman's legs to avoid unnecessary exposure. Make sure that you can see her face whether you are sitting or standing for any part of the examination.

A full bladder makes the abdomen difficult to palpate thoroughly and is uncomfortable for the woman.
An informed woman is more relaxed. She is more likely to cooperate with you throughout the examination. The woman has a right to know what is being done in regard to her body.

This increases her comfort and relaxation. Sometimes women put their hands over their heads during a vaginal examination, which tightens abdominal muscles and makes the examination more difficult or uncomfortable.
The message given to the woman is that you respect her modesty and privacy. This will help her relax. Making sure that you can see her face at all times might reassure her and enable you to note expressions of fear, discomfort, or embarrassment.

6. *Has the mother had any bleeding during the last part of her pregnancy?*

    Do you see signs of bleeding that might be more than just bloody show? Blood running down her legs or bright red bleeding is abnormal.

    If you note any bleeding, do not proceed with the examination.

Vaginal examinations are never done by the nurse if the woman has a history of bleeding. Sometimes the placenta grows partially or completely over the cervix. This condition is called *placenta previa* and happens in 1 of every 200 pregnancies[17] (Fig. 3.18). A vaginal examination might cause severe bleeding and place both mother and fetus in danger.

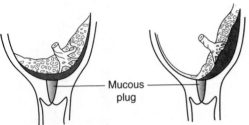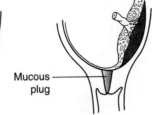

Mucous plug   Mucous plug

FIGURE 3.18 Types of placenta previa.

Getting Ready to Do a Vaginal Examination

7. Wash your hands and put on gloves.

    *   If ruptured membranes are suspected, always use sterile gloves.
    *   If membranes are intact, clean or sterile gloves can be used.

This procedure describes a two-gloved approach. One gloved hand is used to separate the labia (step 13) and the other gloved hand conducts the vaginal/cervical examination.

8. Ask the woman to separate or spread her legs. Do not try to use force or even gently separate her legs.

9. Tell the woman how to relax. If she knows a relaxation and breathing technique learned previously, have her use it. If not, have her do slow, deep, relaxed breathing. Ask her to let herself go limp, to think of herself as a rag doll.

This examination is an intrusive procedure. It should be carried out when the woman is ready for it.

10. Ask the woman if you may proceed now. Watch your facial expression. Remain focused on the woman. Share your findings with her to the extent possible for the situation. Acknowledge the discomfort the examination may be causing her—even offer an apology.

This appropriately gives the woman some control, is empowering, and is humanizing in a difficult situation.

Performing the Examination

If the woman becomes upset or tense during the examination, *stop whatever you are doing.* Do not remove your fingers; simply hold your hand still. Find out what is bothering her. Try to distinguish among discomfort as a result of pressure, fear, or actual pain. Wait until she has regained control, helping her to relax.

11. Generously lubricate the index and middle fingers of your examining hand with lubricating jelly. As you squeeze the tube, let the lubricant drop onto your outstretched fingers. Do not wipe your fingers against the mouth of the tube to obtain the lubricant. The lubricant should be considered clean only—not sterile.

12. Be sure that you have good lighting. A lamp is usually necessary.

If it is uncertain whether the membranes have ruptured and a compelling reason exists for performing the examination, use only sterile water because some substances will interfere with the Nitrazine paper color change.

13. Separate the labia with your gloved fingers (Fig. 3.19). Inspect the general area of the introitus (vaginal opening).

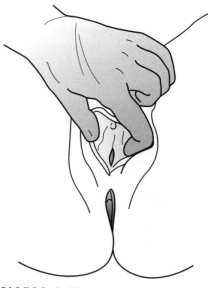

FIGURE 3.19

Look for the following:

- Amount of bloody show
- Wet, glistening perineum
- Malodorous discharge

- Deep yellow or greenish brown discharge

- Ulceration of the labia

- Blisters or raised vesicles on the labia

Elicit signs and symptoms of current infection.

Which might indicate the following:

Labor is advanced.
Membranes have ruptured.
Infection of the amniotic fluid and membranes is present.
Presence of greenish brown fluid indicates fresh meconium. In cephalic presentations, it can indicate that the fetus is in distress.
Syphilis (chancre) or an HSV infection might be present.
HSV infection might be present.

> **STOP THE EXAMINATION. NOTIFY THE PRIMARY CARE PROVIDER IMMEDIATELY.**

The appearance of a raised vesicle or a blistered area can mean that the mother has an active HSV infection. Mothers with herpes virus blisters on the cervix or genitalia can pass the disease on to a newborn delivered vaginally. In primary genital herpes infections, these babies experience high morbidity and mortality.

NOTE: *Herpetic lesions of either type 1 or type 2 can appear anywhere on the body. Sometimes cervical shedding of the virus occurs in a woman who has a herpetic lesion elsewhere on the body. Cervical shedding of the herpes virus can also occur in asymptomatic patients. Current research shows some correlation between HSV infection during pregnancy and cervical shedding at the time of delivery. Fortunately, the incidence of neonatal HSV infection is low when compared with the incidence of known HSV infection in pregnant women.*[5]

Newborns delivered through an infected birth canal should be isolated to protect other newborns in the nursery. The mucous membranes (e.g., eyes, nasopharynx) of the newborn should be cultured at 24 to 48 hours after birth to avoid positive cultures resulting from contamination from the mother.[5]

Current delivery recommendations for pregnant women with genital herpes infection include the following considerations:

- If there are no active lesions at term in a woman with intact membranes who has had active HSV lesions during pregnancy, vaginal delivery is acceptable.[5]
- If there are active lesions near or at term in a woman who is in labor or who has ruptured membranes, cesarean delivery is recommended.[5]

14. Insert the first finger of the other sterile gloved hand and then the second finger gently into the vagina. The hand should be turned sideways in this initial step. Continue to apply downward pressure as you insert the fingers to avoid pressing on the anterior vaginal wall or urethra. The thumb and forefinger on one hand separate the labia widely to expose the vaginal opening and prevent the examining fingers from touching the labia (Fig. 3.20).

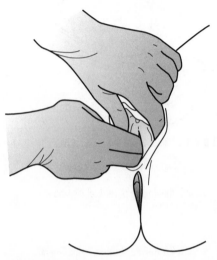

FIGURE 3.20

If you are doing a vaginal examination with one hand, avoid sweeping contaminants into the vagina by separating the labia with the thumb and little finger as you introduce the examining fingers.

15. Move your fingers the full length of the woman's vagina. During the examination, the fourth and fifth fingers should not touch the rectal area. Keep the thumb straight up and stretched out. Keep the fourth and fifth fingers bent inward and touching the palm of your hand (Fig. 3.21).

The length of the vagina varies in women but is usually 3 to 4 cm.

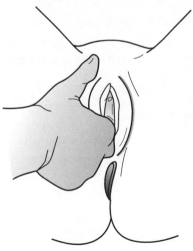

FIGURE 3.21

Assessing Progress in Labor

16. Are the membranes ruptured?

    Palpate for a soft, movable, bulging sac through the cervix (Fig. 3.22). Watch for running fluid during the examination.

If the membranes are not ruptured, they tend to bulge. If they are ruptured, amniotic fluid is likely to leak during the examination.

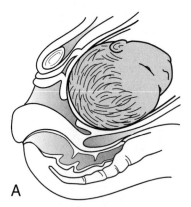

FIGURE 3.22 Membranes. **A.** Watchglass shape. **B.** Bulging into the cervix.

17. What is the degree of cervical dilatation?

Dilatation is measured in centimeters. One finger represents approximately 1.5 to 2 cm dilatation. Measure-ment of dilatation can be from 0 to 10 cm in diameter.

18. What is the degree of cervical effacement?

    Palpate the thickness of the cervix. Estimate the degree of thinness in percentages.

Effacement is measured in percentage. The uneffaced cervix by digital examination is approximately 2 to 2.5 cm (1 inch) thick and would be described as 0% effaced. A cervix measuring approximately 1 cm (0.5 inch) is 50% effaced. Transvaginal ultrasound is often used to measure cervical length in women suspected of cervical incompetency or at risk for preterm labor. The normal cervical length as measured by transvaginal ultrasound at midpregnancy is approximately 4 cm (1.6 inches).

19. What is the presenting part of the fetus?

    Palpate for the presenting part. If you feel:

    • The hard skull with the sagittal suture and follow it to the posterior or anterior fontanelle, it is a *cephalic presentation.*
    • The softer buttocks, it is a *breech presentation.*
    • Irregular, knobby parts like facial features, it is a *face presentation.*

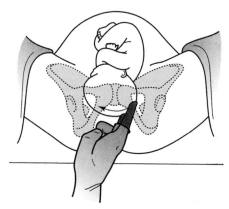

FIGURE 3.23 Identification of the posterior fontanelle.

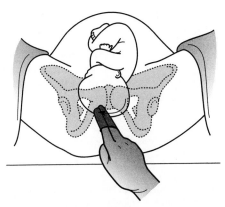

FIGURE 3.24 Identification of the anterior fontanelle.

20. What is the station? Has engagement occurred?

    Locate the lowest portion of the presenting part and then sweep the fingers deeply to one side of the pelvis to feel for the ischial spines (Fig. 3.25). Imagine a straight line from one spine to the other. To determine station, estimate how far (in centimeters) the tip of the presenting part is above or below the ischial spine (see Part III in Module 2). For example, if the fetal head is approximately 1 to 2 cm below the ischial spines, it is at +1 station.

    Engagement occurs when the widest part of the fetal head has entered the inlet of the pelvis. Commonly, this occurs when the tip of the presenting part has reached the level of the ischial spines (i.e., station 0).

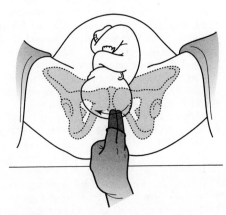

FIGURE 3.25

Station provides some information about the descent of the fetus through the pelvis. If the station is judged to be beyond 0, the pelvis is probably adequate for labor.

Examination between contractions tells you about the degree of dilatation and effacement when the presenting part is not under the pressure of contraction. Examination during a contraction tells you the full extent of dilatation, effacement, and descent. It provides you with a clearer picture of how the laboring woman is doing.

> A vaginal examination can *begin* between contractions but should be *continued* throughout a contraction in the laboring woman.

21. Remove your fingers and discard the glove.

Informing the Mother

22. Tell the woman your findings and relate them to her progress in labor.

    Praise the woman for whatever you can at that point (e.g., working with you during the examination, achieving progress in labor to whatever degree, recognizing the need to come in and be evaluated)

Information can be reassuring and supportive for the woman and for her support system.

Find some words of empowerment from the examination!

You will need to attend a skill session(s) to practice this skill with the help of your preceptor. Mastery of the skill is achieved when you can demonstrate the following:

- Preparation and positioning of the woman for a vaginal examination
- Techniques used in a vaginal examination
- Correct assessment of the status of membranes, cervical dilatation and effacement, fetal presentation, and station

REFERENCES

1. Centers for Disease Control and Prevention. (Spring/Summer, 2000). *Chronic Disease Notes and Reports, 13*(2), 1–4.
2. Maternal and Child Health Bureau, *Child health USA 2000* (p. 20). Washington, DC: U.S. Department of Health and Human Services.
3. Cogswell, M. E., & Yip R. (1995). The influence of fetal and maternal factors on the distribution of birthweight. *Seminars in Perinatology, 19*(3), 222–240.
4. American Academy of Pediatrics and American College of Obstetricians and Gynecologists. (1997). *Guidelines for perinatal care* (4th ed., pp. 214–217). Washington, DC: Author.
5. American College of Obstetricians and Gynecologists. (1999). Management of herpes in pregnancy. ACOG Practice Bulletin Number 8, October (pp. 1–11). Washington, DC: Author.
6. American College of Obstetricians and Gynecologists. (May, 2000). *ACOG committee opinion: Scheduled cesarean delivery and the prevention of vertical transmission of HIV infection, number 234* (pp. 1–5). Washington, DC: Author.
7. Centers for Disease Control and Prevention. (2000) *Tracking the hidden epidemics: Trends in the United States 2000* (pp. 14–17). Atlanta: Author.
8. Cunningham, F. G., Gant, N. F., Leveno, K. J., Gilstrap, L. C., Hauth, J. C., & Wenstrom, K. D. (2001). *Williams obstetrics* (21st ed., pp. 1486–1487). New York: McGraw-Hill.
9. Glantz, J. C., & Woods, J. R. (1999). Significance of amniotic fluid meconium. In R. K. Creasy & R. Resnik (Eds.), *Maternal-fetal medicine* (4th ed., pp. 393–403). Philadelphia: WB Saunders.
10. Tharmaratnam, S. (2000). Fetal distress. *Bailliere's Clinical Obstetrics and Gynecology, 14*(1), 155–172.
11. Schmidt, J. (1999). Prolonged pregnancy. In L. K. Mendeville & N. H. Troiano (Eds.), *High-risk and critical care intrapartum nursing* (p. 129). Philadelphia: Lippincott.
12. Cunningham, F. G., Gant, N. F., Leveno, K. J., Gilstrap, L. C., Hauth, J. C., & Wenstrom, K. D. (2001). *Williams obstetrics* (21st ed., pp. 622–623). New York: McGraw-Hill.
13. Cunningham, F. G., Gant, N. F., Leveno, K. J., Gilstrap, L. C., Hauth, J. C., & Wenstrom, K. D. (2001). *Williams obstetrics* (21st ed., pp. 815–822). New York: McGraw-Hill.
14. Brace, R. A., & Resnik, R. (1999). Dynamics and disorders of amniotic fluid. In R. K. Creasy & R. Resnik (Eds.), *Maternal-fetal medicine* (4th ed., pp. 632–641). Philadelphia: WB Saunders.
15. Campbell, W. A., Nochimson, D. J., & Vintzileos, A. M. (1994). Prolonged pregnancy. In R. A. Knuppel & J. E. Druckker (Eds.), *High-risk pregnancy: A team approach* (2nd ed., pp. 422–432). Philadelphia: WB Saunders.
16. Working Group. (July, 2000). *The National High Blood Pressure Education Program Working Group report on high blood pressure in pregnancy.* Bethesda, MD: National Institutes of Health.
17. Cunningham, F. G., Gant, N. F., Leveno, K. J., Gilstrap, L. C., Hauth, J. C., & Wenstrom, K. D. (2001). *Williams obstetrics* (21st ed., pp. 630–632). New York: McGraw-Hill.
18. Sullivan, C. (1998). Sonographic evaluation of the uterine cervix. *Obstetrics and Gynecology Clinics of North America, 25*(3), 623–627.

SUGGESTED READINGS

American Academy of Pediatrics and American College of Obstetricians and Gynecologists. (1997). *Guidelines for perinatal care* (4th ed.). Washington, DC: Author. (Note: A new edition is published every 5 years.)

American College of Obstetricians and Gynecologists. (1999). Management of herpes in pregnancy. ACOG Practice Bulletin Number 8, October (pp. 1–11). Washington, DC: Author.

Bates, B. (1999). *A guide to physical examination and history taking* (7th ed.). Philadelphia: Lippincott.

Cunningham, F. G., Gant, N. F., Leveno, K. J., Gilstrap, L. C., Hauth, J. C., & Wenstrom, K. D. (2001). *Williams obstetrics* (21st ed.). New York: McGraw-Hill.

Landry, M. L. (1999). Viral infections. In G. N. Burrow & T. P. Duffy (Eds.), *Medical complications during pregnancy* (5th ed.). Philadelphia: WB Saunders.

Lowdermilk, D. L., Perry, S. E., & Bobak, I. M. (Eds.) (2000). *Maternity and women's health care.* St. Louis: Mosby.

Savoia, M. (1999). Bacterial, fungal and parasitic disease. In G. N. Burrow & T. P Duffy (Eds.), *Medical complications during pregnancy* (5th ed.). Philadelphia: WB Saunders.

MODULE 4

Admission Assessment of the Fetus

E. JEAN MARTIN

OBJECTIVES

As you complete this module, you will learn:

1. Methods of determining fetal health
2. How to calculate the date of delivery and gestational age
3. Methods used to obtain an accurate estimated date of confinement (EDC)
4. The relationship of fetal activity to fetal physiology and development
5. What fetal movement tells us about fetal health
6. What to teach expectant mothers about fetal movement counting (maternal assessment measures for fetal activity)
7. The significance of the fetal alarm signal
8. Nursing implications for telephone triage when the expectant mother reports decreased fetal movement
9. Newer appreciations of the true capacities of the developing fetus and how to use this in humanizing the fetus for the mother and father during fetal assessment
10. An organized approach to evaluating fundal height and fetal lie, presentation, and position (Leopold's maneuvers), as well as how to estimate fetal weight and amniotic fluid in its extremes of low and high volumes
11. Clinical issues when findings for fundal height and fetal lie, presentation, and position vary from expected norms
12. The current state of evidence on the effectiveness of two intrapartum fetal surveillance methods: intermittent auscultation (IA) and electronic fetal monitoring (EFM)
13. What can and cannot be assessed with the auscultation method
14. How to apply an organized approach in locating and counting fetal heart rate in intermittent auscultation
15. Definitions for and the significance of variations in fetal heart rate
16. Differentiation of sounds and rates when listening for fetal heart tones
17. Terminology to use when interpreting and charting fetal heart rates heard by the auscultation method
18. Guidelines for fetal surveillance while caring for low- and high-risk laboring women

KEY TERMS

When you have completed this module, you should be able to recall the meaning of the following terms. You should also be able to use the terms when consulting with other health professionals. The terms are defined in this module or in the glossary at the end of this book.

acidosis	hypoxia
ballottement	postterm
fetal bradycardia	oligohydramnios
fetal tachycardia	semi-Fowler's position

Assessing Fetal Health

■ How can you assess fetal health at the time of admission?

As the laboring woman is admitted to the hospital, it is important to keep in mind that two patients are being admitted: the mother and the fetus.

There are several things that you can do to gather important information about fetal health:

- Estimate the gestational age of the fetus using the estimated date of confinement (EDC) or estimated date of delivery (EDD).
- Measure the fundal height of the uterus.
- Evaluate fetal position.
- Ask about fetal movement.
- Listen to fetal heart tones (FHTs).

Gestational Age

■ How is gestational age estimated?

Evaluating fetal size, development, and maturity to identify gestational age depends on the initial determination of when the pregnancy began. Predicting the EDC is another way of looking at gestational age. Follow these two simple steps.

1. Determine the date of the mother's last normal menstrual period (LNMP).
2. Count back 3 months from the date of the LNMP and add 7 days, adjusting the year if appropriate.

EXAMPLE: If the LNMP began August 18, 2002, the EDC is May 25, 2003.

The length of a pregnancy is influenced by factors such as climate, cultural differences, and nutrition. Less than 5% of women deliver on the date predicted, which demonstrates that it is truly an estimation.

■ What can go wrong in estimating the EDC and gestational age?

Many women cannot remember the date of their LNMP. Many also do not realize that an unusually short "period" can occur while they are pregnant because implantation of the fertilized egg with a small amount of bleeding occurs about the same time in the menstrual cycle when bleeding is expected. Occasionally, a pregnancy is achieved during an amenorrheic period when there is no menstruation. Amenorrhea occurs in women experiencing conditions such as diabetes or thyroid problems, obesity, and breastfeeding.

Obtaining an accurate EDC

An EDD or EDC represents a calculation for an average length of gestation in an average woman and appears to be 283 to 284 days, with a standard deviation in humans of 8 to 15 days, rather than the 280 days calculated by Naegele's rule. According to some clinical data, the first pregnancy can be longer than subsequent ones.[1]

The three top predictors with reliable criteria for accuracy in dating pregnancy are as follows[1]:

1. Basal body temperature with a coital record demonstrating ovulation and sustained temperature elevation
2. Serum and urine human chorionic gonadotropin (hCG) levels, which can be detected by 8 to 9 days after ovulation in laboratory testing[2]
3. Ultrasonography[2]
   - The gestational sac can be seen at 4 to 5 weeks' menstrual age (from the LNMP) with transvaginal ultrasound.
   - By 35 days, all normal gestational sacs should be visible with transvaginal ultrasound.
   - The crown-rump length of the fetus can be measured via abdominal ultrasound in the first trimester and is accurate to within 3 to 5 days.
   - The biparietal diameter and femur length are used in the second trimester and are accurate to within 7 to 11 days.

- Third trimester ultrasound assessment of gestational age is much less accurate, with a variation of 14 to 21 days.

A simple way to remember degrees of accuracy when reviewing EDDs by ultrasound follows:

- First trimester—accuracy ± 1 week
- Second trimester—accuracy ± 2 weeks
- Third trimester—accuracy ± 3 weeks

> *NOTE: Using an accurate LNMP for calculating the EDD is as reliable as using ultrasound in the second trimester.*

The following steps are suggested when using a woman's LNMP to calculate her EDD[3]:

- Explore with the woman whether her last menstrual period was normal in length, amount, color, and expected onset.
- If the last menstrual period was abnormal but the previous one was normal, use the first day of the last *normal* period.
- Jog the woman's memory with special dates like holidays, birthdays, and so forth, to help her recall the date of her LNMP.
- If the pregnancy occurred during a period of amenorrhea, determine the approximate EDD by doing the following:
  - Asking the woman about her history of sexual intercourse
  - Questioning the woman about her use of birth control
  - Identifying the date of quickening when the mother first feels the fetus moving (This is generally at 16 to 18 gestational weeks for multigravidas and 18 to 20 gestational weeks for primigravidas.)
  - Noting when FHTs are first heard (Using a Doptone, FHTs can be heard between 10 and 12 weeks. Using a fetoscope, FHTs can be heard between 18 and 20 weeks.)

Fetal Physiology and Movement

■ What does fetal movement tell us about fetal health?

Much of the literature agrees that the five primary situations that place the fetus at risk for intrauterine fetal death are as follows:

- Postterm (beyond 42 weeks' gestation)
- Hypertension
- Diabetes
- Intrauterine growth restriction
- Decreased fetal movement

The widespread use of real-time ultrasound allows for direct measurement of fetal movements. Fetal breathing and body movements are important functions in utero and are necessary for appropriate growth and development.

Fetal activity requires oxygen consumption. When subjected to a hypoxic occurrence, one of the first fetal physiologic adjustments made is to economize movement. Compromise of fetal oxygenation elicits an adaptive response to decrease activity, thereby decreasing oxygen need. This adaptive response can result from a physiologic or a pathophysiologic event.[4]

> *Healthy fetuses have recognizable patterns of movement in utero.*

Adequate functioning of the uteroplacental unit is necessary for the fetus to accomplish and maintain patterns of healthy behavior.

Biologic factors affecting fetal breathing and body movements include the following[4]:

- The maturity level of fetal status in awake/sleep states
- Gestational age
- Time of day
- Relationship to maternal meals (research shows a positive correlation with maternal eating/drinking and breathing movements *but not with body movements*)
- Maternal drug ingestion

> A decrease in fetal activity can be a marker for fetal hypoxia and/or acidosis.

Some clinical situations in pregnancy clearly signal a risk for uteroplacental insufficiency:

- Pregestational diabetes mellitus
- Suspected intrauterine growth restriction
- History of previous intrauterine growth restriction
- Chronic hypertension
- Pregnancy-induced hypertension
- Systemic lupus erythematosus
- Multiple pregnancy
- Oligohydramnios
- Postterm
- Rh disease (less prevalent today)

NOTE:
- *Approximately half of all deaths in near-term fetuses are thought to be associated with hypoxia. Chromosomal abnormalities are found in 5% to 10% of stillbirths, which is a ten-fold increase over live-born infants.[5]*
- *Half of stillbirths occur without obvious causes in otherwise normal pregnancies.[6]*
- *Meconium aspiration and cord accidents are among the most common causes of stillbirth in women having antepartal testing, such as nonstress tests and biophysical profiles.*
- *Studies show that cessation of fetal movement is highly correlated with impending fetal death.*

> Unfortunately, at this time, evidence-based data are inconsistent in demonstrating that fetal movement assessment will result in a reduction in fetal deaths.[7]

In counseling expectant women in fetal movement, it is helpful to appreciate the physiologic development of fetal activity throughout gestation. The following are observations of biophysical activities in the normal fetus[4,8]:

- Fetal breathing movements (FBM) occur episodically and are present 30% of the time from 30 to 40 weeks' gestation.
- FBMs are increased significantly for the first 2 to 3 hours after the mother eats.
- Maternal ingestion of alcohol has a profound inhibitory effect on FBM (e.g., 2 ounces of alcohol ingested by healthy pregnant women at term obliterates FBMs for 3 hours).
- Maternal smoking increases FBM.
- FBMs are decreased during the active phase of labor.
- Gross body movements (GBMs) are present 10% of the time between 30 and 40 weeks of gestation.
- Near term, with increasing fetal maturation, there is an increase in the occurrence and number of GBMs in the late evening, which may be related to increased periods of fetal wakefulness. Maternal perception of these evening movements also increases.
- Premature fetuses less than 28 weeks' gestation are more active and the movements are more sporadic. As the fetus matures, sleep/wake states become better stabilized.
- Small quantities of alcohol appear to have no effect on GBM near term.
- **GBM does not change appreciably in healthy pregnant women before the onset of labor.**
- GBMs, although somewhat reduced, are evident throughout labor.

NOTE: *Women often report "less fetal movement" as term approaches. This change always requires careful evaluation, although what the mother perceives as "less movement" is often a result of less room in utero for the fetus to put "momentum" behind movements. The mother's perception of a significant change always requires further exploration.*

Assessing Fetal Movement

Make time during the prenatal visit to teach the mother how to track fetal movements. Clinical studies show that mothers perceive approximately 80% to 95% of fetal movement.[9]

Maternal attention to fetal movement is a time-honored assessment technique. It is a reliable method that is simple, inexpensive, and noninvasive, and it has no contraindications. Many clinical experts currently recommend that all expectant mothers be taught to carry out this daily assessment. Low-risk mothers are encouraged to begin at 32 to 36 weeks' gestation and high-risk mothers to begin at 28 weeks' gestation.

Many different methods have been devised to assess fetal movement. The objective is that the woman achieve daily awareness of the patterns and level of activity exhibited by her baby in utero.

One method easy to do and popular with mothers is the "count to ten method." This method requires that the mother dedicate 1 hour or less every day to tracking her baby's movements. The short time commitment appears to enhance compliance.[10]

> **Clinical studies indicate that 2 hours is a sufficient period of time for counting fetal movement activity. Maternal perception of 10 distinct movements in up to 2 hours is considered reassuring.[7] When a reassuring count is not obtained, a biophysical means of fetal assessment, such as ultrasound scanning for movement, should be used.[4]**

Instruct the mother to do the following:

1. Select a particular time of day for counting. Mothers often select the time of day when the baby is most active, which is often in the evening.
2. Assume a comfortable position in a chair that allows you to lie on your side. Count each fetal movement until 10 movements are felt. This can take anywhere from a few minutes up to 1 hour. A movement can be a kick, a roll, or a swish. Hiccups or small flutters should not be counted. Mark down the time you feel the baby's first movement. Mark down the time you feel the baby's tenth movement. Note the date.
3. If 10 movements have not been felt after 1 hour, continue counting for as long as an additional hour. Most women will feel 10 movements in 2 hours.
4. If after 2 hours you have not felt 10 movements, call your primary care provider and report your findings. *Do not wait until the next day.*

> Success in promoting fetal movement counting depends more on the staff who teach and supervise the method and less on the method of counting.[11]

Promoting compliance takes into consideration that the expectant mother needs to do the following:

- Appreciate the significance of doing fetal movement counting. **Poor understanding correlates with low compliance in keeping a "kick count."[6]**
- Know normal variations in fetal movements to prevent undue worry.
- Have her fetal activity record reviewed at each visit by the nurse and/or health provider.
- Be made to feel that it is OK to call, and be provided with a designated phone number.

The Fetal Alarm Signal[12]

In several studies, especially those involving high-risk pregnancies, it was found that fetal movements decrease and can cease entirely for up to 12 hours before ending in intrauterine death. *FHTs are heard throughout the 12 hours of movement cessation.*

> **The fetal alarm signal (absence of fetal movement up to 12 hours but with FHTs present) points to a severely distressed fetus and indicates the need for immediate intervention, that is, delivery.**

For high-risk patients: When three or fewer fetal movements are felt in a 12-hour period, the woman must call her primary care provider immediately. Any time an expectant woman calls reporting diminished fetal activity, **it should be followed up.**

A recent clinical study reported that 8% of mothers who phoned in or presented for an unscheduled visit for decreased fetal movement proved to have a stillbirth.[5]

Most of the time, ultrasound and/or EFM reveals a normal FHR and activity pattern. Praise the mother for her vigilance, and as she leaves, offer professional assurance that you or the staff are there to help her in the weeks ahead.

Far too many expectant mothers avoid seeking care because they do not trust what they feel. Many have no prior frame of reference for what they are experiencing, but they also fear being seen as bothersome or a worrier. Anyone who might be a first-line contact for the expectant woman must be sensitized to demonstrate a caring concern.

If a low-risk mother calls reporting decreased fetal movement, explore her background for normalcy. Identify how today's fetal movements compare with those of the previous day and earlier. When movement is present but perceived as lessening, you might instruct the mother as follows:

- Drink two to three glasses of water or juice and then lie down and count fetal movement for 1 to 2 hours. **Either the mother calls to report the results to the nurse (not the secretary) or the nurse calls the mother back. An outcome should be known and a record kept of all calls to and from the unit, practice, or clinic.**

OR

- Come to the appropriate site for further evaluation. If a high-risk mother calls and you are concerned about what she reports, always have the woman come in for further evaluation. Practice on the far side of caution. You will never regret it! The mother will sleep better and so will you, and the baby has a better chance for a good outcome.

Humanizing the Fetus for Parents

The three Skill Units presented in this module not only offer methods to assess fetal health but involve a unique opportunity to help the mother and father or support person perceive the fetus as a developing human. While conducting any of the skills outlined, you can interact with the fetus through abdominal massaging, speaking to and commenting with the fetus and the mother.

Research is revealing amazing true capacities of prenates—(the unborn): "their precocious sensory development, their exquisite sensitivity and responsiveness, and their ability to learn from what is happening in the world of their mother and father."[13]

Modern technologies allow observation of the unborn's behavior throughout the entire period of gestation. Chamberlain, in *Prenatal Body Language: A New Perspective on Ourselves,*[14] describes (1) early and self-initiated spontaneous movement that expresses interest and personality; (2) prenatal pain perception, preferences, learning, memory, and emotional states of fear, anger, and smiling; and (3) interactive movements between twins in utero and between the fetus and parents with play periods.

Reactive movements or behaviors of the fetus are cited by Chamberlain with the following examples:

- Coughing or laughing in the mother brings about movement in nearly all fetuses between 10 and 15 weeks' gestation.
- Fetuses sometimes react to the needle during an amniocentesis by moving away from the needle or even attacking it.
- A bright light shining through the abdominal wall and fixed on the fetal head (vertex) will increase the fetus' heartbeat.
- Some fetuses react to high-volume rock music and violent movies with vigorous movements that can even be painful to the mother.
- Lullabies, children's songs, and melodious classical music sometimes are seen to have a calming effect.

So, as you measure the fundus and palpate the maternal abdomen, talk to the baby and comment to the mother about any response you get. Educate and encourage the mother about fetal hearing and sensory perceptions. Babies will thrive on nuturing attention after birth but what has become clear in the cited studies is that babies thrive with attention *before* birth. See the Suggested Readings for helpful insights into more studies about prenates' amazing development in utero.

PRACTICE/REVIEW QUESTIONS

After reviewing this module, answer the following questions.

1. State four ways to gather information about fetal health when the mother is admitted to the labor unit.

   a. *Fetal heart tones*

   b. *EDC*

   c. *As about movement*

   d. *Measure fundal height*

2. If the LNMP is June 6, 2002, when is the EDC? *3/13/03*

3. Pregnancy can be achieved during an amenorrheic period if the woman has diabetes or thyroid problems.

   A. True

   B. False

4. An estimated date of delivery (EDD or EDC) represents a calculation for the average woman and appears to be _*283-284*_ days rather than _*280*_ days.

5. State three top predictors with reliable criteria for accuracy in dating a pregnancy.

   a. *Basal Bod temp*

   b. *Ultrasound*

   c. *XCG levels*

6. The mother can identify quickening around the twelfth to fourteenth week of pregnancy.

   A. True

   B. False

7. A small amount of bleeding can occur with implantation.

   A. True

   B. False

8. Five primary clinical situations that put the fetus at risk for intrauterine fetal death are:

   a. *Postterm >42 wks gestation*

   b. *↓ fetal movement*

   c. *Diabetes*

   d. *Hypertension*

   e. *Intrauterine growth restriction*

9. When the fetus is deprived of sufficient oxygen, a physiologic adaptive response is:

   ↓ fetal movement

10. A *postdate pregnancy* is defined as one that has gone beyond which gestational week?

    A. 40

    B. 41

    C. 42

11. A critical element required for the fetus to maintain patterns of healthy breathing and body movements is:

    A. Large amounts of amniotic fluid

    B. Mature gestational age

    C. A mother who pays close attention to fetal movement

    D. Good functioning of the uteroplacental unit

12. A significant overall decrease in fetal activity:

    A. Can be related to the awake/sleep state of the fetus

    B. Can signal a sign of maturity

    C. Can be a marker for fetal hypoxia

    D. Should be expected before the onset of labor

13. Name 10 critical situations in which uteroplacental insufficiency can place the fetus at risk:

    a. *Pregestational diabetes mellitus*

    b. *Suspected intrauterine growth restriction*

    c. *H/o previous intrauterine growth restriction*

    d. *Chronic hypertension*

    e. *Pregnancy induced hypertension*

    f. *Lupus*

    g. *Multiple pregnancy*

    h. *Oligohydramnios*

    i. *Post term*

    j. *Rh disease*

14. At what gestational age is it recommended that fetal movement counting begin for the situations you have listed in question 13? *28 wks*

15. Maternal intake of alcohol has a profound effect on fetal gross body movements.

    A. True

    B. False

16. Select *two* statements that reflect what is known about fetal body movement.

    A. The more immature the fetus, the more sporadic the movements.

    B. Between 30 and 40 weeks' gestation, fetal body movement is present 10% of the time.

    C. Movements significantly increase during active labor.

    D. The expectant woman perceives movements more in the afternoons.

17. Maternal perceptions of fetal activity (select two):

    A. Are not reliable

    B. Are influenced by the time of day

    C. Are reliable

    D. Correlate poorly with actual fetal movement

18. A low-risk expectant woman who has been doing fetal movement counting since 36 weeks' gestation is now at 38 weeks' gestation. She phones you with her concern that on doing fetal movement counting this evening, she counted only six movements in 1 hour. She usually has no trouble getting 10 movements in 1 hour. A reasonable response to her would be:

    A. "Come right in and let us evaluate what is going on."

    B. "Drink 1 or 2 glasses of fluids, go to bed this evening, but call your primary care provider in the morning."

    C. "Take a walk and relax. Call tomorrow if you continue to have fewer than 10 movements in 1 hour."

    D. "Drink 1 or 2 glasses of fluids, continue your counting for 1 more hour, and call me back with your results. I'll want to talk with you then."

19. Select your response for question 18 if the mother had a history of stillbirth at 38 weeks' gestation with her last pregnancy and currently has a gestational diabetes. You would choose response:

    A.

    B.

    C.

    D.

20. Describe what the fetal alarm signal is:

    Absence of fetal movement ^ to 10 hrs but c̄ FHTS present

21. An insulin-dependent mother at 35 weeks' gestation calls to state that the baby has been moving a lot less over the past 2 days. When she is placed on the electronic fetal monitor, good fetal activity with fetal heart rate accelerations is seen over 25 minutes. Subsequent to being reassured and sent home, she calls again 4 days later worried because, again, fetal movement appears significantly different. What will you recommend to her?

    Come back in for reevaluation

22. Current research indicates that fetal movement in response to a stimulus is very often not random but truly reactive.

    A. True

    B. False

PRACTICE/REVIEW ANSWER KEY
   1. Any four of the following:
      a. Estimate gestational age of fetus and EDC.
      b. Measure the fundal height of the uterus.
      c. Evaluate fetal position.
      d. Listen to FHTs.
      e. Ask about fetal movement.

2. March 13, 2003

3. A

4. 283 to 284; 280

5. a. Basal body temperature with a coital record demonstrating ovulation and sustained temperature elevation
   b. Transvaginal ultrasound 4 to 5 weeks from the LNMP to identify the gestational sac and/or ultrasound between 7 and 13 weeks (first trimester) using fetal crown-rump length (accurate with 3 to 5 days)
   c. hCG levels in urine or blood serum by 8 to 9 days after ovulation

6. B

7. A

8. a. Postterm
   b. Hypertension
   c. Diabetes
   d. Intrauterine growth restriction
   e. Decreased fetal movement

9. To decrease fetal movement

10 C

11. D

12. C

13. Any 10 of the following:
    a. Pregestational diabetes mellitus
    b. Suspected intrauterine growth restriction
    c. History of previous intrauterine growth restriction
    d. Chronic hypertension
    e. Pregnancy-induced hypertension
    f. Systemic lupus erythematosus
    g. Multiple pregnancy
    h. Oligohydramnios
    i. Previous stillbirth
    j. Postterm
    k. Rh disease (less prevalent today)

14. 28 weeks' gestation

15. A

16. A and B

17. B and C

18. D. **NOTE:** *Some may select A, which is always a safe response. The majority of expectant women, however, will get 10 movements with one additional hour of counting. That is reassuring.*

19. A

20. FHTs are heard throughout several hours of cessation of fetal movement (up to 12 hours).

21. Tell her to come in for evaluation.

22. A

Measuring Fundal Height
SKILL UNIT 1

This section details how to measure the height of the uterine fundus to obtain information about fetal growth and body size. Study this section and then attend a skill practice and demonstration session scheduled with your preceptor. You will need to demonstrate the examination and correctly interpret the results. The steps of the examination are summarized at the end of this unit.

Physical examination techniques used in fetal assessment are structured in the sequence given here, that is, first measuring fundal height, then determining presentation and position, and finally auscultating for FHTs. There is a good reason for this. Measuring fundal height before any abdominal palpation is carried out reduces the likelihood of stimulating contractions or fetal activity, both of which could alter the height of the fundus. Occasionally, when the woman assumes a supine position on the examination table, a contraction is stimulated. This is especially true in the late second trimester and third trimester. Wait until the contraction has subsided before taking the measurement. Moving on to determining fetal lie, presentation, and position will then prepare you to know where to look for FHTs, the last assessment technique.

ACTIONS	REMARKS
Measure the Fundal Height	
1. Ask the woman to empty her bladder. Assist the woman to a supine position on the examination table. Avoid elevating the woman's trunk or flexing her knees, if possible. This may not be a comfortable position for her, so be prepared to move through the assessment without delay. When finished, elevate the examination table to her comfort.	A full bladder will give a false high fundal height of as much as 2 to 3 cm. Maternal position does influence fundal height measurement as seen in the Engstrom et al.[15] study. No research data exist to support the use of a position other than supine for obtaining fundal height measurements.
2. Always inspect the maternal abdomen before beginning fundal height measurements. Look at the abdominal shape. An elongated shape probably denotes a vertical lie; a triangular shape may indicate a transverse lie.	In one study, when the trunk was elevated and knees flexed, the mean difference from measurements obtained in the supine position was 1.69 cm.[15]

ACTIONS	**REMARKS**

Measure the Fundal Height

Facing the woman's head, place your hands on each side of the uterus approximately halfway between the symphysis and the fundus (Fig. 4.1). Feel along the sides of the uterus upward toward the fundus. As you near the top, your hands will begin to come together. They will meet at the top of the fundus.

This assists in identifying exactly where the fundus is located.

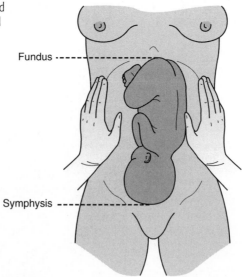

Fundus

Symphysis

FIGURE 4.1

3. Place the zero line of the tape measure on the anterior border of the symphysis pubis and stretch the tape over the midline of the abdomen to the top of the fundus (Fig. 4.2).
   NOTE: *The tape should be brought over the curve of the fundus. The measurement is read at the low-ermost edge of the curved fundus.*

The fundal height is measured in centimeters.

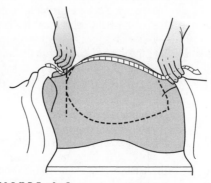

FIGURE 4.2

Slight variations in the way people measure the curve of the fundus result in discrepancies between examiners. **It is essential for clinicians to standardize their fundal height measurement technique so that all measurements are obtained in the same position and use the same anatomic landmarks.**[15]

Interpret the Movement

4. Estimating gestational age from fundal height is based on a simple rule: After the twentieth week of pregnancy, the height of the fundus in centimeters equals the number of weeks of gestation, ± 2 cm. This is a general rule and best applied between the twentieth and thirty-second weeks.

Generally, the height of the uterus increases by approximately 1 cm per week after the twentieth week. It is a way of assessing the growth of the fetus within the uterus when measured regularly.

ACTIONS	REMARKS

Interpret the Movement

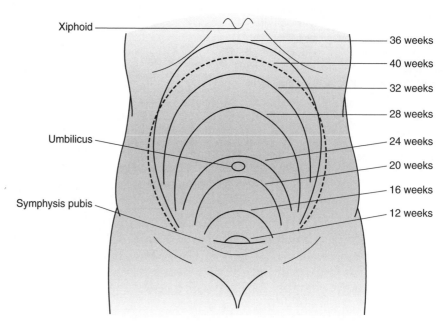

FIGURE 4.3

Week	LOCATION OF THE UTERUS
1–2	The uterus is a pelvic organ for the first 3 months of pregnancy, palpable on vaginal examination.
12	The uterus fills the pelvic cavity. The fundus is felt level with or just above the upper margin of the symphysis pubis. The uterus is the size of a small grapefruit and feels globular and firm.
16	The fundus is halfway between the symphysis pubis and the umbilicus and is ovoid in shape.
20	The fundus is approximately 1 to 2 fingerbreadths below the umbilicus.
24	The fundus is 1 to 2 fingerbreadths above the umbilicus and can rotate to the right; it feels less firm.
28	The fundus is halfway between the umbilicus and the xiphoid, approximately 3 fingerbreadths above the umbilicus.
32	The fundus is three-fourths the distance between the umbilicus and the xiphoid, or approximately 3 fingerbreadths below the xiphoid.
36	The fundus is at or just below the xiphoid.
40	The fundus drops several fingerbreadths, particularly in primigravidas.

Approximate height of the fundus during pregnancy. (Adapted from Carr, K. C. [1976]. *Perinatal nurse clinician program. Maternal-fetal pathway syllabus.* Seattle: University of Washington; as appears in Blackburn, S., & Loper, D. [1992]. *Maternal, fetal and neonatal physiology: A clinical perspective.* Philadelphia: WB Saunders.)

> **NOTE:** *If the fetus is growing abnormally slowly or quickly, the fundal height will be too low or too high to give an accurate gestational age.*

ACTIONS	**REMARKS**

Finding an Abnormal Fundal Height

5. What if you find a *low fundal height* for gestational age? When you measure the mother's abdomen and find it is more than 2 cm less than what would be expected for her due date, it can indicate growth restriction in the fetus.

Consistently low fundal heights can mean that the fetus has a slow growing rate. This is called *intrauterine growth restriction* and can be a cause of serious problems in newborns.

A lack of increase in fundal height over 3 consecutive weeks often indicates fetal growth restriction. *Poor prenatal weight gain in a mother who is average size or smaller adds to the probability of this diagnosis.*

Low fundal height can occur with a transverse lie. Careful abdominal palpation should be done.
The more cigarettes smoked or alcohol used, the greater the growth restriction.
Small women are more likely to have small babies than are large women.

You need to do the following:

- Review the woman's medical and prenatal history for the following:

  –Heart disease
  –Elevated blood pressure
  –Exposure to communicable diseases
  –An incidence of fever, chills, vomiting, or diarrhea
  –Smoking and drinking habits
  –Drug use

- Note the fundal height measurements throughout pregnancy.
- Assess the mother for signs of preeclampsia (hypertension, edema, and proteinuria).
- Consult/notify the care provider.

Twin pregnancies are more likely to result in babies with growth restriction.
The longer a pregnancy goes beyond the due date, the more likely it is that the fetus will not only fail to gain weight but may lose weight.

Severe fetal distress often occurs during labor and delivery in a seriously growth-restricted fetus. If the mother is in a level I hospital, transferring her to a level II or level III hospital for labor and delivery is urgent. Special monitoring and resuscitation equipment must be available throughout the labor and birth of this high-risk infant.

Prompt delivery of the fetus suspected of being severely growth restricted at or near term is recommended. See Module 10 for a detailed discussion of intrauterine growth restriction.

ACTIONS	**REMARKS**

Finding an Abnormal Fundal Height

6. What if a *high fundal height for gestational age* is found?
 	
   A high fundal height of more than 2 cm above the norm for gestational age can mean that the fetus is large but healthy. However, you need to do the following:
 	
• Palpate the mother's abdomen for the presence of an excessive amount of fluid (hydramnios).
• Palpate for the presence of twins.
• Review the mother's prenatal and medical history. Look for the following:
 	
   –The presence of a consistently high fundal height
   –History of diabetes mellitus
	Excessive amounts of fluid are often present in the following:
	
	• Twin gestations
	• Fetuses with congenital anomalies
	• Women who have diabetes mellitus or syphilis
	• Women who have blood incompatibility–Rh isoimmunization
	
	Diabetic mothers have large babies who often look mature but are not. Immature lungs often lead to serious problems for the baby.

> Diabetic screening is recommended for certain populations of pregnant women. See Module 13 for a detailed discussion.

You will need to attend a skill lesson(s) to practice this skill with the help of your preceptor. Mastery of the skill is achieved when you can do the following:

• Identify the anterior border of the symphysis pubis bone as your starting point for measuring fundal height
• Attain the same fundal height measurements as your coordinator
• Correctly interpret your measurements as normal, high, or low
• Describe the implications for management of mothers with low and high fundal height measurements

Evaluating Fetal Lie, Presentation, and Position Using Leopold's Maneuvers
SKILL UNIT 2

This skill unit details how to use a systematic approach in abdominal palpation to determine fetal presentation and position. Study the section and then attend a skill practice and demonstration session scheduled by your preceptor. You will need to demonstrate that you can perform Leopold's maneuvers and correctly identify a variety of fetal lies, positions, and presentations. These steps are summarized at the end of this skill unit.

ACTIONS	REMARKS
Prepare the Mother	
1. Ask the mother to empty her bladder.	
2. Assist the mother onto the examining table. She should lie on her back.	Abdominal muscles are relaxed, and palpating for the fetal parts is generally easier.
3. Slightly elevate her head and shoulders. Ask her to bend her knees so that the soles of her feet rest flat on the table (Fig. 4.4).	Moderately flexed knees decreases abdominal muscle tightening.
	A towel may be placed on one side of the mother's hips and back to induce a lateral tilt. This is especially important if the woman is experiencing supine hypotension (faintness from diminished circulation to heart or brain while supine).

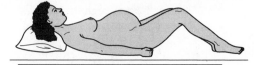

FIGURE 4.4

4. Carry out the examination between contractions if labor has begun.

Determine the Presenting Part and Lie

5. Warm your hands by washing them under warm water or rubbing them together. Cold hands cause abdominal muscles to contract and tighten.

Always inspect the maternal abdomen before beginning any palpation. Look for an elongated abdomen denoting a probable vertical lie or a triangular-shaped abdomen indicating a possible transverse lie.

Use gentle but firm motions.

> Leopold's maneuvers should be done systematically to obtain the best results.

ACTIONS	REMARKS

Determine the Presenting Part and Lie

6. **First maneuver:** Grasp the lower portion of the abdomen just above the symphysis pubis between the thumb and fingers of one hand (Fig. 4.5). Use your other hand to steady the uterus by placing it on the fundus.

   NOTE: *Many authors/diagrams exchange the third maneuver depicted in this skill unit for the first maneuver. Either approach is fine. Beginning the maneuvers by attempting to determine what is in the lower aspect the uterus seems efficient because after 26 weeks' gestation, the hard head is more easily palpated than the softer breech. In 90% of fetal positions, the head can be identified near or in the pelvis.*

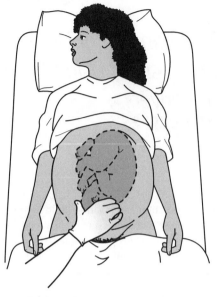

FIGURE 4.5

If the head is identified here, you know that the:
- Lie is *longitudinal*
- Presentation is *cephalic*

7. Attempt to move the head from side to side to see whether it is:

   - Floating—out of the pelvis
   - Dipping—partially into the pelvis
   - Approaching engagement—fixed in the pelvis and unmovable

Locate the Back and Small Parts

8. **Second maneuver:** Move your hands to the sides of the abdomen. Use one hand to steady the uterus and palpate with the other hand for the fetal back or small parts, such as hands and feet (Fig. 4.6).

   Keeping the fingers together, apply firm circular motions with the palmar surface of the hands.

   Avoid any poking motion with the ends of the fingers because this can cause discomfort and will not elicit the information being sought.

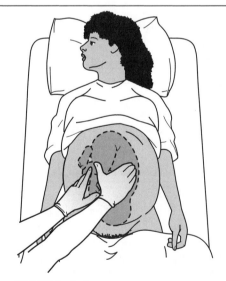

FIGURE 4.6

The side where the fetal back is located will feel firmer and smoother. The side where the fetal hands, elbows, knees, and feet are will feel softer and knobby and have more "give" as you palpate.

ACTIONS	REMARKS

Examine the Fundus

9. **Third maneuver:** Move your hands up the sides of the abdomen to the fundus (Fig. 4.7). Palpate for the breech or head, depending on what you felt in the lower abdomen on the first maneuver. The breech is usually found in the fundus.

   If you think you feel the head in the fundal area, tap it sharply with your fingers to see if it will bounce back.

   Ask yourself if what you are feeling confirms what you felt in the lower abdomen on the first maneuver.

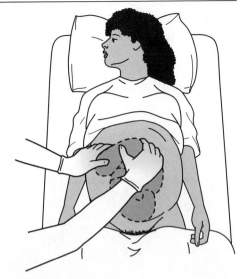

FIGURE 4.7

The breech will feel firm and broad compared with the hard and smaller head. The breech is also less movable.

The head is small and mobile and will bounce or rise up in the amniotic fluid against your fingers. This is called *ballottement.* It might help to confirm your palpation. The breech is not as mobile and does not tap well.

Locate the Cephalic Prominence

10. **Fourth maneuver:** Turn and face the mother's feet. Attempt to locate the cephalic prominence by moving your hands down the sides of the abdomen toward the symphysis pubis (Fig. 4.8).

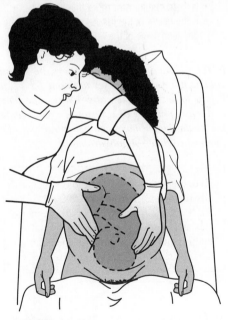

FIGURE 4.8

ACTIONS	**REMARKS**

Locate the Cephalic Prominence

Note whether the head is:

• Free and floating

OR

• Flexed and approaching engagement

The cephalic prominence, or brow, is located on the side where there is greatest resistance to the downward movement of the fingers. When the head is well flexed, it is found on the opposite side from the fetal back (Fig. 4.9). When the fetal head is not well flexed or is hyperextended, the cephalic prominence is found on the same side as the back.

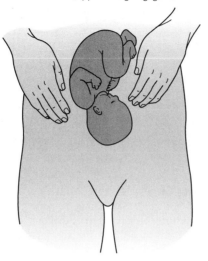

FIGURE 4.9

11. As you carry out the entire procedure, ask yourself the following:

• Is there fetal movement?
• How large is the fetus?
• Is there one fetus or more than one?
• Is the height of the fundus appropriate for the gestational age of the fetus?

NOTE: Throughout the maneuvers, be sensitive to the feel of fluid "fullness." Amniotic fluid volume normally increases to about 1 L (1 quart) or a little more by 36 weeks' gestation but begins to decrease thereafter.[2] With experience, one can sense whether the uterus is very full and tense, possibly as a result of excessive amniotic fluid (hydramnios). On the other hand, if the fundal height has been below normal, the palpation "sense" may be that there is greatly diminished fluid (oligohydramnios).

Hydramnios (polyhydramnios) is generally defined as more than 2,000 mL (2 L). It occurs in about 1% of all pregnancies and is often associated with fetal malformations, especially of the central nervous system or gastrointestinal tract.[2]	In the ACOG Practice Bulletin on Antepartum Fetal Surveillance,[7] oligohydramnios is defined as a nonultrasonographically measurable vertical pocket of amniotic fluid greater than 2 cm or an amniotic fluid volume (AFI) of 5 cm or less.

NOTE: In postterm pregnancy, oligohydramnios is common and associated with increased risk of meconium-stained amniotic fluid and cesarean birth for nonreassuring heart rates. Oligohydramnios has been considered an indication for delivery of a postterm pregnancy, although the effectiveness of this approach has not been established by randomized investigation.[7]

These diagnoses are made with ultrasonography, but using sensitive palpation and the information you bring to it (e.g., a history of intrauterine growth restriction, poor prepregnant weight, poor weight gain in pregnancy, current history of smoking) is essential for assessment of risk.

You will need to attend a skill session(s) to practice this skill with the help of your preceptor. Mastery of the skill is achieved when you can do the following:

- Prepare the woman and yourself for the examination
- Systematically approach abdominal palpation using the first through fourth Leopold's maneuvers
- Correctly identify fetal lie, presentation, and position on three different patients

Auscultation of Fetal Heart Tones
SKILL UNIT 3

This skill unit will teach you how to find and count FHTs and what to do if you hear a fetal heart rate (FHR) that is not reassuring. Study this section and then attend a skill practice and demonstration session scheduled by your preceptor. You will need to demonstrate that you can perform the procedure and correctly interpret the findings. These steps are summarized at the end of this skill unit.

Introduction

The goal during FHR assessment is to detect any signs of fetal compromise.[16] Early intervention can result in healthier neonatal outcomes. Neither auscultation nor electronic FHR monitoring have been effective in predicting the extent of fetal distress in utero. When reassuring signs are present during auscultation or electronic fetal monitoring (EFM), fetal well-bring is a reliable interpretation. (Module 6 discusses in detail the interpretation and physiologic basis of *reassuring* and *nonreassuring* FHR changes.)

Evidence from several randomized controlled trials (RCTs) has shown that intermittent auscultation (IA) and EFM are equivalent methods in conducting fetal surveillance and equivalent in terms of neonatal outcomes.[16]

IA is equivalent to EFM when based on the skill of experienced practitioners who are[16]

- Able to recognize the significance of what is heard in FHR changes
- Experienced in palpating contractions
- Knowledgeable about implementing necessary clinical interventions

Many institutions/providers have obtained EFM tracings on both low- and high-risk women upon admission as a matter of policy or routine. Studies done to date offer conflicting findings on the usefulness of EFM as an admission measure to identify the fetus at risk. More research is needed in this area to guide clinical practice. Until then, Feinstein and others state that decisions regarding the use of IA or EFM should, in the best practice approach, be a mutual one between each woman and her provider and should be shaped by clinical risk situations, preferences, and even staffing.[16]

ACTIONS	REMARKS

Assemble the Equipment

1. The basic types of auscultation devices are as follows:

   a. A modified stethoscope worn on the head of the listener so that bone conduction from the skull increases hearing ability. Sounds associated with the actual opening and closing of fetal ventricular valves can be heard.

a. DeLee-Hillis fetoscope with headpiece (Fig. 4.10)

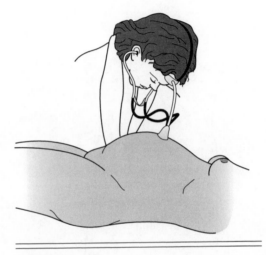

FIGURE 4.10

   b. A large, heavy bell that magnifies fetal heart sounds.

b. Leff stethoscope (Fig. 4.11)

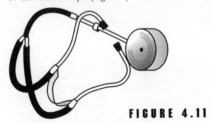

FIGURE 4.11

   c. An electronic device that uses ultrasound technology, which converts heart sounds into a sound that represents cardiac activity.[16]

c. Doptone (ultrasound) (Fig. 4.12)

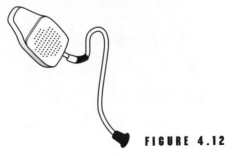

FIGURE 4.12

NOTE: *If the EFM ultrasound transducer (Doppler) is used for FHR auscultation, the paper recorder must not be running. If a tracing of the FHR is produced, it cannot be considered auscultation alone and the tracing will require interpretation.[16]*

Feinstein et al.[16] cite a recent study comparing the fetoscope with Doptone use for intermittent auscultation. Results indicated better neonatal outcomes with the Doptone (Doppler) device.

ACTIONS

REMARKS

Determine Fetal Position and Presentation

2. Raise the head of the bed so that the woman is in a semi-Fowler's position or place a small pillow or rolled towel under the woman so that the woman's side is wedged.

Explain the procedure to the woman and the father or support person.

3. Determine fetal position and presentation through Leopold's maneuvers. Determine where the *fetal back* is.

If the woman is not flat on her back, there is less chance of poor circulation back to the heart and head and, therefore, less risk of her becoming faint (supine hypotensive syndrome).

Begins preparing the woman to attend to the explanation of your examination findings and to turn inward to the unborn.

FHTs are transmitted through the convex portion of the fetus because that is the part in close contact with the uterine wall. In most breech (Fig. 4.13) and cephalic presentations (Fig. 4.14), FHTs are best heard through the fetal back (*).

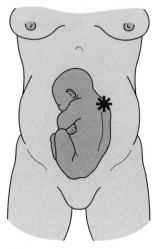

FIGURE 4.13 Breech presentation.

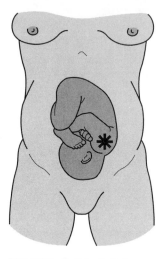

FIGURE 4.14 Cephalic presentation.

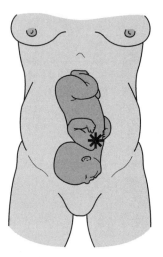

FIGURE 4.15 Face presentation.

In a face presentation (Fig. 4.15), the fetal back becomes concave, and the best place to listen for heart sounds is over the more convex chest.

ACTIONS	REMARKS

Position the Fetoscope

4. Position the fetoscope or Doptone on the appropriate quadrant of the mother's abdomen. Use firm pressure.

   In **ROA** (Fig. 4.16), sounds are best heard in the right lower quadrant.

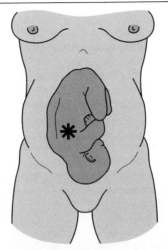

FIGURE 4.16 ROA.

In posterior positions, such as **LOP** (Fig. 4.17) or **ROP** (Fig. 4.18), sounds are best heard at the mother's side.

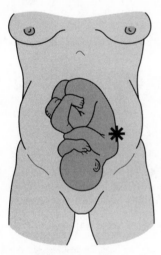

FIGURE 4.17 LOP.

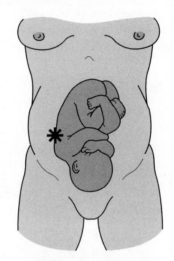

FIGURE 4.18 ROP.

In the breech position (Fig. 4.19), sounds are best heard above the mother's umbilicus on her left side.

> Review common fetal positions discussed in Module 2, Part II.

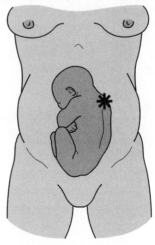

FIGURE 4.19 LSA.

ACTIONS	REMARKS

Guidelines for Listening and Interpretation

5. Guidelines that can aid you in locating the fetal heart beat are as follows[3]:

   a. *Between the tenth and sixteenth weeks of pregnancy, use a Doptone.* Apply a small amount of conduction gel to the contact portion of the Doptone. Begin listening at the upper border of the pubic hair. If you are unable to hear fetal tones, slowly move the instrument up toward the mother's umbilicus. Generally only light pressure is needed. You will need to apply more gel if the search is extensive.

   The ultrasound instrument is more sensitive than the fetoscope. It will pick up FHTs about the tenth week of gestation. Conduction gel aids in the transmission of ultrasound waves.

   b. *Between the sixteenth and twenty-fourth weeks of pregnancy,* measure off 2 fingerbreadths above the pubic hairline and listen along the midline of the abdomen.

   A regular fetoscope can pick up FHTs by the eighteenth or twentieth week of pregnancy.

   c. *After the twenty-fourth week of pregnancy,* search the abdomen in a methodical manner. Place the fetoscope or Doptone at position 1, as shown in Figure 4.20. If nothing is heard, move to position 2 in the lower left quadrant. Continue following the numbered positions.

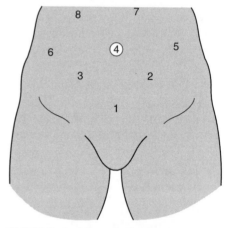

FIGURE 4.20 Methodical search pattern for fetal heart tones. (Adapted with permission from Wheeler, L. A. [1979]. *Fetal assessment. Series 2: Prenatal Care, Module 3* [p 19]. White Plains, NY: The National Foundation–March of Dimes.)

If you do not detect FHTs at these eight positions, begin a systematic search of the abdomen. Place the fetoscope or Doptone at the umbilicus and move it centimeter by centimeter outward along a spokelike pattern. Follow the sequence of numbers in Figure 4.21.

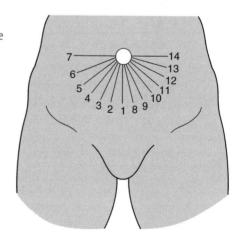

FIGURE 4.21 Systematic search pattern for fetal heart tones. (Adapted with permission from Wheeler, L. A. [1979]. *Fetal assessment. Series 2: Prenatal Care, Module 3* [p 19]. White Plains, NY: The National Foundation–March of Dimes.)

ACTIONS	REMARKS

Differentiating Sounds and Rates

6. Listening for sounds.

   You may hear a soft "blowing" sound of maternal blood coursing through the uterine arteries; this is referred to as *the uterine soufflé.*

   A distinct "swishing" sound may be heard; this is synonymous with blood coursing through the umbilical artery and is referred to as the *funic soufflé.*

   > Fetal heart valve opening and closing have very distinct cardiac sounds—not muffled or swishing sounds as in the uterine or funic soufflé. Check the woman's radial pulse while counting FHR.

   Auscultation can identify the following[16]:

   Baseline fetal heart rate: This is obtained by auscultation between contractions over *at least* a 10-minute period. Baseline FHR is between 110 and 160 beats per minute (bpm) in the normal term infant.

   Fetal bradycardia is defined as a baseline rate below 110 bpm.

   Fetal tachycardia is defined as a baseline over 160 bpm.

   Rhythm is assessed as regular or irregular.

   Decreases or increases from the FHR baseline may be heard with auscultation and should be charted as such (e.g., FHR, 140–144 bpm by auscultation; regular rhythm; acceleration to 160 bpm). *Increases or decreases can be described as accelerations or decelerations, but one cannot type them as done with EFM terms.*

   Dysrhythmia

   Can clarify double or half counting that can occur with EFM as seen on a tracing.

   Can be used to rule out an artifact.

7. Charting: Document each period of auscultation with a description of baseline rate, rhythm, and the occurrence of gradual or abrupt decreases or increases from the baseline.

REMARKS

This is synonymous with the *maternal heart rate.*

This reflects the *FHR.*

The goal in assessing FHR is to search for and count the fetal cardiac sound.
This distinguishes the maternal heart rate from the FHR, which is usually about double the maternal pulse.

Baseline FHR refers to the FHR when the woman is not in labor or is between uterine contractions and when the fetus is not moving. The FHR must be counted long enough to pick up changes in rate and rhythm. Fetal distress during a contraction will be reflected in a lowered FHR immediately following the end of a contraction. If tachycardia or bradycardia is detected, more frequent auscultation should follow.

Irregular rhythms should be further assessed by ultrasound or cardiography but fortunately are usually benign and convert to normal rhythm after birth.

NOTE: Although auscultation allows the listener to hear gradual or abrupt changes from the baseline, neither baseline short-term variability nor the characteristic late, variable, or early deceleration patterns seen with EFM can be identified with auscultation. There is no research to support that the expert listener can make these distinctions.[16]

When an abnormal rhythm is heard using EFM, it should be verified by auscultation because the Doppler device does not generate the actual heart sound.

A clear, organized record of FHR assessments is a professional and legal obligation.

ACTIONS	REMARKS

Intrapartum Guidelines

8. Assessment during labor:

Intermittent auscultation requires a 1:1 nurse:patient ratio.

Support of the laboring woman and her partner should be a significant goal of care regardless of whether intermittent auscultation or EFM is used.

During labor, the Association of Women's Health, Obstetric and Neonatal Nurses (AWHONN) recommends that FHR be counted **after** uterine contractions for at least 30 to 60 seconds.[16]	Fetal well-being during labor is measured by the response of the FHR to uterine contractions.
In the low-risk laboring woman when no maternal or fetal problems exist: The American College of Obstetricians and Gynecologists (ACOG) and AWHONN advise counting the FHR every 30 minutes during active labor. Count every 15 minutes once 10 cm dilatation is achieved and the second stage of labor has begun.[16]	When the mother is pushing during Stage II, counting the FHR after every contraction will enable you to detect abrupt or gradual changes from baseline.
In the high-risk laboring woman: Count the FHR a minimum of every 15 minutes during active labor and every 5 minutes during the second stage of labor.[16] Evaluate FHR characteristics before and after special events during labor (e.g., spontaneous and artificial rupture of membranes, administration of medication, ambulation or a labor-initiating event).[16]	Continuous electronic monitoring of FHR and uterine contractions in the high-risk mother may give a more precise measurement of fetal response to the stress of uterine contractions, showing short- and long-term variability.

Each institution should have a written policy that describes FHR assessment and auscultation guidelines during first and second stages of labor. Readers are urged to study AWHONN's monograph *Fetal Heart Rate Auscultation* (2000), by Feinstein, Sprague, and Trepanier, which provides an excellent overview on the topic.

REFERENCES

1. Merkatz, I. R., & Thompson, J. E. (Eds.) (1990). *New perspectives on prenatal care* (pp. 129–131). New York: Elsevier.

2. Cunningham, F. G., Gant, N. F., Leveno, K. J., Gilstrap, L. C., Hauth, J. C., & Wenstrom, K. D. (2001). *Williams obstetrics* (21st ed., pp. 27, 815–818, 1114–1115). New York: McGraw-Hill.

3. Wheeler, L. A. (1979). *Fetal assessment. Series 2: Prenatal care.* White Plains, NY: The National Foundation—March of Dimes, 19–26.

4. Richardson, B. S., & Gagnon, R. (1999). In R. K. Creasy & R. Resnik (Eds.), *Maternal-fetal medicine* (4th ed., pp. 231–247). Philadelphia: WB Saunders.

5. Weeks, J. W., Asrat, T., Morgan, M. A., Nageotte, M., Thomas, S. J., & Freeman, R. K. (1995). Antepartum surveillance for a history of stillbirth: When to begin? *American Journal of Obstetrics & Gynecology, 172,* 488–492.

6. Grant, A., & Elbourne, D. (1989). Fetal movement counting to assess fetal well-being. In I. Chalmers, M. Enking, & M. Deirse (Eds.), *Effective care in pregnancy and childbirth* (pp. 440–454). Oxford: Oxford University Press.

7. American College of Obstetricians and Gynecologists. (1999). Antepartum fetal surveillance. *ACOG Practice Bulletin, Number 9,* 1–19.

8. Bocking, A. D. (1989). Observations of biophysical activities in the normal fetus. *Clinics in Perinatology, 16*(3), 583–594.

9. Gregor, C. L., Paine, L. L., & Johnson, I. R. B. (1991). Antepartum fetal assessment: A nurse-midwifery perspective. *Journal of Nurse-Midwifery, 36*(3), 155.

10. Rayburn, W. R. (1990). Fetal body movement monitoring. *Obstetrics and Gynecology Clinics of North America, 17*(1), 95–110.

11. Freda, M. C., Mikhail, M., Masioom, E., Palizzotto, R., Damus, K., & Merkatz, I. (1993). Fetal movement counting: Which method? *Maternal Child Nursing, 18,* 314–321.

12. Sadovsky, E., & Polishuk, W. Z. (1977). Fetal movements in utero: Nature, assessment, prognostic value, timing of delivery. *Obstetrics and Gynecology, 50*(1), 49–55.

13. Chamberlain, D. B. (Fall/Winter, 1999). Life in the womb: Dangers and opportunities. *Journal of Prenatal and Perinatal Psychology and Health, 14*(1–2), 31.

14. Chamberlain, D. B. (Fall/Winter, 1999). Prenatal body language: A new perspective on ourselves. *Journal of Prenatal and Perinatal Psychology and Health, 14*(1–2), 173–176, 179–180.

15. Engstrom, J. L., McFarlin, B. L., & Sampson, M. B. (1993). Fundal height measurement. *Journal of Nurse-Midwifery, 38*(6), 318.

16. Feinstein, N. G., Sprague, A., & Trepanier, M. J. (2000). *Fetal heart rate auscultation.* Washington, DC: Association of Women's Health, Obstetric and Neonatal Nurses.

SUGGESTED READINGS

American College of Obstetricians and Gynecologists. (1999, October). Antepartum fetal surveillance. *ACOG Practice Bulletin, Number 9,* 1–14.

Chamberlain, D. B. (Fall, 1994). The sentient prenate: What every parent should know. *Pre- and Perinatal Psychology Journal, 9*(1), 9–31.

Chamberlain, D. B. (Fall/Winter, 1999). Foundations of sex, love, and relationships: From conception to birth. *Journal of Prenatal and Perinatal Psychology and Health, 14*(1–2), 45–64.

Chamberlain, D. B. (Fall/Winter, 1999). Babies don't feel pain: A century of denial in medicine. *Journal of Prenatal and Perinatal Psychology and Health, 14*(1–2), 145–168.

Christensen, F. C., & Rayburn, W. F. (1999). Fetal movement counts. *Obstetrics and Gynecology Clinics of North America, 26*(4), 607–621.

Engstrom, J. L., & Sittler, C. P. (1993). Fundal height measurement. Part 1. Techniques for measuring fundal height. *Journal of Nurse-Midwifery, 38*(1), 5–16.

Engstrom, J. L., McFarlin, B. L., & Sittler, C. P. (1993). Fundal height measurement. Part 2. Intra and interexaminer reliability of three measurement techniques. *Journal of Nurse-Midwifery, 38*(1), 17–22.

Engstrom, J. L., McFarlin, B. L., & Sampson, M. B. (1993). Fundal height measurement. Part 4. Accuracy of clinicians' identification of the uterine fundus during pregnancy. *Journal of Nurse-Midwifery, 38*(6), 318–322.

Maeda, K., Tatsumura, M., & Utsu, M. (1999). Analysis of fetal movements by Doppler actocardiogram and fetal B-mode imaging. *Clinics in Perinatology, 26*(4), 829–851.

Panthuraam, C. (Winter, 1994). How to maximize human potential at birth. *Pre- and Perinatal Psychology Journal, 9*(2), 117–126.

Tharmaratnam, S. (2000). Fetal distress. *Baillieres Clinical Obstetrics and Gynaecology, 14*(1), 155–172.

Wirth, F. (2001). *Prenatal parenting.* New York: HarperCollins Publishers.

MODULE 5

Caring for the Laboring Woman

PATRICIA A. PAYNE AND E. JEAN MARTIN

OBJECTIVES

As you complete this module, you will learn:

1. The goals of intrapartal nursing care
2. To identify cultural needs of the laboring woman
3. To describe the influence of cultural factors on a woman's labor and birth experience
4. Assessment measures necessary for monitoring maternal and fetal health throughout labor
5. Guidelines for effective auscultation of fetal heart tones during labor
6. To identify the normal pattern of labor for the nullipara
7. To identify the normal pattern of labor for the multipara
8. Characteristics, causes, and treatment of abnormal cervical dilatation patterns
9. Characteristics, causes, and treatment of abnormal descent patterns
10. Causes of pain in labor and nonpharmacologic and pharmacologic therapies for pain control
11. The role of a professional doula in providing support to women giving birth
12. Those measures that need to be taken in order to safely use hydrotherapy for women in labor or giving birth
13. Factors to consider in medicating the laboring woman
14. To describe the use of subcutaneous injections of sterile water to treat severe back pain in labor
15. Interventions and rationale for nursing care throughout epidural anesthesia in laboring women
16. Interventions for intrauterine resuscitation
17. Indications, contraindications, and procedural steps for amnioinfusion
18. Indications and procedural steps for fetal pulse oximetry
19. To use graphs to analyze the progress of labor so that you can distinguish normal from abnormal patterns of cervical dilatation and of descent
20. Breathing and pushing techniques to assist the mother in progressing through labor and birth

KEY TERMS

When you have completed this module, you should be able to recall the meaning of the following terms. You should also be able to use the terms when consulting with other health professionals. The terms are defined in this module or in the glossary at the end of this book.

amnioinfusion	hypoxia
conduction anesthesia	lithotomy
doula	spaces used in conduction anesthesia:
epinephrine	arachnoid space
fetal pulse oximetry	extradural space
hyperventilation	subdural space

The Purpose of Intrapartum Care

Intrapartal care is given to ensure a safe passage for both mother and baby, to minimize risks, and to promote a healthy outcome and positive experience. If this basic and reasonable tenet can be accepted, a thoughtful review of other equally important goals can be explored.

Knowledgeable, clinically competent, caring, and skillful individuals are needed in labor and delivery units. The laboring woman requires all that from you—and more. Herein lies the essence of what makes or breaks the marvel and mystique of giving birth for every woman, anywhere in the world: kindness, compassion, and support. Think of this aspect of your caregiving as an art. Every art form asks from the artist something of himself or herself. And so too here. On your busy day, your tired day, the day when sad things happen on the unit, when difficulties occur at home, or when assignments are not to your liking, you must then enter a room and begin giving care that is intimate and demanding with both short- and long-term implications for the family.[1] Nurses have limited time to spend providing supportive care.[2] This requires efficient use of therapeutic support for women and their support person(s) and leads to confidence of the mother in her providers.[3] Nurses may find themselves in conflict with physicians about how to best provide supportive care based on current scientific evidence. The art of "negotiating organizational barriers" requires patience, skill, and knowledge of appropriate evidence-based interventions based on each individual's needs.[4]

Studies indicate that the satisfaction a women experiences during childbirth is related to either her ability to remain in control or to influence what happens to her.[5] Maternal perception of control is closely related to satisfaction, and the issue of control can be seen in terms of power. Both the birth setting and its participants powerfully influence the process of childbirth, shaping the role and amount of control held by a laboring woman, those who support her, and her caregivers. A supportive environment focuses on the woman and her family. An unsupportive environment places the caregivers, with their technologies and procedures, as the primary players and is dehumanizing.[6] Birth has become, in some instances, biologically safe yet psychologically disempowering and unsatisfying.[6]

A risk in the increased application of technology to maternity care is that:

The application becomes "routine" so that . . .
All women are treated alike; therefore . . .
Each woman's physical and emotional response is of less interest to her caregivers. She
then stands a risk of . . .
Having things "done to" rather than "done for" her[6]

The goals of intrapartum care are to do the following:

- Promote maternal coping behaviors
- Provide a safe environment for mother and fetus
- Support the mother and her family throughout the labor and birth experience
- Follow through on the mother's desires and choices throughout labor, whenever possible
- Provide comfort measures and pain relief as needed
- Offer reassurance and information, doing so with attention to the mother's and family's cultural needs

The caregiver should do the following:

- Create an environment sensitive to the psychological, spiritual, and cultural needs of a mother and her family
- Monitor maternal and fetal well-being
- Listen actively
- Recognize that language can have a powerful influence over maternal perceptions of the birth experience[7]
- Use language that is culturally appropriate, provides positive reinforcement, and empowers women and their families
- Touch so as to be therapeutic
- Use knowledge of both nonpharmacologic and pharmacologic therapies for pain relief
- Integrate the mother's support person(s) in all of these responsibilities so that he, she, or they become an essential and valued part of the profound experience of birth.

Cultural Sensitivity

Diversity is the norm in our society, requiring health care providers to be aware of beliefs and cultural practices of the families for which they care. One aspect of quality of care can be measured by cultural competency or the ability of a provider to incorporate knowledge of beliefs and cultural norms as it relates to the birth experience.[8] Women give birth within the context of their cultural background and traditional norms, including factors such as dietary practices and birth rituals. Language represents one example of cultural influences that significantly affect health care needs. The ability to communicate can affect understanding symptoms, preventing errors, and recognizing important home treatment therapies.[9] Other cultural norms surrounding birth need to be addressed by the caregiver. Food intake, positioning, support behaviors, and early infant caretaking all may be influenced by culture. A cultural assessment should be done to ensure adequate knowledge of beliefs about labor support, drug therapies, and taboos.[8,10]

Maternal and Fetal Assessment During Labor: Auscultation and Electronic Fetal Monitoring

Both observation and technical skill are used to identify changes in maternal status, fetal position, presentation, and descent. These, combined with experience in fetal heart rate monitoring techniques, provide the caregiver with the ability to monitor maternal and fetal well-being.

Guidelines for Documentation of Maternal and Fetal Status

The Association of Women's Health, Obstetric and Neonatal Nursing (AWHONN) has established guidelines for documentation during labor and birth, with special consideration of liability issues. "Documentation through the stages of labor includes maternal and fetal physiologic status, labor progression, risk status, and the meeting of educational needs."[11] The caregiver should maintain a flow sheet or written narrative of maternal and fetal status throughout labor. This allows for a permanent record and creates a visual perspective of what transpires during labor; it may also be helpful when identifying potential problems.

Selecting a Fetal Heart Rate Assessment Technique

The goals of fetal heart rate monitoring during labor are to assess fetal well-being and to detect any sign of potential fetal compromise early enough that the most appropriate steps are taken to ensure a good outcome. Once you have studied Module 6, you will recognize that monitoring techniques involve the ability to differentiate reassuring from nonreassuring fetal heart rate changes. Two approaches to this follow:

1. Auscultation with a stethoscope or a Doppler ultrasound device
2. Continuous electronic monitoring

Studies indicate that there is no benefit to continuous electronic fetal monitoring (EFM) for low-risk women[12] and that both approaches are equally effective in predicting outcome. However, a high rate of cesarean birth is associated with EFM.[13] Provided certain criteria are followed, the auscultation technique renders appropriate assessment throughout labor for the low-risk expectant woman.[12] Whichever method is used, nurses must be knowledgeable of protocols and interpretation of findings. Fetal heart rate auscultation requires the nurse to be actively involved during labor, which may result in more supportive behavior but does take more time. Circumstances such as staffing, provider and patient preference, and risk status often dictate the appropriate use of monitoring techniques.

Auscultation technique criteria[14] include the following:

• When fetal heart rate is required every 15 minutes, the nurse:patient ratio is 1:1.
• Clinical skills for auscultation, contraction palpation, and recognition of significant heart rate changes are essential (see Module 4, Skill Unit 3).

Auscultation

Guidelines for the Auscultation Procedure[14]

• Perform Leopold's maneuvers to identify the location of the fetal vertex, buttocks, and back. Fetal heart tones are best heard over the fetal back (in normal fetal flexed positions).

- Palpate for uterine contraction frequency, duration, intensity, and resting tone.
- Take the maternal radial pulse while listening to fetal heart tones to differentiate maternal and fetal heart rates. This helps prevent false conclusions about fetal status.
- *Count the fetal heart rate **after** uterine contractions for at least 30 to 60 seconds. This is helpful in evaluating fetal response to a contraction.*
- When differences are noted between counts, longer periods for recounting should be used to clarify the changes (i.e., type of periodic change and abrupt versus gradual change).
- Recount in multiple periods of 5 to 10 seconds each to clarify accelerations.

Timing of Auscultation During Labor[14]

Low-risk women	Every hour in latent phase
	Every 30 minutes in active labor
	Every 15 minutes in Stage II
High-risk women	Every 30 minutes in latent phase
	Every 15 minutes in active labor
	Every 5 minutes in Stage II

NOTE: Evaluate fetal heart tones:

- *Before artificial rupture of membranes*
- *After artificial and spontaneous rupture of membranes*
- *Before and after ambulation*
- *Before administering medication*
- *At peak times of medication effect*
- *After procedures such as catheterizations and vaginal examinations*

Electronic Fetal Heart Rate Monitoring

Electronic fetal heart rate monitoring offers both visual and auditory monitoring on a continuous basis. External monitoring provides data collection on uterine contraction patterns and timing, as well as fetal heart rate. Continuous electronic monitoring should be considered for the high-risk expectant woman. Meeting the high-risk criteria for auscultation can be disruptive to the woman; external or internal monitoring, if called for, can furnish critical information in a less distracting manner. The decision to use electronic fetal monitoring depends on maternal desires, provider decision by the physician or midwife, staffing, and status of labor progress. *All women with nonreassuring fetal heart rate patterns should have continuous monitoring. Other clinical situations that call for consideration of continuous electronic fetal monitoring are pointed out in this text.*

Evaluating Patterns of Labor

■ **What is the normal pattern of labor for nulliparous women?**

Although each woman's labor and birth experience is unique, the pattern of normal labor is fairly predictable for both the nulliparous and the multiparous woman. In the early 1960s, an obstetrician named Emanuel Friedman published a study showing that *cervical dilatation and descent of the fetus occur within certain time frames, which can be plotted on a graph.* This has been used to measure normal limits for different phases of labor in the nulliparous and the multiparous woman. Using the graph, caregivers can objectively document labor progress. In general, primiparous women will progress an average of 1.2 cm per hour during the first stage of labor; multiparas will progress an average of 1.5 cm per hour. However, Friedman's work was based on 100 "normal labors" that included women with multiple gestations and fetal malpresentations.[15]

Updated information shows that active labor actually varies by race and ethnicity, which should be considered when determining appropriate lengths of labor.[16] In addition, women who have regional anesthesia experience a longer second stage.[17] This information allows better understanding of the variation of length of normal labor, which depends on race, ethnicity, gravidity, and effects of regional anesthesia. Experienced clinicians commonly can predict the stage of labor based on maternal characteristics and fetal heart rate changes. However, inevitably, a vaginal examination will be necessary to confirm the status and progress of labor, and the Friedman graph can be used to indicate potential problems with the *progress of labor. This allows consideration for a variety of factors, including medical and psychological issues that may inhibit labor progress, including anxiety, history of sexual abuse, dehydration, and malpresentation.*

■ What are the elements of a sensitive vaginal examination?

A vaginal examination can provide important information but requires a skillful approach. The technical aspects of vaginal examination are well known and are addressed in Module 3. The manner in which the caregiver approaches and conducts the examination must be sensitive, thoughtful, and woman focused.

A vaginal examination is an extremely invasive procedure. Women can feel violated and demeaned. Impersonalizing the procedure only increases its potential stress.[18] Caregivers who perform vaginal examinations as part of their daily assessments run the risk of becoming "disembodied," desensitized to any pain inflicted during the examination, because "the inflicting of pain requires dissociation from one's own body in order not to suffer with the person in pain."[18]

In addition, the woman being examined might be encouraged to assume a passive role while the caregiver assumes "control." This empowers the caregiver and disempowers the woman. Perhaps the caregiver's sense of power or authority over the woman cannot be eliminated completely, but altering our approach to the procedure can be an impressive improvement.[18] Women who have a history of sexual abuse may find that examinations are difficult and provide a trigger for memories of previous experiences.[19,20]

The caregiver should have the following **maternal history information** before conducting the examination:

- Gravidity
- Parity
- Gestational age
- History of ruptured membranes
- History of bleeding/spotting
- History of the present labor
  - When contractions began
  - When they became regular
  - Frequency and duration

- **Fetal history**
  - Recent movement pattern
  - Lie
  - Presentation
  - Heart rate

- **History of sexual abuse**

During the physical evaluation, the examiner should look for the following findings:

External
- Fluid
- Bloody show

Cervical
- Effacement
- Dilatation
- Position (i.e., anterior, midline, posterior)

Membranes
- Intact
- Ruptured

Presentation
- Leading part
- Degree of flexion
- Molding
- Caput
- Degree of descent

> **NOTE:** *Before performing an initial vaginal examination:*
> - *Do an abdominal palpation for fetal lie and presentation.*
> - *Listen to fetal heart tones.*
> - *Ask about bleeding history.*
> - *Ask about possible ruptured membranes.*

Emotional reactions to the examination associated with history of abuse

- Inability to relax during the examination
- Tightening of vaginal muscles
- Body language that suggests fear and/or anxiety such as covering the eyes or crying

Take care to do the following:

- Introduce yourself.
- Keep vaginal examinations to a minimum. A good reason must exist for doing one. You must make your decision based on the information that needs to be obtained.
- Ensure privacy and draping.
- **Ask the woman's permission to do the examination.** This might require negotiating with her about the examination. Wait for explicit consent; tell her what you want to do and why. If she says "no," wait a while. Give her time to prepare herself. Most women will give consent after a few minutes.
- Consider the optimal position for you and the mother. Experience in performing examinations while mothers are in alternative positions such as squatting or side-lying may optimize her tolerance of the examination.
- Have an organized approach to conducting the examination. If possible, perform the examination between contractions. If an examination is necessary during a contraction, start before the contraction so that the mother does not have to react to both at once; minimize finger/hand movement as much as possible.
- Use solution or lubricant sparingly. Too much lubrication makes the area around the perineum wet and cold. Obtain all cultures and check Nitrazine paper before using lubricants that may interfere with results.
- Take care that you put on gloves discreetly while standing at the bedside; do it as quietly and unobtrusively as possible. Avoid postures such as holding the gloved hand up in a fist as you wait to begin the examination.[18]
- Keep the mother in focus throughout the examination.
- Watch your facial expressions—you are conveying a message.
- Forewarn the mother that the examination might be uncomfortable.
- Pay attention to what the mother says about the pain; acknowledge the discomfort and apologize for it. This can be beneficial for the mother.[18]
- Share your findings with the mother. Use positive language whenever possible ("You are still 5 cm dilated but are now 100% effaced, so some progress has been made."). Avoid using language that describes a diagnosis or disease process such as the "pit patient" or the "section" in room 10.[7]
- Clean and dry the mother's perineum and change bed pads if needed.

Care of the Mother During Active Labor

■ What are the major needs of the woman in active labor?

Assessment of Maternal and Fetal Vital Signs

If, on admission of a mother in early labor, a normal baseline fetal heart rate pattern has been obtained by auscultation or electronic monitoring, fetal heart rate evaluation can be carried out less frequently than every 15 minutes but should be done at least every hour. When active labor begins, evaluation intervals of 15 to 30 minutes are appropriate, as outlined previously. Many providers prefer a "baseline strip" with electronic fetal heart rate monitoring; however, there is no research to suggest a difference in outcome when this strategy is used. See Table 5.1 for a summary of assessment recommendations.

An increased pulse rate often precedes a rise in temperature. Keep this in mind, especially in women who have ruptured membranes.

Support

Women tend to cope better, relax more readily, cooperate with treatment, describe their babies more positively, have a more positive recall of the experience, and adjust more easily to parenthood when they receive kind and sensitive care during their labor. Women who are provided support in labor have shorter labors; use less medication; have less chance of a forceps-assisted,

TABLE 5.1	Assessment of Labor Progress		
	LATENT PHASE	**ACTIVE LABOR**	**STAGE II**
Vital signs	Every 4 hr	Every 4 hr	
Blood pressure	Every 60 min	Every 30 min	
Contractions	Every 30 min to 1 hr	Every 15 min	
Fetal heart rate	Low risk: every hr	Low risk: every 15 min	Low risk: every 15 min
	High risk: every 30 min	High risk: every 15 min	High risk: every 5 min
Show	Every hr	Every 30 min	Every 10 to 15 min

Data from Sleutel, M. R. (2000). Intrapartum nursing care: A case study of supportive interventions and ethical conflicts. *Birth, 27*, 38–45.

vacuum-extraction, or cesarean birth; and have babies with fewer low Apgar scores.[21] Our understanding of physiology shows us that women who are anxious or frightened during labor may experience undue fetal stress as a result of increased catecholamine levels and vasoconstriction. This may contribute to a compromised fetal state in some cases.

Knowledge is empowering. Keeping women informed during labor about what to expect, interpreting the sensations they are experiencing, and explaining their progress in labor are important elements of emotional support.[5,6]

Clinical studies reveal that a woman perceives a supportive caregiver as one who offers detailed or ongoing explanations during labor and who answers a woman's specific questions and avoids giving vague answers.[6]

Information giving relates to the following:

- Helping the woman feel that she can handle the sensations, intensity, and effort required of labor by giving constant feedback, explaining everything, being positive, and validating her efforts
- Reviewing with her how to breathe and how to position herself, placing her hands on the fundus to feel the oncoming contraction, and showing her the baby's progress in a mirror if desired
- Recognizing that the woman might have an unrealistic view of labor and what it involves and following through by anticipating information needs
- Discussing potential barriers to labor progress such as fear or history of sexual abuse or domestic violence
- Being concrete and specific, with an understanding that information might need to be repeated and skills reinforced and validated

In addition, a significant family member or friend should be encouraged to stay and support the mother. The support person will need nursing care too. Show him or her how to offer support and praise his or her efforts. Provide snacks and fluids for the support person if available in the labor area. Be sure to determine whether a support giver has any special medical needs such as diabetes that would require specific nutritional needs.

Ambulation and Positioning

Healthy laboring women should be encouraged to change positions based on their comfort needs and position of the baby. Women who ambulate in labor have shorter labors, less use of anesthesia, and greater satisfaction.[22] Positions that women find helpful in labor include positions listed in Table 5.2 and shown in Figure 5.1.

Positions that may provide comfort and rotate the fetus in a posterior position include the following[23]:

- Knee press
- Lunge
- Pelvic rocks on hands and knees
- Exaggerated lateral

Nurses can be advocates for promoting optimal positioning in labor and for birth. Encourage the laboring woman to select her positions within the bounds of safety and with consideration of fetal monitoring and special procedures such as amnioinfusion. When she is in bed, promote right or left side-lying or sitting.

TABLE 5.2	Maternal Positions for Labor
IN BED	**OUT OF BED**
Upright	Standing/walking/dancing
Semisitting	Sitting on a birth ball
	Sitting on a side chair or rocking chair
	Sitting on the toilet
	Sitting in a tub
Hands and knees	Hands and knees in the shower or tub
Lateral	Side-lying in a tub
Exaggerated lateral	
Squatting	Squatting in the shower or on the floor

From Simkin, P. (1995). Reducing pain and enhancing progress in labor: A guide to nonpharmacologic methods for maternity caregivers. *Birth, 22*(3), 161–170.

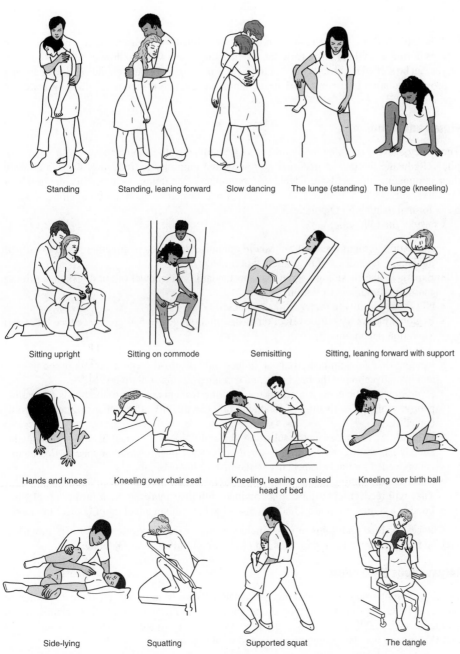

FIGURE 5.1 Maternal positions for labor and birth. *Top row.* Upright positions. *Second row.* Sitting positions. *Third row.* Kneeling positions. *Fourth row.* Second-stage positions. (Adapted with permission from Simkin, P. [1995]. Reducing pain and enhancing progress in labor: A guide to nonpharmacologic methods for maternity caregivers. *Birth* 22[3], 161–170.)

As a result:

- In 1% to 15% of women, blood pressure (BP) is lowered and hypotension results.
- Collateral circulation by blood vessels in the vertebral canal is facilitated. These vessels become distended and the sizes of the extradural and arachnoid spaces in the vertebral canal are reduced. THIS REQUIRES SMALLER ANESTHETIC DOSES IN WOMEN RECEIVING REGIONAL ANESTHESIA.

> Supine positions result in the heavy uterus resting on the major veins leading back to the heart, diminishing cardiac input. This is greatest when a lithotomy position is assumed.

> Laboring women should be encouraged to avoid remaining on their backs for long periods.

It is unlikely that a supine position must be maintained for a reason; however, if such is the case as during a cesarean birth, raise the woman's right hip with a pillow or wedge so that the uterus can be shifted to the left. Raising the right hip relieves pressure on the vena cava and may improve circulation to the maternal heart, lungs, uterus, and placenta, resulting in fewer low Apgar scores.[23]

Fluids and Food

The policy of NPO (nothing by mouth) is, regrettably, a well-established routine in many hospitals. Reducing the risk of maternal morbidity and mortality by reducing stomach contents, thus eliminating the acidic contents for pulmonary aspiration, is given as the rationale. However, surveys of literature from anesthesia and obstetrics show no compelling scientific basis for maintaining NPO policies.[24,25]

Consider the following:

- Aspiration during general anesthesia in operative deliveries is directly related to difficult intubation, regardless of the patient's oral intake.
- Experts in anesthesiology agree that substandard management of anesthesia is a primary cause of pulmonary aspiration.
- NPO status results in increased gastric acidity.
- Regional blocks have little effect on gastric emptying time and greatly reduce the risk of aspiration pneumonia.
- A regional block is appropriate for most emergency cesarean deliveries.
- Routine IV fluid administration can induce fluid overload, hyperglycemia in the fetus, and hypoglycemia in the newborn, and can alter plasma sodium levels.[26]
- Hydration and the energy needs of the laboring woman are akin to the needs of a competitive athlete. Deprivation of food and fluid can directly affect labor progress and outcome.[26]
- IV fluids are an unreasonable substitute for oral fluids in a normal healthy woman, who already has approximately 2 L of stored body water in extravascular spaces. IV therapy is not needed routinely, especially in the first 12 hours of labor.[27]
- Nausea and vomiting can be experienced in labor by a certain percentage of women. They will recover and usually can continue with their intake without further problems.
- Food is a source of comfort and can also give the woman a feeling of control in labor.

Choices for food and fluids in labor include water or ice, juices (less acidic are preferable; may be frozen in ice cubes), popsicles, and hydrating fluids such as Gatorade.

Intravenous Hydration

IV fluids (usually dextrose and water or lactated Ringer's solution) are indicated when the mother is NPO status and should be run at a rate of 125 mL per hour, which ensures that the mother receives 1,000 mL of fluid every 8 hours. Encourage policy changes from routine NPO and IV fluids to one that promotes eating and drinking.

Bladder Status

Provide the woman with the opportunity to empty her bladder every 2 hours. A full bladder can halt progress in labor, especially descent of the presenting part. If she is ambulating, urination is much more likely to be addressed by the mother because of increased pressure from the presenting part that is evident with upright positions.

Assessing Progress in Labor

Friedman's plotting and analysis of labor in the nulliparous and multiparous woman has provided a norm for evaluating progress in labor for many years. Recent studies indicate that progress throughout active labor varies by race and ethnicity.[16] Although Friedman's norms are cited here, it is important to refrain from using these norms as rigid criteria for judging the adequacy of progress in every woman. Maternal positions affecting gravity during labor, race, ethnicity, and the use of regional anesthesia need to be considered.[16]

■ **If plotted on a graph, what does the normal labor pattern look like?**

Two major physiologic and anatomic events occur during labor:

1. Cervical dilatation
2. Fetal descent

Cervical Dilatation

Friedman found that most women in labor for the first time (nulliparas) experienced a cervical dilatation rate that, when plotted on a graph, looked like Figure 5.2.

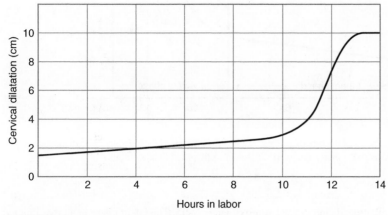

FIGURE 5.2 Labor progress of nulliparas. (Adapted from Friedman, E. A. [1967]. *Labor: Clinical evaluation and management* [p. 40]. New York: Appleton-Century-Crofts.)

Notice that during the fourth hour of labor, exactly 2 cm of dilatation has been achieved; at 10 hours, 3 cm of dilatation has occurred. Dilatation then progresses rapidly. The graph shows that the nulliparous woman achieves full dilatation after *14 hours* of labor.

For the multiparous woman, cervical dilatation occurs more quickly. The graph looks like Figure 5.3.

The multiparous woman reaches full dilatation after an average of *8 hours* of labor.

The normal labor patterns of cervical dilatation have an S-shaped curve. Friedman found that this curve could be divided into two major phases: *latent* and *active*. If the S curve is marked to show the occurrence of these phases, it looks like Figure 5.4.

The *latent phase* (preparatory phase) extends from the onset of regular contractions to the beginning of the active phase, when dilatation occurs more rapidly. It usually extends over several hours and appears as a nearly flat line on the graph. At the end of the latent phase, the

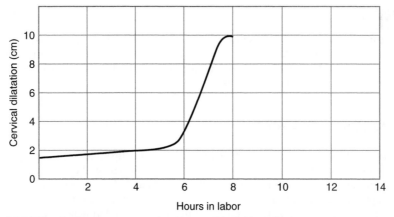

FIGURE 5.3 Labor progress of multiparas. (Adapted from Friedman, E. A. [1967]. *Labor: Clinical evaluation and management* [p. 38]. New York: Appleton-Century-Crofts.)

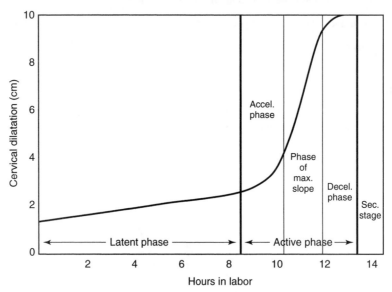

FIGURE 5.4 Phases of the cervical dilatation pattern in nulliparas. (Adapted from Friedman, E. A. [1967]. *Labor: Clinical evaluation and management* [p. 30]. New York: Appleton-Century-Crofts.)

cervix is soft, well effaced, and dilated approximately 3 cm. The latent phase can be prolonged if the laboring woman is given heavy sedation.

The *active phase* (dilatational phase) begins at the end of the latent phase, with a sharp upswing in the curve as the rate of dilatation increases rapidly. This phase ends at complete dilatation. Effective labor begins with the active phase.

The active phase is subdivided into three parts:

1. *Acceleration phase*—when the cervix begins to dilate rapidly
2. *Phase of maximum slope*—when the incline on the graph is very steep because most of the cervical dilatation happens at this time
3. *Deceleration phase*—when the rate of cervical dilatation slows (This happens just before complete dilatation; sometimes it is short or not present at all.)

The *rate of cervical dilatation* during the active phase is as follows:

- 1.2 cm or more per hour in *nulliparas*
- 1.5 cm or more per hour in *multiparas*

Overall, the *length of the first stage of labor* is shown in Table 5.3.

TABLE 5.3	Length of the First Stage of Labor	
	AVERAGE (hr)	**UPPER NORMAL (hr)**
Nulliparas	13.3	28.5
Multiparas	7.5	20

■ What can go wrong with the progress of cervical dilatation in labor?[a]

Certain factors can affect cervical dilatation. Some women have a dilatation pattern that, when graphed, differs from the normal S-shaped curve. Four major abnormal labor dilatation patterns have been identified. They are referred to as patterns of *dysfunctional labor*. Each pattern can be easily distinguished when plotted (Fig. 5.5).

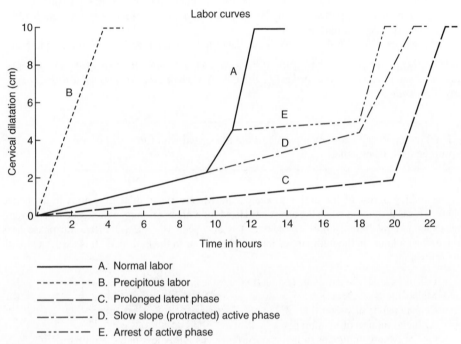

— A. Normal labor
- - - - - B. Precipitous labor
— — — C. Prolonged latent phase
—·—·— D. Slow slope (protracted) active phase
—··—··— E. Arrest of active phase

FIGURE 5.5 Labor patterns of nulliparous women. (Reproduced with permission from Malinowski, J. S. [1983]. *Nursing care of the labor patient* [2nd ed., p. 109]. Philadelphia: FA Davis.)

Dysfunctional Labor Patterns for Nulliparas

Dysfunctional labor patterns occur in both the latent phase (prolonged latent phase) and the active phase. Active phase disorders fall into two categories:

1. Progressing too slowly (protraction)
2. Failing to progress (arrest)

Both dilatation and/or descent can be involved. Protraction and arrest disorders must be separated because treatment differs for each. Both are associated with increased perinatal morbidity.

A **prolonged latent phase** is longer than 20 hours in the nullipara and 14 hours in the multipara. It is associated with the following:

- An unripe cervix
- Too-early use of analgesics or sedatives
- Too-early use of conduction anesthesia
- Nearly one third of abnormal labors in nulliparas and more than half in multiparas

Treatment consists of the following:

- Support and therapeutic rest with sedation
- Oxytocin stimulation

[a]Recommendations for treatment of dysfunctional labor patterns in this text are according to those outlined in Friedman, E. A. (1978). *Labor: Clinical evaluation and management* (2nd ed., Chap. 9 and 13). New York: Appleton-Century-Crofts.

NOTE: Artificial rupture of membranes as a treatment method usually is not effective.

A **protracted active phase** occurs when dilatation is less than 1.2 cm per hour in the nullipara and less than 1.5 cm per hour in the multipara. It is associated with the following:

- Cephalopelvic disproportion
- Minor malpresentations, such as posterior or transverse occiput
- Amniotomy before or at onset of labor
- Administration of conduction anesthesia before active labor is well established

Treatment consists of the following:

- Cesarean section for women with confirmed cephalopelvic disproportion
- Support
  –Explain the situation of slow progress to the woman and her family.
  –Ensure adequate fluid and electrolyte intake.
  –Anticipate with the woman and her family the course that labor is likely to take, explaining that progress will likely be slow but steady; cooperation is given more readily when full explanations are offered
- Avoidance of forceps delivery to shorten labor unless there is serious reason for doing so

NOTE: This pattern cannot be improved by amniotomy or oxytocin stimulation. Excessive sedation or use of conduction anesthesia can actually slow or stop (arrest) what little progress has been made.

Fetal mortality and neurologic problems are associated with forceps delivery in protracted labor patterns.

Secondary arrest of the active phase occurs when cervical dilatation stops in the active phase. This is diagnosed when the arrest has lasted for 2 hours or more, as assessed by two vaginal examinations done 2 hours apart. Arrest is also seen when the deceleration phase lasts longer than 3 hours in the nullipara or longer than 1 hour in the multipara. It is associated with the following:

- Use of excessive sedation or conduction anesthesia
- Malpositions
- Cephalopelvic disproportion
- Artificial rupture of membranes
- One of twenty nulliparas in labor; occurrence is slightly less in the multipara

---

Current studies show a good outcome for babies born after secondary arrest occurs *if delivered by a spontaneous vaginal birth.* A good outcome is less likely when a forceps delivery is done.

Treatment consists of the following:

- Immediate cesarean section for cephalopelvic disproportion
- Oxytocin stimulation if the pelvis is diagnosed as adequate
- Depending on the diagnosis and cause of the arrest, sedation for therapeutic rest, fluid and electrolyte therapy, and watchful waiting

NOTE: Artificial rupture of membranes is not effective, although this can be done to begin internal fetal monitoring.

Precipitous labor occurs when cervical dilatation is faster than 5 cm per hour (or 1 cm every 12 minutes) in nulliparas and 10 cm per hour (1 cm every 6 minutes) in multiparas. It is associated with the following:

- A normal latent phase in nulliparas
- Oxytocin administration
- Twice as many multiparous labors as nulliparous labors
- Uncomplicated and spontaneous vaginal deliveries

Heavy sedation, minor fetal malpositions, and conduction anesthesia do not prevent precipitous dilatation from occurring.

Treatment: *The best treatment for precipitous labor is to anticipate the rapid descent of the fetus and a spontaneous delivery. Anticipate the potential for a stressed newborn.*

Fetal Descent

■ How does the pattern of descent appear on a graph?

Changes in the progressive descent of the fetus can be plotted by noting the fetal station. Friedman analyzed many labors to determine averages for descent of the fetus in nulliparas and multiparas. A definite relationship exists between dilatation and descent pattern.[15] *Descent in the nullipara occurs at approximately 1 cm per hour in the active phase.*

The *right side* of the graph in Figure 5.6 has the station marked from −1 to +5 (Friedman uses the −5 to +5 station range). The distance between each point is 1 cm. Notice that descent begins well before Stage II of labor starts. The rate of descent increases late in the first stage of labor. By using the graph, you can determine whether the pattern of descent is normal or abnormal. The descent curve can also be divided into latent, accelerated, and maximum slope phases.

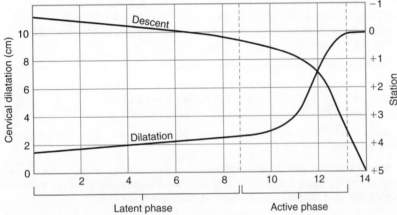

FIGURE 5.6 Dilatation and descent patterns in nulliparas. (Reproduced with permission from Friedman, E. A. [1970]. An objective method of evaluating labor. *Hospital Practice, 5*[7], 83. © 1970, The McGraw-Hill Companies. Illustration by Albert Miller.)

Figure 5.7 illustrates the normal dilatation and descent pattern in the multipara. *Descent in the multipara occurs at approximately 2 cm per hour or faster in the active phase.*

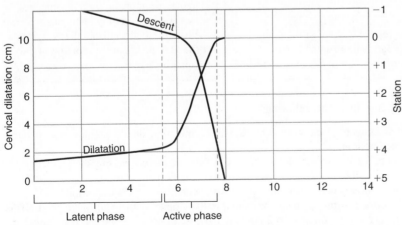

FIGURE 5.7 Dilatation and descent patterns in multiparas. (Adapted from Friedman, E. A. [1970]. An objective method of evaluating labor. *Hospital Practice, 5*[7], 82. Illustration by Albert Miller.)

THE TWO FRIEDMAN GRAPHS SHOWING PATTERNS OF DESCENT CLEARLY IL-
LUSTRATE THAT THE MOST PROGRESS IN DILATATION AND THE ONSET OF AC-
CELERATION IN DESCENT OCCUR DURING MAXIMUM SLOPE OF THE ACTIVE
PHASE IN BOTH THE NULLIPARA AND THE MULTIPARA.

Both the rates of descent and dilatation are faster in the multipara than in the nullipara.

Abnormal descent patterns occur twice as often in the nullipara as in the multipara.

Two major abnormal descent patterns can occur: protracted descent and arrest of descent.

A protracted descent pattern occurs when the rate of descent in the active phase is less
than 1.0 cm per hour in the nullipara or less than 2.0 cm per hour in the multipara. This pattern
is associated with the following:

- Protracted dilatation in the active phase
- Cephalopelvic disproportion
- Minor fetal malpositions, such as occiput posterior
- Excessive sedation
- Conduction anesthesia

Treatment consists of the following:

- Cesarean section is indicated if cephalopelvic disproportion is diagnosed.
- Avoid oxytocin stimulation because it is generally ineffective with this pattern.
- Provided the fetus is tolerating labor well, permit labor to continue with spontaneous
  vaginal delivery. Avoid forceps delivery if possible.

Higher incidences of depressed infants and perinatal deaths occur when oxytocin stimulation is given in protracted labors, especially with forceps delivery.

- Careful attention must be given to hydration and electrolyte needs, as well as emotional
  support for the woman and her family.

Arrest of descent occurs during the *active phase*, when there is no progress (as documented
by two well-spaced vaginal examinations) for 1 hour or more in the nullipara or for $^1/_2$ hour or
more in the multipara. This pattern is associated with the following:

- Advanced gestational age
- Infants weighing more than 2,500 g (especially with infants weighing more than 4,000 g)
- Cephalopelvic disproportion
- Fetal malpositions (e.g., persistent occiput transverse or occiput posterior)
- Coexistent labor disorders (e.g., protraction disorders)

When progressive descent of the fetal
presenting part is interrupted late in
labor, a serious problem can exist.

Vaginal examination for assessment of
descent must carefully distinguish
between true descent and the occurrence
of fetal scalp edema or molding of the
cranial bones.

Treatment consists of the following:

- Careful assessment of the woman by vaginal examination should be done in all patterns
  of protraction or arrest.
- If cephalopelvic disproportion does not exist, rule out factors causing the problem that
  might be reversible (e.g., excessive sedation, conduction anesthesia).
- Cesarean section is performed on women with cephalopelvic disproportion.
- Careful oxytocin stimulation can be started in the woman with an adequate pelvis. This
  should be carried out for at least 2 hours in the case of arrested descent, beginning from
  the time of an established contraction pattern.

NOTE: If arrest of descent occurs during oxytocin stimulation, continued use of such stimulation is ineffective.

- Infrequently, allowing excessive sedation or conduction anesthesia to wear off or allowing therapeutic rest for the exhausted woman will result in return of progressive labor.

Pain Control

Pain is a subjective experience. Pain is whatever someone says it is—for him or her. Physical, psychological, and cultural factors play important roles in the response women have to the childbirth experience. Pain control is managed in different ways, varying according to the stage of labor; the rate of progress; the condition of the mother and fetus; the skill, experience, and attitude of members of the obstetric team; and the requests and attitudes of the mother and her family.

Methods of pain management include the following:

- Breathing and relaxation techniques
- Comfort measures
- Nonpharmacologic pain relief (e.g., water therapy)
- Analgesia
- Anesthesia

Comfort Measures

- *Do not leave a woman in active labor alone.*
- Promptly change soiled and damp linen.
- For mothers who are NPO status, provide frequent mouth care, give ice chips, lubricate lips, and/or encourage frequent mouth rinses.
- Suggest ambulation, position change, or the use of a shower or hot tub, if available.
- Apply massage to abdomen, back, and legs as desired.
- Ensure good ventilation in the room.
- Control the labor room environment according to the mother's wishes (e.g., lights, music, quiet, privacy).
- Promote the participation of a coach or significant family member.
- Offer support from a professional doula.

"Doula refers to a supportive companion professionally trained to provide labor support."[28] A doula is not trained to do clinical tasks and may provide support during labor and the postpartum period. Women who have a doula have been shown to have improved outcomes of birth with fewer epidurals and more positive feelings about their birth experience.[29,30] This may be particularly useful in busy birth units where individualized care by a nurse or midwife is not possible.

■ What causes pain in labor?

Pain can be physical, physiologic, and psychological and is affected by a variety of factors, including level of anxiety, environment, support, and previous experience with painful stimuli.

Physical and physiologic causes are thought to include the following:

- Hypoxia of the uterine muscle because of diminished blood supply to the uterus during a contraction
- Stretching of and pressure on the cervix, vagina, and perineal floor muscles
- Distension of the lower uterine segment
- Traction on reproductive structures, such as the fallopian tubes, ovaries, and uterine ligaments
- Pressure on skeletal muscles
- Pressure on the bladder, urethra, and rectum
- Distension of the pelvic floor with tearing of the subcutaneous fascial tissue

NOTE: Factors that undoubtedly influence the degree and character of pain include the following:

- *Nature of contractions (intensity and duration)*

- *Degree of cervical dilatation*
- *Degree of perineal distension*
- *Maternal age, parity, and general health*
- *Maternal position*
- *Fetal size and position (e.g., posterior positions are usually accompanied by intense back pain)*

Other factors that determine a mother's response to pain include the following:

- Anxiety and fear
- History of abuse or previous traumatic birth or hospital experience[19]
- Cultural influences and upbringing
- Value system and education level
- Lack of knowledge or preparation
- Absence of supportive significant person
- Lack of motivation

■ Can pain in labor have harmful effects on the mother or fetus?

Besides the memory of an unhappy, painful experience for both mother and family (and, sometimes, the staff), pain has the following harmful effects[30]:

- Rapid breathing associated with pain leads to oxygen and carbon dioxide imbalance in maternal blood and lungs. This hyperventilation results in decreased blood flow to the uterus and brain. Breathing changes can also lead to fetal acidosis.
- Poorly coordinated uterine activity, regulated by the sympathetic nervous system, worsens.
- When the mother is stressed, epinephrine is released and uterine blood vessels constrict, decreasing blood flow to the placenta and fetus.
- Epinephrine also causes high glucose levels in the mother's blood, leading to an increase of glucose in fetal blood and, therefore, in brain tissue. Such high glucose levels decrease the fetal brain cells' ability to handle hypoxia and render those cells susceptible to damage.
- Cardiac output and BP increase considerably during painful periods.
- Severe pain can change cardiac rhythms and decrease blood flow to the coronary arteries.
- Muscle tightening of the perineal floor makes delivery difficult.
- Fear, tension, and anxiety are greatly aggravated by pain.

■ What nonpharmacologic pain relief measures can be used with the laboring woman?

Many techniques and therapies can be used to provide nonpharmacologic pain relief for labor and birth. These can be used alone or in combination with pharmacologic options or in an effort to delay the use of pharmacotherapy.

Commonly used therapies include the following:

- Acupressure
- Heat and cold therapy
- Hydrotherapy
- Massage
- Intradermal injections of sterile water

Nurses can use the following techniques, which have been found to be useful for women in labor:

- Help mothers identify the most comfortable position(s) and encourage frequent position changes.
- Provide hot and cold therapy with ice packs or hot packs.
- Use acupressure points.
- Encourage the use of a tub or shower.
- Provide or train support person to use massage techniques.
- Apply counterpressure with tennis balls or other firm objects, particularly with women who have a baby in posterior position.

- Use the double hip squeeze to increase the outlet diameter and decrease pain. Hands are placed over the gluteus muscles with mothers assuming a position with hip joints flexed. Using the palms, pressure is given toward the center of the pelvis.[22]
- Use intradermal injections of sterile water for severe back pain.[31]
- Encourage support by a professional doula.

■ What measures should be taken to safely use hydrotherapy for women in labor and/or for birth?[23,32]

Actions	Remarks
Rule out any contraindications for hydrotherapy in labor.	Any mothers requiring electronic fetal monitoring are not appropriate candidates.
	Dissatisfied mothers may be able to get out of the tub or shower quickly if necessary.
	Thick meconium is a contraindication to the use of tubs for labor and/or birth.
	Maternal fever is a contraindication.
Use established protocols for the following:	Jets must be cleaned according to infectious disease protocols.
• Cleaning of tubs	
• Use of long gloves for vaginal examinations	
• Fetal heart rate monitoring	
Use water at normal body temperature. Determine baseline fetal heart rate and maternal vital signs before initiation of hydrotherapy.	High water temperatures can result in elevated maternal temperatures and rapid fetal heart rate.
Cover IV lines or heparin locks with plastic.	Intermittent fetal heart rate monitoring can be accomplished when the mother is out of the water or by using a waterproof Doptone or a fetoscope.
Provide a stool and/or pillow or a birth ball for maternal comfort.	Many women prefer to sit or lean in the shower.
Constant support must be available for women using hydrotherapy.	Neck pillows provide neck support for women using tubs.
Discontinue hydrotherapy at any time if requested by the mother or if unsafe conditions occur.	If water birth is anticipated, follow specific protocols established by a practice or institution.
	Care must be given to ensure that babies are lifted out of the water immediately after birth.

■ What measures should be taken when giving pain medication to the laboring woman?[32]

- Be sure that the mother has given informed consent to her health care provider.
- Know the mother's medical and obstetric history; check for allergies.
- Take vital signs, BP, and fetal heart rate before and after administration of any medications.
- Know the status of labor and anticipated delivery at the time the medication is given.
- Consider the mother's requests.
- Be aware of the therapeutic effects, contraindications, and side effects of the drug being given.
- Use a large-bore (18-gauge) catheter when starting an IV infusion, which permits rapid fluid or blood administration if needed.

- Consider the mother's weight, the progress of labor, the maturity and size of the fetus, and the dosage of medicine being prepared.
- Give all IV medications at the beginning of a contraction, when the blood vessels of the uterus and placenta are somewhat constricted. If possible, inject the medicine over a few minutes. Because the medication is concentrated in bolus form, this technique enables a smaller amount of the drug to cross the placenta during the first few minutes of circulation so that the fetus does not receive a large amount of the drug all at once.
- Aspirate the syringe before giving any medication.
- Use filters with all IV medications and epidural catheters. Filters help screen out glass particles and bacteria that are sometimes present in ampules after they have been broken open.
- Do not give any drug with which you are unfamiliar.

Nursing Responsibilities in Performing Subcutaneous/Intracutaneous Injections of Sterile Water

Sterile water injections have been used to relieve acute pain such as pain associated with renal colic and other types of musculoskeletal pain.[31,33] Possible theories that explain the reason for its effectiveness include blocked pain pathways according to the gate theory and release of endogenous endorphins.[31,33] This technique is particularly appropriate for women in labor who are experiencing acute back pain. A period of pain relief provided by this procedure gives an opportunity for rest and comfort and time for position changes to facilitate rotation of a posterior vertex to anterior.[34]

Actions	Remarks
1. Secure informed consent.	
2. Explain steps in the procedure.	Emphasize to mothers that they will feel an acute "stinging" sensation associated with injection.
3. Assist the obstetric provider with injection.	Use 0.1 mL sterile water in four sites in the lumbar-sacral region area adjacent to the Michaelis rhomboid.[33]
4. Document the time of injection and pain relief.	Most women report relief soon after the injection and for up to 60 to 90 minutes. Use this time to reposition mothers to optimize rotation of the fetus to an anterior position.

Figure 5.8 shows the location of the injection sites.

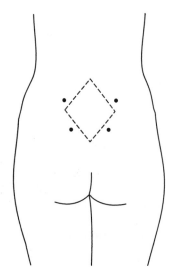

FIGURE 5.8 Location of injection sites in relation to the Michaelis rhomboid for intradermal injections of sterile water. (Adapted with permission from Martensson, L., & Wallin, G. [1999]. Labor pain treated with cutaneous injections of sterile water: A randomized controlled trial. *British Journal of Obstetrics and Gynecology* *106*[7], 634.)

Nursing Responsibilities in Monitoring and Maintaining Epidural Anesthesia in the Laboring Woman

Epidural anesthesia entails threading a catheter into the epidural space to administer local anesthetics. Located between the dura mater and the enclosing vertebrae, the epidural space provides a passageway for nerve roots leaving the spinal cord. The nerves are bathed in the anesthetic instilled into the epidural catheter, providing pain relief for the particular areas of the body that they innervate (Fig. 5.9).

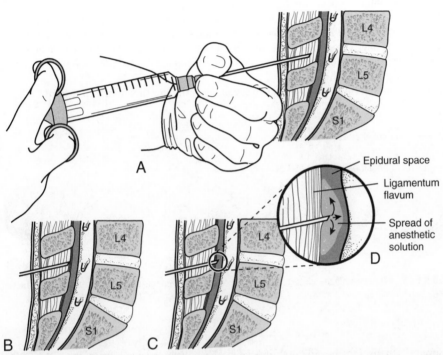

FIGURE 5.9 Technique of epidural block. **A.** Proper position of insertion. **B.** Needle in the ligamentum flavum. **C.** Tip of needle in epidural space. **D.** Force of injection pushing dura away from tip of needle. (Reprinted with permission from Taylor, T. [1993, March/April]. Epidural anesthesia in the maternity patient. *Maternal-Child Nursing Journal, 18*[2], 86.)

Currently, there are no reliable statistically significant data showing a cause-and-effect relationship between the use of epidural anesthesia and adverse effects; however, prolonged labor, increased use of oxytocin, malrotation, assisted vaginal birth, cesarean birth, and maternal fever associated with neonatal procedures have all been cited as possible effects.[11,17,35,36] Little research in the nursing literature is available to contribute to guidelines for care. The AWHONN has identified key components related to the procedure and the physiologic effects of specific medications. There continue to be areas of controversy because of insufficient data, including effects on labor, such as maternal fever. There is concern that epidural anesthesia may be associated with prolonged stages of labor, increased use of assisted techniques for delivery (e.g., vacuum extraction, forceps), and higher rates of cesarean births. Some clinicians believe that these effects may be related to individual styles of obstetric management (e.g., early labor assessment, Pitocin augmentation) and have just as much influence on the incidence of perceived effects of epidural anesthesia as does the procedure itself.[17] There is unclear evidence to guide protocols for maternal blood pressure and fetal heart rate monitoring. However, the AWHONN guidelines include accumulated research to determine a model for practice.[35] There is no question that increased technology is associated with the use of epidurals, including IV therapy and electronic fetal heart rate monitoring.

Women need to give informed consent before the procedure, before the effects of labor make it difficult to discuss.[37,38] Consent may be obtained as a component of prenatal care to allow sufficient time for education, discussion, and feedback.

Adequate nursing support is essential to the safe provision of an epidural. Evidence is lacking regarding the safety of nurses administering bolus medications during labor. However, the significance of potential side effects has necessitated standards that preclude this activity from nursing functions currently. It is important that a registered nurse evaluate maternal and fetal status before, during, and intermittently after the epidural procedure. The AWHONN position statement maintains that the insertion of epidural catheters and injection or rebolus of regional analgesic/anesthetic agents remains within the scope of the licensed, credentialed anesthesia care provider.[35]

Continuous low-dose lumbar epidural infusion is the anesthetic used most often. Sensory blockage gives uninterrupted pain relief with minimal motor blockade.

During the first stage of labor, anesthetic dosages are given to limit the block to the lower thoracic (T10) and upper lumbar segments. This allows perineal tone to be maintained to avoid interfering with internal rotation of the fetal head to the occiput anterior position. When Stage II labor is reached, the block can be extended to the sacral area to promote perineal relaxation, delivery, and episiotomy repair.

Levels of anesthesia for vaginal and cesarean deliveries are shown in Figure 5.10.

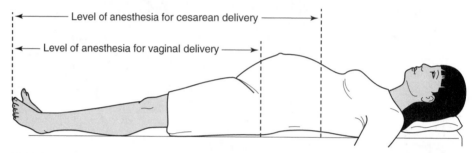

FIGURE 5.10 Levels of anesthesia for vaginal and cesarean deliveries. (Adapted with permission from Taylor, T. [1993, March/April]. Epidural anesthesia in the maternity patient. *Maternal-Child Nursing Journal, 18*[2], 92).

Several actions for the epidural procedure have been adapted from the AWHONN's *Evidence-Based Clinical Practice Guideline, Nursing Care of the Woman Receiving Regional Analgesia/Anesthesia in Labor.*[35] Readers are encouraged to read this document for further details and explanation of the scientific evidence surrounding this procedure.

Actions Before the Procedure[35,36]	**Remarks**
1. Consult with anesthesia and obstetric providers when epidural anesthesia is requested.	The physician, anesthesiologist, or nurse-anesthetist is responsible for explaining complications. The nurse clarifies and elaborates on information regarding the purpose, the desired effect, possible side effects, the procedure itself, and recovery.
2. Document informed consent by the woman.	
3. Note contraindications, such as maternal fear or refusal, local infection at the injection site, coagulation defects, and maternal hypotension or shock.	Sympathetic blockade worsens some of these.
4. Move the crash cart to an area nearby.	This provides for any emergency.
5. Obtain maternal baseline BP, pulse rate, respiratory rate, and fetal baseline heart rate and variability. Confirm a reassuring fetal heart tracing before the procedure.	Anesthetic effects include vascular vasodilatation, decreased BP, and possible fetal heart rate accelerations that could exacerbate a preexisting problem.
6. Have the woman void before the procedure.	The epidural block can reduce or eliminate bladder sensation.

7. Administer an IV fluid bolus of 500 to 1,000 mL balanced saline or lactated Ringer's solution 10 to 30 minutes before the epidural procedure.

A preprocedure bolus will help prevent hypotension caused by vasodilatation from the anesthetic.
NOTE: IV glucose solutions are not recommended because of the potential impact of fetal hyperglycemia with subsequent and rebound newborn hypoglycemia.

Never leave a mother unattended during the first 20 minutes following administration of the initial anesthetic or any bolus dose.

Actions During the Procedure[35,36]

8. Assist the woman to a side-lying position with legs slightly flexed or to a sitting position with the mother's head flexed forward, elbows resting on her knees, and feet supported on a chair.

9. Support the mother throughout the procedure of local infiltration and catheter threading.

10. A high-pressure volumetric pump is required for continuous epidural infusion. Check frequently to ensure that the proper hourly rate is according to the prescribed orders. Ensure that all connections along the epidural route are secure.

11. Note maternal BP and pulse rate before and after the test dosage. Repeat at least every 5 minutes throughout administration of the anesthetic dose and for 15 minutes afterwards. Thereafter, record BP, pulse, and respiration rate regularly based on institutional protocol and patient's status.

Remarks

This promotes moderate spinal flexion to assist in locating the appropriate vertebrae.

Breathing techniques appropriate to the phase of labor can be encouraged to promote relaxation.
This is important to overcome catheter resistance.

Epinephrine is added to the test dosage. If the catheter is misplaced and is in the dilated epidural vein, maternal pulse rate will increase 20% to 30%. A normal rate reflects that the drug was not injected intravascularly. Systolic drops below 90 mm Hg are considered inadequate to maintain uterine blood flow for fetal oxygenation.

Actions Following the Procedure[35-37]

12. May need to reassure the mother if she feels a warm tingling sensation down her legs when the initial bolus loading dose is given.

13. Avoid maternal hypotension by promoting uterine displacement with a pillow/wedge or placing the mother in a full lateral position or in a supine position, with the head of the bed elevated. Assist the mother in turning every hour.

14. Evaluate the mother's bladder every 30 minutes.

15. Periodically assess for level of anesthesia before administration of any bolus dose.

Remarks

This is a normal preanesthetic effect.

This allows the drug to defuse bilaterally.

Avoid excessive pressure in one area.
The woman can lose the sensation to void. A full bladder not only is subject to trauma but also can impede descent of the fetus.
This is important to avoid potentially high levels of anesthesia.

(One way to do this is to move an ice cube from the mother's groin area upward. Mark with a skin marker the level at which the mother becomes aware of the cold; repeat on other side.)

16. Determine the level of pain relief using institutional pain assessment scales.

This is done to assess the fading of anesthesia. Avoid anesthesia receding too far before a "top off" (bolus dose) is needed.

17. Continually monitor for maternal complications.

18. During Stage II of labor, in preparation for delivery, assist the mother to a semiupright position, an upright position, or a side-lying position.

This allows the anesthetic to migrate into the sacral area. However, if the epidural is associated with a rapid second stage or if fetal heart rate decelerations occur, a lateral position may optimize blood flow to the fetus and prevent a rapid birth.

19. Administer narcotics: Morphine sulfate or fentanyl for analgesic effect can be given by way of the epidural catheter. Observe for potential side effects.

Nausea, vomiting, itching, and urinary retention are possible.

Can be rapidly reversed by administering naloxone hydrochloride (Narcan).

20. Document the following per institutional policy:

This documentation is placed on the fetal monitor strip and becomes part of the medical record. Document the same information in the nursing notes, including description of the following:

- Times, types, and amounts of anesthetic
- Maternal BP and pulse rates
- Position changes
- Oxygen administration
- IV rate changes
- Maternal response
- Use of oxygen
- Other supportive interventions, should they be necessary

- The woman's responses to the procedure
- Any complications

Actions to Respond to Complications[35-37]

Remarks

21. Evaluate and document maternal pain levels using standard assessment tools such as visual and verbal analog scales

Special techniques include the following:
- Patient-controlled epidural anesthesia (PCEA): allows the patient to self-titrate periodic amounts of anesthetic
- Walking epidural: patients who have intentional motor function and mobility with a bolus or continuous infusion via an indwelling epidural catheter preceded by an injection of local anesthetic into the subarachnoid space

22. *Maternal Hypotension*
- Maternal hypotension is defined as a systolic blood pressure less than 100 mm Hg or a 20% decrease from preanesthesia levels.[35]

Maternal hypotension may result in a fetal hypotensive response showing fetal bradycardia and/or late decelerations. These supportive measures are intended to restore uterine blood flow.

- Place the mother in a full lateral or upright position.
- Give oxygen by face mask.
- Give 250 to 500 mL IV bolus of non–glucose-balanced saline solution.
- If vasopressors are needed, 5 to 10 mg IV ephedrine is recommended.[35]

23. Pruritus, a common and mild reaction to anesthetic, usually begins within 10 to 30 minutes of epidural initiation and medication administration.

24. *Urinary retention* is a side effect of epidural anesthesia in a large percentage of women.

Promote and maintain uterine displacement. Avoid the supine position.

Nausea and vomiting can occur in up to 50% of women having epidural anesthesia.[35]

This is the vasopressor of choice because it targets cardiac muscle, thus increasing uterine blood flow by enhancing cardiac output.

The use of opioids may increase the risk of pruritus by 40% to 90%. Less than 20% of women require medication to alleviate it. Diphenhydramine or naloxone is used for treatment. Usually, the pruritus resolves within an hour of onset.[35] 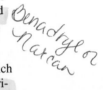 *Benadryl or Narcan*

Assessment of bladder status is critical to avoid overdistension of the bladder, which the mother cannot feel. Urinary catheterization will be necessary in some women.

> *Observe for signs of fetal bradycardia and/or late decelerations in response to maternal hypotension.*

25. *High Spinal*
    - Prevailing symptom: profound motor and sensory block within 1 to 5 minutes of the epidural injection
    - Severe hypotension
    - Cessation of respirations
    - Cardiac arrest

    Take steps to do the following:
    - Establish a patent airway.
    - Give 100% oxygen at a high flow rate.
    - Intubate if necessary.
    - Administer vasopressors.
    - Manually push the gravid uterus to one side.

26. *Intravascular Injection of Local Anesthetic*

    Signs of this include the following:
    - Change in maternal heart rate (tachycardia or bradycardia)
    - Maternal hypertension
    - Dizziness, tinnitus, or metallic taste
    - Loss of consciousness

Urinary displacement relieves pressure on the vena cava and aorta, promoting better venous return to the heart.

Inadvertent dural punctures occur in approximately 2% of pregnant women, and inadvertent intravenous catheter placements can occur in up to 5% of pregnant women.[35]

> Intravascular injection of a local anesthetic may result in seizure or cardiac arrest and requires an immediate response, including cardiopulmonary resuscitation, O_2 administration, and assisted ventilation.

27. *Spinal Headaches*
    - If the dura is accidentally punctured, women may experience

Headaches develop in 1% to 3% of women who receive epidural anesthesia.[35] As cere-

spinal headaches 24 to 48 hours after the puncture.
- Conservative treatment involves maintaining a flat position, hydration, and an abdominal binder and administering analgesics.
- A blood patch is used to seal the puncture site, using 15 mL of the patient's unanticoagulated blood. As the blood clots, it "patches" the area, usually affording quick relief.

brospinal fluid is lost, pressure is diminished throughout that compartment and the brain descends somewhat, especially when the mother is in an upright position.

Actions During Recovery From Epidural/Delivery

Remarks

28. During the mother's recovery, keep the side rails up and the bed in a low position.
29. Remove the catheter once the placenta has been delivered and the mother begins her recovery period. It is preferable to remove the catheter with the mother in the same position used during placement. A registered nurse with training may remove the catheter. Inspect the catheter carefully to make sure it is intact. If you suspect breakage, alert the anesthesiologist immediately. Always save the catheter for the anesthesiologist's inspection. Assess for motor and sensory return by asking the mother to move her legs up and down and side to side; perform plantar flexion and dorsiflexion of the feet. The mother must be able to support her knees in an upright position, as in a standing position.

The maternal position increases the intervertebral space.

Under the influence of epidural anesthesia, Stage II of labor is sometimes delayed. The American College of Obstetricians and Gynecologists (ACOG) defines a prolonged Stage II as being greater than 3 hours in a nullipara with regional anesthesia and greater than 2 hours without regional anesthesia. For the multipara, a prolonged Stage II is greater than 2 hours with regional anesthesia and greater than 1 hour without regional anesthesia.

Actions to Assess Effects on the Neonate

Remarks

30. Neonatal respiratory depression as a result of opioids can be treated with narcotic antagonists.
31. Monitor neonates for signs of neurobehavioral change associated with the use of epidurals.

Effects on the neonate may be observed up to 24 hours of age.

All neonatal care providers should be aware of anesthetic/analgesic agents used by a mother in labor.

Neonatal effects may interfere with breastfeeding. Such an effect could be decreased neonatal motor tone. If severe effects occur, separation of mother and baby might be necessary.

Intrauterine Resuscitation

■ What is intrauterine resuscitation?

Interventions undertaken to improve uteroplacental blood flow and fetal oxygenation are referred to as intrauterine resuscitation. These include the following:

- Positioning the mother laterally to improve blood flow to the uterus
- Repositioning the mother to alleviate cord compression
- Discontinuing oxytocin or using tocolysis to moderate uterine activity and improve blood flow
- Increasing intravenous (IV) fluids to enhance maternal blood flow volume
- Administering oxygen to the mother in an effort to promote oxygen flow across the placental membrane
- Performing amnioinfusion—fluid instillation into the amniotic cavity through a catheter; usually performed transcervically during the intrapartum period.[39]

Variable or prolonged decelerations caused by cord compression are common in the second stage of labor. However, cord compression brings about reduction in blood flow and therefore oxygenation, leading to fetal heart rate decline. Cord compression often occurs in clinical events that result in oligohydramnios, such as premature rupture of membranes, postmaturity, and uteroplacental insufficiency. Replacement of amniotic fluid can be used to reduce cord compression and the frequency and intensity of decelerations in the presence of these risk factors.[39] Approximately 10% of fetuses pass meconium before birth.[40] Clinical researchers now believe that this event alone might not indicate fetal distress; however, thick meconium leading to meconium aspiration syndrome (MAS) is associated with increased perinatal mortality and morbidity. Amnioinfusion results in improved Apgar scores among these newborns by thinning the meconium and decreasing the incidence of MAS.[41]

Amnioinfusion

The amnioinfusion procedure is used to[39,42–44]:

- Replace lost or absent amniotic fluid
- Dilute any impurities (e.g., meconium) in the amniotic fluid to prevent adverse effects on the fetus

Indications for amnioinfusion include the following:

- Meconium-stained amniotic fluid that is thick or contains particulate matter
- Suspected cord compression (e.g., nuchal cord)
- Oligohydramnios
- Nonreactive fetal heart rate pattern
- Repetitive variable decelerations with increasing intensity

Contraindications to amnioinfusion include the following:

- Nonvertex presentation
- Any situation in which placement of an intrauterine pressure catheter is not advisable (e.g., placenta previa)
- Absent or diminished fetal heart rate variability
- Chorioamnionitis
- Fetal anomalies incompatible with life
- Fetal malpresentation
- Fetal scalp pH less than 7.20 (delaying delivery to perform amnioinfusion can introduce unnecessary risks)
- Impending delivery
- Repetitive late decelerations (*do not delay delivery*)
- Multiple gestation
- Persistent nonreactive fetal heart rate pattern (*delaying delivery to perform amnioinfusion can introduce unnecessary risks*)
- Undiagnosed third trimester bleeding
- Uterine anomalies

Figure 5.11 shows the overall system used for amnioinfusion.

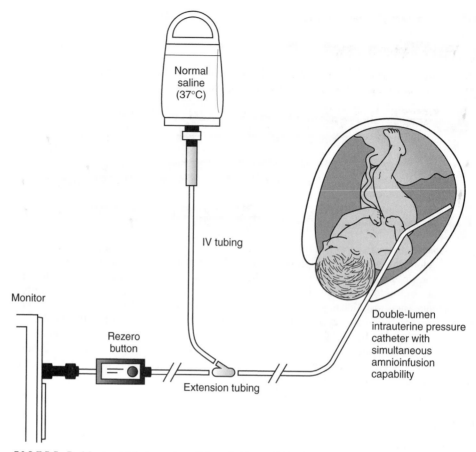

FIGURE 5.11 Amnioinfusion system. (Adapted with permission from Strong, T. H., & Phelan, J. P. [1991]. Amnioinfusion for intrapartum management. *Contemporary Obstetrics and Gynecology, 36*[5], 18.)

Guidelines for the Amnioinfusion Procedure[39,43,44]

- Obtain informed consent, including purpose, risks, and benefits, and explain the procedure to the mother.
- With the mother's permission, perform a vaginal examination to rule out cord prolapse. Determine cervical dilatation, effacement, station, status of membranes, and presentation.
- Ask the woman to position herself on her side.
- With the mother's consent, insert a fetal scalp electrode and an intrauterine pressure catheter. New-generation pressure catheters are equipped with dual lumens, internal transducers, and amnioports (sites for injecting the amnioinfusion fluid). Connect the catheter to the amnioinfusion system. Double-lumen uterine catheters permit monitoring of uterine activity while amnioinfusion is being performed. Otherwise, use a separate uterine catheter to monitor uterine activity throughout the procedure.
- Prepare the infusion (an initial bolus of normal saline or lactated Ringer's), by either gravity flow or an infusion pump.

NOTE: A literature survey revealed no demonstrable benefits using infusion pumps or solution warmers during amnioinfusion. Warming is accomplished by using a standard blood-warming unit. Extremes of temperature should be avoided.[44] **Do not use a microwave oven to warm the fluid.**[39]

- Infuse the stipulated infusate at the rate determined by protocols and by primary care provider orders. Infusion rates vary among recent reports in the literature. An initial bolus of 250 to 600 mL and an hourly maintenance rate of 150 to 180 mL has been suggested.[39] Recent studies show initial bolus ranges from 250 to 600 mL followed by a maintenance infusion rate of 150 to 180 mL per hour. Observe for fluid return; if 250 mL infuses with no evidence of return, discontinue the infusion and wait to see fluid.[44]
- Continue the infusion until either the variable decelerations cease or 800 mL of normal saline or lactated Ringer's has been infused. **Resolution of variable decelerations**

might not occur. **The woman's primary care provider should be contacted if resolution is not achieved within the time frame stipulated in nursing protocols.**
- Reduce the infusion rate to the hourly maintenance rate designated by nursing and institutional protocols.
- Carefully monitor uterine activity throughout the procedure.
  - **–Artificially increased uterine resting pressures higher than the preinfusion baseline can occur.**
  - **–A resting baseline pressure of less than 25 mm Hg should be maintained.**
- Carefully calculate fluid output during the amnioinfusion. Iatrogenic polyhydramnios can occur if the fetal head is pressed closely against the cervix. Too much fluid may result in maternal symptoms of shortness of breath, hypotension, or tachycardia.[45] Fluid output can be evaluated by comparing a dry-weight item with a wet-weight item; 1 mL of fluid is equal to 1 g of weight.[44] Therefore, all vaginal fluid should be captured in whatever padding is kept under the mother.
- Watch uterine resting tone.
- Be attentive to other possible complications in association with amnioinfusion.
  - –Signs and symptoms of abruptio placentae include a hard, boardlike abdomen; vaginal bleeding; and pain. *NOTE: Vaginal bleeding does not always occur with abruptions of the placenta.*
  - –Umbilical cord prolapse
- Document the procedure on the fetal monitor tracing and in nursing progress notes.

Fetal Pulse Oximetry

■ What is fetal pulse oximetry?

Current techniques for evaluating fetal status in labor are limited in their ability to predict outcome. Fetal oxygen saturation monitoring is used to provide additional information when a nonreassuring fetal heart rate pattern occurs and a management decision cannot be made without benefit of additional information regarding fetal oxygenation.[45–47] This procedure provides a continuous measure of fetal oxygenation and is used to evaluate peripheral tissue perfusion.[48] A sensor is inserted into the uterus and placed next to a fetal vascular bed (e.g., temple, cheek, forehead)[45] (Fig. 5.12). Measurements are based on a fraction that represents the rate of hemoglobin that is oxygenated (oxyhemoglobin), as measured by differences in light absorption, and are displayed on the electronic fetal monitoring strip providing continuous real-time data[44,45] (Fig. 5.13).

The normal range of fetal oxygenation in labor is between 30% and 70%. Values *greater than 30%* provide reassurance and may prevent unnecessary birth and cesarean birth.[20] Institutional protocols will dictate nursing priorities in caring for women who undergo this new monitoring technique.

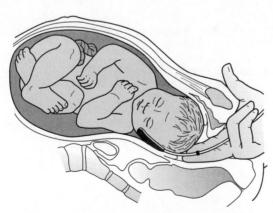

FIGURE 5.12 Fetal oxygen sensor in place. (Modified with permission from Nellcor Puritan Bennett, Inc. Copyright 1998.)

Indications for fetal pulse oximetry include the following[44,45]:

- Single fetus at term
- Vertex presentation
- Nonreassuring fetal heart rate pattern
- Ruptured membranes
- Cervix dilated at least 2 cm with station −2 or below

Contraindications for fetal pulse oximetry include the following[44]:

- Placenta previa
- Nonreassuring fetal heart rate pattern necessitating immediate delivery
- Infectious diseases that preclude internal fetal heart rate monitoring (e.g., HIV; active herpesvirus; hepatitis B, C, and E)

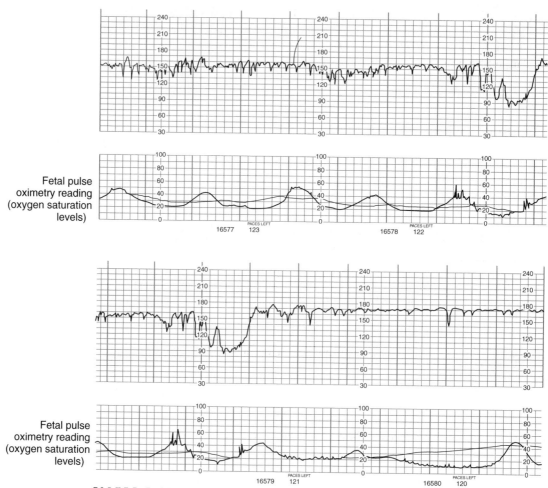

FIGURE 5.13 Examples of electronic fetal monitoring tracings with oxygen saturation continuously recorded. (Courtesy of Nellcor Puritan Bennett, Inc.)

PRACTICE/REVIEW QUESTIONS

After reviewing this module, answer the following questions.

1. There are many goals in intrapartum care. List at least four.
   a. *Promote maternal coping behaviors*
   b. *Provide a safe environment for mother + fetus.*
   c. *Support mother/family through birthing process*
   d. *Provide comfort measures and pain relief*

2. What steps can the caregiver take to promote achievement of the goals stated in question 1?
   a. *Listen actively to the pt.*
   b. *Provide a good environment for the laboring mother*
   c. *Touch as to be therapeutic*
   d. *Use knowledge of pharmocologic + non pharmocologic therapies for pain relief.*

3. Name the two major techniques for monitoring fetal status during labor.
   a. *Auscultation*
   b. *Electronic fetal heart Monitoring*

4. What is the appropriate nurse:patient ratio if fetal heart rate is being assessed every 15 minutes by auscultation? *1:1*

5. What is the correct procedure for auscultating a fetal heart rate during any active labor contraction? Why?
   Count the fetal ♡ rate p̄ Ctx for a least 30-60 sec. This is helpful in evaluating fetal response to a contraction

6. How is the average fetal baseline assessed by auscultation?
   Count fetal ♡ rate for 30-60 secs p̄ contraction

7. How can a distinction be made between maternal and fetal heart rates during auscultation?
   By taking the mothers pulse @ the same time.

8. State five situations in which fetal heart rate should be assessed.
   a. *Before AROM or SROM (after)*
   b. *Before + after medication administration*
   c. *Before + after ambulation*
   d. *Before + after and exam or other procedures*
   e. *At peak times of the medication*

9. How might caregivers conduct a vaginal examination so that a laboring woman is empowered?
   Gently, quickly, explain the procedure wait for consent

Give at least four elements of a sensitive vaginal examination.

a. *Explain your findings*

b. *Acknowledge that the exam might be painful*

c. *Pay attention to what the women says about her pain*

d. *Apologize if you cause pain*

10. What physical examination component should always precede your initial vaginal examination of a pregnant woman?

Fetal heart tones / leopolds

11. For the low-risk woman in active labor who is dilated 8 to 10 cm, BP should be taken every ___*30*___ minutes; contractions should be monitored every ___*15*___ minutes; fetal heart rate, every ___*15*___ minutes; and show, every ___*30*___ minutes.

12. The best bed rest position for the laboring woman is probably the *lateral position*

13. Maintaining the supine position for a long time sometimes results in *supine hypotensive syndrome*

14. Discuss six ways that you, as a nurse, can help make the laboring woman more comfortable.

a. *Do not leave her alone*

b. *Give frequent mouth care – face ice, lip balm*

c. *Massage*

d. *Be sure room is well ventilated*

e. *Control environment – room temp, noise, privacy*

f. *Promote participation from the support p*

15. What activities do caregivers engage in that laboring women perceive as "supportive"?

a. *helping the women feel she can handle her Ctx herself*

b. *Showing her how to breath + position*

c. *Anticipating her information needs*

d. *Reinforcing information + being concrete*

16. The nulliparous woman experiencing normal labor progress will achieve full dilatation after approximately ___*14*___ hours.

17. The multiparous woman having normal labor progress will achieve full dilatation after approximately ___*8*___ hours.

18. The dilatation curve can be divided into two major phases: *latent* and *active*.

19. At the end of the latent phase, the cervix is *soft* and dilated approximately ___*3*___ cm in a normal labor pattern.

20. During the active phase of labor, the *rate* of cervical dilatation in nulliparas should occur at ___*1.2*___ cm or more per hour; in multiparas, cervical dilatation should occur at ___*1.5*___ cm or more per hour.

21. The *average* length of the first stage of labor for nulliparas is _____13.3_____ hours; in multiparas, the average length of the first stage of labor is _____7.5_____ hours.

22. Identify the dysfunctional cervical dilatation patterns in the following graph.

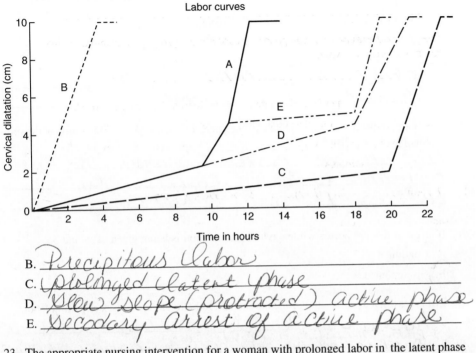

Labor curves

B. _Precipitous labor_
C. _Prolonged latent phase_
D. _Slow slope (protracted) active phase_
E. _Secodary arrest of active phase_

23. The appropriate nursing intervention for a woman with prolonged labor in the latent phase is _Emotional support and position changes._

24. Protracted labor in the active phase can be associated with:
   a. _Cephalopelvic disproportion_
   b. _Minor fetal male presentation_
   c. _Amniotomy before the onset of labor_
   d. _Administration of conduction anesthesia before active labor is well established_

25. Secondary arrest of labor in the active phase occurs when _cervical dilation_ stops.

26. The outcome is good for babies born after secondary arrest of labor if delivered by _spontaneous vaginal birth_ .

27. Precipitous labor occurs when cervical dilatation is faster than _____5_____ cm per hour in nulliparas and __5 10__ cm per hour in multiparas.

28. Descent normally begins well before the _____2nd_____ stage of labor starts in both nulliparas and multiparas.

29. The rate of descent and dilatation is _faster_ in the multipara than in the nullipara.

30. Abnormal descent patterns occur _twice_ as often in the nullipara as in the multipara.

31. Protracted descent occurs when the rate of descent in the active phase is _<1.0_ cm per hour in the nullipara or _<2.0_ cm per hour in the multipara.

32. It is important to avoid use of _____*pit*_____ and/or _____*forceps*_____ when protracted descent occurs.

33. Arrest of descent occurs when there is no progress for _____*1 hour*_____ in the nullipara or for _____*1/2*_____ in the multipara.

34. List four factors associated with arrest of descent.
    a. *Advanced gestational age*
    b. *Large Babies*
    c. *fetal mal positions ex OP*
    d. *Coexistent labor disorders*

35. What careful distinctions must be made when performing a vaginal examination of the presenting part for descent?
    true descent of fetal part and the occurance of scalp edema or molding of cranial Bones

36. If arrest of descent occurs while oxytocin stimulation is being given, it should be:
    A. Continued
    B. Discontinued

37. List at least five theories and/or factors thought to be related to causes of pain in labor.
    a. *Hypoxia of the Uterine Muscle because of ↓ Blood supply during Contraction*
    b. *Stretching and pressure of the cervix, vagina, perineal floor muscle*
    c. *Distension of the lower Uterine Segment*
    d. *Pressure on skeletal Muscles*
    e. *Pressure on the Bladder, Urethra, + rectum*

38. What are three therapies commonly used for nonpharmacologic pain relief in labor?
    a. *Acupressure*
    b. *Heat and cold*
    c. *Hydrotherapy, Intradermal Sterile Inji. Massage*

39. Why should IV medications be given at the beginning of a contraction and slowly over several minutes?
    To see how the fetal responds to the drug / the Blood vessels in the Uterus+ placenta Constrict giving Less Med to Bab

40. Discuss the measures you should take when administering pain medication to the laboring woman.
    Informed Consent; Medical + OB HX; AX; Vital Signs; Status of labor; Mother's request Be aware of the Medications Side effects, therapeutic effects + Contraindications; Use 18 G IV

41. What are two reasons to provide sterile water injections in labor for women with a baby in a posterior position?
    a. *Gives the Mother pain relief for 60-90 Min.*
    b. *Relaxes the Mother so the Baby can rotate (with different position changes)*

42. Epidural anesthesia is intended to provide complete blockade of _sensory_ nerves and minimal blockade of _motor_.

43. During the first stage of labor, the anesthetic dose is given so that the sensory block is limited to the lower _thoracic_ and the upper _lumbar_ segments. This allows _perineal tone_ to be maintained to avoid interfering with internal rotation of the fetal head.

44. Who is responsible for explaining to the mother the essentials of the epidural procedure and possible complications? _Doctor and anesthesiologist_

45. State three contraindications to epidural anesthesia.
    a. _Maternal fear or refusal_
    b. _Coagulation defects_
    c. _Maternal hypotension_

46. Why are IV glucose solutions not recommended for fluid loading before epidural administration?
    a. _Fetal hyperglycemia_
    b. _Rebound hypoglycemia_

47. Why is fluid loading done before epidural administration?
    to help c̄ hypotension

48. The mother's bladder status should be evaluated every _30 minutes_.

49. The most common complication with an epidural is _hypotension_

50. List three steps to take in a maternal hypotensive episode with epidural anesthesia.
    a. _Position ∆ (lateral (L) or (R) side)_
    b. _Fluid Bolus_
    c. _give O₂_

51. What are three signs associated with intravascular injection of local anesthetic?
    a. _∆ in Maternal heart rate_
    b. _Metallic taste, ringing in ears_
    c. _Loss of consciousness_

52. The epidural catheter can be removed by a trained nurse.
    A. True (circled)
    B. False

53. There are no known neonatal effects associated with maternal use of epidurals during labor and delivery.
    A. True
    B. False (circled)

54. What is intrauterine resuscitation?
    Measures taken to improve uteroplacental blood flow and oxygenation

55. Give five examples of intrauterine resuscitation.

    a. *Position Δ*

    b. *Fluid Bolus*

    c. *Oxygen*

    d. *DC Pit*

    e. *Amnio infusion*

56. State at least two situations in which amnioinfusion can be helpful.

    a. *PROM   Late* ✓

    b. *Cord Compression*

57. Should amnioinfusion be carried out in the case of repetitive late decelerations? **Why or** why not? State your reason.

    no delaying delivery is not in the best interest of the fetus.

58. Amnioinfusion requires that the fetal heart rate be monitored internally.

    (A.) True

    B. False

59. Select the appropriate solution(s) to use during amnioinfusion.

    (A.) Lactated Ringer's

    B. 5% dextrose and water

    C. Sterile water

    (D.) Normal saline

60. Variable decelerations will definitely resolve after the initial bolus of amnioinfusate.

    A. True

    (B.) False

61. During amnioinfusion, the uterine resting baseline pressure should be:

    A. Above 25 mm Hg

    B. At 0 mm Hg

    (C.) Less than 25 mm Hg

    D. It does not matter

62. List three serious potential complications that can occur during an amnioinfusion.

    a. *Iatrogenic polyhydramnios*

    b. *Abruption*

    c. *Cord prolapse*

63. Fetal pulse oximetry provides additional information when nonreassuring fetal heart rate patterns occur.

    (A.) True

    B. False

PRACTICE/REVIEW ANSWER KEY

1. Any four of the following:
   a. Ensure a safe passage for mother and baby.
   b. Promote maternal coping behaviors.
   c. Support the mother and her family.
   d. Follow through on the mother's choices and desires whenever possible.
   e. Provide pain relief.
   f. Offer reassurance and information.

2. a. Create a quiet environment.
   b. Listen actively.
   c. Touch in a therapeutic manner.
   d. Integrate the support person.

3. a. Auscultation
   b. Continuous electronic fetal monitoring

4. 1:1

5. Count the fetal heart rate after uterine contractions and for at least 30 to 60 seconds. This is necessary to evaluate the fetal response to contractions.

6. Count between uterine contractions for 30 to 60 seconds.

7. Take the mother's radial pulse while counting fetal heart rate.

8. a. Before artificial rupture of membranes
   b. After artificial rupture of membranes
   c. Before and after ambulating the woman
   d. Before administering medication
   e. After procedures such as catheterizations

9. Explain why the examination is necessary, and ask the woman if you may perform the examination. Wait for her consent. Remain focused on the woman and maintain eye contact.
   a. Explain your findings.
   b. Acknowledge that the examination might be painful.
   c. Pay attention to what the woman says about any pain.
   d. Apologize for causing her any pain.

10. Leopold's maneuvers and fetal heart rate assessment

11. 30; 15; 15; 30

12. Lateral (right or left) position

13. Supine hypotensive syndrome (i.e., lowered BP and hypotension)

14. a. Do not leave the mother alone while she is in active labor.
    b. Give frequent mouth care: give ice chips, lubricate lips, and encourage mouth rinses.
    c. Massage abdomen, back, and legs.
    d. Be sure the room is well ventilated.
    e. Control the environment so that quiet, privacy, and appropriate lighting are provided.
    f. Promote participation of a support person.

15. a. Helping the woman feel that she can handle her contractions
    b. Showing her how to breathe or position herself
    c. Anticipating her information needs
    d. Reinforcing information and being concrete

16. 14

17. 8

18. Latent; active

19. Soft, well effaced; 3

20. 1.2; 1.5

21. 13.3; 7.5

22. B. Precipitous labor
    C. Prolonged latent phase
    D. Slow slope (protracted) active phase
    E. Secondary arrest of active phase

23. Emotional support and rest

24. a. Cephalopelvic disproportion
    b. Minor fetal malpresentations
    c. Amniotomy before or at onset of labor
    d. Administration of conduction anesthesia before active labor is well established

25. Cervical dilatation

26. Spontaneous vaginal birth

27. 5; 10

28. Second

29. Faster

30. Twice

31. Less than 1.0; less than 2.0

32. Oxytocin stimulation; forceps delivery

33. 1 hour or more; $1/2$ hour or more

34. a. Advanced gestational age
    b. Large babies
    c. Fetal malpositions, such as occiput posterior
    d. Coexistent labor disorders, such as protraction disorders

35. Vaginal examinations must carefully distinguish between true descent of the fetal part and the occurrence of fetal scalp edema or molding of the cranial bones.

36. B

37. Any five of the following:
    a. Hypoxia of the uterine muscle because of diminished blood supply to the uterus during a contraction
    b. Stretching of and pressure on the cervix, vagina, and perineal floor muscles and perineum
    c. Traction on reproductive structures such as the fallopian tubes, ovaries, and uterine ligaments
    d. Pressure on the bladder, urethra, and rectum
    e. Nature of contractions (intensity and duration)
    f. Degree of cervical dilatation and perineal distension
    g. Maternal age, parity, and general health
    h. Fetal size and position (e.g., posterior positions are usually accompanied by intense back pain)
    i. Cultural influences and upbringing
    j. Value system and education level
    k. Anxiety and fear
    l. Lack of knowledge or preparation
    m. Absence of supportive significant person
    n. Lack of motivation

38. Any three of the following:
    a. Acupressure
    b. Heat and cold therapy
    c. Hydrotherapy
    d. Massage
    e. Intradermal injections of sterile water

39. Because the medicine is concentrated in a bolus. Giving medication at the beginning of a contraction and over a few minutes will reduce the amount of the drug crossing the placenta so that the fetus does not receive a large amount of the drug all at once.

40. Know the mother's medical and obstetric history; check for allergies. Take vital signs, BP, and fetal heart rate readings before administering any medications. Know the status of labor and anticipated delivery at the time medication is given. Consider the mother's request. Be aware of the therapeutic effects, contraindications, and side effects of the drug being given. Use a large-bore (18-gauge) catheter when starting an IV infusion, which permits rapid fluid or blood administration if needed. Consider the mother's weight, the progress of labor, the maturity and size of the fetus, and the dosage of medicine being prepared. Give all IV medications at the beginning of a contraction, when the blood vessels of the uterus and placenta are somewhat constricted. If possible, inject the medicine over a few minutes. Because the medication is concentrated in bolus form, this technique enables a smaller amount of the drug to cross the placenta during the first few minutes of circulation so that the fetus does not receive a large amount of the drug all at once. Aspirate the syringe before giving any medication. Use filters with all IV medications and epidural catheters. Filters help screen out glass particles and bacteria that are sometimes present in ampules after they have been broken open. Do not give any drug with which you are unfamiliar. Provide pain relief. Allow the mother to assume other optimal positions for fetal rotation.

41. a. Blocked pain pathways according to the gate theory
    b. Release of endogenous endorphins

42. Sensory; motor

43. T10 (thoracic); lumbar; perineal tone

44. The physician and anesthesiologist

45. Any three of the following:
    a. Refusal
    b. Maternal fear
    c. Coagulation defects
    d. Maternal hypotension

46. Because of possible fetal hyperglycemia with subsequent and rebound newborn hypoglycemia

47. The epidural induces vascular vasodilatation with resultant decreased BP. Adequate plasma volume helps offset hypotensive effects.

48. 30 minutes

49. Hypotension

50. a. Place mother in a full lateral position.
    b. Give oxygen.
    c. Give 250 to 500 mL IV bolus non–glucose-balanced saline solution.

51. Any three of the following:
    a. Change in maternal heart rate
    b. Metallic taste
    c. Loss of consciousness
    d. Seizures
    e. Tinnitus
    f. Maternal hypertension

52. A

53. B

54. Interventions undertaken to improve uteroplacental blood flow and fetal oxygenation

55. a. Positioning the mother laterally to improve blood flow
    b. Administering oxygen
    c. Discontinuing oxytocin or tocolytics
    d. Increasing IV fluid
    e. Performing amnioinfusion

56. Any two of the following:
    a. When meconium-stained fluid is present
    b. When a nuchal cord is suspected
    c. Oligohydramnios
    d. Repetitive variable decelerations

57. No, delaying delivery is not in the best interest of the fetus.

58. A

59. A and D

60. B

61. C

62. a. Iatrogenic polyhydramnios
    b. Abruptio placentae
    c. Cord prolapse

63. A

Friedman Graph: Plotting and Analysis
SKILL UNIT 1

This section details how to plot and analyze dilatation and descent patterns of labor using the Friedman graph. Study this section and then attend a skill practice and demonstration session scheduled with your preceptor. You will need to demonstrate that you can plot various labor patterns and correctly analyze them.

ACTIONS	REMARKS
Prepare the Graph Paper	

1. Use basic graph paper. Mark off time in hours, centimeters of dilatation, and fetal station (Fig. 5.14).

   The time is marked in 2-hour intervals on every other grid. Timing starts at the hour labor began.

Graphic recordings of cervical dilatation and fetal descent provide a guide for early detection of abnormal labor.

It is sometimes difficult to assign a definite time to the beginning of labor. It is generally determined from the point at which contractions occur at regular intervals, usually 3 to 5 minutes apart for the multipara. Sometimes it is necessary to assign a time to the beginning of labor in retrospect.

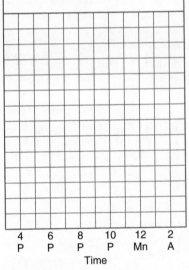

FIGURE 5.14

2. Cervical dilatation is marked on the *left vertical side* of the grid using a key symbol, such as ⊙ (Fig. 5.15).
3. Station of the fetal presenting part is marked on the *right vertical side* of the grid using a key symbol, such as ×.

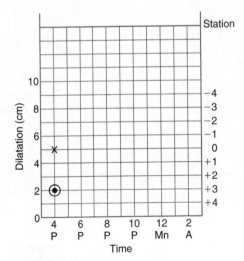

FIGURE 5.15

Plot the Graph

Mrs. Joy's contractions began occurring regularly 5 minutes apart at 12 noon. To prepare and plot the labor graph of Mrs. Joy, a nullipara, the following information is given:

TIME	CERVICAL DILATATION (cm)	STATION
12:00 noon	1	−1 to 0
4:00 PM	1	−1 to 0
6:00 PM	2–3	0
9:00 PM	3	0
10:00 PM	4	0 to +1
12:00 midnight	5	0 to +1
2:00 AM	6	0 to +1
3:00 AM	7	+1
4:00 AM	7	+1
4:30 AM	8	+2
5:00 AM	10	+3

4. *Station* at 12 noon is −1 to 0 and is indicated by × (Fig. 5.16).

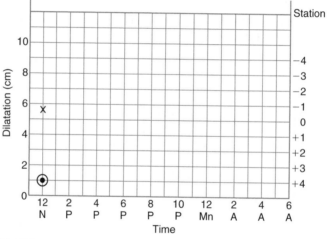

FIGURE 5.16

Dilatation at 12 noon is 1 cm and is shown by ⊙. *Time* labor begins starts at 12 noon, and 2 hours are marked on every other grid.

5. Mrs. Joy is not examined again until 4 PM and then again at 6 PM. Each finding is plotted and connected by a line (Fig. 5.17).

6. The findings from each vaginal examination are plotted (Fig. 5.18). Although this labor is slightly longer than the average 14 hours for a nullipara, the characteristic phases appear.

Latent phase is seen as straight line. If time is counted off to the point of the upward swing of dilatation, the latent phase lasts from 12 noon until 4 PM.

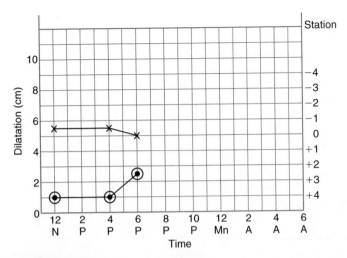

FIGURE 5.17

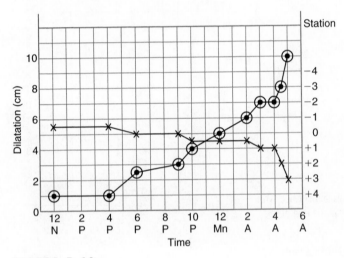

FIGURE 5.18

Active phase begins approximately 4 PM and lasts through full dilatation at 5 AM, approximately 13 hours.

Phase of maximum slope of dilatation occurs from 9 PM to 5 AM.

Note that the dilatation and descent lines cross, forming an "X" where the maximum slope begins (see Fig. 15.18).

The *deceleration phase,* when dilatation slows, often goes unnoticed and cannot be seen.

The rate of *cervical dilatation* during the active phase can be calculated. At 4 PM, when the active phase begins, Mrs. Joy is dilated 1 cm. At the end of the active phase, 13 hours later, she is dilated 10 cm. She dilated 9 cm in 13 hours, or $9 \div 13 = 0.69$ cm/hr. Mrs. Joy had an abnormal protracted active phase. The nullipara's normal rate of cervical dilatation during the active phase is 1.2 cm or faster.

The *rate of descent* of the presenting part during the active phase is slow also. The normal descent rate in the nullipara during the active phase is 1 cm/hr or more, and in the multipara, 2 cm/hr or more.

At 4 PM, the station was −1 to 0 and by 5 AM, +3. If −1 is used as the starting station, a total of 4 cm of descent during the active phase is achieved in 13 hours, or 4 ÷ 13 = 0.3 cm/hr. This is a protracted descent pattern.

Practice Plotting Labor Patterns

7. Graph the labor data provided for a *nulliparous* patient.

TIME	CERVICAL DILATATION (cm)	STATION
1:00 AM	2	−2
6:30 AM	3	−1
7:00 AM	3	0
8:00 AM	7	+1
8:30 AM	9	+2
9:00 AM	10	+3

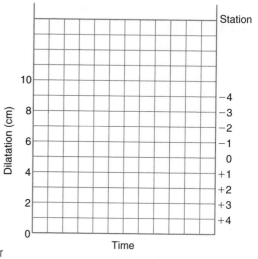

How would you interpret this labor? Check your answer with the answer key at the end of this Skill Unit.

8. Graph the labor data provided for a *multiparous* patient. Contractions became fairly regular at approximately 3 PM.

TIME	CERVICAL DILATATION (cm)	STATION
3:00 PM	3	−1
4:00 PM	6	0
5:00 PM	7	0
7:00 PM	7	+1
8:00 PM	7	+1
9:00 PM	8	+2
10:00 PM	10	+3

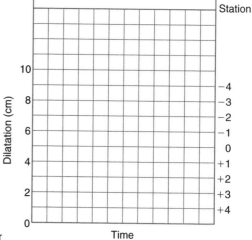

How would you interpret this labor? Check your answer with the answer key at the end of this Skill Unit.

ANSWERS TO SKILL PRACTICE

7. Your graph pattern for the nulliparous patient should appear like Figure 5.19.

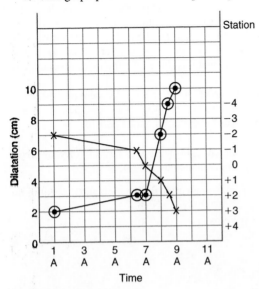

FIGURE 5.19

Interpretation

Assume that labor began at approximately 1 AM. Ordinarily, this is determined at the point when contractions begin to occur regularly. Because the average duration of labor for a nullipara is approximately 14 hours, this 8-hour labor is faster than usual. The *latent phase* occurred from 1 to 7 AM. The *active phase* began at 7 AM with a sharp maximum slope and ended at 9 AM when the patient reached 10 cm. There was no deceleration phase. The rate of cervical dilatation during the active phase was 7 cm in 2 hours, or 3.5 cm per hour. This rate is faster than the average of 1.2 cm per hour for the nullipara.

When looking at the descent pattern, note that the fetus descended during the active phase from 0 station to 13 station in 2 hours, or at a rate of 3 cm in 2 hours or 1.5 cm per hour. This is well within normal limits for the nullipara. A *protracted descent* occurs in the active phase when descent is less than 1 cm per hour in the nullipara.

This labor contained no protractions or arrests. Dilatation and descent occurred more rapidly than the average rates for the nullipara.

8. Your graph pattern of the multiparous patient should appear like Figure 5.20.

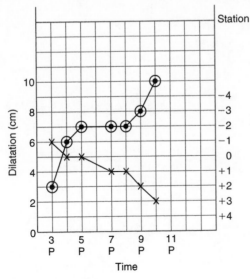

FIGURE 5.20

Interpretation

Assume that labor began at 3 PM. No latent phase was seen. Labor occurred over 7 hours with a cervical dilatation rate of 3 to 10 cm in a 7-hour period, or 7 cm in 7 hours = 1 cm per hour. This is slightly less than the average rate of 1.5 cm per hour for the multipara. Arrest of the active phase began at 7 cm at approximately 5 PM. Arrest is diagnosed when dilatation stops for 2 hours or more, as assessed by two vaginal examinations done 2 hours apart. It occurs more frequently in nulliparas than in multiparas.

Fortunately, this patient went on to dilate at a good rate after 8 PM. Descent of the fetus occurred from −1 station to +3 station in 7 hours. This is 4 cm per 7 hours or 0.57 cm per hour, a much slower rate than the normal 2 cm per hour for the multiparous patient.

You will need to attend a skill session(s) to practice this skill with the help of your preceptor. Mastery of the skill is achieved when you can demonstrate the following:

- Graphing of at least three different labors showing cervical dilatation and descent of the presenting part
- Accurate analysis of the graphed labor patterns

Techniques for Breathing and Effleurage
SKILL UNIT 2

This section details two breathing techniques and a massage technique called effleurage, which can be taught to the laboring woman and her coach if they have had no childbirth preparation. Study this section and then attend a skill practice and demonstration session scheduled with your preceptor. You will need to demonstrate that you can perform and teach the techniques listed at the end of this section.

ACTIONS	REMARKS

Begin the Breathing Technique

These techniques are done only during contractions. Rest and sleep between contractions is important. Instruct the laboring woman to do the following:

- Assume a comfortable position.
- Try to maintain a relaxed state throughout the contraction.
- Concentrate on a focal point while doing the breathing (e.g., a pretty picture, a button on someone's shirt).
- Begin and end each breathing technique with a cleansing breath. This is simply a deep quick breath, like a big sigh. Inhalation is through the nose; exhalation is through slightly pursed lips.

Every woman beginning labor must be taught simple techniques for coping with labor.
The use of a specific breathing pattern during labor contractions has two objectives:

1. Helping the woman relax by distracting her from the intense contraction sensations
2. Ensuring a steady, adequate intake of oxygen

Slow Chest Breathing (Lamaze Technique: Slow-Paced Breathing)

This technique can be used in early labor and for as long as the mother is comfortable with it. For some women, this may last throughout the entire first stage of labor.

1. Take a cleansing breath as soon the contraction begins.
2. Breathe slowly and deeply in through the nose and out through slightly pursed lips or the nose over the duration of the contraction.
3. Maintain a steady rate of approximately 6 to 9 breaths during a 60-second contraction (the cleansing breaths do not count) (Fig. 5.21).

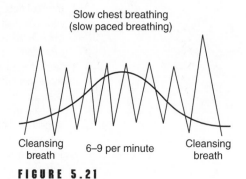

Slow chest breathing
(slow paced breathing)

Cleansing breath | 6–9 per minute | Cleansing breath

FIGURE 5.21

4. Use a focal point throughout.
5. Finish the contraction with a cleansing breath.

This technique is suggested for early and active labor up to transition. However, some women use it throughout the entire labor.

In addition, the woman may gradually increase her rate of breathing as labor intensifies. This might work well for her as long as the intensification is not rapid.

Effleurage

This is a light massage over the abdomen with the fingertips. It can be done along with the breathing technique during a contraction.

1. Starting at the pubic bone, move the hands slowly up the sides of the abdomen in a wide circular sweep (Fig. 5.22).
2. During exhalation, move the fingertips down the center of the abdomen.
3. Effleurage can be done with one hand if a side-lying position is assumed.

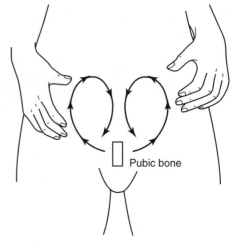

FIGURE 5.22

Effleurage often has a soothing effect and provides a distraction for the mother when she concentrates on a stimulus that is not painful. Coaches can be encouraged to do this for the mother. This technique can be used to help mothers slow their breathing and match the rhythm of effleurage.

Pant-Blow Breathing (Lamaze Technique: Patterned, Paced Breathing)

1. Begin with a cleansing breath.
2. Take four shallow breaths *through the mouth,* making a "hee" or "heh" sound. The exhalation is emphasized to give a sense of rhythm to this breathing.
3. Blow out through the mouth one time at the end of the four shallow breaths (Fig. 5.23). *The blow should be a short puff,* not a prolonged exhalation.
4. Keep an even and steady rhythm. The rate should not exceed 1 breath per second.
5. These rhythms can vary from two pants and one blow to three pants and one blow, or even six pants and one blow. Use whatever rhythm feels most comfortable.
6. Take a cleansing breath at the end of the contraction.
7. Effleurage is usually not used with this technique.

Pant-blow breathing
(patterned paced breathing)

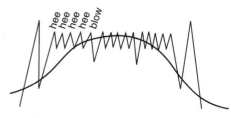

FIGURE 5.23

This is an effective technique to use during strong contractions and is particularly recommended for transition labor of 7 to 10 cm. However, some women might wish to begin using it earlier, especially those who experience a premature urge to push or those with rapid labor

You will need to attend a skill session(s) to practice this skill with the help of your preceptor. Mastery of the skill is achieved when you can demonstrate the following:

- Slow chest breathing technique
- Effleurage
- Pant-blow breathing technique

M O D U L E 5

Techniques for Second Stage and Birth
SKILL UNIT 3

Stage II of labor is a normal physiologic event that progresses to delivery usually without intervention. Instead of defining the beginning of Stage II solely by attaining 10 cm of dilatation, take into account the onset of the spontaneous urge to push and the station of the presenting part. Many women experience an urge to push or begin spontaneous pushing before full cervical dilatation.

When the pelvic floor is distended by the descending fetal presenting part, stretch receptors activate the release of endogenous oxytocin, resulting in the urge to push. This is called the Ferguson reflex. It appears that the urge to push is influenced more by fetal station than by cervical dilatation.[37] Women often have given birth in the position of choice as determined by obstetric provider preference, which may have no relationship to maternal desire of efficiency of labor.[49,50] Women have given birth using a variety of positions for centuries and should be encouraged to use the position(s) of their choosing for Stage II, provided they are not contraindicated for medical reasons. Although upright positions may be associated with an increase in blood loss, gravity may increase the pelvic diameter as much as 30% and facilitate descent and rotation, resulting in decreased use of vacuum and forceps and a shorter second stage; painful sensations may be minimized and the incidence of perineal trauma reduced. Maternal satisfaction with the birth experience may be enhanced.[51,52]

"Laboring down" is a concept and clinical practice that promotes maternal rest and nondirected pushing once 10 cm of cervical dilatation is achieved. Instead of instructing the mother to push immediately upon reaching full dilatation, the traditional approach, she is encouraged to rest until involuntary urges are experienced. During the maternal rest period, uterine contractions may facilitate further descent of the fetal head; if an epidural is used, the anesthetic effect is allowed to taper down and rectal pressure is eventually felt.[53,54]

Spontaneous maternal bearing-down efforts are found to be more effective and satisfying, resulting in less maternal fatigue.[55] As long as progress is being made and fetal signs are reassuring, no specific time limits on the duration of second stage are deemed necessary.[53] The practice of "laboring down" is appropriate for women in whom fetal compromise neither exists nor is the cause for the need to hasten delivery.

Guidelines for Second Stage

1. Let the mother rest if she does not feel any urge to push as she approaches full dilatation.

> **Promote spontaneous pushing.**

2. Respond to cues from the mother and support her short pushes if this occurs at approximately 8 or 9 cm of dilatation. Suggestions like "push when you feel the urge" will help mothers begin Stage II with minimal coaching.

> **Avoid prolonged bearing-down efforts. Encourage 4- to 6-second pushes.**

Clinical studies show that when women rely on their own bodies, they tend to push for less than 6 seconds and often take several breaths between pushes. This applies to using breath holding (closed glottis) or short pushes with release of air (open glottis).

3. Encourage pushing from different positions (e.g., side-lying, hands and knees).

   NOTE: *When the fetal position is posterior, it may be useful to position a mother in alternate positions, such as on hands and knees, to facilitate rotation. By doing so, she can do pelvic rocks during the contraction to provide additional pressure on the heaviest presenting part (the head) to rotate. Other positions such as the lateral position, squatting, or sitting on the birth ball may also assist with rotation. An exaggerated side-lying position may assist with rotation of the presenting part for mothers with epidural anesthesia.*[22]

4. Carefully monitor fetal heart tones.
5. Keep the mother hydrated, the perineal area clean, and the underpad dry. Perineal care remains an important comfort and hygiene measure.
6. When an epidural is used, the urge to bear down can diminish. More active coaching will be needed and/or the epidural effect allowed to wear off.[56]

   NOTE: *Although evidence regarding the benefits of perineal massage is conflicting, some women may receive comfort/benefit from warm compresses to the perineum. Using a mirror to view the perineum and encouraging the mother to touch the fetal head when it is visible at the perineum may promote effective pushing.*[57]

7. When no urge to push occurs after a rest period, the mother can be encouraged to move into an upright position in bed or in squatting or sitting on a toilet.
8. Keep the mother informed.[50,51,58]

   • Let her know when she is being effective in her efforts.
   • Use terminology that she can understand (e.g., not all women will understand "station +1").
   • Avoid negative statements (e.g., "That baby's head is way up there!").

9. Tell the mother when you are going to do a vaginal examination. Tell the her your findings and avoid talking across the bedside (over the mother) when sharing results of the examination with another caregiver.[56,58]
10. Avoid raising your voice when supporting a woman during the second stage.

ACTIONS	REMARKS (PICTORIAL)

Positions for Stage II

A woman may choose several positions during Stage II, depending on the intensity of contractions, the urge to push, and the length of Stage II. Stage II provides an opportunity for support person(s) to assist women as they move closer to birth and need reassurance and sensitivity. Vaginal examinations can be disruptive, uncomfortable, and discouraging. They should be used when specific information is necessary and not done routinely with indication.[18]

1. **Semisitting**

   Head and shoulders should be elevated at least 30 to 45 inches (Fig. 5.24). The head of the bed

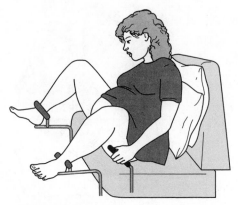

FIGURE 5.24

can be rolled up. If in the delivery room, use pillows to prop up the mother. Mothers may grasp the legs with the hands behind or in front of the knees or have their partners sit behind them and hold their legs (Fig. 5.25).

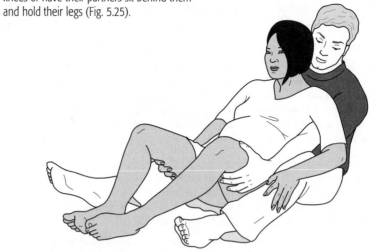

FIGURE 5.25

Flex the thighs on the abdomen by grasping the legs behind the knees, in front of the knees (Fig. 5.26), or at the ankles.

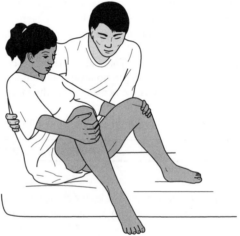
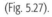

FIGURE 5.26

Variation: Permit the legs to relax in a frog-leg position with pillows under each knee (Fig. 5.27).

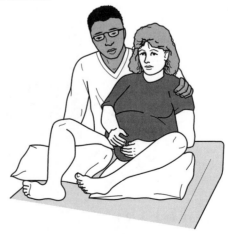

FIGURE 5.27

2. **Squatting**

The squatting position is extremely effective. Pushing efforts are maximized in this position, and the force of gravity assists the mother's efforts (Fig. 5.28).

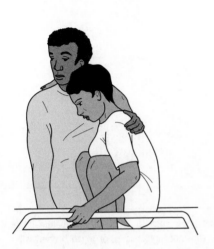
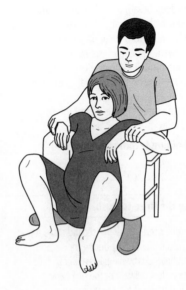

FIGURE 5.28

3. **Side-Lying**

The side-lying position (Fig. 5.29) is useful for women who need to lie on their side for medical reasons or who are experiencing a rapid second stage and benefit from increased spacing of contractions that can occur in a lateral position.

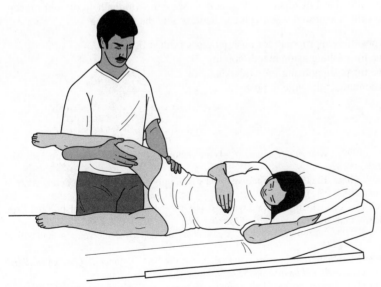

FIGURE 5.29

Technique for Physiologic Pushing (Open Glottis)

Encourage the mother to do the following:

1. Assume the position of choice.
2. Take two cleansing breaths.
3. Take a slow, deep breath in and begin to expel the breath slowly through slightly pursed lips.
4. Exhale slowly over 4 to 6 seconds. Grunting may occur toward the end of the exhalation. This is fine and provides effective effort in pushing. Remember to keep the perineal muscles relaxed.
5. Take a cleansing breath at the end of the contraction and relax.

Any breath-holding technique should be avoided!

Counteracting the Urge to Push

This method can be used before the second stage for intensive pelvic/rectal pressure or during the second stage as the fetal head is crowning. Less intense pushing may facilitate a slow delivery of the head and avoid tears and/or the need for an episiotomy.

Blow out with short, forceful exhalations. An equal amount of air is taken in after each exhalation. Take caution that this is not done too rapidly, causing dizziness and numbness in fingers and lips from hyperventilation. This is sometimes called "feather blowing."

Sometimes the urge to push is truly premature. If the cervix is not approaching 9 or 10 cm, pushing will only tire the mother. In order to push, the diaphragm is fixed and the breath held. Repeated blowing attempts help counteract this tendency to push prematurely.

This technique is used only during that part of the contraction where the urge to push is felt.

You will need to attend a skill session(s) to practice this skill with the help of your preceptor. Mastery of the skill is achieved when you can demonstrate the following:

- A variety of positions appropriate for pushing during Stage II of labor
- The technique for pushing using breath holding
- The technique for pushing using forceful exhalation
- Breathing to counteract the urge to push

REFERENCES

1. Mackey, M. C. (1998). Women's evaluation of the labor and delivery experience. *Nursing Connections, 11*(3), 19–32.
2. Gagnon, A. J., & Waghorn, K. (1996). Supportive care by maternity nurses: A work sampling study in an intrapartum unit. *Birth, 23*(1), 1–6.
3. Walker, J., Brooksby, A., McInerny, J., & Taylor, A. (1998). Patient perceptions of hospital care: Building confidence, faith and trust. *Journal of Nursing Management, 4,* 193–200.
4. Sleutel, M. R. (2000). Intrapartum nursing care: A case study of supportive interventions and ethical conflicts. *Birth, 27*(1), 38–45.
5. Gennero, S. (1998). The childbirth experience. In F. H. Nichols & S. S. Hummenick (Eds.), *Childbirth education: Practice research and theory* (pp. 52–68). Philadelphia: WB Saunders.
6. McKay, S. C. (1991). Shared power: The essence of humanized childbirth. *Pre- & Perinatal Psychology Journal, 5*(4), 283–295.

7. Zeidenstein, L. (1998). Birth language: A renewed consciousness [Editorial]. *Journal of Nurse-Midwifery, 43*(2), 75–76.

8. Mattson, S. (2000). Providing culturally competent care. *AWHONN Lifelines, 4*(5), 37–39.

9. Brasch, C., & Fraser, I. (2000). Can cultural competency reduce racial and ethnic health disparities? A review and conceptional model. *Medical Care Research and Review, 57*(99), 181–217.

10. Willis, W. O. (1999). Culturally competent nursing care during the perinatal period. *Journal of Perinatal and Neonatal Nursing, 13*(3), 45–59.

11. Rostant, D. M., & Cady, R. F. (1999). *AWHONN liability issues in perinatal nursing* (p. 101). Philadelphia: Lippincott Williams & Wilkins.

12. Thacker, S. B., & Stroup, D. F. Continuous electronic heart rate monitoring versus intermittent auscultation for assessment during labor (Cochrane Review). Cochrane Library, Issue 4, Oxford: Update Software.

13. Thacker, S. B., Stroup, D. F., & Chang, M. Continuous electronic heart rate monitoring for fetal assessment during labor. *Cochrane Review).* In: The Cochrane Library, Issue 4, 2001. Oxford: Update Software.

14. Feinstein, N. F., Sprague, A., & Trepanier, M. J. (2000). *Fetal heart rate auscultation* (p. 22). Washington, DC: The Association of Women's Health, Obstetric and Neonatal Nurses.

15. Friedman, E. A. (1978). *Labor: Clinical evaluation and management* (2nd ed.). New York: Appleton-Century-Crofts.

16. Albers, L. L., Schiff, M., & Gorwoda, J. G. (1996). The length of active labor in normal pregnancies. *Obstetrics and Gynecology, 87*(3), 355–359.

17. Howell, C. J. Epidural versus non-epidural analgesia for pain relief in labour. *(Cochrane Review).* In: The Cochrane Library, Issue 2, 2000. Oxford: Update Software.

18. Bergstrom, L., Roberts, J., Skillman, L., & Seidel, J. (1992). "You'll feel me touching you, sweetie": Vaginal examinations during the second stage of labor. *Birth, 19*(1), 10–18.

19. Holz, K. A. (1994). A practical approach to clients who are survivors of sexual abuse. *Journal of Nurse-Midwifery, 39*(1), 13–18.

20. Rhodes, N., & Hutchinson, S. (1994). Labor experiences of childhood sexual abuse survivors. *Birth, 21*(4), 213–219.

21. Hodnett, E. D. Caregiver support for women during childbirth. *(Cochrane Review).* In: The Cochrane Library, Issue 4, 2000. Oxford: Update Software.

22. Shermer, R. H., & Raines, D. H. (1997). Positioning during the second stage of labor: Moving back to basics. *Journal of Obstetric, Gynecologic, and Neonatal Nursing, 26*(6), 727–34.

23. Simkin, P. (1995). Reducing pain and enhancing progress in labor: A guide to nonpharmacologic methods for maternity caregivers. *Birth, 22*(3), 161–170.

24. Ludka, L. M., & Roberts, C. C. (1993). Eating and drinking in labor: A literature review. *Journal of Nurse-Midwifery, 38*(4), 199–207.

25. Tourangeau, A., Carter, N., Tansil, N., McLean, A., & Downer, V. (1999). Intravenous therapy for women in labor: Implementation of a practice change. *Birth, 26*(1), 31–35.

26. American College of Nurse-Midwives (ACNM). (1999). Clinical Bulletin No. 3: Intrapartum nutrition. *Journal of Nurse-Midwifery, 44*(2), 124–128.

27. Enkin, M., Kierse, M. J. N. C., Neilson, J., Crowther, C., Duley, L., Hodnett, E., & Hofmeyr, J. (2000). *A guide to effective care in pregnancy and childbirth* (3rd ed.). New York: Oxford University Press.

28. Doulas of North America (DONA). *What is a doula?* Available at: www.dona.org/faq.html.

29. Simkin, P., & Way, K. (1998). *Doulas of North America position paper: The doula's contribution to modern maternity care.* Available at: www.dona.org/positionpapers.html.

30. Perez, R. H. (1981). *Protocols for perinatal nursing practice* (pp. 193–198, 217–221). St. Louis: Mosby.

31. Reynolds, J. L. (2000). Sterile water injections relieve back pain of labor. *Birth, 27*(1), 58–60.

32. Bachman, J. A. (2001). Management of discomfort. In D. L. Lowdermilk, S. E. Perry, & I. M. Bobak (Eds.), *Maternity and women's health care* (7th ed., pp. 463–487). St. Louis: Mosby.

33. Martensson, L., & Wallin, G. (1999). Labour pain, treated with cutaneous injections of sterile water: a randomized, controlled trial. *British Journal of Obstetrics and Gynecology, 106*(7), 633–637.

34. Hansson, B., & Wallin, G. (1990). Parturition pain treated by intracutaneous injections of sterile water. *Pain, 41*(2), 133–138.

35. Association of Women's Health, Obstetric and Neonatal Nursing (AWHONN). (2001). *Evidence-based clinical practice guideline: Nursing care of the woman receiving regional analgesia/anesthesia in labor.* Washington, DC: AWHONN.

36. Taylor, T. (1993). Epidural anesthesia in the maternity patient. *Maternal-Child Nursing Journal, 18*(2), 86–93.

37. Vincent, R. D., Jr., & Chestnut, D. H. (1998). Epidural analgesia during labor. *American Family Physician, 58*(8), 1785–1792.

38. Mann, O. H., & Albers, L. L. (1997). Informed consent for epidural analgesia in labor. *Journal of Nurse-Midwifery, 42*(5), 389–392.

39. Wallerstedt, C., Higgins, P., Kasnic, T., & Curet, L. B. (1995). Amnioinfusion: An update. *Journal of*

Obstetric, Gynecologic, and Neonatal Nursing, 23(7), 573–577.

40. Ash, A. K. (2000). Managing patients with meconium-stained amniotic fluid. *Hospital Medicine, 61*(12), 844–848.

41. Hofmeyr, G. J. Amnioinfusion for umbilical cord compression in labour. *(Cochrane Review).* In: The Cochrane Library, Issue 2. 2001. Oxford: Update Software.

42. Major, C. A., & Garite, T. J. (1991). Amnioinfusion: Prophylaxis and therapy. *The Female Patient, 16,* 83–86.

43. Strong, T. H., & Phelan, J. P. (1991). Amnioinfusion for intrapartum management. *Contemporary Obstetrics and Gynecology, 36*(5), 15–24.

44. King, T. L., & Simpson, K. R. (2001). Fetal assessment during labor. In K. R. Simpson & P. A. Creehan (Eds.), *Perinatal nursing* (pp. 406–414). Philadelphia: Lippincott Williams & Wilkins.

45. Tucker, S. M. (2000). Pocket guide to fetal monitoring (4th ed.). St. Louis: Mosby.

46. Simpson, K. R. (1998). Fetal oxygen saturation monitoring during labor. *Journal of Perinatology and Neonatal Nursing, 12*(3), 26–37.

47. Yam, J., Chua, S., & Arulkumaran, S. (2000). Intrapartum fetal pulse oximetry. Part 1: Principles and technical issues. *Obstetrical and Gynecological Survey, 55*(3), 163–172.

48. Yam, J., Chua, S., & Arulkumaran, S. (2000). Intrapartum fetal pulse oximetry. Part 2: Clinical application. *Obstetrical and Gynecological Survey, 55*(3), 173–183.

49. Fraser, W. D., Turcot, L., Krauss, I., & Brisson-Carrol, G. Amniotomy for shortening spontaneous labour. *(Cochrane Review).* In: The Cochrane Library, Issue 2, 2000. Oxford: Update Software.

50. Varney, H. (Ed.) (1997). *Varney's midwifery* (pp. 433–445). Boston: Jones and Bartlett.

51. AWHONN. (2000). *Evidence-based clinical practice guideline, nursing management of the second stage of labor* (pp. 1–29). Washington, DC: Author.

52. Gupta, J. K., & Nikodem, V. C. (2000). Woman's position during second stage of labour. *Cochrane Database System Review,* (2), CD002006.

53. Roberts, J., & Woolley, D. (1996). A second look at the second stage of labor. *Journal of Obstetric, Gynecologic and Neonatal Nursing, 25*(5), 415–423.

54. Mayberry, L. J., Gennaro, S., Strange, L., Williams, M., & De, A. (1999). Maternal fatigue: Implications of second stage labor nursing care. *Journal of Obstetric, Gynecologic and Neonatal Nursing, 28*(2), 175–181.

55. Sampselle, C. M. (1999). Spontaneous pushing during birth. *Journal of Nurse-Midwifery, 44*(1), 36–39.

56. Mayberry, L. J., Hammer, R., Kelly, C., True-Driver, B., & De, A. (1999). Use of delayed pushing with epidural anesthesia: Findings from a randomized, controlled trial. *Journal of Perinatology 19*(1), 26–30.

57. Albers. L. L., Anderson, D., Cragin, L., Daniels, S. M., Hunter, C., Sedler, K. D., & Teaf, D. (1996). Factors related to perineal trauma in childbirth. *Journal of Nurse-Midwifery, 41*(4), 269–276.

58. McKay, S., & Smith, S. Y. (1993). "What are they talking about? Is something wrong?" Information sharing during the second stage of labor. *Birth, 20*(3), 142–147.

SUGGESTED READINGS

Albers, L. L. (1999). The duration of labor in healthy women. *Journal of Perinatology, 19*(2), 114–119.

Association of Women's Health, Obstetric and Neonatal Nursing (AWHONN). (2001). *Evidence-based clinical practice guideline: Nursing care of the woman receiving regional analgesia/anesthesia in labor* (pp. 1–35). Washington, DC: AWHONN.

Association of Women's Health, Obstetric and Neonatal Nursing (AWHONN). (2000). *Evidence-based clinical practice guideline: Nursing management of the second stage of labor* (pp. 1–29). Washington,

Barrett, J., & Pitman, T. (1999). *Pregnancy and birth: The best evidence* (pp. 130–178). Toronto: Key Porter Books.

Enkin, M., Kierse, M. J. N. C., Neilson, J., Crowther, C., Duley, L., Hodnett, E., & Hofmeyr, J. (2000). *A guide to effective care in pregnancy and childbirth* (3rd ed.). New York: Oxford University Press.

Kardong-Edgren, S. (2001). Using evidence-based practice to improve intrapartum care. *Journal of Obstetric, Gynecologic, and Neonatal Nursing, 30*(4), 371–375.

Lowdermilk, D. L., Perry, S. E., & Bobak, I. M. (2001). *Maternity and women's health care* (7th ed.). St. Louis: Mosby.

Mandeville, L. K., & Troiano, N. H. (Eds.) (1999). *High-risk & critical care* (2nd ed.). Philadelphia: Lippincott.

Mayberry, L. J., Gennaro, S., Strange, L., Williams, M., & De, A. (1999). Maternal fatigue: Implications of second stage labor nursing care. *Journal of Obstetrics, Gynecologic and Neonatal Nursing, 28*(2), 175–181.

Nolan, M. (1998). *Being pregnant, giving birth. A national childbirth trust guide.* Cambridge, England: National Childbirth Trust.

Ratcliffe, S. D., Baxley, E. G., Byrd, J., & Sakornbut, E. (2001). *Family practice obstetrics.* Philadelphia: Hanley & Belfus.

Rooks, J. (1999). Evidence-based practice and its application to childbirth care for low risk women. *Journal of Nurse-Midwifery, 44*(4), 355–369.

Sampselle, C. M. (1999). Spontaneous pushing during birth. *Journal of Nurse-Midwifery, 44*(1), 36–39.

Simpson, K. R., & Creehan, P. A. (2001). *Perinatal nursing* (2nd ed.). Philadelphia: Lippincott Williams & Wilkins.

Simkin, P., & Ancheta, R. (2000). *The labor progress handbook: Early interventions to prevent and treat dystocia.* Malden, MA: Blackwell Science.

MODULE 6

Intrapartum Fetal Monitoring

MEEGAN D. PAGE

Introduction to Fetal Monitoring

OBJECTIVES

As you complete Part 1 of this module, you will learn:

1. How intermittent auscultation is used to monitor the fetus during labor
2. Standards related to intrapartum auscultation
3. The definition of *electronic fetal monitoring*
4. To describe three variations of electronic fetal monitoring
5. Indications for both methods of fetal monitoring during labor
6. How to use monitoring equipment
7. Advantages and disadvantages of external fetal monitoring
8. Advantages and disadvantages of internal fetal monitoring
9. Mechanics involved in strip use and interpretation

KEY TERMS

When you have completed Part 1 of this module, you should be able to recall the meaning of the following terms. You should also be able to use the terms when consulting with other health professionals. The terms are defined in this module or in the glossary at the end of this book.

auscultation	internal fetal monitoring
baseline fetal heart rate	Montevideo units
baseline uterine tone	noninvasive fetal monitoring
direct fetal monitoring	spiral electrode
external fetal monitoring	strip graph
fetal monitoring	tocodynamometer
indirect fetal monitoring	ultrasonic transducer
intrauterine pressure catheter	

Introduction to Fetal Monitoring

■ What is fetal monitoring?

Fetal monitoring is a method of assessing fetal status both before and during labor. The fetal heart tones (FHTs) are obtained and evaluated to identify any abnormalities that can affect fetal well-being. This evaluation can be done at intervals (by intermittent auscultation) or continuously (by minute-to-minute electronic fetal monitoring). Although fetal monitoring is an important element in the assessment of fetal status, it is only one aspect of evaluation and must be used in conjunction with other parameters, such as laboratory data, patient medical and obstetric history, and clinical judgment. All laboring patients should have some kind of fetal monitoring to assist in identifying potential problems and adequately planning for further care. Many factors, such as availability of equipment, patient preference, unit staffing, and knowledge and skill level of personnel, combine to determine the method of fetal monitoring used in a particular setting. Regardless of which method of monitoring is chosen, each unit should have written policies for both electronic fetal monitoring (EFM) and intermittent auscultation (IA) that meet minimum guidelines set by national professional organizations, such as the Association of Women's Health, Obstetric and Neonatal Nurses (AWHONN) and the Association of Obstetricians and Gynecologists (ACOG). In addition, it is essential that the fetal surveillance method chosen be performed in accordance with the policies and guidelines of the institution.

Intermittent Auscultation

■ What is intermittent auscultation?

Fetal assessment may be successfully accomplished by using either auscultation or electronic monitoring. IA involves monitoring the fetal heart, through the use of either a fetoscope or Doppler, at specified intervals. This method of fetal assessment not only assists in identifying heart rate abnormalities but also provides greater mobility and often is more comfortable for the laboring woman. IA is a safe and practical alternative if correctly performed by a skilled practitioner; that is, someone who[1-5]:

- Is experienced in the labor and delivery setting
- Can discern, by auditory means, significant changes in the fetal heart rate (FHR)
- Is practiced in palpating uterine contraction and relaxation
- Is capable of initiating appropriate interventions when indicated

Research with well-controlled studies has demonstrated that IA is equivalent to continuous electronic monitoring when IA is performed at specific intervals with a 1:1 nurse:patient ratio.[1] Research also indicates that the cesarean birth rate and rate of general anesthesia are lower with IA compared with rates seen with EFM.[6] ACOG and AWHONN guidelines for FHR auscultation are shown in Table 6.1.

TABLE 6.1	Guidelines for Auscultation of Fetal Heart Tones[1,2,6-8]	
	ACOG	**AWHONN**
Low Risk		
Latent phase	No standard set	qh
Active phase	q30min	q30min
Second stage	q15min	q15min
High Risk		
Latent phase	No standard set	q30min
Active phase	q15min	q15min
Second stage	q5min	q5min

■ What can be assessed with intermittent auscultation?

In general, baseline rate and baseline rhythm can both be evaluated using IA. Baseline rate is assessed using the same method employed when EFM is performed, that is, between contractions and during periods when the fetus is not active. In addition, baseline variations such as tachycardia and bradycardia can be readily identified using IA. Because baseline rate is determined by assessing the FHR over a 10-minute period, deviations from the normal baseline range require more frequent auscultation. Auscultation can also assist in identifying changes in the fetal heart baseline. It is effective in detecting accelerations and decelerations, although there is no research at present that indicates that the practitioner can differentiate between kinds of decelerations[7,8].

Baseline rhythm can also be ascertained with auscultation and is best heard using a device such as a stethoscope, fetoscope, or Pinard device. Actual heart sounds can be heard with use of these instruments. Doppler can also be used to identify rhythm and rate; however, the sound produced from this device is a mechanical representation, not the actual heart sounds. Even though an irregular rhythm or dysrhythmia is usually benign and does not require intervention, assessment using other methods (e.g., visual ultrasound) may be indicated to rule out artifact or to determine the kind of dysrhythmia present[3,7,8].

■ How is intermittent auscultation performed?

Follow these steps in sequence[1,2,4,5]:

1. Determine fetal position using Leopold's maneuvers.
2. Apply the fetoscope or Doppler to the maternal abdomen where the fetal back is located.
3. Palpate the uterus to determine uterine activity. This assists the practitioner in determining the relationship of FHR to uterine activity.
4. Auscultate the FHR between contractions, beginning immediately after the end of the contraction and listening for at least 30-second intervals to determine fetal response to the contraction, rate, and rhythm.
5. Occasionally count maternal pulse to differentiate between fetal and maternal heart rates.
6. Document your observations.

It is recommended that FHR assessment be performed **before:**

- Induction or augmentation of labor (administration of Pitocin or amniotomy)
- Administration of medications, including analgesia and initiation of anesthesia
- Ambulation
- Transfer or discharge

Assessment of the FHR should be performed **after:**

- Rupture of membranes
- Ambulation
- Vaginal examination
- Abnormal uterine activity
- Change in oxytocin administration
- Change in analgesia and anesthesia
- Patient admission

Advantages/Benefits of Auscultation[2,3,8]

Patient comfort—The woman may be up and about and may move easily in bed. Sometimes, the abdominal area and the lower back of a laboring woman is extremely sensitive. Belts and other equipment can cause irritation and discomfort and interfere with her ability to concentrate and relax.

Facilitation of ambulation—Ambulation often contributes to greater patient comfort and perhaps more rapid progress in labor. Freedom of movement (i.e., the ability to walk and stand) is supported by IA.

Requirement of caregiver to be at the bedside—This provides many benefits, such as comfort, support, and encouragement. A critical component of intrapartum care is support in labor. With IA, close, frequent contact between the patient and caregiver occurs.

Fewer interventions—Women who desire an atmosphere in which birth is viewed as a normal, natural event might prefer this method of monitoring.

Neonatal outcomes—Outcomes are comparable to those with EFM.

Lower cesarean birth rates—Cesarean birth rates are lower in comparison with EFM.

Equipment—Required equipment is less costly than that necessary for EFM.

No automatic documentation on paper—No documentation is automatically produced with IA, in contrast to EFM, in which differences of opinion in interpretation of strips may lead to legal problems.

Disadvantages/Limitations of Auscultation[2,3,8]

Practitioner skilled in auscultation—Strong auscultation skills and patience are required to differentiate subtle changes in the FHR. Errors can be made by those less experienced by subconsciously normalizing the rate.

Nurse:patient ratio of 1:1—The nurse:patient ratio must be 1:1. However, nursing shortages sometimes preclude this capability.

Invasion of personal space—Because very frequent, close personal contact is required to provide adequate assessment through IA, some patients feel as if their personal space is being invaded.

Rapid heart rates (greater than 160 bpm)—These are difficult to accurately count.

Inability to evaluate certain aspects of the FHR—Examples include variability, deceleration types.

Physical limitations of equipment—Maternal size (obesity), position, and polyhydramnios may interfere with the practitioner's ability to adequately assess the FHR by IA.

Documentation of FHR by Auscultation

Documentation of the findings of each auscultation must be performed regardless of the method used to assess the FHR. The form chosen for documenting the FHR may vary among institutions; however, its most important aspect is that every record must be clear and precise. Each chart should reflect baseline rate, rhythm, and the presence of gradual or abrupt increases or decreases from baseline. In addition, patient status, interventions, staff consultations, and communication with health care providers should be included as part of the documentation process.[1,2,4,5,7]

Electronic Fetal Monitoring

■ What is electronic fetal monitoring?

EFM is an electronic method of providing a continuous visual record of the FHR and obtaining information about the laboring woman's uterine activity (Fig. 6.1). This information is recorded on *graph paper,* allows an ongoing minute-to-minute assessment of fetal well-being during labor, and provides a permanent record for the medical chart. It is useful for screening or surveillance, but it is not intended as a diagnostic tool. There is also a general agreement that a normal, reactive EFM tracing is highly predicative of a well-oxygenated fetus.[9,8–11] However, the problem lies in the correlation of the strip with fetal status when the tracing is not reassuring. A nonreassuring tracing does not necessarily mean that the fetus is in trouble.[12,13] In fact, the predictive value of a nonreassuring strip for poor fetal outcome is not strong.

NOTE: At the onset of EFM, validation of the equipment should be performed by auscultation of the FHTs with a nonmechanical means such as the fetoscope and by testing of the internal circuitry by pushing the "test" button on the monitor and examining the test lines on the graph paper.[14]

■ What are indications for electronic fetal monitoring?

Many factors may make the desirability for using a continuous method of fetal monitoring during labor more pronounced. Factors appearing before the woman is in labor are considered *antepartal risk factors.* Other indications for monitoring that do not appear until the woman is already in labor are *intrapartal risk factors.* Note that fetuses in at-risk pregnancies can also be followed in labor by IA according to guidelines set forth by AWHONN and ACOG; however, many practitioners have become more comfortable using EFM to assist in the assessment of fetal status.

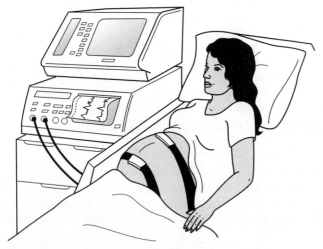

FIGURE 6.1 The electronic fetal monitor.

Antepartal risk factors include the following:

Hypertension
Pregnancy-induced hypertension
Diabetes mellitus
Chronic renal disease
Congenital or rheumatic heart disease
Sickle cell disease
Rh isoimmunization
Preterm infants (less than 37 weeks' gestation)
Age factors (younger than 15 years of age or older than 35)

Postmature infants (more than 42 weeks' gestation)
Multiple gestations
Grandmultiparity
Anemia
Intrauterine growth restriction (IUGR) or small for gestational age (SGA)
Genital tract disorders/anomalies
Poor obstetric history

Intrapartal risk factors include the following:

Prolonged rupture of membranes
Premature rupture of membranes
Failure to progress in labor or dysfunctional labor
Meconium-stained amniotic fluid
Abnormal FHR detected during auscultation

Abnormal presentations
Pitocin augmentation/induction
Premature labor
Possible cephalopelvic disproportion (CPD)
Previous cesarean section in labor
Hypotensive episodes in labor
Bleeding disorders—abruptio placentae, placenta previa

■ Should the electronic fetal monitor be used routinely during labor?

Whether the fetal monitor should be used routinely during labor is controversial. Its use can limit mobility, interfere with the use of comfort techniques, and potentially contribute to the mother having negative feelings about the experience. Some women might believe that "something is wrong" even if an explanation is given about the routine use of the equipment. This is especially true for women whose pregnancies are low risk. Although EFM is an excellent means of predicting fetal well-being, it is much less accurate in predicting fetal stress. In fact, mistaken diagnoses of fetal distress have contributed to the increased rates of cesarean sections and forceps deliveries. Ominous-looking FHR patterns can present a much worse picture of fetal condition than actually exists.[15] Another consideration is the change in the level of support, which is widely recognized to play an extremely important role in labor. When EFM replaces IA, the nurse's focus shifts from the patient to machinery, reducing physical contact and the level of intimacy between the patient and caregiver. Research has shown that many factors are affected by the personal support given to the patient during labor, such as shorter labors, decreased need for oxytocin augmentation, fewer epidurals, and fewer operative deliveries.[13,15]

There is no doubt that support during labor has a significantly positive effect on fetal and maternal well-being.[2,16–19] In addition, EFM technology increases accountability and exposure to legal risk due to difference in opinion related to strip interpretation. Knowledge of machine operation, troubleshooting, and maintenance, as well as interpretation of the tracings, represents additional skill that are essential and are legal expectations when EFM is used.[20-24] In view of the evidence supporting the reliability of IA, its benefit in conjunction with promoting labor support, and the legal implications related to strip interpretation, perhaps we should reconsider our choice of methods for evaluation of fetal status during labor.[20,25]

■ How is the electronic monitor used to determine fetal well-being?

The electronic fetal monitor may be used in three different ways:

1. *External fetal monitoring* is also called *indirect fetal monitoring,* or *noninvasive fetal monitoring.* This method involves the use of an ultrasonic transducer to monitor the fetal heart while the contraction pattern is monitored with a tocodynamometer. Both are placed on the woman's abdomen and are secured in place by belts or adhesive patches (Fig. 6.2).

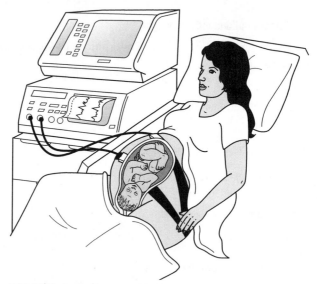

FIGURE 6.2 The external fetal monitor.

The *ultrasonic transducer,* more commonly known as an *ultrasound,* or *Doppler,* transmits high-frequency sound waves that detect movement within the fetal heart. The signal, which is similar to sonar used in submarines, is reflected back from moving structures and is recognized by the machine as a cardiac event. The movement detected is both ventricular contraction and the actual opening and closing of valves within the heart.

The *tocodynamometer,* more commonly known as a *toco,* provides information about the laboring woman's contraction pattern by detecting changes in the shape of the abdominal wall directly over the uterine fundus. These changes in shape are the direct result of the effects of the uterine contraction on the maternal abdomen.

As a result of the manner in which the data are obtained, these methods are referred to as *indirect* or external monitoring because the techniques are performed external to the fetus and uterus. Because the vagina, cervix, and uterus are not invaded when applying an external monitor, the technique is also termed *noninvasive.*

2. *Internal fetal monitoring* is also called *direct fetal monitoring,* or *invasive fetal monitoring.* With this method, the FHR is monitored by the use of a *helix/fetal spiral electrode (FSE),* which is applied directly to the presenting part of the fetus. The laboring woman's contraction pattern is monitored by the use of an *intrauterine pressure catheter (IUPC),* which is inserted vaginally directly into the uterine cavity through the

cervix (Fig. 6.3). Information is obtained *internally* from the laboring woman by the use of *invasive* methods, which *directly* monitor the fetus and the uterine activity.

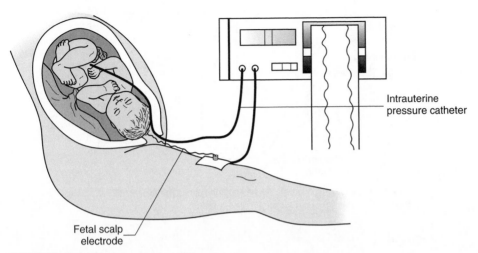

FIGURE 6.3 The internal fetal monitor.

3. *A combination of internal and external fetal monitoring* has become one of the most common ways to monitor the fetus. Usually, the FHR is monitored internally by the use of an *electrode,* and the laboring woman's contraction pattern is monitored externally by the use of a tocodynamometer (Fig. 6.4). However, the opposite may also be used. The FHR can be monitored externally by the use of an *ultrasound transducer,* and the laboring woman's contraction pattern can be monitored internally by the use of an *IUPC* (Fig. 6.5).

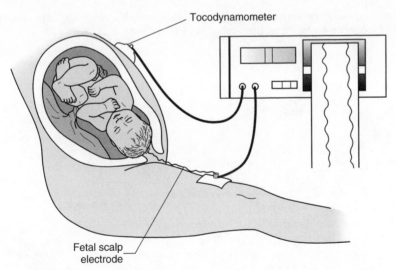

FIGURE 6.4 Combination of external and internal monitoring. The tocodynamometer and helix/fetal scalp electrode are used together.

■ How is the fetal spiral electrode used?

The electrode tracks the FHR by picking up *R waves* on the fetal electrocardiogram (ECG). The interval between each R wave is measured and processed by internal circuitry and calculated to a rate in beats per minute (bpm); the result is printed on graph paper (Fig. 6.6).

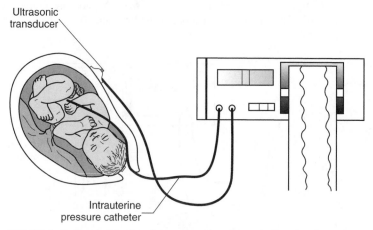

FIGURE 6.5 Combination of external and internal monitoring. The ultrasonic transducer and intrauterine pressure catheter are used together.

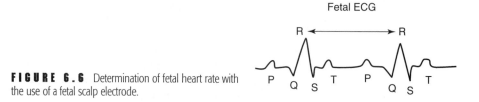

FIGURE 6.6 Determination of fetal heart rate with the use of a fetal scalp electrode.

During a vaginal examination, the examiner attaches the *spiral electrode,* or *fetal scalp electrode (FSE),* directly to the presenting part of the fetus (Figs. 6.7 and 6.8).

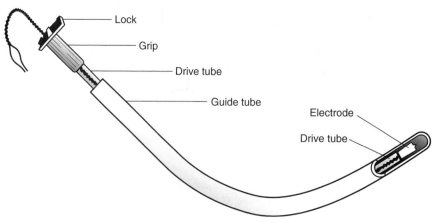

FIGURE 6.7 Components of the fetal scalp electrode.

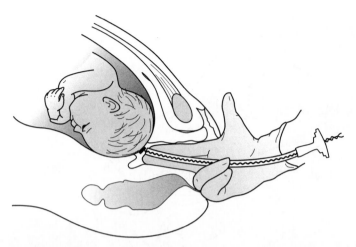

FIGURE 6.8 Application of a fetal scalp electrode to the presenting part of the fetus.

The FSE is then connected to a leg plate/pad, which has been attached to the woman's thigh by a belt or adhesive patch (Fig. 6.9). If a leg plate is used, a small amount of ECG paste is applied to that part of the leg plate in contact with the mother's thigh. This assists with conduction and transmission of the FHR.

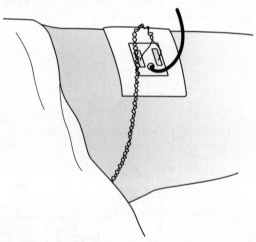

FIGURE 6.9 Fetal scalp electrode attached to an adhesive patch.

Clinical situations in which an FSE is the monitoring mode of choice include the following:
- A satisfactory tracing cannot be obtained externally.
- There is limitation of patient movement resulting from difficulty in obtaining a tracing when the woman changes position.
- FHR variability must be determined or assessed more completely (see Part 2 of this module).
- The fetus has a prenatally identified problem that might be adversely affected by labor.

■ How is the intrauterine pressure catheter used?

During a sterile vaginal examination, the intrauterine pressure catheter, often called a *pressure catheter* or *IUPC,* is inserted through the cervix into the uterus beside the presenting part of the fetus (Fig. 6.10).

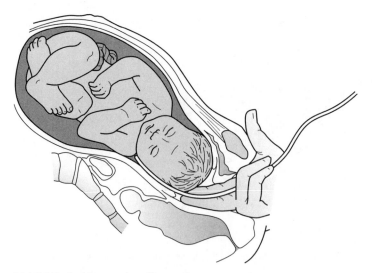

FIGURE 6.10 Insertion of intrauterine pressure catheter.

The IUPC is used to determine the actual pressure inside the uterus during contractions (Fig. 6.11). Changes in pressure at the tip of the catheter (inside the uterus) are transmitted along the catheter. These pressure changes are caused by the force or intensity of the contractions and are translated into an electrical signal that is converted to a pressure reading expressed in millimeters of mercury (mm Hg). This measurement is then displayed on the monitor.

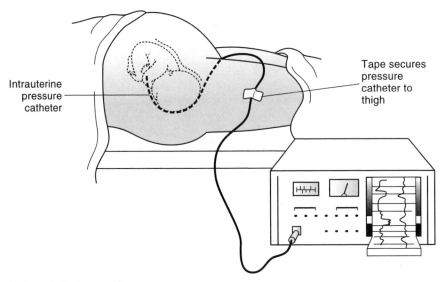

Intrauterine pressure catheter

Tape secures pressure catheter to thigh

FIGURE 6.11 Intrauterine pressure catheter.

Clinical circumstances in which an internal pressure catheter might be the preferred method of uterine monitoring consist of situations that require accurate measurement of contraction intensity. Examples of these situations *might* include the following:

- Pitocin use for induction/augmentation
- Labor abnormalities, including prolonged labor and arrested labor
- Suspected CPD
- The need to accurately define relationships between decelerations and contractions
- Individuals who have had previous cesarean sections who are attempting vaginal birth (vaginal birth after cesarean [VBAC])

- Uterine anomalies (e.g., bicornuate uterus, fibroid)
- Prior uterine surgery

Points to remember when using the IUPC include the following:

- When the IUPC is inserted, if resistance is met, the catheter must be slightly withdrawn and repositioned before insertion is attempted again.
- IUPCs must be "zeroed" to calibrate the instrumentation. (*Zeroing* means that the instrument is calibrated to air pressure so that pressure changes in the uterus can be compared against a baseline measurement.) Most IUPCs should be zeroed before insertion, as the transducer is in the catheter tip; however, some can be recalibrated after insertion.

Advantages of External/Indirect Fetal Monitoring[26–28]

- The patient can be monitored at any time, regardless of whether the cervix has dilated or the membranes have ruptured.
- It is convenient.
- It is noninvasive (does not involve a vaginal examination).
- Minimal training is required to apply the external monitor.
- A continuous tracing allows health care providers to continuously assess fetal reaction to labor stresses.
- Certain aspects of contractions are more easily assessed. Determination of frequency and duration of contractions is simpler and can be accomplished at a glance. Intensity, however, might not be fully appreciated with a tocodynamometer.
- Changes in the FHR, such as accelerations, decelerations, tachycardia, and bradycardia, can be easily detected.
- No fetal or maternal complications are associated with the use of an external fetal monitor.
- Relationships between some patterns (decelerations) can often be assessed earlier and more definitively than with auscultation alone.
- Long-term FHR variability can be assessed (see Part 2 of this module).

Disadvantages of External/Indirect Fetal Monitoring[26–28]

- It is often difficult to obtain a readable tracing if the patient is obese or is active during labor.
- The ultrasonic transducer may pick up and trace extraneous sounds. For example, the maternal pulse might be detected by the Doppler and traced instead of the FHR, causing the heart rate to appear bradycardic. Other sounds, such as bowel sounds, hiccups, fetal movement, or the rumpling of sheets, might also be detected by the machine, which can result in an inaccurate tracing. The tracing that these sounds cause is called *artifact*.
- The FHR can temporarily be lost or difficult to follow continuously if the fetus is active or changes position.
- Sometimes the FHR is detected only when the laboring woman stays in one position. Not only is this uncomfortable for the woman, but some positions (e.g., the woman lying on her back) can adversely affect blood flow to mother and fetus.
- The heart rate tracing *does not* give information about FHR short-term variability (see Part 2 of this module).
- The contraction tracing *does not* give information about the quality or intensity of the contractions. Therefore, the fundus *must* be palpated during a contraction to determine contraction intensity.
- The baseline tone (resting tone between contractions) of the uterus cannot be determined.

Advantages of Internal/Direct Monitoring[26–28]

- Internal monitoring allows the patient greater freedom of movement (e.g., standing, pushing alternatives, sitting in a chair) without compromising the quality of the monitor tracing.
- Internal monitoring accurately measures the intensity of the contractions. Uterine pressure is measured in millimeters of mercury (mm Hg).
- Complete assessment of FHR variability (short and long term) can be performed.
- Internal monitoring measures the pressure of the uterus between contractions (baseline tone, resting tone).
- Internal monitoring is not usually affected by artifact.

Disadvantages of Internal/Direct Fetal Monitoring[26–28]

- Partial dilatation of the cervix and ruptured membranes are required for application of the FSE and IUPC.
- Application of the FSE and IUPC requires skill.
- Insertion of the IUPC is often uncomfortable for the woman because considerable pressure and cervical manipulation might be necessary for proper placement.
- Materials used must be sterile, and most are disposable, resulting in increased cost.
- If the presenting part of the fetus is at a low pelvic station, it might not be possible to insert the IUPC.
- Maternal and/or fetal morbidity is associated with the FSE and the pressure catheter

Morbidity Associated With Internal Fetal Monitoring

The following complications associated with the use of a FSE have been reported[29,30]:

Fetal
- Cerebrospinal fluid leak
- Hydrocephalus
- Meningoencephalitis
- Injuries to eyelids or genitalia
- Scalp abscess and/or necrosis
- Osteomyelitis
- Ventriculitis

Maternal
- Endometritis
- Uterine perforation
- Placental injury, separation

Interpreting the Fetal Monitor Strip

■ **How do you read a fetal monitor strip?**

Figure 6.12 illustrates monitor paper. This graph is marked in specific time intervals of 3 minutes to allow easy readability (paper speed should be set at 3 cm per minute).

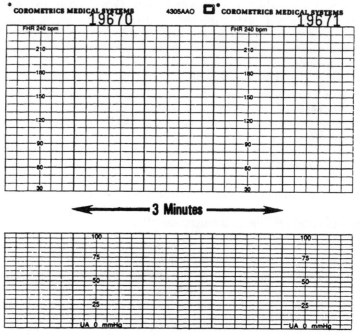

FIGURE 6.12 Graph monitor paper.

The numbers at the top of the strip in Figure 6.13 are reference numbers. They are sequential and appear at set intervals. On newer machines, these numbers may be located just above the uterine graph. These numbers assist in charting specific events by identifying their location on the strip. They also assist in chronologically reassembling a strip that has been separated for closer inspection.

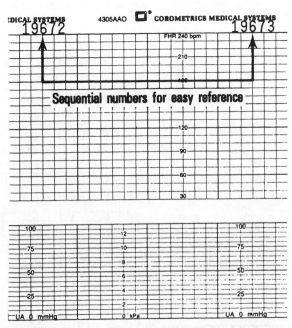

FIGURE 6.13 Sequential numbering of strip graph paper.

The strip is divided into two sections: an upper and a lower section (Fig. 6.14). The *upper* section is the portion of the graph on which the *FHR* appears. The *lower* section is the portion of the graph on which the *contractions,* or uterine activity, are recorded.

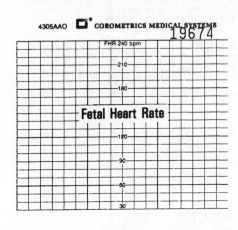

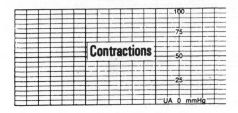

FIGURE 6.14 Strip graph monitor paper provides sections for tracing fetal heart rate and uterine activity.

The FHR (upper) section of the graph is divided vertically by dark lines, with five light, vertical lines between every two dark lines (Fig. 6.15). The time interval between any two dark lines is *1 minute;* therefore, the time interval between any two light lines is *10 seconds.* This section of the graph is also divided *horizontally* by dark lines, with two light, horizontal lines between every two darker lines (Fig. 6.16). There is a horizontal column of numbers ranging from 30 to 240. These are reference numbers used in determining the FHR and are labeled *bpm.* The distance between any two darker lines is *30 bpm;* therefore, the distance between any two lighter lines is *10 bpm.*

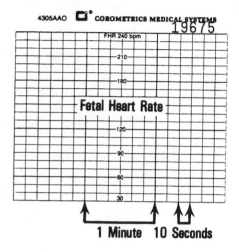

FIGURE 6.15 Division of fetal heart rate section into time intervals.

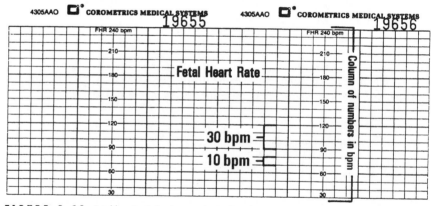

FIGURE 6.16 Fetal heart rate beats per minute (*bpm*).

The contraction or uterine activity (lower) section of the graph is divided *vertically* by dark lines, with five light, vertical lines between every two dark lines (Fig. 6.17). The time interval between any two dark lines is *1 minute;* therefore, the time interval between any two light lines is *10 seconds.*

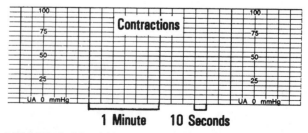

FIGURE 6.17 Division of uterine activity section into time intervals.

This portion of the graph is also divided *horizontally* by dark lines, with five light, horizontal lines between every two dark lines (Fig. 6.18). The numbers ranging from 0 to 100 in the horizontal column are reference numbers that are used to determine the intensity of contractions when a pressure catheter is used; they are labeled *mm Hg*. The abbreviation *UA* stands for "uterine activity."

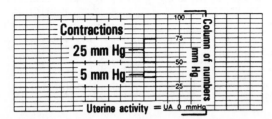

FIGURE 6.18 Uterine activity in millimeters of mercury (*mm Hg*).

Fetal Heart Rate

■ What is the baseline fetal heart rate, and how is it determined?

The baseline FHR is determined *between* contractions. It does not include periodic changes (decelerations or accelerations). It is assessed and reported in a range, not as one number, because there is normally a slight fluctuation or irregularity from one heartbeat to the next. A more accurate assessment of the FHR results from charting the baseline in a *range*. In addition, a 10-minute window of the strip is reviewed to accurately determine baseline FHR. The FHR range occurring during the 10-minute strip is charted as the baseline rate. The normal FHR baseline range is indicated in Figure 6.19.

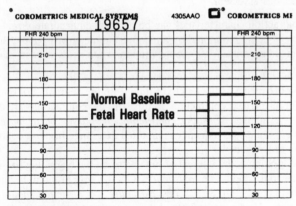

FIGURE 6.19 Normal baseline fetal heart rate.

On the strip in Figure 6.20, look at the FHR occurring between contractions. The baseline FHR is approximately 148 to 160 bpm.

Characteristics of the Baseline Fetal Heart Rate[2,19,24,25]

- Normal fetal heart baseline in a term or postterm fetus: 110 to 160 bpm
- Does not include accelerations or decelerations
- Decreases as the fetal nervous system matures and the parasympathetic nervous system becomes more dominant[24]
- Is determined between contractions

In the absence of nonreassuring elements, a fetal heart baseline of 100 to 110 bpm is also usually considered normal.

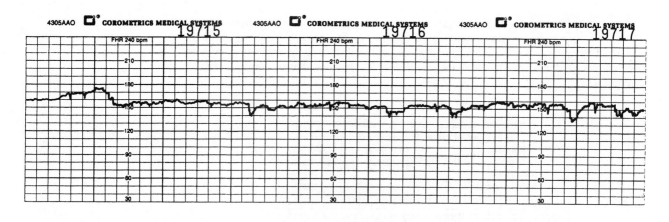

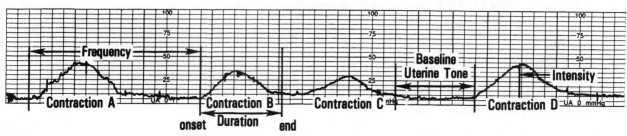

FIGURE 6.20 Pertinent information about the contraction pattern.

Contraction Pattern

■ How are contractions assessed?

The following contraction characteristics can be determined accurately *regardless* of whether the uterine activity is being monitored by a tocodynamometer or by a pressure catheter (refer to Fig. 6.20). Remember to use a 10-minute window when assessing the characteristics of the contractions.

- **Frequency**—Frequency is the length of time from the beginning of one contraction to the beginning of the next contraction. In this strip the contractions are occurring approximately every 2 minutes. *Normally, contractions should not occur more frequently than every 1½ to 2½ minutes.* Frequency is reported in a range because contractions are seldom uniform in frequency.
- **Duration**—Duration is the interval of time between the beginning (onset) and the end (offset) of the contraction. For *contraction B* on the strip graph in Figure 6.20, the duration is approximately 70 to 80 seconds. *Normally, a contraction should last no longer than 90 seconds.* (Uteroplacental blood flow decreases dramatically during the contraction, resulting in a reduction of available oxygen for the fetus. Contractions that last longer than 90 seconds might affect fetal oxygenation and reserve.) Contraction duration is also recorded in a range because duration is usually different from one contraction to the next.

The following assessments can be obtained from the strip only if an IUPC is being used to monitor contractions (refer to Fig. 6.20):

- **Baseline uterine tone**—Baseline uterine tone (tone, tonus, baseline tone) is the amount of tone, or degree of muscular tension, in the uterus *between* contractions. *Normally, baseline uterine tone is 5 to 15 mm Hg.* Baseline tone often increases just as contraction strength increases as labor progresses. This normal increase in tone is usually slight, and tone should always remain within normal limits regardless of progress in labor. Persistently elevated uterine tone represents a significant decrease in placental perfusion and fetal oxygenation. **Never accept as normal a uterine tone of greater than**

30 mm Hg. Blood flow to the placenta at this level of tension is significantly decreased (approximately 30% to 40%). A uterine pressure of 40 mm Hg results in the complete cessation of blood flow through the uterus to the placenta. Increased tone can also indicate complications such as abruptio placentae or uterine hyperstimulation. The use of *Pitocin,* synthetic oxytocin, for induction/augmentation can also increase baseline uterine tone. Baseline tone is determined by identifying the numerical range of uterine pressure between contractions. It is reported and documented in a range. Baseline tone can change between each contraction. In Figure 6.20, the baseline uterine tone is 5 to 10 mm Hg.

If the catheter reveals a baseline tone of 0 mm Hg or a negative number, the system should be recalibrated according to manufacturer's specifications. A tone of 0 mm Hg or less is an indication of a malfunctioning internal pressure system. Situations in which this can occur include the following:

–The catheter may not be attached securely to the monitor. The internal pressure system should be checked to ensure proper attachment of all parts.

–The catheter may have curled on itself during insertion, with the tip coming near or out of the cervix in the vagina.

–The catheter may not have been accurately calibrated or zeroed before or after insertion.

–The catheter might be wedged against the uterine wall. Gently withdraw the catheter slightly to release any wedging.

–The catheter might have migrated from the uterine cavity into the vagina. The primary care provider should be notified so that a sterile vaginal examination can be performed to verify placement and/or to replace the catheter. Make no attempt to reinsert the catheter.

NOTE: *Uterine rupture/dehiscence of a scar can cause general failure of the IUPC to pick up contractions.*

• **Intensity**—Intensity is also measured in mm Hg. It is calculated by subtracting the baseline tone from the peak pressure of the contraction. For *contraction A* in Figure 6.20, the contraction intensity is 40 mm Hg. The strength of a mild contraction is approximately 15 to 30 mm Hg, the strength of a moderate contraction is approximately 30 to 50 mm Hg, and the strength of a strong contraction is 50 to 75 mm Hg (Figs. 6.21 and 6.22).

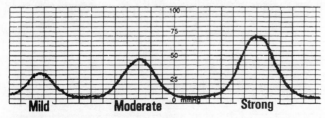

FIGURE 6.21 Contraction intensity.

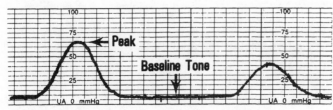

FIGURE 6.22 Determination of contraction intensity.

In Figures 6.23 and 6.24, notice the difference in appearance of the contraction curve using an external and internal monitor. The contractions were actually much stronger when internal monitoring was instituted than they appeared in the external tracing.

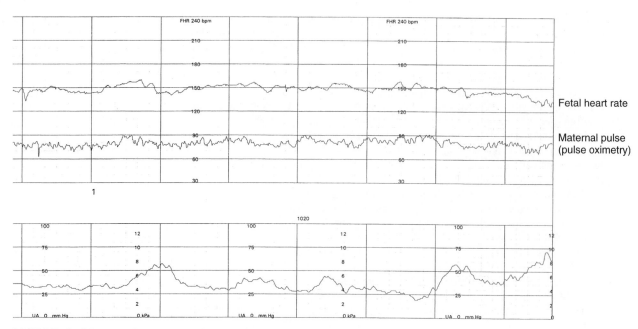

Fetal heart rate

Maternal pulse (pulse oximetry)

FIGURE 6.23 External (toco) contraction monitoring.

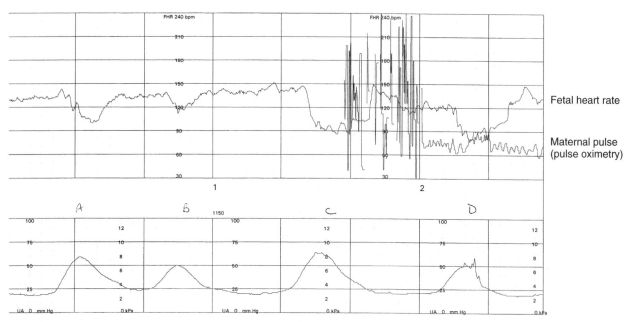

Fetal heart rate

Maternal pulse (pulse oximetry)

FIGURE 6.24 Internal (IUPC) contraction monitoring and FSE. Note the difference in the clarity of the contraction pattern with the IUPC as opposed to the contraction pattern in Figure 6.23 using the toco.

An obese or multiparous patient with lax abdominal muscle tone and/or increased layers of tissue between the tocodynamometer and the abdominal muscles might be experiencing strong contractions that can appear mild when external monitoring is used. Conversely, a thin or nulliparous patient with good abdominal muscle tone might experience mild contractions, which, when monitored externally, appear strong. Remember that the external tocodynamometer is registering *only* changes in abdominal shape dependent on abdominal muscle tone as the fundus contracts. **When using a tocodynamometer, contraction intensity must be assessed by palpation.**

To review terms associated with contraction pattern description of a normal contraction pattern, see Figure 6.25.

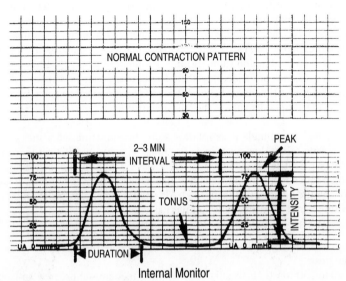

FIGURE 6.25 Normal contraction pattern.

The uterine activity on the strip in Figure 6.26 should be interpreted as follows:

Interval (frequency)	Approximately 2 to 3 minutes
Duration	60 to 90 seconds
Tonus	10 mm Hg
Intensity	40 to 60 mm Hg

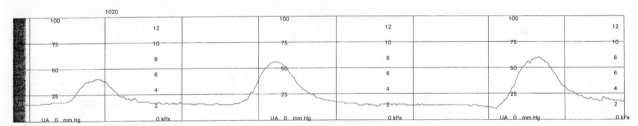

FIGURE 6.26 Internal contraction monitoring.

■ How is contraction intensity documented during external monitoring?

Manual assessment of the uterine contraction and baseline tone must be performed if the external mode of monitoring is used. This kind of assessment is accomplished by palpating the fundus with the fingertips. The strength of the contraction is measured at its most intense point. In general, if the fundus is easily indented with the tips of the fingers, the contraction is considered "mild." If more pressure is needed to indent the fundus, the contraction is "moderate." The contraction is "strong" if the fundus cannot be indented at the contraction peak. **When contraction strength exceeds 40 mm Hg, the uterine wall becomes difficult to depress with the fingertips.**

■ How is uterine tone measured during external monitoring?

Manual assessment of the uterine tone is also an important consideration in external monitoring. The fingertips are sensitive to pressures beginning at approximately 15 mm Hg, so baseline tones above this level can be identified and appropriate action can be taken.

■ When is labor adequate?

The simplest way to know that a contraction pattern is effective is to see progress in labor (the cervix dilates and the presenting part of the fetus descends further into the pelvis). Regardless of the characteristics of the contractions, if progress continues, labor is adequate.

If cervical dilatation is not progressing at the expected rate, another method of uterine monitoring using an IUPC may be employed to assess adequacy of labor. When contractions do not produce progression of labor, adequacy of the contraction pattern can be evaluated by a measurement standard called *Montevideo units (MVUs)*. MVUs are calculated by identifying the peak pressure of each contraction (mm Hg) in a 10-minute section (window) of the strip. All peak contraction pressures are added together. The baseline tone is determined by adding together the resting tone of the uterus between each contraction in the same 10-minute window. The final step is to subtract the sum of the baseline tone from the sum of the peak contraction intensity.

In simpler terms, the formula is as follows: sum of contraction intensities (in a 10-minute strip) minus the sum of baseline tone (in a 10-minute window) = Montevideo units.

MVUs may be calculated in a slightly different way by multiplying the average intensity by the contraction frequency in 10 minutes minus tone. Other units of measurement are also sometimes used to measure adequacy of labor (e.g., Alexandria units, planimeter units), but the most common measurement for quantification of uterine activity is MVUs.

MVU guidelines are as follows:

- Less than 150 MVUs indicates that the contraction pattern might be inadequate to affect labor progress.
- From 180 to 250 MVUs is usually sufficient to affect normal progress in labor.
- More than 300 MVUs indicates hyperstimulation.

PRACTICE/REVIEW QUESTIONS

After reviewing Part 1, answer the following questions.

1. List at least 10 risk conditions that may indicate a need for increased fetal surveillance in labor.

   a. _____

   b. _____

   c. _____

   d. _____

   e. _____

   f. _____

   g. _____

   h. _____

   i. _____

   j. _____

2. What is the normal FHR range in the term fetus? _____

3. Describe the parameters of IA for low-risk women and women with risk factors:

   Low-risk women: _____

   Women with risk factors: _____

4. Describe the advantages and disadvantages of IA.

   _____

   _____

   _____

   _____

5. What is recommended before beginning EFM with regard to validating the machine?

   _____

6. Clinically, what might indicate the need for internal monitoring?

   _____

   _____

   _____

7. What unit is used to measure uterine pressure with an IUPC? _____

8. List three disadvantages of the external fetal monitor.

   a. _____

   b. _____

   c. _____

9. Which of the following are advantages of external fetal monitoring?

   A. The mother may lie in any comfortable position.

   B. There are no fetal complications associated with its use.

   C. All necessary information can be obtained.

   D. Minimal training is necessary for application of equipment.

10. Define *uterine hypertonus.*

    _____

11. List three disadvantages of the internal fetal monitor.

    a. _____

    b. _____

    c. _____

12. Study the following strip and then answer the following questions. This tracing is taken using internal fetal monitoring. The patient was receiving Pitocin.

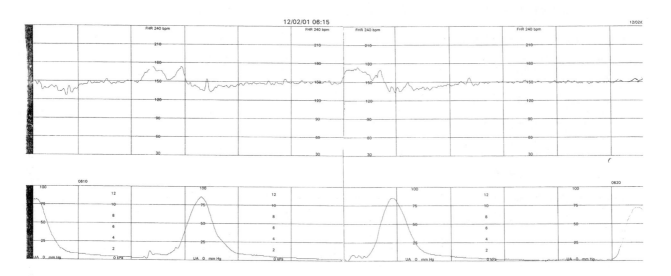

a. What is the baseline FHR? _____

   Is it in the normal range? _____

b. What is the frequency of the contractions? _____

   Is it in the normal range? _____

c. What is the duration of the contractions? _____

   Is it in the normal range? _____

d. What is the baseline uterine tone? _____

   Is it in the normal range? _____

e. What is the intensity of the contractions? _____

f. Are these contractions mild, moderate, or strong? _____

13. How is the baseline FHR determined?

   _____

   _____

   _____

14. The tocodynamometer measures contraction duration, frequency, and intensity.

   A. True

   B. False

15. What uterine pressure is considered abnormal as a baseline tone? _____

16. What are Montevideo units, and how are they calculated?

   _____

   _____

   _____

PRACTICE/REVIEW ANSWER KEY

1. Any 10 of the following:
    a. Hypertension
    b. Pregnancy-induced hypertension
    c. Diabetes mellitus
    d. Chronic renal disease
    e. Congenital or rheumatic heart disease
    f. Sickle cell disease
    g. Rh isoimmunization
    h. Preterm infants (less than 37 weeks' gestation)
    i. Postmature infants (more than 42 weeks' gestation)
    j. Multiple gestations
    k. Grandmultiparity
    l. Anemia
    m. Intrauterine growth-restricted infants or small-for-gestational-age infants
    n. Genital tract disorders/anomalies
    o. Poor obstetric history
    p. Age factors (younger than 15 years or older than 35 years of age)
    q. Prolonged rupture of membranes
    r. Premature rupture of membranes
    s. Bleeding disorders—abruptio placentae, placenta previa
    t. Premature labor
    u. Previous cesarean section in labor
    v. Hypotensive episodes in labor

2. 110 to 160 bpm

3. Low-risk women: FHTs obtained every 30 minutes during active labor and every 15 minutes during second stage. FHTs assessed during a contraction and for 30 seconds after its end.

    Women with risk factors: FHTs obtained every 15 minutes during active labor and every 5 minutes during the second stage. FHTs are assessed during a contraction and for 30 seconds after it is over.

4. Advantages of IA: patient comfort; allows ambulation, which assists in labor progression; provides a more natural experience. Disadvantages of IA: a 1:1 nurse:patient ratio is needed; nurses must have extensive experience with auscultation to pick up subtle changes in the FHR; human error in counting the heart rate can be made; maternal movement might make it difficult to locate and follow the heart rate during contractions; it might take longer to detect subtle or early changes in the FHR.

5. Auscultation of FHR with a fetoscope and the pressing of the "test" button to check the internal circuitry of the monitor

6. The presence of risk factors either antepartal or intrapartal might show the need for closer surveillance of the fetus by internal monitoring. Labors that do not progress at the expected rate might require assessment of contraction strength to help identify the cause of the delay.

7. Millimeters of mercury (mm Hg)

8. Any three of the following:
   a. It is often difficult to obtain a readable tracing if the patient is obese or is active during labor.
   b. The ultrasonic transducer might pick up and trace artifacts.
   c. The FHR might be lost if the fetus is active or changes position. Sometimes, the FHR is picked up only when the laboring woman is on her back—this is not the preferred position for labor, and the woman might experience backache from continually lying on her back.
   d. The heart rate tracing does *not* give information about FHR variability.
   e. The contraction tracing does *not* give information about the quality or intensity of the contractions; therefore, the fundus *must* be palpated during a contraction to determine intensity.
   f. The baseline tone of the uterus cannot be determined.

9. B and D

10. Resting tone greater than 30 mm Hg

11. Any three of the following:
    a. It requires partial dilatation of the cervix and ruptured membranes for application of the FSE and IUPC.
    b. It requires a skilled examiner to apply the FSE and pressure catheter.
    c. Insertion of the IUPC is often uncomfortable for the patient because much pressure and cervical manipulation might be necessary.
    d. It requires sterile, disposable equipment.
    e. If the presenting part of the fetus is at a low station, it might not be possible to insert the IUPC.
    f. Maternal and/or fetal morbidity is associated with the FSE and the pressure catheter.

12. a. 145 to 152 bpm (approximate); yes
    b. Every 3½ to 4½ minutes; yes
    c. 50 to 80 seconds; yes
    d. Approximately 2 to 5 mm Hg; yes
    e. 70 to 80 mm Hg; strong

13. Baseline FHR is determined by assessing a 10-minute FHR strip between contractions. It is reported in a range and should not include any periodic changes (accelerations or decelerations).

14. B

15. More than 30 mm Hg

16. The MVU is a standard of measurement used to denote the strength and adequacy of the contraction pattern. It is calculated by the following method: sum of contraction intensities (in a 10-minute strip) minus the sum of baseline tone (in a 10-minute window) = Montevideo units.

Fetal Heart Rate Variability

OBJECTIVES

After you complete Part 2 of this module, you should be able to:

1. Outline the regulatory factors of the fetal heart
2. Describe fetal heart rate variability
3. Differentiate between short- and long-term variability
4. Explain the characteristics and significance related to changes in variability
5. Identify appropriate responses to nonreassuring variability and describe the rationale for these interventions

KEY TERMS

When you have completed Part 2 of this module, you should be able to recall the meaning of the following terms as they relate to FHR. You should also be able to use the terms when consulting with other health professionals. The terms are defined in this portion of the module or in the glossary at the end of this book.

absent variability	moderate variability
baroreceptors	parasympathetic nervous system
chemoreceptors	pH
fetal reserve	short-term (beat-to-beat) variability
long-term variability	sympathetic nervous system
marked variability	variability
minimal variability	

Overview of Fetal Heart Rate Variability

■ How is the fetal heart regulated?

The fetal heart is influenced by many factors, but it is primarily regulated by the autonomic nervous system (parasympathetic and sympathetic branches), chemoreceptors, and barorecep-tors.

■ What are the effects of the autonomic nervous system on fetal heart rate?

The effects of the autonomic nervous system on the fetal heart depend on which of its branches is stimulated at a particular time. The two parts of the autonomic nervous system are the parasympathetic and sympathetic branches. Their characteristics and effects are outlined in Display 6.1.

| **DISPLAY 6.1** | Characteristics of the Parasympathetic Nervous System and Sympathetic Nervous System |

PARASYMPATHETIC NERVOUS SYSTEM (PSNS)

- It is the cardiodecelerator, slowing heart rate.
- Its influence on the FHR increases as gestation progresses. This means that, as gestational age increases, the FHR gradually decreases. The parasympathetic branch is not fully mature until relatively late in gestation at ap-proximately 28 to 32 completed weeks' gestation. As a result of the late maturity of the PSNS, extremely prema-ture infants (less than 20 weeks) can have a higher-than-normal heart rate.
- It is the primary factor that influences short-term variability.
- It is extremely sensitive to decreased levels of oxygen and lowered pH. pH is a measurement of acidity or alka-linity. A low pH indicates acidity, and high pH indicates alkalinity.

SYMPATHETIC NERVOUS SYSTEM

- It is the cardioaccelerator. It increases heart rate, cardiac output, and myocardial contractility.
- Its primary influence is on long-term variability.
- It matures earlier in gestation and therefore has more of an impact on FHR before 32 weeks' gestation.

■ How do baroreceptors and chemoreceptors affect fetal heart rate?

Baroreceptors are located in the carotid arch and the aortic sinus. Cells in these areas are sen-sitive to the stretching of surrounding tissue (changes in arterial wall diameter) caused by in-creased or decreased blood pressure. When fetal blood pressure increases, it is sensed by the baroreceptors, which transmit the message to the brainstem, where the parasympathetic nerv-ous system is stimulated to decrease or increase the fetal blood pressure.

Chemoreceptors are located in the aortic and carotid bodies and in the medulla oblongata. They are sensitive to changes in oxygen, carbon dioxide, and pH of fetal blood. Reduction in blood oxygen and pH and/or increases in CO_2 are recognized by the chemoreceptors. This causes an initial increase in heart rate in an attempt to increase circulation and thereby increase oxygen levels and stabilize pH. Prolonged stimulation of the chemoreceptors, along with hy-poxia of the cardiac muscle, eventually results in a drop in heart rate to bradycardic levels. This drop can be gradual; however, it is often sudden.

■ What is fetal heart rate variability?

FHR variability is described as the normal changes and fluctuations in the FHR over time. The time interval addressed can be short, from one beat to another beat. This is called *short-term variability* (STV) and appears as the roughness or smoothness of the tracing (Fig. 6.27). Variability can also be evaluated over a longer period. This is called *long-term variability* (LTV) and looks like small hills or fluctuations on the strip baseline. Variability is a character-istic of the baseline and does not include accelerations or decelerations (Fig. 6.28).

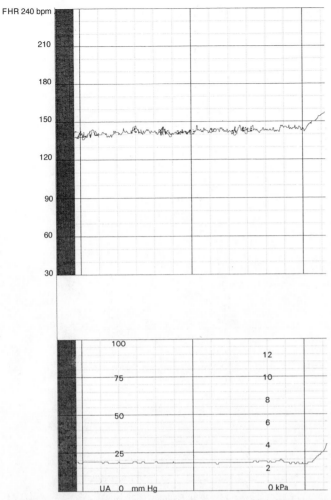

FIGURE 6.27 Short-term variability (assessed only with an FSE).

■ What causes variability, and why is it important?[11,31-34]

- Changes in variability are primarily transmitted along the parasympathetic nerves in primates. It is believed to be a result of multiple sporadic impulses from various areas of the cerebral cortex and lower centers of the medulla. These impulses are then transmitted down the vagus nerve to the heart. Variability evidences the balance and interplay of a normal sympathetic and parasympathetic relationship. Largely controlled by the autonomic nervous system, it indicates central nervous system (CNS) status and is the most important factor in characterizing the FHR.

- Variability is sensitive to hypoxia and decreased pH. The usual fetal heart response to these events is a decrease in variability, but occasionally these stimuli can cause variability to increase. Decreased variability occurs because of the fetus' limited ability to compensate for reduced oxygenation. The effect of oxygen deprivation is a decrease in the number of impulses from the cerebral cortex. The reduction of impulses results in decreased variability.

- *Variability represents a mature, intact nervous pathway through the brain, vagus nerve, and cardiac conduction system. It is believed to be the most significant indicator of fetal well-being. Variability also indirectly reflects fetal reserve.*

- Its appearance can be influenced by drugs, hormonal regulation, fetal sleep–wake states, oxygenation, hemodynamic changes, and abnormalities of the CNS (a fetus with anencephaly or hydrocephaly may exhibit absent or minimal variability). *Variability is a marker for fetal acid-base balance.*

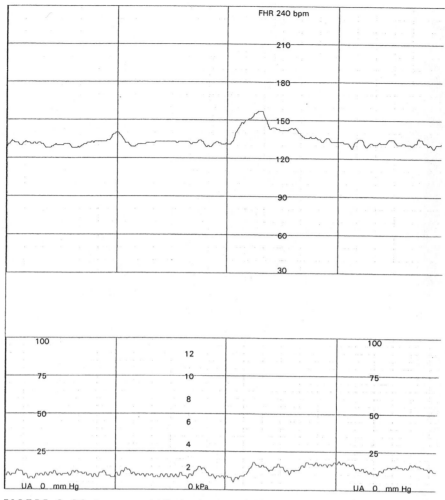

FIGURE 6.28 Long-term variability (can be assessed with internal or external monitoring).

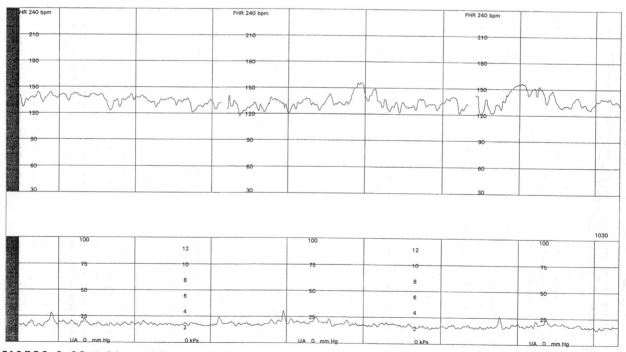

FIGURE 6.29 Both long- and short-term variability.

■ What is fetal reserve?

The fetus uses a certain amount of oxygen to carry out basic metabolic functions. Normally, more oxygen is delivered to the fetus, by way of the placenta, than is required to meet these basic needs. The difference between the oxygen supplied and the oxygen required or consumed equals the fetal reserve. If there is only enough oxygen available to meet minimal needs, reserve will quickly disappear. Fetal reserve illustrates fetal ability to deal with stress related to reduced oxygen levels in the tissues (hypoxia).

$$O_2 \text{ delivery} - O_2 \text{ required} = \text{Fetal } O_2 \text{ reserve}$$

■ How is variability evaluated and documented?

The type of variability is identified by its appearance on the monitor strip. It is evaluated between contractions, decelerations, and accelerations. It cannot be evaluated by auscultation.[4,25] There continues to be some controversy in the medical community as to how variability should be identified and documented. Some experts believe that variability should be considered as a single entity, not as LTV or STV, because in the clinical setting that is how this information is interpreted and used in the evaluation of fetal status and in planning intervention.[11,28] Other sources, such as AWHONN, identify two kinds of variability to be identified and documented.[4,6] Most authorities separate variability into two categories, and for the purposes of this text, the AWHONN classification will be used. There is an international movement to define and classify terms related to EFM, but at the time of this writing, a consensus of opinion has not been finalized.

Long-Term Variability

LTV, as previously stated, represents wavelike or cyclic changes in the heart rate over several (usually 15 to 20) minutes. LTV resembles hills rising from the baseline. LTV is primarily governed by the sympathetic nervous system. Because this branch of the autonomic nervous system matures earlier, LTV appears sooner than STV. LTV is evaluated between contractions and does not include accelerations or decelerations. LTV is classified in the following categories depending on the range of change of the FHR from the baseline: *decreased/minimal* (Fig. 6.30), *moderate/normal* (Fig. 6.31), and *marked/salutatory* (Fig. 6.32). LTV can be determined by **both** external and internal EFM.

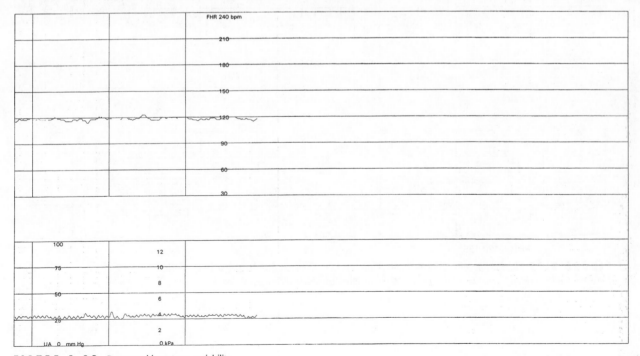

FIGURE 6.30 Decreased long-term variability.

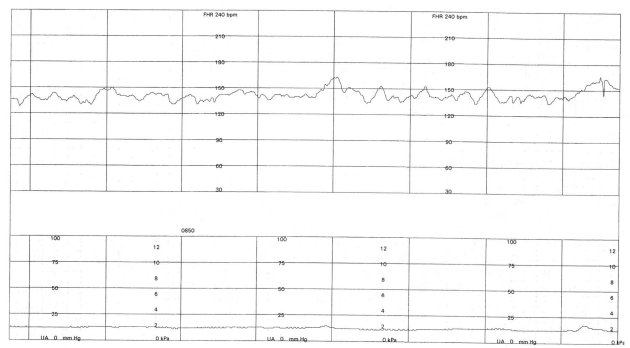

FIGURE 6.31 Moderate long-term variability.

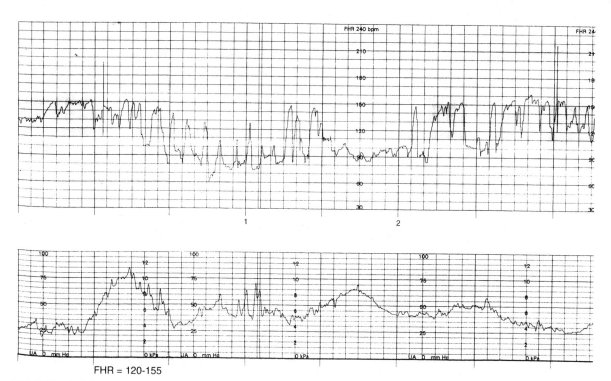

FHR = 120-155

FIGURE 6.32 Saltatory pattern. (Reprinted with permission from Menihan, C. A., & Zottoli, E. K. [2001]. *Electronic fetal monitoring: Concepts and applications.* Philadelphia: Lippincott Williams & Wilkins.)

Decreased/Minimal Long-Term Variability

Characteristics/Causes
- Range of 0 to 5 bpm
- Fetal behavioral state can influence variability (fetal sleep states—decreased variability—may last up to 90 minutes)
- Hypoxia
- Dysrhythmia (SVT or complete heart block)
- Medications (e.g., CNS depressants)
- Fetal anemia
- Congenital brain anomaly
- Maternal temperature elevation
- Hypovolemia
- Maternal hypotension

Some experts further separate this category into *absent LTV* (range of 0 to 2 bpm) and *minimal LTV* (range of 3 to 5 bpm). AWHONN states that interventions for persistent decreased variability are the same, so it is clinically appropriate to consider the range of 0 to 5 bpm as one category.[4,6]

Interventions
- Evaluate behavioral state and response to stimulation (fetal scalp stimulation by vaginal examination abdominal palpation)—total clinical overview.
- Administer oxygen per mask at 10 L per minute.
- Change maternal position—Turn patient to her left or right side to maximize uteroplacental blood flow.
- Check maternal vital signs and take appropriate action to rectify abnormalities (e.g., fluid bolus, antibiotics).
- Provide immediate intervention and notify the provider if persistent decreased LTV in the absence of medications or a known anomaly is noted.

Moderate/Normal Long-Term Variability

Characteristics/Causes
- Range of 6 to 25 bpm
- Fetal wake state
- Fetal responsiveness results in the wide range of values

Interventions
- Continued surveillance

Marked/Saltatory Long-Term Variability [12,31,32]

Characteristics/Causes
- Range greater than 25 bpm
- Baseline that "jumps" up and down
- Highly chaotic baseline
- Rare in preterm fetuses
- Higher incidence in postterm fetuses—probably because of neurologic maturation
- Compensatory response to a hypoxic event
- May follow ephedrine administration
- Frequently seen during second stage of labor
- Seen during delivery with assistance of vacuum

Interventions
- Check maternal vital signs and treat abnormalities.
- Perform VE to assess for impending birth.
- Administer O_2 per mask if hypoxia is suspected.
- Communicate findings to the provider.

Short-Term Variability

STV is either *absent* (Fig. 6.33) or *present* (Fig. 6.34) and is based on the beat-to-beat fluctuation of the fetal heart. It can be evaluated *only* when internal monitoring is used. STV is primarily regulated by the parasympathetic nervous system (PSNS) and is not fully mature until approximately 28 to 32 weeks' gestation. STV is very sensitive to hypoxia. When the medulla is hypoxic, poor impulse transmission results, causing loss of STV. Loss of STV occurs before loss of LTV.

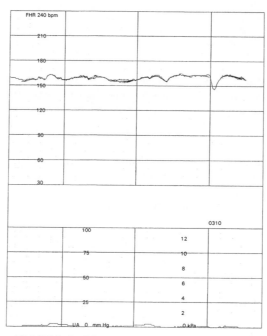

FIGURE 6.33 Absent short-term variability.

Decreased and Increased Variability

Causes of Decreased Variability

- **Hypoxia/acidosis**—Reduced oxygen decreases impulses from the cerebral cortex, as previously discussed.
- **Drugs**—CNS depressants, barbiturates, sedatives, narcotics, alcohol, magnesium sulfate, atropine, and anesthetic agents can cause decreased variability.
- **Fetal sleep**—Decreased LTV can occur during fetal sleep; however, fetal sleep cycles should not affect STV. Fetal sleep cycles last approximately 20 to 40 minutes. During this time, LTV is often diminished. When the cycle is over, LTV usually resumes its normal appearance.
- **Congenital anomalies**—Anomalies that affect the central nervous system often affect variability.
- **Extreme prematurity**—Immature parasympathetic nervous system affects the appearance of variability.
- **Fetal tachycardia and other dysrhythmias**—Nodal rhythm and complete heart block affect cardiac control mechanisms and therefore variability.

Causes of Increased Variability

- **Increased fetal movement**—Greater oxygen demands and increased catecholamines for an extremely active fetus produce this variability change. When fetal activity returns to more moderate levels, variability usually returns to normal if this is the causal factor.

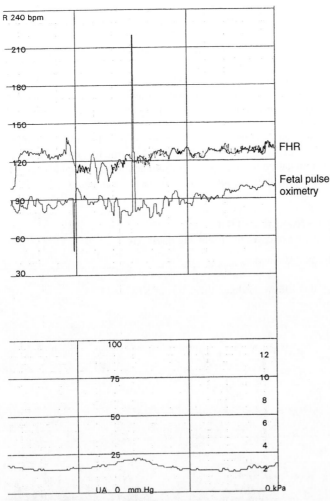

FIGURE 6.34 Present short-term variability. Note that lower tracing on the upper graph represents fetal oxygenation saturation (oximetry).

- **Hypoxia**—Variability is affected by a surge of catecholamines during stress (hypoxic episode). The fetus has some reserves at this point and is attempting to compensate somewhat for the insult.
- **Vaginal examinations**—Stimulation of the fetal presenting part can elicit a catecholamine surge, causing increased variability. Excessively vigorous stimulation can cause a vagal response, resulting in a decreased FHR.
- **Second stage/pushing**—This is because of the reduced availability of oxygen with maternal breath holding. This is especially true when the closed glottis technique is used.

Interventions

■ What is the treatment for decreased variability?[37,38]

Decreased variability might be an indication of fetal stress, unless another cause can be identified (e.g., medications, prematurity) as a potential factor in its appearance. It is especially ominous if seen in conjunction with late, prolonged, or repetitive variable decelerations (see Part 3 of this module).

Management consists of the following:

- **Turn patient to her side**—This displaces the gravid uterus to the side, reducing pressure on the maternal vena cava and aorta. The result optimizes fetal oxygenation by improvement of maternal cardiac output and placental perfusion.

- **Provide oxygen**—Begin oxygen therapy by face mask at 10 to 12 L per minute. This action optimizes the O_2 saturation of the woman's blood so that more O_2 is available to the fetus.
- Treat the underlying cause of any decelerations occurring with the decreased variability (see Part 3 of this module).
- Notify the primary care provider promptly!
- Chart time of occurrence, treatment, notification of primary care provider, and any associated factors such as decelerations or the presence of meconium. *Write the treatment on the strip graph.*
- Attempt to stimulate the fetus. This is the first step in determining whether this a true problem with variability or just fetal sleep. Fetal stimulation may be accomplished by fetal scalp stimulation during a vaginal examination or by fetal acoustic stimulation.
- Assess maternal hydration. Administer a bolus of IV fluids.

PRACTICE/REVIEW QUESTIONS

After reviewing Part 2, answer the following questions.

1. FHR variability is defined as _____.

2. On the strips that follow, evaluate the status of STV and LTV.

Strip A

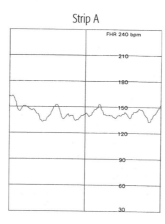

Strip B

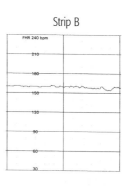

3. How should decreased variability in FHR be treated?

a. _____

b. _____

c. _____

d. _____

e. _____

f. _____

g. _____

4. List at least three possible causes for decreased variability and at least three possible causes of marked variability.

   Decreased:

   a. _____

   b. _____

   c. _____

   Increased:

   a. _____

   b. _____

   c. _____

5. Identify the branch of the autonomic nervous system (parasympathetic = P; sympathetic = S) that is responsible for the following:

   a. ____ Cardioaccelerator

   b. ____ Slows the heart rate

   c. ____ Primary influence is on STV

   d. ____ Primary influence is on LTV

   e. ____ Sensitive to low O_2 levels and low pH

   f. ____ Matures earlier in gestation

6. _____ are located in aortic sinus and carotid arch and are sensitive to blood pressure changes.

7. _____ are located in the aortic and carotid bodies and medulla and are sensitive to oxygen and carbon dioxide content and pH of the blood.

8. _____ is a marker for acid-base balance.

9. What does *fetal reserve* mean?

   _____

PRACTICE/REVIEW ANSWER KEY

1. The normal changes and fluctuations in the FHR over time

2. Strip A: Absent STV

            Present LTV

   Strip B: Present STV

            Absent LTV

3. a. Try to identify cause (medication?); check temperature.
   b. Begin oxygen therapy by face mask at 10 to 12 L per minute.
   c. Put the patient in the lateral position.
   d. Notify primary care provider.
   e. Chart time of occurrence, treatment, notification of primary care provider, and any associated factors such as decelerations or the presence of meconium.
   f. Attempt fetal stimulation.
   g. Ensure maternal hydration by giving a bolus of IV fluids.

4. Decreased (any three of the following):
   a. Hypoxia/acidosis
   b. Drugs
   c. Fetal sleep
   d. Congenital anomalies
   e. Extreme prematurity
   f. Fetal tachycardia and other dysrhythmias

   Increased (any three of the following):
   a. Increased fetal movement
   b. Hypoxia
   c. Vaginal examinations
   d. Second stage/pushing

5. a. S
   b. P
   c. P
   d. S
   e. P
   f. S

6. Baroreceptors

7. Chemoreceptors

8. Variability

9. The difference between the oxygen supplied and the oxygen required or consumed equals the fetal reserve.

Fetal Heart Rate Baseline, Periodic, and Nonperiodic Patterns

OBJECTIVES

As you complete Part 3 of this module, you will learn:

1. To identify and name fetal heart rate baseline patterns
2. Causes of abnormal baseline fetal heart rate patterns
3. Nursing interventions appropriate for abnormal baseline changes
4. Effects of uterine contractions on fetal heart rate
5. To identify periodic patterns and explain the physiologic basis of each pattern
6. Characteristics of accelerations and their importance related to fetal well-being
7. Characteristics of early, variable, late, and prolonged decelerations
8. Interventions appropriate in the treatment of late, variable, and prolonged decelerations

KEY TERMS

When you have completed Part 3 of this module, you should be able to recall the meaning of the following terms. You should also be able to use the terms when consulting with other health professionals. The terms are defined in this portion of the module or in the glossary at the end of this book.

early decelerations
fetal accelerations
fetal bradycardia
fetal tachycardia
late decelerations
nonperiodic heart rate changes

periodic heart rate changes
prolonged decelerations
sinusoidal pattern
uteroplacental insufficiency
variable decelerations

Baseline Fetal Heart Rate Patterns

FHR patterns are referred to in terms of being reassuring or nonreassuring. *Reassuring* patterns illustrate fetal well-being and ability to compensate for stresses. *Nonreassuring* patterns are associated with loss of fetal reserve, hypoxia, and/or acidosis.

Nurses are accountable for understanding and using nationally determined definitions and interventions for baseline and periodic patterns. They must also know how and when to institute interventions and be able to name the identified patterns in the patient chart. Abnormal baseline characteristics are tachycardia, bradycardia, and sinusoidal.[4,6,37]

Fetal Tachycardia

■ What is fetal tachycardia, and what causes it?[1,6,37,38]

Fetal tachycardia is an increase in the baseline FHR above 160 bpm for 10 minutes or longer (Fig. 6.35). Fetal tachycardia is associated with decreased variability when the FHR is especially rapid or following prolonged periods of hypoxia. It represents an increase in sympathetic tone and a decrease in parasympathetic tone.

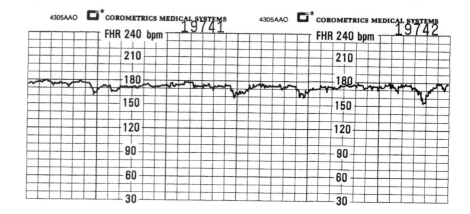

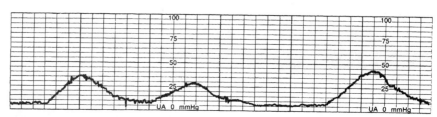

FIGURE 6.35 Fetal tachycardia.

Causes

- **Fetal hypoxia**—Tachycardia is often an *early* sign of hypoxia. The fetus attempts to increase heart rate to compensate for a decrease in oxygen supply.
- **Infection**
- **Prolonged fetal activity or stimulation**
- **Drugs**—Parasympatholytic drugs such as *atropine* and *scopolamine* block the parasympathetic nervous system, resulting in an increase in heart rate. Illicit drugs such as methamphetamine, cocaine, and PCP can also increase the heart rate. Drugs used to prevent or stop premature labor, such as *terbutaline* (beta-adrenergics), have a stimulating effect on the fetal heart, which increases the rate.
- **Maternal anxiety**—During periods of maternal stress and anxiety, *epinephrine* is released into the mother's circulation. Small amounts of this epinephrine will cross the placenta, resulting in an increase in FHR. The heart rate increase because of this factor is usually only slightly elevated.

- **Maternal/fetal temperature elevation**—During periods of maternal hyperthermia, both the mother's and the fetus' metabolism are elevated. The pH decreases as a result of lactic acid formation, and oxygen demands are increased. This, in turn, causes chemoreceptor stimulation and increased activity of the sympathetic nervous system. The effect of this process is to increase heart rate. Tachycardia can be an early sign of an intrauterine infection (chorioamnionitis), especially in the presence of decreased variability. Prolonged rupture of membranes can lead to uterine and/or fetal infection and temperature elevation.
- **Fetal anemia**—Reduced oxygen-carrying capacity of the fetal blood, resulting from anemia (decreased hemoglobin), can result in tachycardia. Causal factors for anemia might be related to placental abnormalities, such as partial abruption or previa and twin-to-twin transfusion.
- **Fetal cardiac tachyrhythmia**—This generally occurs intermittently, and most often is identified as supraventricular tachycardia (SVT) and atrial flutter. Cardiac rates of greater than 200 are almost always a result of a dysrhythmia. Nonimmune hydrops can result from cardiac failure.
- **Maternal hyperthyroidism**—Just as a patient with hyperthyroidism often exhibits an increased pulse rate, so does her fetus. Long-acting thyroid-stimulating hormones cross the placenta and stimulate the fetal thyroid, causing an elevated FHR.
- **Idiopathic causes**—In some fetuses, tachycardia has no apparent cause. Perhaps in these fetuses, the sympathetic nervous system becomes dominant in its regulatory action over the fetal heart.

Interventions

The treatment of fetal tachycardia is aimed at the specific cause:

- Begin oxygen therapy by face mask, 100% O_2 at 10 to 12 L per minute. This maximizes oxygen perfusion of the blood.
- Take the laboring woman's temperature. This helps identify an infection process.
- Turn the patient to the lateral position. This displaces the uterus from the aorta and the vena cava and increases placental perfusion.
- Administer a bolus of 200 mL of intravenous (IV) fluids. This enhances hydration and improves cardiac output, resulting in improved uterine blood flow.
- Validate the heart rate obtained on the monitor by auscultation with a fetoscope.
- Notify the primary care provider.

Fetal Bradycardia

■ What is fetal bradycardia, and what causes it?[1,6]

Fetal bradycardia is a decreased fetal heart baseline of less than 110 or 120 bpm that persists for 10 minutes or longer (Fig. 6.36). *An FHR baseline that is only slightly below (100 bpm) the normal range is usually well tolerated for prolonged periods if normal variability is present.* A baseline rate that is between 90 and 110 bpm in the absence of nonreassuring changes is not considered indicative of fetal compromise.[6,39,40] Because the fetus has only a limited ability to increase cardiac output if bradycardia persists, chances of inadequate oxygenation are increased. *Bradycardia is usually a late event in the development of hypoxia and acidosis.*

Causes

- **Fetal hypoxia**—Bradycardia is a *late* sign of fetal hypoxia. The fetus, after initial attempts to normalize the oxygen level by increasing heart rate, can no longer compensate. The increased heart rate cannot be maintained in the presence of continued hypoxia and falling pH. The heart rate slows in response to these changes because they cause direct depression of heart muscle and sinoatrial (SA) node due to acidosis.
- **Drugs**—Drugs such as *propranolol* cause a decrease in heart rate by *preventing* receptor sites in the fetal heart muscle from accepting epinephrine. (Epinephrine increases heart rate.) Anesthetic agents such as medications used in *epidurals, spinals, caudals,* and *pudendal blocks* can decrease heart rate indirectly as a result of a reflex mechanism or as a result of hypotension. Drugs used in *paracervical blocks* can produce bradycardia approximately 5 minutes after the block is given, with the FHR dropping to 60 bpm for as long as 10 minutes. The FHR will gradually increase, sometimes overshooting the

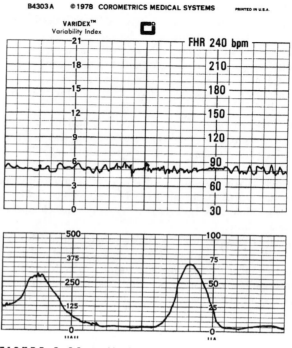

FIGURE 6.36 Fetal bradycardia.

baseline rate and producing temporary tachycardia before returning to its normal rate. *Synthetic oxytocin (Pitocin)* can indirectly produce bradycardia by causing a hyperstimulation of the uterine muscle (myometrium), reducing placental perfusion, which results in hypoxia.

- **Hypothermia**—Maternal hypothermia similarly affects the fetal temperature. The temperature reduction decreases metabolism of the fetal myocardium. The lowered myocardial activity lowers oxygen requirements of the fetus, resulting in bradycardia.
- **Fetal cardiac dysrhythmias**—Fetal dysrhythmias resulting in bradycardia might be caused by congenital cardiac lesions. Fetal congenital heart block can be seen in women who have connective tissue disease such as systemic lupus erythematosus.
- **Reflex events**—Occurrences including prolonged cord compression can precipitate bradycardic episodes. Increased blood pressure from obstructed blood flow stimulates baroreceptors to reduce heart rate. As long as the cord remains occluded, the heart rate remains low
- **Idiopathic causes**—In some fetuses, bradycardia has no apparent cause. Perhaps in these fetuses, the parasympathetic nervous system becomes dominant in its regulatory action over the fetal heart. As long as variability is within normal limits, the fetal outcome is usually good.

Interventions[4,37,38]

The treatment of fetal bradycardia is aimed at the specific cause to correct the precipitating event:

- Begin oxygen therapy by face mask at 10 to 12 L per minute.
- Perform a vaginal examination to check for cord prolapse.
- Change maternal position.
- Administer a bolus of 200 mL (nonglucose) IV fluids.
- If during second stage of labor:
  – Limit bearing-down efforts—gentle pushing rather than breath-holding pushing; use squatting or upright positions.
  – Discontinue oxytocics.
- Notify the primary care provider immediately.

The bradycardia that is sometimes seen at the end of labor just before delivery is called *end-stage bradycardia. Terminal bradycardia,* on the other hand, is a pattern that is often seen just before fetal death. It is associated with absent variability, a declining baseline, acidosis, and hypoxia. These two terms should not be confused.

Sinusoidal Patterns

■ What are sinusoidal patterns, and what causes them?[1,4,6,41]

Pathologic Sinusoidal Pattern

The true sinusoidal pattern is a regular, persistent sine wave variation of the baseline, which is within the normal FHR range (110 to 160 bpm). Changes in this baseline are seen as uniform undulations, sawtoothed or wavelike, with an amplitude of 5 to 15 bpm (Fig. 6.37). It is seen in about 2% of patients and is usually continuous; however, it may also occur intermittently. In general, the wave frequency is approximately 2 to 5 cycles per minute. Higher-amplitude oscillations (more than 25 cycles per minute) have been associated with a greater perinatal mortality than that in fetuses with lower-amplitude oscillations. STV is absent; LTV is uniform, and there are no accelerations in the sinusoidal pattern.

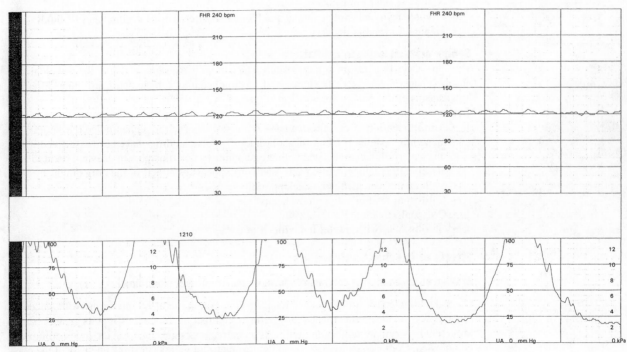

FIGURE 6.37 Sinusoidal pattern seen in a laboring patient with a partial placental abruption. Note uniform long-term variability and absent short-term variability.

Causes

- **Severe fetal anemia**—Causes of fetal anemia are erythroblastosis fetalis, twin-to-twin transfusion, fetomaternal hemorrhage, vasa previa, abruptio placentae, placenta previa, umbilical vein thrombosis, cytomegalovirus, and human parvovirus. Sinusoidal patterns associated with fetal anemia are not often seen in the intrapartum period but develop during the antepartal period (Fig 6.38).
- **Severe fetal hypoxia and acidosis**—Severe and prolonged hypoxia and metabolic acidosis that has resulted in damage to the higher centers of the brain can result in a sinusoidal FHR.

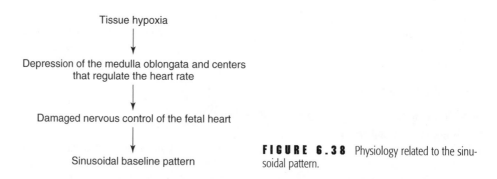

FIGURE 6.38 Physiology related to the sinusoidal pattern.

Interventions[1,4,6]

- Rule out benign pattern—recent drug administration, fetal activity, accelerations, risk factors for anemia, bleeding, twins, condition of fetus before onset, review of history for risk factors.
- Check vital signs.
- Administer O_2 per mask.
- Notify provider immediately.
- Promote maternal cardiac output and blood pressure—lateral position and IV fluids
- Prepare for prompt delivery.

Benign or Pseudosinusoidal Pattern

The appearance of a benign or pseudosinusoidal pattern is the same as that of the pathologic sinusoidal pattern; however, its causes and the implications for the fetus are quite different. Mechanisms of this pattern are not clear (Fig. 6.39).

Causes

- **Administration of certain drugs**—Common drugs such as alphaprodine (Nisentil), meperidine (Demerol), butorphanol (Stadol), and street drugs have been associated with this pattern. When associated with drug administration, this pattern does not seem to adversely affect fetal condition and usually disappears as effects of the drug diminish.
- Sucking movements/thumb-sucking of the fetus
- Clusters of fetal breathing movements[42]
- CNS malformations[43]
- Gastroschisis **with a fetal hematocrit of 65%**[41]

Effects of Uterine Contractions

■ What effect do uterine contractions have on maternal/fetal blood flow?

Normal uterine contractions produce repeated stress on the fetus by interfering with placental blood flow from the mother to the fetus. Before a contraction, blood flow is at its greatest, moving freely between the mother and fetus. As a contraction begins, *veins* in the myometrium are compressed. Compression of *arteries* in the myometrium will occur if the intensity of the contraction is greater than the mean arterial blood pressure of the mother. With the compression of the myometrial arteries, blood flow ceases and the fetus in essence "holds its breath." The point at which blood flow stops is at approximately 40 mm Hg and is referred to as *physiologic isolation.* In a normal contraction, this physiologic isolation is brief, and the fetus is able to withstand this stress and maintain the heart rate. As the contraction subsides, the myometrial *arteries* open first, followed by an opening of the myometrial *veins.* Blood flow through the uterus to the placenta and fetus is restored.

Abnormal Uterine Activity (Increased)

Tetanic contractions are contractions that last longer than 2 minutes. These contractions result in decreased blood flow through the uterus for an extended period. An already-compromised fetus might be unable to tolerate these contractions. The degree of effect on the fetus is related to fetal health, the persistence of the contractions, and/or contraction length. Even the healthy fetus can be adversely affected under these circumstances.

In Figure 6.40, baseline is quickly affected by the contraction pattern. The first contraction lasts 130 seconds, and the second contraction lasts 190 seconds; both are tetanic contractions. The fetus has only a brief time for reoxygenation between the contractions and can no longer

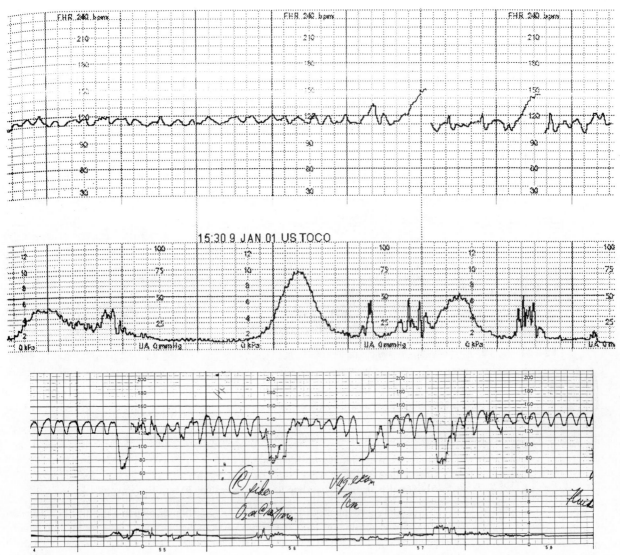

FIGURE 6.39 Sinusoidal pattern. (Reprinted with permission from Menihan, C. A., & Zottoli, E. K. [2001]. *Electronic fetal monitoring: Concepts and applications.* Philadelphia: Lippincott Williams & Wilkins; and Freeman, R. K., Gante, T. J., & Nageotte, M. P. [1991]. *Fetal heart rate monitoring* [2nd ed., p.90]. Philadelphia: Lippincott Williams & Wilkins.)

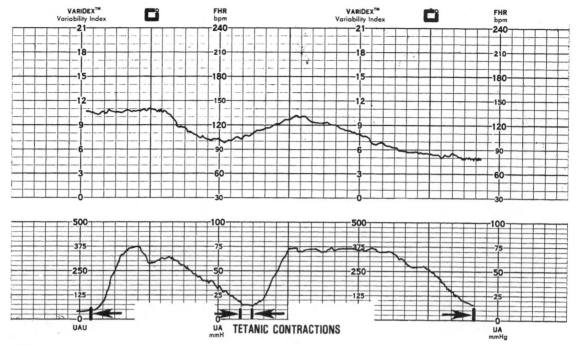

FIGURE 6.40 Effect of tetanic contractions on fetal heart rate.

compensate for the hypoxic stress. The onset of the FHR drop will depend on the degree of fetal reserve and the persistence of the insult.

Hyperstimulation occurs in any one of the following circumstances:

- More than five contractions in 10 minutes
- Greater than 300 MVUs
- Abnormally increased baseline tone (greater than 30 mm Hg)

These patterns pose threats to adequate fetal oxygenation by reducing the time between contractions or by decreasing the amount of blood flow to the placenta. These contraction patterns can be related to uterine hypoxia (from hypotension, blood loss, maternal hypoxia) or oxytocin stimulation.

When any of the events listed occur, blood flow through the uterus is diminished and the potential for fetal hypoxia and related heart rate patterns is present. ***The administration of Pitocin is perhaps the most frequently identified cause of hyperstimulation and resulting stress on the fetus.***

In Figure 6.41, the FHR progressively shows signs of stress in the form of decelerations and decreasing fetal heart baseline in response to contractions that occur too frequently.

Treatment for Hyperactive Uterine Activity[6,38]

Treatment is based on increasing blood flow to and through the uterus.

- Turn the patient to either her left or right side. This displaces the gravid uterus off the aorta and vena cava, thus promoting venous return and improving blood pressure and cardiac output, resulting in better uterine perfusion.
- Administer a bolus of 200 mL of IV fluids. This increases blood volume and improves blood pressure and perfusion.
- Turn off Pitocin if it is infusing. This assists in promoting uterine relaxation by removing the effects of the uterine stimulant.
- Prepare to administer tocolytics if other measures are not successful.
- Notify the provider.

Imagine holding your breath for a few seconds. This is a brief stress, but one that can be easily withstood. But what if you are ill? You might not be able to withstand the stress of holding your breath even for a few seconds. Whether or not you can withstand this stress depends on

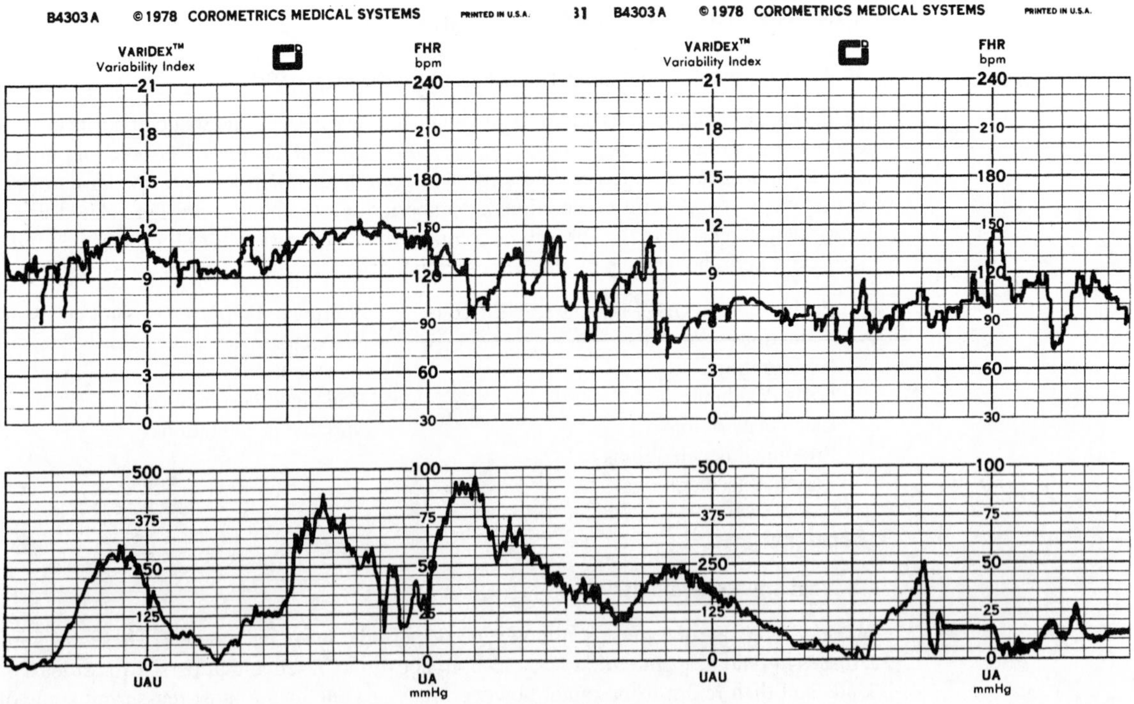

FIGURE 6.41 Effect of Pitocin-induced uterine hyperstimulation on the fetal heart rate.

your reserve or status. The same holds true for the fetus. Minimal or average labor might prove too stressful in a fetus whose reserve is poor. On the other hand, too frequent uterine contractions might cause no distress in a fetus who has good reserve.

In summary, with each contraction, blood flow from the fetus to the mother is initially affected as the myometrial veins are compressed. (Venous walls are less muscular, so they are more easily compressed.) If the contraction pressure is greater than the mother's mean arterial blood pressure, blood flow from the mother to the fetus ceases as the myometrial arteries are compressed. At this point, the mother and fetus are physiologically separated from each other. As the contraction begins to subside, the myometrial arteries reopen, allowing blood carrying oxygen and nutrients to flow from the mother to the fetus. As the contraction continues to subside, the myometrial veins open, allowing blood carrying fetal waste products to flow from the fetus to the mother.

■ How do uterine contractions affect fetal heart rate?

Uterine contractions can affect FHR by increasing or decreasing that rate in association with any given contraction. The three primary mechanisms by which uterine contractions can cause a decrease in FHR (refer to Fig. 6.42) are by compression of the following:

- Fetal head
- Umbilical cord
- Myometrial vessels

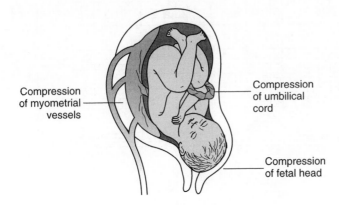

Compression of myometrial vessels

Compression of umbilical cord

Compression of fetal head

FIGURE 6.42 Three mechanisms by which uterine contractions may decrease fetal heart rate. (Adapted with permission from Barden, T. [1975]. *Intrapartum labor monitoring: A slide/lecture series.* [Slide 4]. Wallingford, CT: Corometrics Medical Systems.)

Periodic and Nonperiodic Patterns

■ What are periodic and nonperiodic heart rate changes?[1,4,6,12,38]

FHR changes that are transient in nature and occur at intervals and that can occur in relation to contractions are termed *periodic* or *nonperiodic* heart rate changes. Periodic and nonperiodic changes are separated into accelerations and decelerations. Periodic rate changes are related to contractions (occur with contractions). Nonperiodic rate changes are not related to contractions; they can occur in the absence of contractions. The interventions for the same kind of pattern, be it periodic or nonperiodic, are essentially the same.

Periodic patterns—associated with contractions
Accelerations
Early deceleration
Late decelerations
Prolonged decelerations
Variable decelerations

Nonperiodic patterns—not necessarily associated with contractions
Accelerations
Prolonged decelerations
Variable decelerations

Accelerations

■ What are accelerations?[1,5]

Accelerations are the most common type of periodic heart rate change. These are abrupt increases in fetal heart rate of at least 15 bpm above the baseline that persist for at least 15 seconds and then return to baseline; however, they are one of the most reassuring signs of fetal well-being (Fig. 6.43). Accelerations are the normal response of an intact CNS and reflect fetal well-being. They are associated with a low probability of fetal compromise or death. *Accelerations often occur during contractions (periodic) as a result of maternal abdominal manipulation, fetal acoustic stimulation, fetal scalp stimulation, or fetal movement, or they may not be associated with contractions (nonperiodic).* The premature fetus at less than 32 weeks' gestational age, which has not yet developed neurologic maturity, may not have the ability to produce the 15 × 15 rule. In this case a transient increase from the baseline of 10 bpm lasting for at last 10 seconds may be satisfactory.[12] Regardless of the cause (spontaneous or induced), they are indicative of a normal fetal pH and rule out metabolic acidemia.

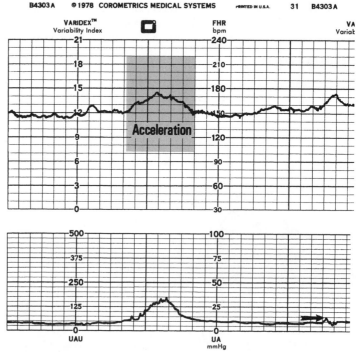

FIGURE 6.43 Fetal heart rate accelerations.

No treatment is necessary for accelerations. They are a normal part of the FHR. However, it should be noted in the labor record that accelerations are present.

Decelerations

■ What are decelerations?

Decelerations are decreases in the FHR baseline, which can be abrupt or gradual. The three main categories of decelerations are uniform, prolonged, and variable (Fig. 6.44).

1. *Uniform* decelerations are so named because they have a uniform shape. These decelerations consist of a gradual drop from the baseline, followed by a gradual return to the baseline. Uniform decelerations are further divided into two groups: late and early decelerations.
2. *Prolonged* decelerations last longer than other kinds of decelerations (between 2 and 10 minutes).
3. *Variable* decelerations are variable in shape, onset, and frequency.

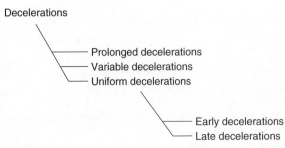

FIGURE 6.44 Categories of decelerations.

Uniform Decelerations

■ What are early decelerations, and what do they mean?[1,6]

***Early decelerations* are one kind of uniform deceleration.** This deceleration always occurs with a contraction, so they are always periodic. They are caused by pressure on the fetal head from pelvic structures as the contraction pushes the fetus further into the pelvis. This causes vagal stimulation, resulting in a decreased heart rate, and is a normal reflexive response of the fetus to vascular pressure changes (Figs. 6.45 and 6.46). They are not associated with the level of fetal oxygenation.

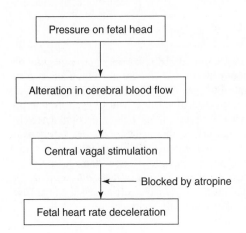

FIGURE 6.45 Mechanism of early deceleration (head compression). (Adapted with permission from Freeman, R. K., Garite, T. J., & Nageotte, M. P. [1991]. *Fetal heart rate monitoring* [2nd ed., p. 13]. Baltimore: Williams & Wilkins.)

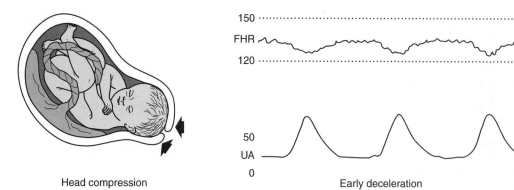

Head compression   Early deceleration

FIGURE 6.46 Head compression leading to early decelerations. (Adapted with permission from Hon, E. H. [1973]. *An introduction to fetal heart rate monitoring* [p. 29]. Los Angeles: Postgraduate Division, University of Southern California.)

Early decelerations, which are often repetitive, occur most often in the following clinical situations:

- In primigravidas
- *In association with CPD,* especially when seen in early labor
- With occiput posterior presentations
- During vaginal examinations
- *In the late active phase and the second stage of labor during pushing*
- *During application of FSE or IUPC*
- *After membranes have ruptured*

Characteristics of early decelerations

- **Uniform shape**—Early decelerations have a uniform shape and appearance that changes little during labor. They are typically shallow, usually falling no more than 15 bpm from the baseline.
- **Timing**—"Mirrors the contraction." The deceleration begins with the onset of the contraction. It gradually deepens as the contraction gains intensity and then slowly returns to baseline as the contraction intensity decreases. The deceleration mirrors the contraction. The deceleration also *always* returns to baseline by the end of the contraction.
- **Depth**—The depth of the deceleration reflects the intensity of the contraction. The stronger the contraction, the more pressure on the fetal head and therefore the lower the heart rate.
- **Amplitude**—These decelerations rarely fall below 100 bpm.
- **Variability**—FHR variability is usually normal. (Refer to Part 2 of this module.)

No treatment is necessary for early decelerations. However, continue to watch the FHR pattern closely and *make sure the decelerations are early decelerations and not late decelerations,* because implications for each of very these are different. Chart the presence of early decelerations in the patient chart.

■ What are late decelerations, and what do they mean?[1,4,6,38]

Late decelerations are periodic uniform decreases in the FHR caused by *uteroplacental insufficiency* (Fig. 6.48). Uteroplacental insufficiency means that blood flow to the fetus is compromised, resulting in a reduction in the amount of oxygen available for fetal use. Late decelerations indicate that the fetus is affected by decreased blood flow and oxygen availability during the contraction, when the uterine vessels are compressed. The heart rate is influenced by a relatively short period of hypoxia because fetal reserve is diminished. *Late decelerations in general are nonreassuring patterns.* They are associated with metabolic acidemia when paired with absent STV and decreased LTV. Maternal diseases that cause vessel damage and affect blood supply are commonly associated with these decelerations. *Late decelerations are a sign of fetal stress.* The hypoxia seen in uteroplacental insufficiency adversely affects the fetal CNS and myocardium. Late decelerations are *always* associated with contractions.

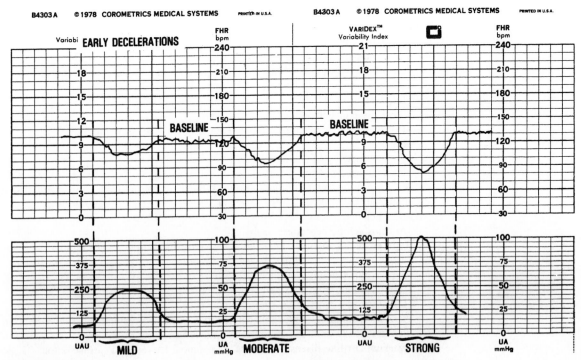

FIGURE 6.47 Early decelerations. Notice that as the intensity of the contraction improves, the depth of the early deceleration increases.

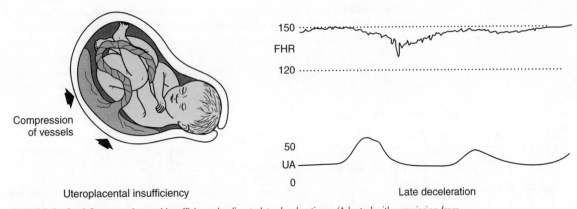

FIGURE 6.48 Uteroplacental insufficiency leading to late decelerations. (Adapted with permission from Hon, E. H. [1973]. *An introduction to fetal heart rate monitoring* [p. 29]. Los Angeles: Postgraduate Division, University of Southern California.)

Late decelerations occur most frequently in the following clinical situations:

- **Hematologic disorders**—Affect the oxygen-carrying capacity of the blood, contributing to hypoxia.
  - –Anemia
  - –Sickle cell disease
  - –Rh isoimmunization
- **Bleeding disorders**—Contribute to hypovolemia and resulting hypoxia.
  - –Abruptio placentae
  - –Placenta previa

- **Hypertensive disorders**—Interferes with oxygen transfer as a result of changes at the site of gas exchange in the placenta.
  - –Chronic hypertension
  - –Pregnancy-induced hypertension
- **Placental dysfunction**—Contributes to fetal hypoxia through diminished sites for gas exchange.
  - –Infarcted placentas
  - –Postmature placentas
  - –Placentas from small-for-gestational-age or growth-restricted fetuses
  - –Maternal smoking
  - –Premature aging of placenta
  - –Placental calcification
- **Disorders affecting the blood vessels**—Thickening of the walls of intervillous spaces diminishes the efficiency of gas exchange.
  - –Diabetes mellitus
  - –Arteriosclerotic heart disease
- **Hypotensive problems**—Reduced maternal cardiac output results in poor placental perfusion.
  - –Supine hypotension syndrome
  - –Complications from anesthetic procedures
  - –Dehydration
- Uterine hyperstimulation/tetanic contractions—Produces extended periods of hypoxia related to vascular compression during contractions.
- **Maternal cardiac disease**—Creates the potential for reduced cardiac output.

Characteristics of late decelerations

- **Uniform shape**—Late decelerations have relatively the same uniform shape throughout labor. They begin with a gradual descent from the baseline and end with a gradual ascent back to the baseline.
- **Timing**—The deceleration usually begins after the onset of the contraction but *always* ends after the offset of the contraction. The deceleration can begin at any point in the contraction; however, it often coincides with the peak of the contraction, and the nadir of the deceleration usually occurs after the peak of the contraction.[12]

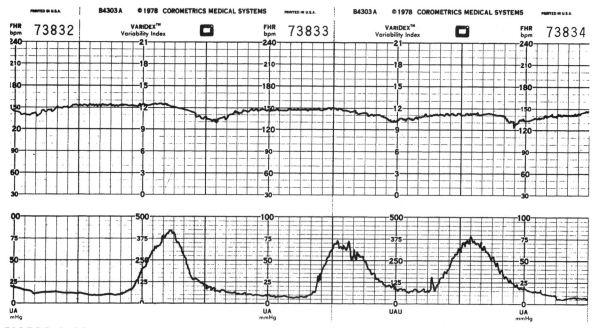

FIGURE 6.49 Late decelerations.

- **Amplitude**—The deceleration rarely falls below 100 bpm.
- **Variability**—These decelerations are associated with loss of short-term variability. (Refer to Part 2, FHR Variability.)
- **Depth**—The depth of the deceleration is NOT proportional to the severity of the hypoxia and acidemia. In fact, the subtle late deceleration (barely drops from the baseline) can indicate the reduced capacity of the fetus to respond to hypoxia (Fig. 6.50).
- **Frequency**—The presence of repetitive late decelerations, especially when combined with a loss of variability, is an ominous sign.

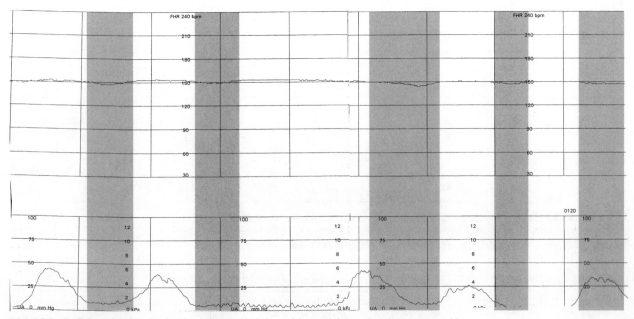

FIGURE 6.50 Subtle late decelerations seen on admission to labor and delivery in a G1 P0 30-year-old woman with a blood pressure reading of 180/106 mm Hg.

Reflex late decelerations *(Fig. 6.51) occur as a result of fetal response to hypoxia and are associated with hypotensive events in the fetus with good reserve. These late decelerations occur in the presence of moderate LTV and present STV. Present variability demonstrates fetal reserve and fetal ability to compensate. Patients can be allowed to labor with this kind of late deceleration; however, close attention must be paid to the variability of the baseline (Fig. 6.52).*

Interventions for Late Decelerations

- Place the woman in the lateral position. This position decreases pressure on the inferior vena cava, aorta, and renal and uterine arteries by displacing the pressure caused by the weight of the gravid uterus. The decrease in pressure improves blood flow, placental perfusion, and fetal oxygenation.
- Turn off Pitocin. This action decreases uterine activity and as a result maximizes blood flow from the mother to the fetus.
- Begin oxygen therapy by mask at 10 to 12 L per minute. This will help increase the oxygen saturation of maternal blood, making more oxygen available for the fetus.
- Correct hypotension. Increase IV fluids with a bolus of 200 mL. This will increase the woman's blood volume, which contributes to better perfusion.
- Notify the primary care provider. Indicate time of occurrence, frequency, variability, association with other factors, and treatment.
- Document in the labor record and on the monitor strip. Note time, frequency, interventions, and notification of the primary care provider. *Write on the strip any treatment but not a diagnosis.*
- Consider performing a vaginal examination. This examination provides information about progress in labor and a basis for estimating the time of delivery.

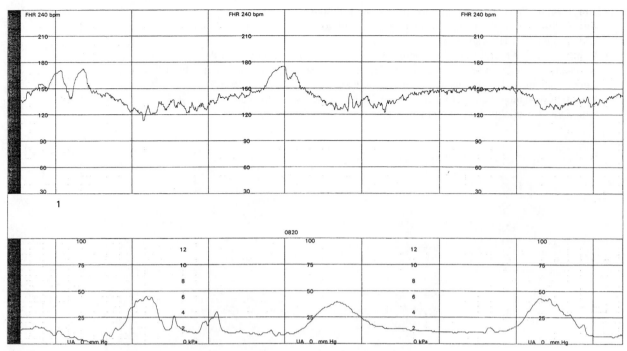

FIGURE 6.51 Reflex late decelerations. At 38 weeks' estimated gestation, this patient was a 29-year-old G2 P0 smoker who was lying in a supine position. When the patient was turned to the left lateral position, these decelerations resolved. At delivery, the placenta was small, with multiple infarcts and calcification.

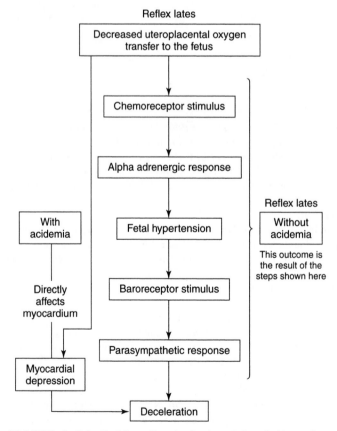

FIGURE 6.52 Physiology of late decelerations. (Adapted with permission from Freeman, R. K., Garite, T. J., & Nageotte, M. P. [1991]. *Fetal heart rate monitoring* [2nd ed., p. 17]. Baltimore: Williams & Wilkins.)

Variable Decelerations[1,4,6]

■ What are variable decelerations, and what do they mean?

Variable decelerations are transient decreases in FHR believed to be caused by *umbilical cord compression* (Fig. 6.53). Variable decelerations are a relatively common occurrence. In fact, if a fetus was continuously monitored throughout pregnancy, these decelerations could be seen occasionally as the fetus grabs the umbilical cord or the cord gets compressed between the fetus and the uterine wall during fetal movement. Approximately 80% of fetuses experience variable decelerations during labor. As long as the deceleration returns to baseline promptly, the baseline FHR remains stable, and the variability remains good, these decelerations are *not* associated with poor fetal outcome.

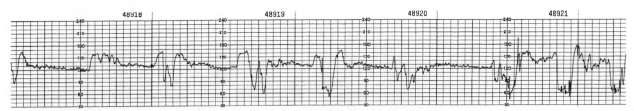

FIGURE 6.53 Reassuring variable decelerations. (Reprinted with permission from Freeman, R. K., Garite, T. J., & Nageotte, M. P. [1991]. *Fetal heart rate monitoring* [2nd ed., p. 116]. Baltimore: Williams & Wilkins.)

Characteristics of Variable Decelerations

- **Variable shape**—Variable decelerations can assume *any* shape. They can appear V-, W-, or U-shaped. It is not unusual for several variable decelerations on the same laboring woman's strip graph to appear different. *There is no consistent shape.*
- **Variable onset**—Variable decelerations can begin at any time with or without the presence of contractions. If they do occur with a contraction, they can begin at the beginning, peak, or end of the contraction. There is no consistent timing of onset.
- **Variable offset**—Variable decelerations can return to the baseline quickly, or the return can be gradual. If the deceleration occurs with a contraction, it can start at any point during the contraction and can return to baseline during or after the contractions end. However, if the deceleration has occurred in relation to a contraction, it will often be resolved by the contraction's end because the contraction might have been the cause of the cord pressure. There is no consistent offset.
- **Variable depth (amplitude)**—Variable decelerations vary in the depth to which the FHR will drop. Often, they will fall below 90 bpm. It is not unusual for variable decelerations on the same strip to vary in depth. This is because the depth of the deceleration is a reflection of the amount of pressure increase in the fetal system. The heart rate will decrease as much as needed to prevent vascular pressure from becoming too great. There is no consistent depth.
- **Variable duration**—Variable decelerations can last for any length of time, from a few seconds up to 2 minutes. It is not unusual for variable decelerations on the same strip to have different durations. *There is no consistent duration.*
- **Variability**—The decelerations are usually associated with normal or increased variability unless nonreassuring characteristics are present.
- **Implications**—Not associated with fetal acidosis unless the variable decelerations are severe or prolonged and/or associated with other nonreassuring features.

Variable decelerations occur most frequently in the following clinical situations:

- **Late labor**—As the fetus descends through the birth canal, the umbilical cord is more likely to be stretched and compressed.
- **Nuchal cord**—One or more loops of the umbilical cord can become wrapped around the fetal neck or shoulder.
- **Cord occlusion**—A true knot can occur in the umbilical cord.
- **Body cord**
- **Prolapsed cord**
- **After rupture of membranes**—There is no longer the protective fluid cushion of fluid.

■ How are variable decelerations classified?

Variable decelerations can be classified as either reassuring or nonreassuring. Strip characteristics of the reassuring variable include *shouldering, rapid return to baseline, good variability,* and *accelerations.* Nonreassuring variable patterns include *reduced variability, loss of shouldering, slow return to baseline, continuation of baseline at a lower rate,* and *overshoots.*

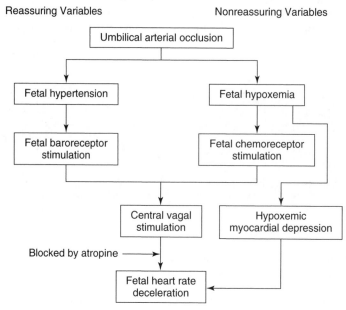

FIGURE 6.54 Physiology of variable decelerations. (Reprinted with permission from Freeman, R. K., Garite, T. J., & Nageotte, M. P. [1991]. *Fetal heart rate monitoring* [2nd ed., p. 16]. Baltimore: Williams & Wilkins.)

Characteristics of Reassuring Variable Decelerations
- **Resolves quickly**—A rapid return to baseline following the deceleration demonstrates that the fetus is able to return to its normal heart rate quickly, has had minimal exposure to a hypoxic episode, and has good reserve.
- **Normal variability and baseline**—As previously stated, normal variability is always a reassuring strip characteristic and is indicative of normal oxygenation and normal pH, indicating a fetus that is maintaining homeostasis.
- **Short duration**—The deceleration lasts no more than 30 to 45 seconds. Variables of short duration yield minimal time of reduced oxygen and a shorter time for carbon dioxide buildup in the fetal blood.
- **Presence of shoulders**—*In reassuring variable decelerations there is a brisk increase in the FHR just before and immediately after the deceleration.* These increases are referred to as *preshoulders* and *postshoulders.* Shouldering, a normal physiologic mechanism, is believed to be a result of the initial partial occlusion of the umbilical cord at the beginning of the deceleration, causing a reduction in blood flow to the fetus. This mild hypoxia and increased blood pressure cause stimulation of the chemoreceptors and baroreceptors, which results in an increase in the heart rate (shoulders). As the umbilical cord is completely occluded, there is increased fetal blood pressure. This increased pressure is sensed by the baroreceptors, which respond by causing a dramatic decrease in the FHR (deceleration). As the cord compression diminishes and as circulation resumes, there is a further increase in amount of carbon dioxide in the fetal system. The increased levels of carbon dioxide and reduced fetal blood pressure combine to cause stimulation of both chemoreceptors and baroreceptors, which produce an increase in the FHR. This helps increase blood flow so that the excess carbon dioxide can be more rapidly removed from fetal circulation and restore fetal blood pressure to normal levels.

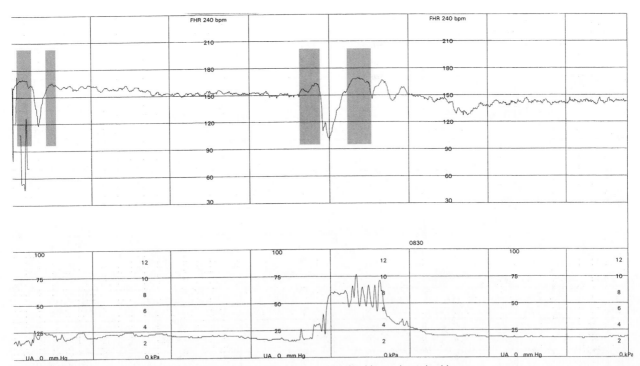

FIGURE 6.55 Reassuring variable decelerations. Note the presence of preshoulders and postshoulders and normal variability.

Shouldering emphasizes the fetal ability to prepare for and recuperate quickly from the deceleration. When shoulders are present, variability is usually normal and in most cases their presence is indicative of a rapid return to a normal baseline.[4,11,43,44]

Characteristics of Nonreassuring Variable Decelerations Nonreassuring variable decelerations are associated with a high incidence of low Apgar scores and usually possess more than one nonreassuring feature.

- **Loss of initial and/or secondary shoulder**—When the fetus starts to be adversely affected by these decelerations, the normal physiologic responses of shouldering begin to disappear. In most cases, preshoulders are the first to disappear. *Variable decelerations become nonreassuring as the shoulders are lost* (Figs. 6.56 to 6.58). *At this point, fetal pH probably becomes acidotic.* This pH change results from cord compression and the consequent buildup of carbon dioxide in fetal circulation caused by the frequent, complete occlusion of the umbilical cord. Loss of shoulders indicates the loss of fetal compensatory ability.[4,43]
- **Overshoots**—Overshoots are a prolongation of the postshoulder and are an exaggerated response to fetal hypoxia and increased levels of carbon dioxide. At the end of the deceleration, instead of the brief increase (usually 20 seconds or less) in FHR and return to baseline as expected, the FHR remains elevated above the baseline heart rate for an extended period (Fig. 6.59). This represents a fetus that must work harder and longer to restore a level of homeostasis. It is evidence of a stressed, decompensating fetus.[4,43]
- **Loss of variability**—The loss of variability is consistent with fetal stress and is often associated with a high incidence of low Apgar scores (see Fig. 6.49). The combination of variable decelerations with a loss of variability, biphasic deceleration (the fetal heart rate drops, increases, and then drops again), slow return to baseline, a baseline rate change, loss of shoulders, and overshoots is especially ominous, indicating fetal acidosis and poor fetal outcome.

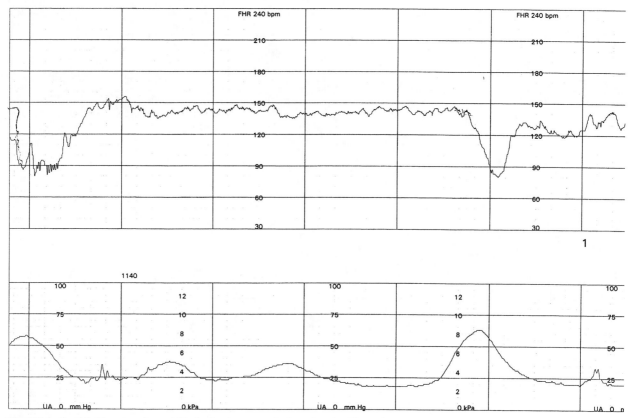

FIGURE 6.56 Nonreassuring variable decelerations. Note the loss of preshoulder and postshoulder, overshoot after first deceleration, and slow return to baseline with second deceleration.

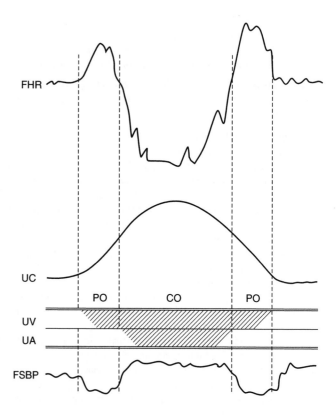

FIGURE 6.57 Blood pressure changes during variable decelerations. This figure represents fetal heart rate and fetal systemic blood pressure (*FSBP*) occurring during compression of the umbilical vein (*UV*) and the umbilical artery (*UA*). UC, uterine contraction. (Reprinted with permission from Lee, C. V., Loreto, P. C., & O'Lane, J. M. [1975]. A study of fetal heart rate acceleration patterns. *Obstetrics and Gynecology, 45,* 142.)

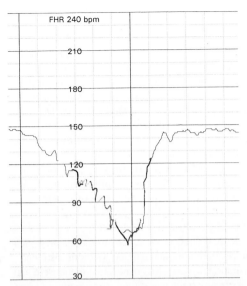

FIGURE 6.58 Loss of preshoulders and postshoulders.

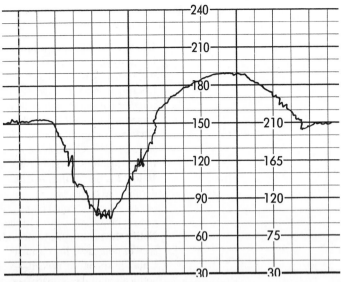

FIGURE 6.59 Variable deceleration with overshoots.

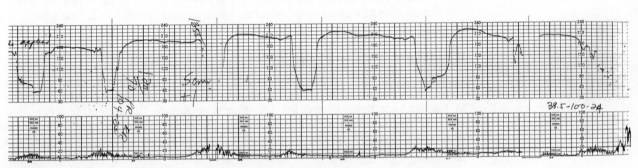

FIGURE 6.60 Variable decelerations with loss of variability and overshoots. (Reprinted with permission from Freeman, R. K., Garite, T. J., & Nageotte, M. P. [1991]. *Fetal heart rate monitoring* [2nd ed., p. 80]. Baltimore: Williams & Wilkins.)

- **Rising baseline**—A rising baseline often indicates decreasing fetal ability to tolerate hypoxic episodes. After the deceleration the fetal heart may need to increase its rate to reoxygenate the tissues and maintain adequate level of homeostasis (Fig. 6.60).•
  Prolonged return to baseline and/or bradycardia following variable decelerations—This lengthens the hypoxic episode, indicates that there is a problem resuming the original heart rate, is commonly associated with hypoxemia, and is an ominous event.
- **Development of tachycardia**—Tachycardia indicates that the fetal heart is working harder to maintain adequate oxygen levels.[39]
- **Persistent decreases to less than 70 bpm and lasting longer than 60 seconds**—Variable decelerations of this magnitude create increasing stress on the fetus by decreasing the interval for reoxygenation.[1]

Interventions

■ **What treatment is necessary to alleviate variable decelerations?**

Many variable decelerations return to the FHR baseline quickly, and no treatment is necessary. However, if the deceleration lasts longer than 30 seconds or the recovery to the baseline is slow, treatment should begin. The treatment of variable decelerations is aimed at alleviating the cause of the compression.

- **Change the laboring woman's position**—Try side-lying, one side and then the other, followed by the semi-Fowler's position. The knee–chest position can also be used; however, it is generally reserved as the last position to be tried because it is uncomfortable for the laboring woman. *Remember to wait several seconds after each position change to assess whether the change has reduced cord compression and improved the heart rate.* This is sometimes difficult to do when the deceleration is especially severe.
- **Perform a vaginal examination**—This is done to rule out a prolapsed cord, to assess the stage of labor, and to assist in estimating the time of delivery.
- **If the variables persist or are nonreassuring, begin oxygen therapy by face mask at 10 to 12 L per minute**—Although the blood flow to the fetus is compromised or stopped during cord compression, oxygen therapy improves the oxygen saturation of maternal blood. When the cord compression is relieved, the fetus will have access to a richer oxygen supply, which can assist the fetus in a quicker recovery.
- **Notify the primary care provider**—Include time of occurrence, duration, frequency, presence of nonreassuring characteristics of the decelerations, and any interventions instituted.
- **Chart in the labor record**—Note time, duration, severity, frequency, treatment used, and notification of the primary care provider. *Write any treatment on the strip graph.*
- **Turn off Pitocin if the decelerations are persistent or nonreassuring**—Although Pitocin has not caused the variable decelerations, it might be contributing to the problem, especially if the decelerations are occurring with the contractions.
- **Administer a bolus of IV fluids.**
- **Consider amnioinfusion according to protocols**—This done to assist in relieving cord compression by reintroducing fluid into the uterus, thus providing a cushioning effect.

Prolonged Decelerations

■ **What are prolonged decelerations?**[1,4,6,38]

Prolonged decelerations are nonperiodic decelerations that last 2 minutes or longer and whose duration does not exceed 10 minutes.[11] That means that they remain below, and do not return to, baseline for at least 2 minutes but they return to baseline by 10 minutes (Fig. 6.61). There is *no one specific event* associated with these decelerations. In fact, any of several different stimuli can cause prolonged decelerations. However, these decelerations are associated with dramatic changes in the fetal environment.

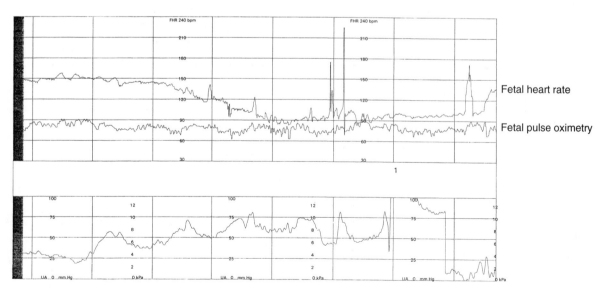

Fetal heart rate

Fetal pulse oximetry

FIGURE 6.61 Prolonged deceleration associated with uterine hyperstimulation.

Precipitating factors of prolonged decelerations include the following:

- Cord compression
- Anesthetic agents that are associated with maternal hypotension
- Vigorous fetal scalp stimulation
- Placental insufficiency
- Abruption
- Uterine hypertonus or hyperstimulation
- Maternal death
- Cord problems—short cord, thrombosis, knots, prolapse
- Uterine rupture
- Maternal seizure
- Maternal cardiac collapse

Characteristics of Prolonged Decelerations

- **Onset**—The onset of the prolonged decelerations can be abrupt or gradual because this deceleration can be caused by many different factors. The onset of a particular deceleration might present a clue to the possible origin of the precipitating event (e.g., an abrupt drop in the FHR can indicate cord compression).
- **Duration**—This deceleration lasts at least 2 minutes (often lasts much longer) but no more than 10 minutes.
- **Offset**—The offset can be abrupt or gradual.

Interventions

The interventions for this kind of deceleration are the same as those used in the treatment of variable decelerations.

The documentation of a prolonged deceleration must be completed in the patient chart using a narrative format. This description must include information about the onset (gradual or abrupt), nadir (lowest point of the FHR), return to baseline (gradual or rapid), and the length of the deceleration. Interventions must also be recorded on both the chart and the strip.

Summary

Periodic or nonperiodic changes in the FHR are transient excursions from the baseline. They can be reassuring or nonreassuring depending on their characteristics. These patterns provide clues to fetal oxygen status and reserve during labor. The data that these patterns provide should be used in planning and conducting interventions.

PRACTICE/REVIEW QUESTIONS

After reviewing Part 3, answer the following questions.

1. Define *fetal tachycardia.*

2. Define *fetal bradycardia.*

3. For each of the following terms, indicate whether the condition might be a cause of fetal tachycardia (FT), fetal bradycardia (FB), or both (B).
   a. _____ Fetal hypoxia
   b. _____ Atropine
   c. _____ Propranolol
   d. _____ Pitocin
   e. _____ Maternal anxiety
   f. _____ Prolapsed umbilical cord
   g. _____ Fetal infection
   h. _____ Maternal hypothermia
   i. _____ Prematurity
   j. _____ Fetal movement
   k. _____ Idiopathic causes
   l. _____ Maternal fever

245

4. Describe the nursing interventions appropriate for fetal tachycardia.

a. _____

b. _____

c. _____

d. _____

e. _____

f. _____

5. Describe the nursing interventions appropriate for fetal bradycardia.

a. _____

b. _____

c. _____

d. _____

e. _____

f. _____

g. _____

6. List the three primary ways in which uterine contractions can decrease FHR.

a. _____

b. _____

c. _____

7. Study the following strip.

a. Is the baseline rate normal? _____

b. What periodic pattern is present? _____

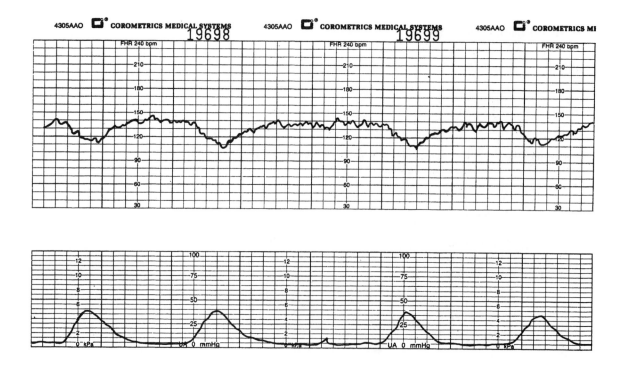

8. Describe the sinusoidal baseline pattern.

   _____

   _____

9. Name three possible causes of a sinusoidal pattern.

   a. _____

   b. _____

   c. _____

10. Identify and describe two kinds of abnormally increased uterine activity.

    a. _____

    b. _____

11. State the nonpharmacologic interventions for abnormally increased uterine activity.

    a. _____

    b. _____

    c. _____

12. Define *periodic heart rate changes.*

    _____

    _____

13. Indicate whether the following statements are true (T) or false (F).

    a. _____ Contractions have no effect on FHR.

    b. _____ Accelerations are a reassuring sign of fetal well-being.

    c. _____ Accelerations are a sign of fetal distress.

    d. _____ Early decelerations are *not* a sign of fetal distress.

    e. _____ Early decelerations usually do not fall below 100 bpm.

14. Define the following terms:

    a. Accelerations: _____

    b. Early decelerations: _____

15. List three situations in which early decelerations might occur.

    a. _____

    b. _____

    c. _____

16. Study the following strip. What **FHR** pattern(s) is (are) present? _____

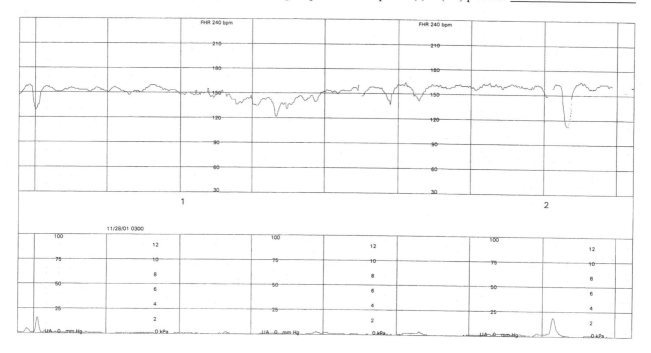

17. Variable decelerations are caused by _____.

18. Indicate whether the following statements are true (T) or false (F).
    a. _____ Variable decelerations always have the same shape and appearance.
    b. _____ Variable decelerations always begin at the peak of a contraction.
    c. _____ A variable deceleration might or might not occur with contractions.
    d. _____ There is no consistent depth to a variable deceleration.
    e. _____ It is unusual for several variable decelerations on the same patient's strip graph
       to have different durations.
    f. _____ Variable decelerations are commonly seen in labor.

19. List the actions used to alleviate variable decelerations.
    a. _____
    b. _____
    c. _____
    d. _____
    e. _____

20. Late decelerations are caused by _____.

21. Indicate whether the following statements are true (T) or false (F).
    a. _____ Late decelerations are a sign of fetal stress.

    b. _____ Late decelerations are uniform in shape throughout labor.

    c. _____ Labor may be allowed to continue when late decelerations are present if the
       variability is reassuring.

    d. _____ Late decelerations are often associated with a loss in variability.

22. List the treatment indicated for late decelerations.

    a. _____

    b. _____

    c. _____

    d. _____

    e. _____

    f. _____

23. Study the following strip graph. Describe the FHR pattern. _____

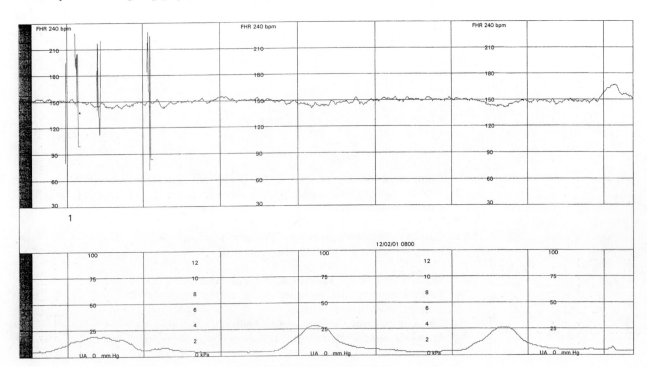

24. Describe the appearance of late decelerations.

    _____

    _____

25. The deeper the late deceleration falls, the more ominous the tracing.

    A. True

    B. False

26. Name four nonreassuring characteristics of variable decelerations.

    a. _____

    b. _____

    c. _____

    d. _____

27. What are overshoots? _____

    _____

28. What are prolonged decelerations? _____

_____

PRACTICE/REVIEW ANSWER KEY

1. Fetal tachycardia is a heart rate above 160 bpm that is sustained for 10 minutes or longer.

2. Fetal bradycardia is a heart rate below 110 or 120 bpm (depending on your institutional policy) that is sustained for 10 minutes or longer.

3. a. B
   b. FT
   c. FB
   d. FB
   e. FT
   f. FB
   g. FT
   h. FB
   i. FT
   j. FT
   k. B
   l. FT

4. a. Begin oxygen therapy via mask at 10 L per minute.
   b. Take the mother's vital signs, especially the temperature.
   c. Turn the patient to her side.
   d. Validate monitor with a fetoscope.
   e. Consider administering a bolus of IV fluids if patient is febrile.
   f. Notify the primary care provider immediately.

5. a. Begin oxygen therapy via mask at 10 L per minute.
   b. Take the mother's vital signs.
   c. Turn the patient to her side.
   d. Consider administering a bolus of IV fluids.
   e. Attempt to increase FHR by performing scalp stimulation.
   f. Listen to FHTs with a fetoscope.
   g. Notify the primary care provider immediately.

6. a. Compression of the myometrial vessels
   b. Compression of the fetal head
   c. Compression of the umbilical cord

7. a. Yes
   b. Early decelerations

8. A sinusoidal baseline is characterized by a regular, undulating baseline pattern that is within the normal heart rate range.

9. a. Severe fetal anemia
   b. Fetal asphyxia
   c. Drugs

10. Any two of the following:
    a. Tetanic contractions (i.e., contractions that last longer than 90 seconds)
    b. More than 300 MVUs in 10 minutes or more than 5 contractions in 10 minutes
    c. Increased baseline tone of greater than 30 mm Hg

11. a. Give bolus IV fluids.
    b. Turn the patient to her side.
    c. Administer oxygen per mask at 10 to 12 L per minute.

12. Periodic heart rate changes are FHR changes that are transient and associated with contractions.

13. a. F
    b. T
    c. F
    d. T
    e. T

14. Accelerations: brisk increases in the FHR of at least 15 beats above the baseline rate and lasting at least 15 seconds

    Early decelerations: caused by head compression, mirror the contraction, and always resolve by the end of the contraction

15. Any three of the following:
    a. In primigravidas
    b. During vaginal examinations
    c. In the late active phase and the second stage of labor during pushing
    d. During application of FSE or IUPC
    e. With CPD
    f. After amniotic sac has ruptured
    g. With occiput posterior presentations

16. Variable decelerations

17. Umbilical cord compression

18. a. F
    b. F
    c. T
    d. T
    e. F
    f. T

19. a. Change the patient's position.
    b. Perform a vaginal examination.
    c. Administer oxygen if variables are consistent or prolonged or if there is decreasing variability.
    d. Notify the primary care provider.
    e. Turn off Pitocin if decelerations are severe or prolonged or if there is decreasing variability.

20. Uteroplacental insufficiency

21. a. T
    b. T
    c. T
    d. T

22. a. Ask the patient to lie on her side.
    b. Turn off Pitocin if infusing.
    c. Administer oxygen.
    d. Correct hypotension (increase IV fluids).
    e. Perform a vaginal examination to estimate point in labor.
    f. Notify the primary care provider.

23. Early decelerations

24. Late decelerations usually start after contraction onset but *always* last longer than the contraction. They are uniform in shape and rarely drop below 100 bpm.

25. B (Subtle late decelerations are thought to mean the fetus is barely able to respond to the hypoxic insult.)

26. a. Overshoots
    b. Loss of shoulders
    c. Loss of variability
    d. Slow return to baseline

27. Overshoots are a prolongation of the posterior shoulder of a variable deceleration. They are nonreassuring and are considered a sign of progressing stress.

28. Prolonged decelerations are decelerations that last longer than 2 minutes and less than 10 minutes.

Fetal Homeostasis and Dysrhythmias

As you complete Part 4 of this module, you will learn:

1. Normal fetal umbilical cord blood gas values
2. Cord blood gas results according to guidelines presented
3. "How to determine metabolic or respiratory "shifts" and implications of these shifts" to the fetus and care provider
4. Common terms used in acid-base analysis
5. To identify fetal heart rate patterns associated with abnormal and normal fetal cord gas results
6. To identify the clinical significance to the fetus and provider when abnormal tracings indicate acidosis
7. Common fetal dysrhythmias and their clinical significance
8. Necessary adjustments to monitoring equipment that allows documentation of fetal heart tones during dysrhythmic patterns

Fetal Homeostasis and Acid-Base Balance[16,27,28,45]

> **■ What is the connection between the appearance of fetal heart tracings and the acid-base status of the fetus?**

The pH of the blood and tissues has an impact on all enzymes and proteins in the body, affecting organ function and infant status at birth. Acid-base status of the fetus is reflected in the characteristics of the fetal heart tracings. Certain patterns are associated with normal pH while other patterns are associated with pH reduction and acidosis. These relationships allow the practitioner to determine/predict fetal status by evaluating the characteristics of the tracing.

Terms Associated With Acid-Base Analysis

Acidemia—the buildup of acid (reduced pH) in the *blood*[a]
Acidosis—the buildup of acid (reduced pH) in the *tissues*
Base deficit (BD)—represents the amount of bases used by the body in an attempt to normalize a reduced pH (neutralize the acid); illustrates the degree of change in the bicarbonate concentration in the body; the more base used in attempting to normalize the pH, the larger the number becomes and the greater the deficit
Hypoxemia—reduction of oxygen in the *blood*
Hypoxia—reduction of oxygen in the *tissues*
pH—a representation of the hydrogen ion concentration
P_{CO_2}—the partial pressure of carbon dioxide (quantity of CO_2 in the blood)
P_{O_2}—the partial pressure of oxygen (quantity of O_2 in the blood)

> **■ What are the normal values for fetal blood gases?**

Normal values are as follows:

pH	≥ 7.10
P_{O_2}	≥ 20 mm Hg
P_{CO_2}	≤ 60 mm Hg
BD	≤ 10

Metabolic Acidemia/Acidosis

> **■ What is metabolic acidemia/acidosis?**

Each fetus reacts to periods of reduced oxygen in a unique way. "Healthy" fetuses with good reserves that are the products of uncomplicated pregnancies initially respond to the stress of hypoxia with little or no change in the heart rate pattern. Fetuses with little or no reserve will often be quickly affected by even a small reduction in oxygen availability. Reduction of the pH in fetal blood below normal range (*acidemia*) can result when oxygen levels in fetal circulation fall below certain values. The pH values of the fetal blood are an indication of the pH found in the tissues; however, tissue pH tends to be even lower than the pH levels found in the blood. The kind of acidosis (decreased pH in the tissues) linked to decreased O_2 has its basis in metabolic processes and is called *metabolic acidosis*.

At the cellular level, as glucose is used for energy, this metabolic process results in the formation of lactic acid. Normally, oxygen combines with lactic acid to produce CO_2 and H_2O, which are easily excreted by the fetus. If fetal oxygen is limited, the process stops at the formation of lactic acid, resulting in a buildup of this strong acid in the tissues and blood. The importance of oxygen in the acid-base schema is outlined in Figure 6.62.

> **■ What acid-base values identify metabolic acidemia?**

Changes in values that identify the process of metabolic acidemia are as follows:

pH	<7.20 **REDUCED**
P_{O_2}	<20 mm Hg **REDUCED**
P_{CO_2}	<60 mm Hg **NORMAL**
BD	>10 **INCREASED**

---

[a]The pH of the tissues is generally lower than the pH found in the blood. As a result, the terms *acidosis* and *acidemia* are often used interchangeably. When blood values demonstrate a decreased pH, it can be assumed that the tissues are affected in the same manner.

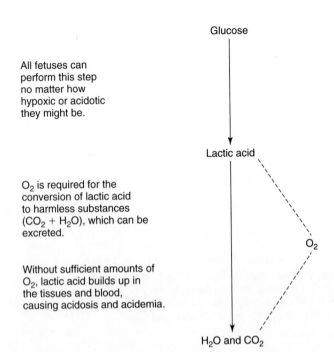

FIGURE 6.62 The importance of O_2 in normal metabolic processes.

The flow diagram shows:

Glucose

All fetuses can perform this step no matter how hypoxic or acidotic they might be.

Lactic acid

O_2 is required for the conversion of lactic acid to harmless substances ($CO_2 + H_2O$), which can be excreted.

O_2

Without sufficient amounts of O_2, lactic acid builds up in the tissues and blood, causing acidosis and acidemia.

H_2O and CO_2

■ What FHR monitor strip characteristics indicate metabolic acidemia/acidosis?

- **Absent STV**—As the fetus becomes more oxygen deprived and the pH falls, variability decreases and can vacillate between periods of minimal and absent variability. The periods of decreased variability become longer. Hypoxic effects on the autonomic nervous system, especially its parasympathetic branch, cause this change in variability, which is the identifying characteristic of metabolic acidosis. **If STV is absent and LTV is decreased, prepare for an aggressive resuscitation at delivery.**
- **Late decelerations**—Late decelerations are associated with hypoxia and metabolic acidosis. They are often seen in conjunction with poor variability. The presence of late decelerations alone does not mean that acidosis is present but might indicate a shift toward that direction. In this case the Po_2 is decreased, but the pH remains in the normal range. These late decelerations are associated with absent STV and decreased LTV (Fig. 6.63).

  A "shift" toward metabolic acidosis means that there is a reduction in the oxygen content of the fetal blood but that the pH remains within normal limits, as do the other blood gas values. If oxygenation does not improve, there is a risk of progression to metabolic acidosis. Evidence of this shift might be seen on the tracing in the following characteristics: normal variability with late decelerations.

Blood gases values expected in a shift toward metabolic acidosis are as follows:

pH	**NORMAL**
Po_2	**REDUCED**
All other values	**NORMAL**

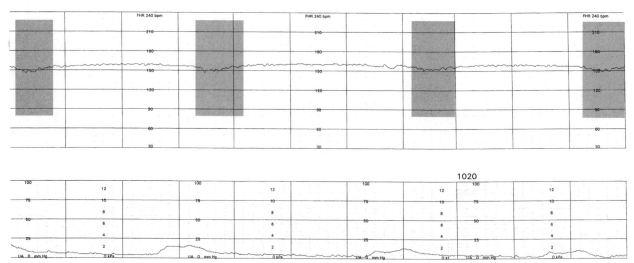

FIGURE 6.63 Repetitive subtle late decelerations. Note decreased variability. If you look closely, the baseline appears to be sinusoidal. The patient, a 33-year-old G3 P1, had been diagnosed with partial placenta previa before the onset of labor. She was admitted in early labor at 36 weeks' estimated gestation with vaginal bleeding. This pattern is indicative of metabolic acidemia/acidosis. An emergency cesarean section was performed. Apgar scores were 1, 3, and 7.

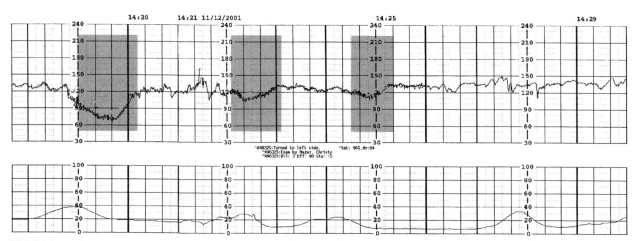

FIGURE 6.64 Late decelerations with moderate long-term variability and present short-term variability. A 26-year-old G1 P0 at 41 weeks' estimated gestation was admitted for induction of labor. The fetus demonstrated poor tolerance to mild contractions, which worsened as contractions became stronger. During the cesarean section, a very small placenta and abnormal cord were found. There was almost a complete absence of Wharton's jelly, with only a sheath covering cord vessels.

Respiratory Acidemia/Acidosis

■ What is respiratory acidemia/acidosis?

Fetal acid-base status can also be affected by increased levels of CO_2. Because CO_2 is acidic, elevated levels of CO_2 in the fetal blood cause a reduction in pH and can result in acidosis and acidemia. This kind of acidemia is called respiratory acidemia because it is concerned with CO_2 buildup. Increased levels of CO_2 in fetal circulation are associated with variable decelerations.

■ What acid-base values identify respiratory acidemia?

Changes in values that identify the process of respiratory acidemia are as follows:

pH	<7.2 **REDUCED**
Po_2	>20 mm Hg **NORMAL**
Pco_2	>60 mm Hg **INCREASED**
BD	<10 **NORMAL** (no buildup of lactic acid)

■ What FHR monitor strip characteristics indicate respiratory acidemia/acidosis?

- **Variable decelerations with loss of one shoulder**—Variable decelerations, the pattern identified with cord compression, results in CO_2 buildup (lowers pH) in fetal circulation. When CO_2 levels rise high enough, fetal pH is affected and the outcome is an increase in acidity of tissues and blood. *The most probable indicator of the onset of acidosis is the point at which one shoulder of the variable deceleration is lost.* The preshoulder is most often the first to disappear, and this is the identifying characteristic (Fig. 6.65).

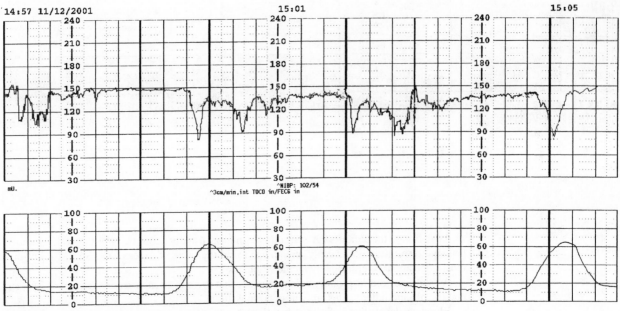

FIGURE 6.65 Variable decelerations with loss of shouldering. At delivery, this baby had a true knot in its cord. This strip probably indicates respiratory acidosis in the fetus.

- **Overshoots**—When the deceleration has resolved, an extended period of increased heart rate above the baseline can occur. This represents the extra effort and time required by the fetus to compensate for the hypoxic event. Overshoots are often associated with respiratory acidosis. This is an effort to increase circulation and rid the fetal circulation of excess Pco_2. The presence of variable decelerations (no loss of shoulders) with or without overshoots represents a shift toward respiratory acidosis. In this case the Pco_2 is elevated but the pH remains within normal limits (Fig. 6.66).

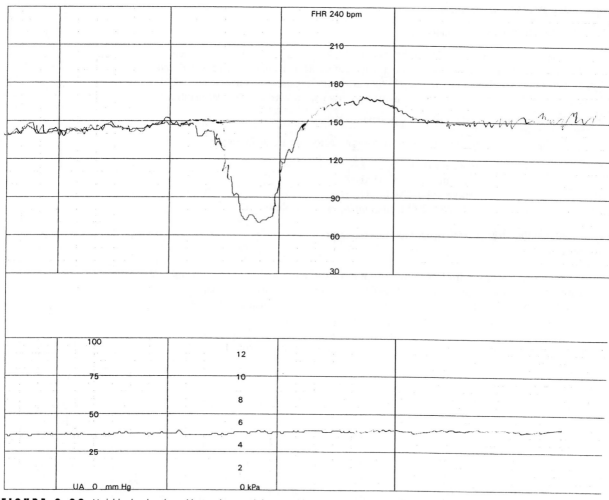

FIGURE 6.66 Variable deceleration with overshoot and decreased long-term variability, probably associated with respiratory acidosis.

At delivery, the infant with respiratory acidosis usually requires only the stimulation of neonatal respiration (i.e., crying, breathing) to rid the body of excess CO_2. Successful efforts most often are accomplished by tactile stimulation.

A "shift" toward respiratory acidosis means that there is an increase in the level of CO_2 but that the pH and other values are within normal limits.

Blood gas levels that indicate a shift toward respiratory acidosis are as follows:

P_{CO_2}	**INCREASED**
pH	**NORMAL**
Other values	**NORMAL**

Mixed Acidosis

■ **What is mixed acidemia/acidosis?**

Mixed acidosis occurs when both metabolic and respiratory acidoses are present. The pH and P_{O_2} are reduced, and P_{CO_2} and base deficit are increased. **Be prepared:** A baby born at this time will probably be severely depressed, and resuscitation can be extremely difficult.

■ **What acid-base values are associated with mixed acidosis?**

All cord gas values are abnormal.

pH	<7.10 **REDUCED**
Po_2	>20 mm Hg **REDUCED**
Pco_2	>60 mm Hg **INCREASED**
BD	>10 **INCREASED**

■ **What FHR monitor strip characteristics indicate mixed acidosis?**

The strip characteristics of the fetus with mixed acidosis might show the following:

- **Absent STV**—must be present
- **Variable decelerations with loss of at least one shoulder**—must be present
- **Late decelerations**—*might* be present in mixed acidosis
- **Overshoots**—*might* be seen in this state of acid-base balance
- **Decreased/absent LTV** (Fig. 6.67)

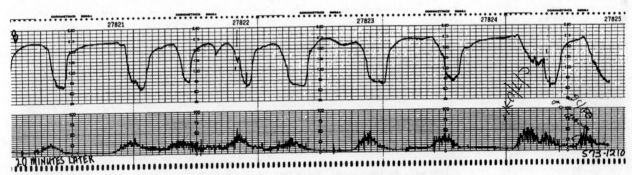

FIGURE 6.67 Mixed acidosis pattern. Note absent short-term variability, decreased long-term variability, variable decelerations with loss of shoulders, and overshoot on first deceleration and late deceleration. (Reprinted with permission from Freeman, R. K., Garite, T. J., & Nageotte, M. P. [1991]. *Fetal heart rate monitoring* [2nd ed., p. 117]. Baltimore: Williams & Wilkins.)

Variable decelerations combined with minimal decreased LTV and absent STV demonstrates a decreased pH and Po_2, increased Pco_2, and probably *mixed acidosis*.

■ **What is a shift toward mixed acidosis?**

A "shift" toward mixed acidosis means that although the pH is normal, the other values are abnormal. Usually, the abnormal values are only slightly affected, and the pH can be on the low end of the normal range.

pH	**NORMAL**
Po_2	**DECREASED**
Pco_2	**INCREASED**
BD	**INCREASED**

Characteristics of the monitor strip that indicate a fetus with a shift toward mixed acidosis are those that demonstrate both metabolic and respiratory shifts (i.e., absent STV, normal LTV [possibly late decelerations], and variable decelerations) (Fig. 6.68).

Interventions

Fetuses whose tracings indicate an acidotic state require interventions aimed at promoting oxygenation.

- Change the maternal position to the lateral.
- Administer oxygen per mask at 10 to 12 L per minute.
- Administer a bolus of IV fluids if hypotension is suspected.

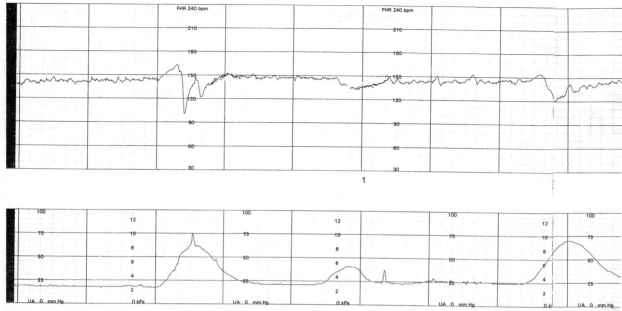

FIGURE 6.68 Shift toward mixed acidosis. Note variable and late decelerations, presence of shoulders, presence of short-term variability, and decreased long-term variability.

- Perform a vaginal examination to determine the status of labor and the estimated time of delivery.
- Decrease uterine activity—stop Pitocin and consider a tocolytic agent.
- Notify the primary care provider.

Summary: Acid-Base Balance

Certain FHR patterns and characteristics of patterns are related to fetal academia/acidosis. Fetal metabolic acidosis is associated with hypoxia. The heart rate pattern indicative of this kind of acidosis is absent variability. The related pattern is late decelerations. Fetal respiratory acidosis is associated with CO_2 buildup in the fetal system. The fetal pattern indicative of this pH alteration is variable decelerations with the loss of at least one shoulder. Associated pattern characteristics are increasing frequency and duration of variables and the presence of overshoots. Both kinds of acidoses can be present simultaneously (mixed acidosis) with characteristics of each present on the strip. It is important to recognize some of these patterns as serious threats to fetal well-being. It is also essential to understand causes and implications of these patterns so that appropriate measures can be instituted to improve fetal status and provide for emergency treatment after delivery.

Fetal Heart Dysrhythmias

■ How can the presence of a fetal heart dysrhythmia be determined?

Normally, the electrical impulse that governs heart rate and rhythm originates in the SA node located in the right atrium. Once initiated, the impulse then spreads downward to the atrioventricular (AV) node, the bundle of His, and Purkinje fibers. These impulses cause muscular contraction of the heart. Each part of this electrical system has the capacity for initiating cardiac contraction if the preceding mechanism fails. If abnormalities of the system exist, heart rate can be affected by dropped/skipped beats or premature contractions that can cause deviations in cardiac rhythm and rate. Deviations can also occur as a result of cardiac injury. These deviations are called dysrhythmias. *The causal mechanism or kind of dysrhythmia can be identified only by its characteristics on an ECG* (Fig. 6.69).

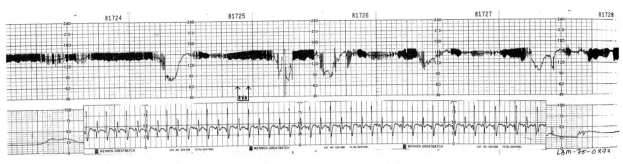

FIGURE 6.69 This tracing shows the fetal heart rate pattern above and fetal electrocardiograph below. (Reprinted with permission from Freeman, R. K., Garite, T. J., & Nageotte, M. P. [1991]. *Fetal heart rate monitoring* [2nd ed., p. 98]. Baltimore: Williams & Wilkins.)

Incidence of Fetal Dysrhythmias

Approximately 1% to 10% of fetuses demonstrate a dysrhythmic pattern during labor. Most dysrhythmias (99%) disappear shortly after birth and pose no long-term consequences to the fetus or infant.[40] Causes include electrolyte imbalance, congenital malformations of the heart, infection, acidosis, and hydrops fetalis. Most of these patterns are premature beats. Fortunately, most dysrhythmias are benign; however, certain patterns can indicate more serious problems that might require intervention before and/or after delivery.

Dysrhythmic Patterns

■ **What types of dysrhythmias are seen in the fetus, and what is their significance to fetal well-being?[46–48]**

- **Premature atrial contractions (PACs) and premature ventricular contractions (PVCs)**—These are the most common sources of heart rate irregularity in the fetus. They are usually benign and require no intervention. They are not a sign of hypoxia. Even

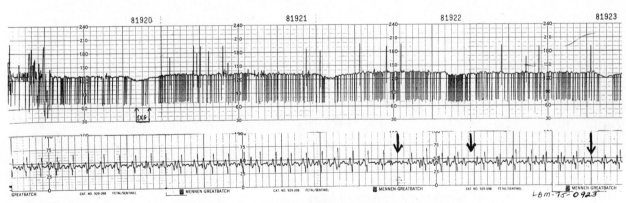

FIGURE 6.70 This tracing shows a series of downward deflections of the fetal heart rate in the upper tracing; the simultaneous fetal electrocardiograph in the lower tracing shows absent QRS complexes or dropped beats. (Reprinted with permission from Freeman, R. K., Garite, T. J., & Nageotte, M. P. [1991]. *Fetal heart rate monitoring* [2nd ed., p. 101]. Baltimore: Williams & Wilkins.)

though the atrial extrasystoles appear benign, there is a possibility that they might trigger supraventricular tachycardia, which is a concerning finding.[41]

- **Supraventricular tachycardia (SVT)**—This is the most commonly encountered tachy-dysrhythmia and should be evaluated carefully because these dysrhythmias are associated with underlying cardiac disease. SVT is usually identified in the second trimester. The rate is often greater than 200 bpm but can exceed 250 bpm and can lead to fetal congestive heart failure, hydrops, and death. Paroxysmal atrial tachycardia can be intermittent, which can allow for fetal self-resuscitation, growth, and development. Management can include medications such as digoxin, beta-blocking agents, or calcium channel blockers (Fig. 6.70).
- **Heart block**—Causes of heart block in the fetus can be congenital or genetically inherited problems and can be secondary to myocarditis or maternal systemic lupus erythematosus. In the latter case, antibodies that damage the heart's conductive system are capable of crossing the placenta and attacking cardiac tissue. Approximately 50% to 65% of mothers whose fetuses have complete heart block will have evidence of connective tissue disease. If the block is severe, immediate cardiac pacing is necessary and that capability must be available at delivery. The incidence of heart block is 1 in 20,000 births, and approximately 50% of these babies have congenital heart anomalies. If this is suspected, consultation is recommended with a maternal–fetal medicine specialist (Fig. 6.71).
- **Vagal cardiac arrest**—During deep variable decelerations, the fetal heart can pause (skip a few beats). This is the result of baroreceptor stimulation by fetal hypertension during cord compression and is a completely normal physiologic response to hypertension.

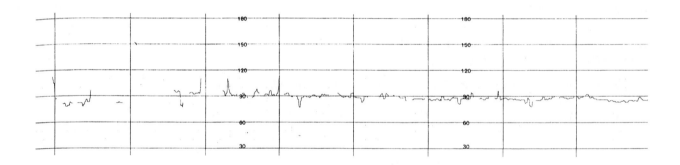

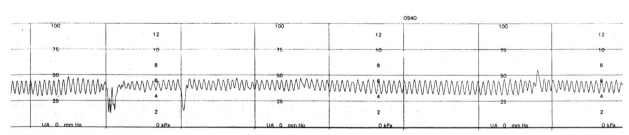

FIGURE 6.71 Fetal bradydysrhythmias. (From Menihan, C. A., & Zottoli, E. K. [2001]. *Electronic fetal monitoring: Concepts and applications.* Philadelphia: Lippincott Williams & Wilkins.)

Characteristics

■ **What FHR monitor strip characteristics indicate that a dysrhythmia might be present?**

The appearance of the tracing when a dysrhythmia is present is unique. It can be described as an irregular but organized pattern. Excursions can be either below or above the baseline and look like "hatch marks." *Auscultation with a fetoscope must be performed to verify the presence of a fetal heart irregularity (dysrhythmia).*

Interventions

■ **What interventions are necessary when a dysrhythmic pattern is suspected?**

- *If the monitor has a logic switch, turn it to the off position.* During the dysrhythmia, variability is no longer controlled by the fetal brain. Guidelines programed into the computer provide information that allows FHTs to be logically analyzed and evaluated. Because dysrhythmias are not logical (i.e., they do not fit the programmed norms for the FHR), the machine cannot adequately interpret the dysrhythmic signals and will often try to normalize what does not logically fit programmed parameters.
- *Evaluate the FHTs with a fetoscope when a dysrhythmic process is suspected.* This validates that there is an irregularity in the fetal heartbeat (a dysrhythmia). Hearing it through the monitor is not enough to validate its presence.
- *Evaluate variability between dysrhythmic episodes.* Variability cannot be accurately evaluated during the dysrhythmia, so it is important to auscultate the fetal heart if a dysrhythmia is suspected.
- *Identify causal factors that can contribute to dysrhythmic development* (e.g., hypoxia, infection, maternal collagen disease).
- *Notify the primary care provider of the findings.*

Summary: Dysrhythmias

Fortunately, most fetal dysrhythmias are benign; however, it is important to understand that some can be potentially life threatening either during pregnancy or after delivery. The presence of a suspected dysrhythmia must be verified by auscultation of the FHT with a fetoscope. The provider should be notified of these findings. If a dysrhythmia associated with serious fetal/neonatal effects is suspected, measures must be instituted to ameliorate these complications.

PRACTICE/REVIEW QUESTIONS

After reviewing Part 4, answer the following questions.

1. Determine the acid-base status demonstrated in the following fetal cord gases. (Acidosis or shift and kind [i.e., metabolic, respiratory, or mixed].)

   a. pH, 7.22; P_{O_2}, 18 mm Hg; P_{CO_2}, 48 mm Hg; BD, 7 _____

   b. pH, 7.19; P_{O_2}, 22 mm Hg; P_{CO_2}, 70 mm Hg; BD, 7 _____

   c. pH, 7.17; P_{O_2}, 16 mm Hg; P_{CO_2}, 81 mm Hg; BD, 11 _____

   d. pH, 7.28; P_{O_2}, 26 mm Hg; P_{CO_2}, 40 mm Hg; BD, 5 _____

   e. pH, 7.16; P_{O_2}, 24 mm Hg; P_{CO_2}, 78 mm Hg; BD, 12 _____

2. Evaluate the following strips in terms of your expectations of the acid-base status of the fetus.

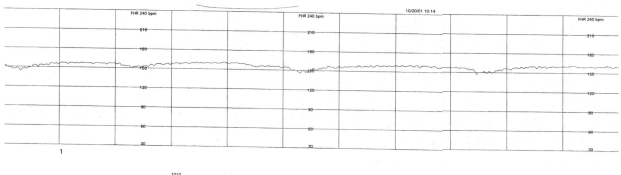

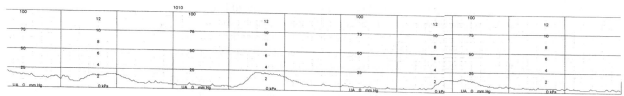

a. _____

_____

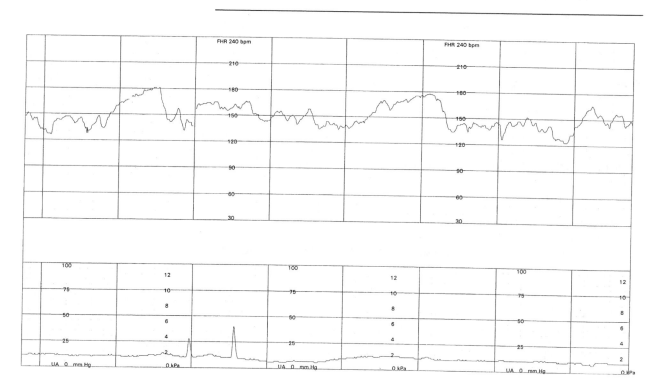

b. _____

_____

3. Describe the necessary interventions if you suspect that a fetus has metabolic acidosis.

    a. _____

    b. _____

    c. _____

    d. _____

4. Where would you expect the pH to be lower (more acidic): in the blood or in the tissues?

    _____

5. State the identifying characteristic of the fetus with respiratory acidosis.

    _____

6. State the identifying characteristic of the fetus with metabolic acidosis.

    _____

7. What is the primary cause of metabolic acidosis?

    _____

8. What is the primary cause of respiratory acidosis?

    _____

9. What is meant by a "shift" toward acidosis?

    _____

    _____

    _____

10. Match the following terms in Column A with their meanings in Column B.

    Column A

    Column B

    1. _____ Hypoxia   a. Used by the body in an attempt to normalize a reduced pH

    2. _____ Acidemia   b. Buildup of acids in the tissues

    3. _____ Acidosis   c. Partial pressure of oxygen

    4. _____ Hypoxemia   d. Reduced amount of oxygen in the blood

    5. _____ pH   e. Representation of the hydrogen ion concentration

    6. _____ Po_2 f. Partial pressure of carbon dioxide

    7. _____ Pco_2 g. Buildup of acids in the blood

    8. _____ Base deficit h. Reduction of oxygen in the tissues

11. Explain the importance of pH in the biologic function of the body.

    _____

    _____

12. If you suspect a fetal cardiac dysrhythmia, how can you confirm this assessment?

    a. _____

    b. _____

13. What is the only definitive method available for diagnosing the kind of dysrhythmia that is present? _____

14. Most fetal dysrhythmias represent grave consequences for the baby when it is born.

    A. True

    B. False

15. What is the most common dysrhythmia, and what are the implications of the dysrhythmia for the fetus?

    _____

    _____

PRACTICE/REVIEW ANSWER KEY

1. a. Normal with a shift toward metabolic acidosis
   b. Respiratory acidosis
   c. Mixed acidosis
   d. Normal
   e. Respiratory acidosis

2. a. Metabolic acidosis—late decelerations, absent STV, and decreased LTV
   b. Normal gases—moderate LTV, present STV and accelerations

3. a. Administer O_2 per mask at 10 to 12 L per minute.
   b. Place the mother in the lateral position.
   c. Give bolus of IV fluids.
   d. Notify the provider (also consider discontinuation of Pitocin if infusing).

4. In the tissues

5. Variable decelerations with the loss of one shoulder

6. Absent STV

7. Hypoxia (i.e., insufficient oxygen supply to the fetus)

8. CO_2 buildup

9. A shift toward acidosis means that the pH is normal but other characteristics are present that are associated with developing acidosis. Compensation is possible at this time because reserve is present; however, the body is utilizing necessary resources to maintain a normal pH.

10. 1. h
    2. g
    3. b
    4. d
    5. e
    6. c
    7. f
    8. a

11. The pH of the blood and tissues has an impact on all enzymes and proteins in the body, affecting tissue, enzyme, and organ function.

12. a. Auscultation with a fetoscope
    b. ECG

13. ECG

14. B

15. Premature atrial contractions (PACs). They are usually benign and require no intervention.

P A R T   5

Documentation

OBJECTIVES

As you complete Part 5 of this module, you will learn:

1. Rationale for documentation on the monitor strip
2. Essential information that must be documented on the strip
3. Information that should be documented on the patient chart
4. Rationale for maintaining a current knowledge base related to fetal monitoring

Documentation[38,49]

■ What information *must* be charted on the monitor strip?

The fetal monitor strip is a permanent part of the mother's medical record, and like any other legal document, it can be used as evidence in malpractice suits. In fact, fetal injury suits can be instituted and strips used as evidence up to the time the fetus reaches adulthood. Therefore, pertinent, precise information must be noted on the strip, preferably at the time of assessment or intervention. When an emergency arises and it is not possible to formally chart, interventions and assessments are written on the strip at the time they occur. Following the resolution of the emergency, this information may be transcribed and documented in detail, following an accurate time line, on the patient chart. Data charted on the monitor strip and on the chart demonstrate that health care providers have been assessing, interpreting, and acting on these findings on a regular basis throughout the course of labor. In turn, *if no supporting data or interventions are recorded on the strip, it is assumed that no action was taken.* In other words, **if it is not documented, it was not done.** Inaccurate or missing information can present serious legal consequences and ethical dilemmas.

■ What information *should* be charted on the monitor strip?

The fetal monitor strip must provide a well-documented picture of a woman's labor course, from admission through delivery of the newborn (Fig. 6.72).

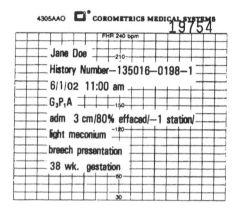

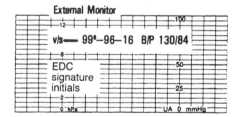

FIGURE 6.72 Identifying information noted on the fetal monitor strip.

The following information should be included on the monitor strip:
- **Identifying information about the woman** (Display 6.2)—Several monitor companies provide gummed labels that list information topics and provide space for recording the information. This assists in ensuring that a complete database is obtained and documented at admission. Many monitoring systems today are computer based, so data may be entered directly on the strip by means of a keyboard.
- **Change in monitor mode**—Any time a change in monitor mode is made, that change must be noted on the strip. If a change is made from external to internal monitoring or vice versa, the notation may simply read "external monitor applied" or "internal monitor applied." However, if a combination of external and internal monitoring is used, the specific parts of each type of monitor should be listed, such as FSE and tocodynamometer

or Doppler and pressure catheter. Identifying the method of monitoring provides the reviewer with information required to make an accurate and thorough assessment of fetal status and uterine activity. Most newer machines automatically print the mode when it changes and at regular intervals thereafter (Fig. 6.73).

| **DISPLAY 6.2** | Identifying Information About the Laboring Woman to Be Entered on the Strip |

Name, history and patient number

Gravidity and parity

Gestational age of fetus at admission and estimated date of confinement status at admission—This information includes cervical dilatation; effacement and station; status of amniotic membranes; if membranes are ruptured, include when rupture occurred, character of rupture (leak or gush), color, consistency, and odor of fluid. Admission vital signs should also be noted on the strip graph.

Presence of complications—Information including abnormal presentations, significant medical history, meconium-stained fluid, or other complications should be noted on the strip graph.

Date and time monitor applied

Monitoring method used (newer monitors automatically print the current mode of monitoring)

Signature and initials of the person applying the monitor

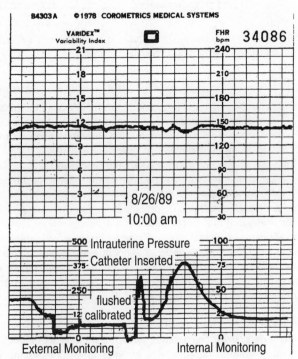

FIGURE 6.73 Changes in monitor mode should be noted on the strip.

- **Test of internal circuitry**—This should be performed before initiating the use of EFM and should be documented in the nursing notes.
- **Vital signs**—Any time vital signs are obtained, regardless of whether they are routine or emergent, they must be documented on both the strip and the labor record (Fig. 6.74). Current maternal vital signs placed directly on the strip often provide clues to the origin of changes in FHR pattern. Two examples of vital signs are as follows:
  –Maternal hyperthermia and related fetal tachycardia
  –Maternal hypotension resulting in late decelerations

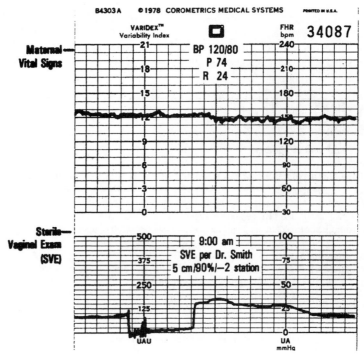

FIGURE 6.74 By identifying the association between vital signs and fetal heart rate, measures can be implemented to treat causative factors.

- **Vaginal examinations**—All vaginal examinations, treatments, and findings should be documented. These examinations provide information related to the progress or status of labor and the assessment of fetal status and/or the basis for a nonreassuring baseline pattern or onset of decelerations. Examples include the following:
  –Checking for a prolapsed cord following variable decelerations
  –Performing scalp stimulation following a bradycardic episode or prolonged deceleration
  –Assessing for station following the onset of early decelerations
  –Determining scalp pH, sampling amniotic fluid, or performing amnioinfusion
- **Treatment for abnormal heart rate patterns**—*All* interventions in the treatment of abnormal heart rate patterns, as they are performed, *must* be noted on the strip (Fig. 6.75). Failure to document these actions means that nothing was done to correct or relieve stress-causing factors affecting the fetus or mother. In the event of poor fetal or maternal outcome, there is no defense because there is no evidence of any treatment measures. (Refer to Part 3 of this module for treatment of nonreassuring periodic changes in the FHR.)
- **Administration of medications and IV fluids**—All drugs administered during labor must be charted on the strip. The notation on the strip graph should include the drug or fluid name, route of administration, rate (if given by infusion pump this must also be charted), dosage, and time given. When drugs are administered throughout labor, such as Pitocin, Apresoline, or ritodrine, *each change in the dosage* must be charted on the strip. The administration of anesthetic agents, such as medications used in epidural anesthesia, must also be noted on the strip.
- **Occurrences causing an alteration in the strip tracing**—Many occurrences can momentarily alter or cause the loss of a tracing, especially when using an external monitor. These occurrences include maternal vomiting, restlessness, or sitting on the bedpan; such occurrences can affect not only the quality of the FHR tracing but the uterine activity graph as well (Fig. 6.76). A belt that is too loose or too tight can also alter the uterine activity graph. The cause of the tracing alteration should be noted on the strip graph.
- **Delivery information** (Display 6.3 and Fig. 6.77)—Some monitor companies provide gummed labels with printed delivery information and space for recording that information.

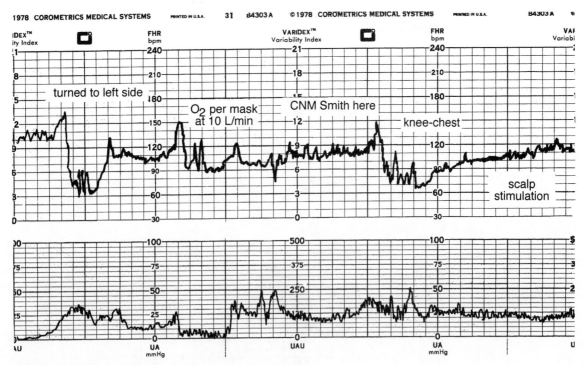

FIGURE 6.75 Documentation for abnormal fetal heart rate pattern.

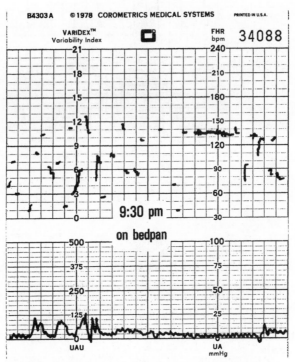

FIGURE 6.76 Placing a laboring woman on the bedpan can cause the fetal heart rate to be lost or distorted.

DISPLAY 6.3	Delivery Information to Be Entered on the Strip

Date and time of delivery
Type of delivery (e.g., spontaneous, low forceps, breech)
Sex and birth weight
Apgar score and cord gases
Presence of delivery complications:
- Abnormal presentations
- Nuchal cord
- Shoulder dystocia
- Placental condition (e.g., infarcts, calcification)
- True knot in the cord
- Anesthesia and kind, if used

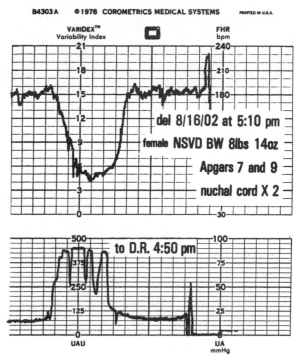

FIGURE 6.77 Delivery information, including complications, should be noted at the end of the laboring woman's strip.

- **Initialing of the strip**—When the strip is evaluated or interventions are done, the strip should be initialed by the person performing the evaluation or interventions. Policies regarding charting and assessment should include a notation in the form of initialing the strip as evidence that strip review and assessment was performed at regular intervals.

NEVER CALL ATTENTION TO A NONREASSURING FHR PATTERN OR A UTERINE ACTIVITY ABNORMALITY ON THE STRIP BY:

- Circling an abnormal event
- Writing a fetal heart pattern or uterine activity diagnosis on the strip

A monitor tracing that is unreadable has little value in determining fetal or maternal status (Fig. 6.78). To obtain a better tracing, change the location of the external Doppler and tocodynamometer. Make sure the internal water-filled pressure catheter is flushed and calibrated and the FSE is still attached. If the FHR tracing is temporarily lost, chart on the strip the rate obtained by using a fetoscope.

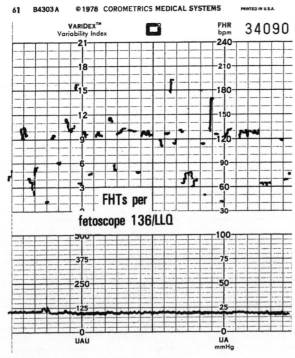

FIGURE 6.78 Unreadable tracing.

General Guidelines for Institutional Documentation and Continuing Education

- Use uniform terminology based on national standards and definitions to describe FHR patterns and uterine activity. This ensures that communications are clearly understood.
- Follow written guidelines for documentation. Formulate institutional guidelines with respect to meeting national standards.
- Ensure that *all caregivers and providers* are current in their knowledge of standards, terminology, and interpretation of fetal monitoring by requiring competency validation at set intervals and by providing resources and opportunities for both formal and informal continuing education.
- Encourage staff consultation of nonreassuring and/or questionable patterns. Document these consultations. Good documentation is the best defense available for all staff members if a lawsuit occurs. Make sure correct terminology is used and that it represents a thorough accounting of what occurred during labor, delivery, and recovery.

PRACTICE/REVIEW QUESTIONS
After reviewing Part 5, answer the following questions.

1. Why is it necessary to write information on the strip? _____

_____

_____

2. List some of the kinds of information that should be included on the strip.

    a. _____

    b. _____

    c. _____

    d. _____

    e. _____

    f. _____

    g. _____

    h. _____

3. What should never be documented on a strip?

    _____

    _____

    _____

4. Why is initialing of the strip recommended?

    _____

    _____

    _____

5. Why is documentation on the strip during emergency situations important?

    _____

    _____

    _____

PRACTICE/REVIEW ANSWER KEY

1. The graph is a permanent part of the mother's medical record. Also, data on the strip ensure that health care providers are reading, interpreting, and utilizing the tracing in planning care and interventions for the patient in labor.

2. a. Identifying information
   b. Change in type of monitor
   c. Routine vital signs
   d. Findings of vaginal examinations
   e. Treatment of abnormal heart rate patterns
   f. Medications given
   g. Occurrences that can alter the tracing
   h. Delivery information

3. Never call attention to a nonreassuring FHR pattern or a uterine activity abnormality on the strip by circling an abnormal event or writing a fetal heart pattern or uterine activity diagnosis on the strip.

4. Initialing the strip is important in determining who reviewed the strip and to ensure that it was reviewed on a regular basis.

5. When an emergency arises and it is not possible to formally chart, interventions and assessments are written on the strip at the time they occur. Following the resolution of the emergency, this information may be transcribed and documented in detail, following an accurate time line, on the patient chart.

Practice With Strip Graph Interpretation

For each of the strip graphs presented, you should be able to:

1. Determine the baseline fetal heart rate and evaluate variability
2. Determine frequency, duration, and intensity of the contraction patterns
3. Determine the baseline tonus of the uterus
4. Correctly identify any periodic heart rate patterns
5. Describe the appropriate treatment for any abnormal tracings
6. Estimate cord gases

For each strip represented, answer the set of questions following the strip. **The monitoring mode for both FHR and contractions is internal unless otherwise stated.**

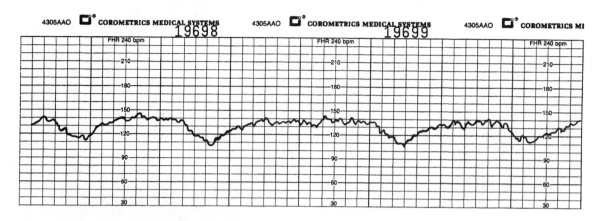

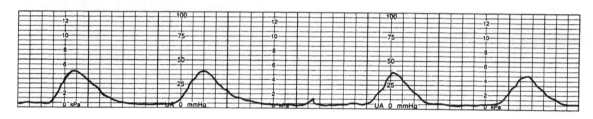

FIGURE 6.79 Practice strip 1.

1. What is the baseline FHR? _____

   Is it within normal limits? _____

2. Describe frequency, duration, and intensity of the contraction pattern.

   Frequency: _____

   Duration: _____

   Intensity: _____

   Is the contraction pattern within normal limits? _____

3. What is the baseline tonus of the uterus? _____

   Is the tonus within normal limits? _____

4. What is the heart rate variability? _____

   Is the variability considered:

   A. Decreased

   B. Normal

   C. Increased

   D. Unable to be assessed

5. Are any periodic or nonperiodic changes present? _____ If so, are they:

   A. Accelerations

   B. Early decelerations

   C. Variable decelerations

D. Late decelerations

E. Prolonged deceleration

6. Based on your interpretation of **practice strip 1,** what treatment, if any, would you administer?

_____

_____

7. Estimate blood gas results, if done at this time. (Acidemia? What kind? Shift? Normal?)

_____

_____

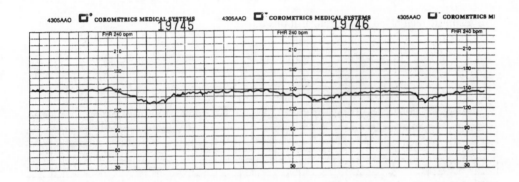

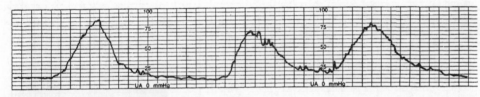

FIGURE 6.80 Practice strip 2.

1. What is the baseline FHR? _____

   Is it within normal limits? _____

2. Describe frequency, duration, and intensity of the contraction pattern.

   Frequency: _____

   Duration: _____

   Intensity: _____

   Is the contraction pattern within normal limits? _____

3. What is the baseline tonus of the uterus? _____

   Is the tonus within normal limits? _____

4. What is the heart rate variability? _____

   Is the variability considered:

   A. Decreased

   B. Normal

   C. Increased

   D. Unable to be assessed

5. Are any periodic changes present? _____ If so, are they:

    A. Accelerations

    B. Early decelerations

    C. Variable decelerations

    D. Late decelerations

    E. Prolonged deceleration

6. Based on your interpretation of **practice strip 2,** what treatment, if any, would you administer?

_____

_____

7. Estimate fetal blood gases, if done at this time.

_____

_____

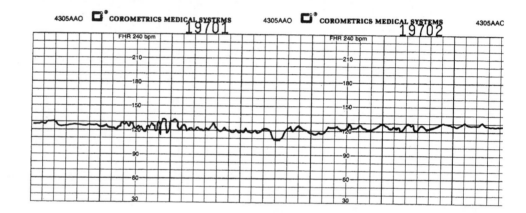

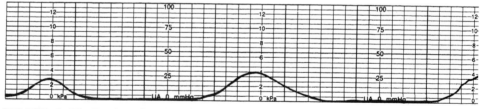

FIGURE 6.81 Practice strip 3.

1. What is the baseline FHR? _____

    Is it within normal limits? _____

2. Describe frequency, duration, and intensity of the contraction pattern.

    Frequency: _____

    Duration: _____

    Intensity: _____

    Is the contraction pattern within normal limits? _____

3. What is the baseline tonus of the uterus? _____

   Is the tonus within normal limits? _____

4. What is the heart rate variability? _____

   Is the variability considered:

   A. Decreased

   B. Normal

   C. Increased

   D. Unable to be assessed

5. Are any periodic or nonperiodic changes present? _____ If so, are they:

   A. Accelerations

   B. Early decelerations

   C. Variable decelerations

   D. Late decelerations

   E. Prolonged deceleration

6. Based on your interpretation of **practice strip 3,** what treatment, if any, would you administer?

   _____

   _____

7. Estimate fetal blood gases, if done at this time.

   _____

   _____

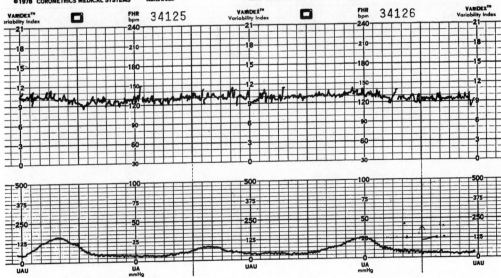

FIGURE 6.82 Practice strip 4.

1. What is the baseline FHR? _____

   Is it within normal limits? _____

2. Describe frequency, duration, and intensity of the contraction pattern.

   Frequency: _____

   Duration: _____

   Intensity: _____

   Is the contraction pattern within normal limits? _____

3. What is the baseline tonus of the uterus? _____

   Is the tonus within normal limits? _____

4. What is the heart rate variability? _____

   Is the variability considered:

   A. Decreased

   B. Normal

   C. Increased

   D. Unable to be assessed

5. Are any periodic or nonperiodic changes present? _____ If so, are they:

   A. Accelerations

   B. Early decelerations

   C. Variable decelerations

   D. Late decelerations

   E. Prolonged deceleration

6. Based on your interpretation of **practice strip 4,** what treatment, if any, would you administer?

   _____

   _____

7. Estimate fetal blood gases, if done at this time.

   _____

   _____

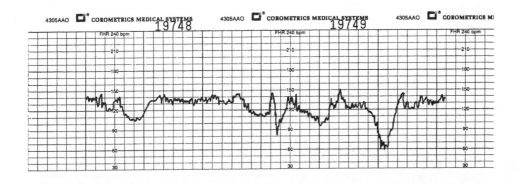

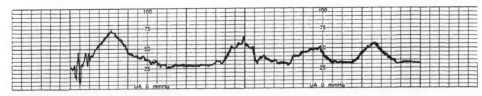

FIGURE 6.83. **Practice strip 5.**

1. What is the baseline FHR? _____
   Is it within normal limits? _____

2. Describe frequency, duration, and intensity of the contraction pattern.
   Frequency: _____
   Duration: _____
   Intensity: _____
   Is the contraction pattern within normal limits? _____

3. What is the baseline tonus of the uterus? _____
   Is the tonus within normal limits? _____

4. What is the heart rate variability? _____
   Is the variability considered:
   A. Decreased
   B. Normal
   C. Increased
   D. Unable to be assessed

5. Are any periodic or nonperiodic changes present? _____ If so, are they:
   A. Accelerations
   B. Early decelerations
   C. Variable decelerations
   D. Late decelerations
   E. Prolonged deceleration

6. Based on your interpretation of **practice strip 5,** what treatment, if any, would you administer?

_____

_____

7. Estimate fetal blood gases, if done at this time.

_____

_____

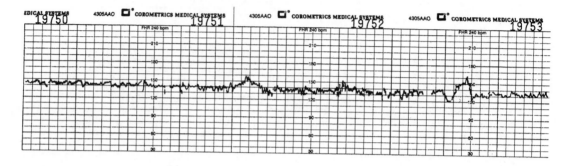

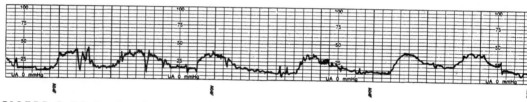

FIGURE 6.84 Practice strip 6.

1. What is the baseline FHR? _____

   Is it within normal limits? _____

2. Describe frequency, duration, and intensity of the contraction pattern.

   Frequency: _____

   Duration: _____

   Intensity: _____

   Is the contraction pattern within normal limits? _____

3. What is the baseline tonus of the uterus? _____

   Is the tonus within normal limits? _____

4. What is the heart rate variability? _____

   Is the variability considered:

   A. Decreased

   B. Normal

   C. Increased

   D. Unable to be assessed

5. Are any periodic or nonperiodic changes present? _____ If so, are they:

   A. Accelerations

B. Early decelerations

C. Variable decelerations

D. Late decelerations

E. Prolonged deceleration

6. Based on your interpretation of **practice strip 6,** what treatment, if any, would you administer?

_____

_____

7. Estimate fetal acid-base status at this time.

_____

_____

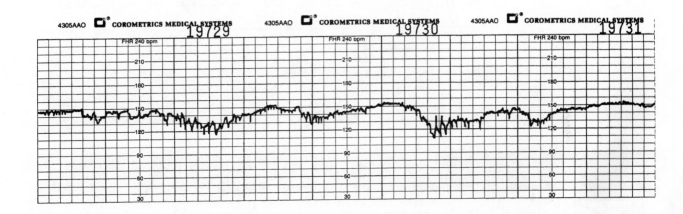

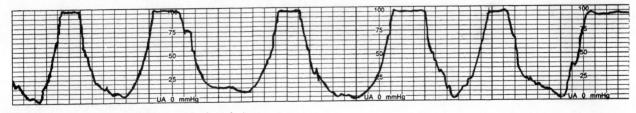

FIGURE 6.85 Practice strip 7 (external monitor).

1. What is the baseline FHR? _____

   Is it within normal limits? _____

2. Describe frequency, duration, and intensity of the contraction pattern.

   Frequency: _____

   Duration: _____

   Intensity: _____

   Is the contraction pattern within normal limits? _____

3. What is the baseline tonus of the uterus? _____

   Is the tonus within normal limits? _____

4. What is the heart rate variability? _____

Is the variability considered:

A. Decreased

B. Normal

C. Increased

D. Unable to be assessed

5. Are any periodic or nonperiodic changes present? _____ If so, are they:

A. Accelerations

B. Early decelerations

C. Variable decelerations

D. Late decelerations

E. Prolonged deceleration

6. Based on your interpretation of **practice strip 7,** what treatment, if any, would you administer?

_____

_____

7. Estimate fetal acid-base status at this time.

_____

_____

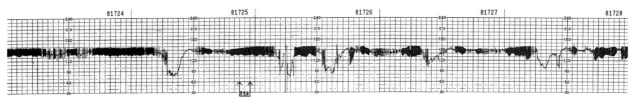

F I G U R E 6 . 8 6 **Practice strip 8** (external monitor).

1. What is the baseline FHR? _____

   Is it within normal limits? _____

2. What is the heart rate variability? _____

   Is the variability considered:

   A. Decreased

   B. Normal

   C. Increased

   D. Unable to be assessed and why

3. Are any periodic or nonperiodic changes present? _____ If so, are they:

   A. Accelerations

   B. Early decelerations

   C. Variable decelerations

   D. Late decelerations

   E. Prolonged decelerations

4. Based on your interpretation of **practice strip 7,** what treatment, if any, would you administer?

_____

_____

5. Estimate fetal acid-base status at this time.

_____

_____

6. What do you think is happening in this strip? How would you confirm this?

_____

_____

PRACTICE STRIP REVIEW ANSWER KEY

Practice Strip 1
1. 130 to 140 bpm
   Yes

2. Frequency: 2 to 3 minutes
   Duration: 50 to 60 seconds
   Intensity: 35 to 40 mm Hg
   Yes

3. 3 to 5 mm Hg
   Yes

4. 5 to 10 bpm; present STV and moderate LTV
   B

5. Yes
   B

6. No treatment is necessary. May consider a vaginal examination if this is a new pattern, if it has become more pronounced, or if the woman feels vaginal or perineal pressure, because fetal descent might be occurring. Continue to watch tracing.

7. Within normal limits

Practice Strip 2
1. 146 to 150 bpm
   Yes

2. Frequency: 2 to 3 minutes
   Duration: 70 to 90 seconds
   Intensity: 70 to 85 mm Hg
   Yes

3. 10 to 20 mm Hg
   Yes

4. 0 to 2 bpm; absent STV and decreased LTV
   A

5. Yes
   D

6. Start oxygen therapy per face mask at 10 L per minute. Turn woman to the lateral position. Administer a bolus of IV fluids. Turn off Pitocin, if on. Notify primary care provider.

7. Metabolic acidosis

Practice Strip 3
1. 120 to 130 bpm
   Yes

2. Frequency: 3 to 31/2 minutes
   Duration: 60 to 90 seconds
   Intensity: 20 to 30 mm Hg
   Yes

3. 0 mm Hg
   No; below lower limit (calibrate or replace pressure catheter)

4. Absent STV, decreased LTV
   A

5. No
   Not applicable

6. Look for cause of decreased variability—medications, etc. Change maternal position to the side-lying. Perform scalp stimulation—watch for acceleration. If no cause can be isolated and variability does not improve with these interventions, begin oxygen therapy per face mask at 10 L per minute and notify primary care provider.

7. Within normal limits but shift toward metabolic acidosis

Practice Strip 4
1. 120 to 135 bpm
   Yes

2. Frequency: 21/2 minutes
   Duration: 70 to 80 seconds
   Intensity: 18 to 37 mm Hg
   Yes

3. 5 to 10 mm Hg
   Yes

4. Present STV and decreased LTV
   B—in general

5. No
   Not applicable

6. Possibly VE to stimulate fetus for better assessment

7. Within normal limits

Practice Strip 5

1. 128 to 145 bpm
   Yes

2. Frequency: 1 to 2^1/$_2$ minutes
   Duration: 50 to 70 seconds
   Intensity: 65 to 70 mm Hg
   No; hyperstimulation, last three contractions occur too frequently

3. 25 to 30 mm Hg
   No; tone is increased, hypertonus

4. Present STV, decreased LTV
   B

5. Yes
   C

6. Change position (preferably to the side to attempt to alleviate pressure on the cord, improve perfusion, and decrease contraction frequency). Begin oxygen therapy per face mask at 10 L per minute. Discontinue Pitocin, if infusing, to decrease frequency of contraction pattern and to decrease baseline uterine tone. Notify primary care provider. Perform vaginal examination to assess for cord prolapse. Administer a bolus of IV fluids.

7. Progression to respiratory acidosis; loss of preshoulder with the last deceleration

Practice Strip 6

1. 125 to 148 bpm
   Yes

2. Frequency: 1 to 2 minutes
   Duration: 50 to 80 seconds
   Intensity: 35 to 40 mm Hg
   No; contractions too frequent, hyperstimulation

3. 10 to 20 mm Hg
   Yes

4. Present STV decreased LTV
   B

5. No, increases in FHT do not meet the 15 × 15 criteria

6. No treatment is necessary at this point for fetal heart pattern; however, that could quickly change if this contraction pattern continues. Discontinue Pitocin. Turn the patient to her side to increase CO, improve uterine perfusion, and decrease the frequency of contractions. Notify the primary care provider.

7. Normal cord pH

Practice Strip 7

1. 145 to 155 bpm
   Yes

2. Frequency: 80 to 110 seconds
   Duration: 70 to 90 seconds
   Intensity: cannot interpret without palpating fundus
   No; most of the contractions are too frequent

3. Cannot interpret on external monitor
   Cannot interpret

4. LTV decreased; STV cannot be interpreted with the external monitor
   Cannot interpret completely; certainly decreased LTV

5. Yes
   Probably B, but is somewhat difficult to assess

6. No treatment for diagnosis of early decelerations. Consider vaginal examination for assessment of labor progress. Early decelerations and flattening at the top of contractions can indicate fetal descent and pushing. If labor is early or progress is abnormal, consider applying an internal monitor to more accurately assess contraction strength and FHR pattern.

7. Normal cord gases (pH)

Practice Strip 8

1. Difficult to determine based on this strip, appears to be within normal range, at approximately 150 bpm.
   Yes

2. D; unable to assess because there is almost no portion of the strip that is free of "hatch marks," so variability cannot be assessed.

3. C

4. Auscultate with a fetoscope, reposition to promote fetal oxygenation, and notify the primary care provider.

5. Variable decelerations with loss of shoulders and respiratory acidosis; however, because variability cannot be assessed, there is a potential for problems with hypoxia metabolic acidosis and respiratory acidosis.

6. Fetal cardiac dysrhythmia
   Auscultate with a fetoscope and/or obtain a fetal ECG.

REFERENCES

1. American College of Obstetricians and Gynecologists (ACOG). (1995). *Fetal heart rate patterns: Monitoring, interpretation, and management.* ACOG Technical Bulletin No. 207. Washington, DC: Author.
2. Society of Obstetricians and Gynecologists of Canada (SOGC). (1995). Fetal surveillance in labor. SOGC Policy Statement. *Journal of SOGC, 17,* 865–901.
3. Nurses Association of the American College of Obstetricians and Gynecologists (NACOG). (1990). *Fetal heart auscultation. OGN Nursing Practice Resource.* Washington, DC: Author.
4. Feinstein, N. F., & McCartney, P. (Eds.). For the Association of Women's Health, Obstetric and Neonatal Nurses (AWHONN). (1997). *Fetal heart monitoring principles and practices* (2nd ed.). Dubuque, IO: Kendall/Hunt Publishing.
5. American College of Obstetricians and Gynecologists (ACOG). (1995). Induction of labor. Technical Bulletin No. 217. Washington, DC: Author.
6. Association of Women's Health, Obstetric and Neonatal Nurses. (1997). *Fetal heart monitoring principles and practices* (2nd ed.). Dubuque, IA: Kendall Hunt.

7. Neilson, J. P. (1994). Electronic fetal heart rate monitoring during labour: Information from randomized trials. *Birth, 21,* 101–104.

8. Paine, L. L., Benedict, M. I., Strobino, D. M., Gregor, C. L., & Larsen, E. C. (1992). A comparison of the auscultated acceleration test and the non stress test as predictors of perinatal outcomes. *Nursing Research, 41,* 87–91.

9. Rosen, M., & Dickenson, J. (1993). The paradox of electronic monitoring: More data may not enable us to predict or prevent infant neurologic morbidity. *American Journal of Obstetrics and Gynecology, 76,* 812–816.

10. Zuspan, F. P., Quilligan, E. J., Ians, J. D., & Van Geign, H. P. (1999). National Institute of Child Health and Human Development (NICHD) Consensus Development Task Force report: Predictors of intrapartum fetal distress—The role of electronic fetal monitoring. *The Journal of Pediatrics, 95*(6), 1026–1030.

11. Parer, J. T. (1997). *Handbook of fetal heart rate monitoring.* Philadelphia: WB Saunders.

12. National Institute of Child Health and Human Development (NICHD) Research Planning Workshop. (1999). Electronic fetal heart rate monitoring: Research guidelines for interpretation. *American Journal of Obstetrics and Gynecology,177,* 1385–1390.

13. Haggerty, L. A. (1999, July/August). Continuous electronic fetal monitoring: Contradictions between practice and research. *Journal of Obstetric, Gynecologic, and Neonatal Nursing, 28*(4), 409–416.

14. National Institute of Child Health and Human Development (NICHD) Research Planning Workshop. (1999). Electronic fetal heart rate monitoring: Research guidelines for interpretation. *Journal of Obstetric, Gynecologic and Neonatal Nursing, 26,* 635–640.

15. Vintzileos, A. M., Nochimson, D. J., Antsaklis, A., Varvarigos, I., Guzman, E. R., & Knuppel, R. A. (1995). Comparison of electronic fetal monitoring versus intermittent auscultation: A meta-analysis. *Obstetrics and Gynecology, 85,* 149–155.

16. Hodnett, E. (1997). Support from caregivers during childbirth (Cochrane Review). In *The Cochrane Library,* Issue 2. Oxford: Update Software.

17. Albers, L.L. (1994). Clinical issues in electronic fetal monitoring. *Birth, 21,* 108–110.

18. Thacker, S. B., & Stroup, D. F. Continuous electronic fetal monitoring for assessment during labor. (*Cochrane Review*). In: The Cochrane Library Issue 2, 2000. Oxford: Update Software.

19. Kennell, J., Klauss, M., McGrath, S., Robertson, S., & Hinckley, C. (1991, May). Continuous emotional support during labor in a U.S. hospital: A randomized controlled trial. *Journal of the American Medical Association, 265*(17), 2197–2201.

20. Parer, J., & King, T. (2000). Fetal heart rate monitoring: Is it salvageable? *American Journal of Obstetrics and Gynecology, 182,* 282–287.

21. McRae, M. J. (1999). Fetal surveillance and monitoring: legal issues revisited. *Journal of Obstetric, Gynecologic, and Neonatal Nursing, 28*(3), 310–319.

22. Umstad, M. P., Permezel, M., & Pepperell, R. J. (1995). Litigation and the intrapartum cardiotocograph. *British Journal of Obstetrics and Gynaecology, 102,* 89–91.

23. Schrifrin, B. S. (Ed.) (1993). Fetal surveillance during labor: The role of the expert witness. *Journal of Perinatology, 13*(2), 151–152.

24. Schrifrin, B. S., Weissman, H., & Wiley, J. (1985, June). Electronic fetal monitoring obstetrical malpractice. *Law, Medicine and Health Care, 13,* 100–105.

25. Feinstein, N. F., Sprague, A., & Tre'panier, M. J. (2000). *Fetal heart rate auscultation.* Washington, DC: Association of Women's Health, Obstetric and Neonatal Nurses.

26. Murray, M. L., & Urbanski, P. (2000). *Essentials of fetal monitoring.* Albuquerque: Learning Resources International.

27. Murray, M. (1997). *Antepartal and intrapartal fetal monitoring* (2nd ed.). Albuquerque: Learning Resources International.

28. Menihan, C. A., & Zottoli, E. K. (2001). *Electronic fetal monitoring, concepts and applications.* Philadelphia: Lippincott.

29. Wagener, M. M., Rycheck, R. R., Yee, R. B., McVaay, J. F., Buffenmyer, C. L., & Harger, J. H. (1984, July). Septic dermatitis of the neonate, and maternal endometritis with intrapartum internal fetal monitoring. *Pediatrics, 74*(1), 81–85.

30. Overturf, G. D., & Balfour, G. (1975, February). Osteomyelitis and sepsis: Severe complications of fetal monitoring, *Pediatrics, 55*(2), 244–247.

31. Tourmaine, M., Sturbeis, G., Zorn, J. R., Breart, G., & Sureace, C. (1980). Fetal monitoring before and during labor. In S. Aladjem, A. K. Brown, & C. Sureau (Eds.), *Clinical perinatology* (pp. 146–156). St. Louis: Mosby.

32. Rudolf, A. M. (1998). Circulation in the fetal-placental unit. In R. M. Crowlett (Ed.), *Principles and of perinatal-neonatal metabolism* (2nd ed., pp. 851–485). New York: Springer.

33. Ries, E., Gabbe, S., & Petrie, R. (1999). Intrapartum evaluation. In S. Gabbe, J. Niebyl, & J. L. Simpson (Eds.), *Obstetrics: Normal and problem pregnancies* (pp. 397–421). New York: Churchill Livingstone.

34. Cunningham, F. G., Gant, N. F., Leveno, K. J., Gilstrap, L. C., Hauth, J. C., & Wenstrom, K. D. (2001). *Williams obstetrics* (21st ed.). New York: McGraw-Hill.

35. Cibils, L. A. (1979, December 15). Clinical significance in fetal heart rate patterns during labor. *American Journal of Obstetrics and Gynecology, 169*(1), 113–115.

36. O'Brien-Abal, N. E., & Benedetti, T. J. (1992). Saltatory fetal heart rate pattern. *Journal of Perinatology, 12*(1), 13–17.

37. Penning, S., & Garite, T. J. (1999, June). Management of fetal distress. *Obstetrics and Gynecology Clinics of North America, 26*(2), 259–274.

38. Association of Women's Health, Obstetric and Neonatal Nurses. (1998). *Clinical competencies and education guide. Antepartal and intrapartal fetal surveillance.* Washington, DC: Author.

39. Freeman, R. K., Garite, T. J., & Nagrotte, M. P. (1991). *Fetal heart rate monitoring* (2nd ed.). Baltimore: Williams & Wilkins.

40. Parer, J. (1999). Fetal heart rate. In R. K. Creasy & R. Resnik (Eds.), *Maternal fetal medicine: Principles and practice* (4th ed., p. 314). Philadelphia: WB Saunders.

41. Elliot, J. P., Castro, R. J., & O'Keefe, D. F. (1988, July 1). Sinusoidal fetal heart rate associated with gastroschisis. *American Journal of Perinatology, 5*(3), 295–296.

42. Sherer, D. M., D'Amico, M. L., Arnold, C., Ron, M., & Abramowicz, J. S. (1993, July). Physiology of isolated long-term variability of the fetal heart rate. *American Journal of Obstetrics and Gynecology, 169*(1), 113–115.

43. Gimovsky, M. L., & Bruce, S. L. (1986, March). Aspects of fetal heart rate tracing as warning signals. *Clinical Obstetrics and Gynecology, 29*(1), 51–63.

44. Schrifrin, B. (1990). *Exercises in fetal monitoring.* St. Louis: Mosby.

45. Gilstrap, L. (1999). Fetal acid-base balance. In R. K. Creasy & R. Resnik (Eds.), *Maternal-fetal medicine* (4th ed., pp. 331–340). Philadelphia: WB Saunders.

46. Copel, J. A., Friedman, A. H., & Kleinman, C. S. (1997). Management of fetal cardiac arrhythmias. *Obstetrics and Gynecology Clinics of North America, 24*(1), 201–211.

47. Clement, D., & Schrifrin, B. (1987). Diagnosis and management of fetal arrhythmias. *Perinatal/Neonatal, 11,* 9–20.

48. Copel, J., Liang, R., Demasio, K., Oozeren, S., & Kleinman, C. (2000). The clinical significance of the irregular fetal heart rhythm. *American Journal of Obstetrics and Gynecology, 182,* 813–819.

49. Association of Women's Health, Obstetric and Neonatal Nurses. (1992). *Nursing responsibilities in implementing intrapartum fetal heart rate monitoring* (Position Statement). Washington, DC: Author.

SUGGESTED READINGS

American Academy of Pediatrics and American College of Obstetricians and Gynecologists. (1997). *Guidelines for perinatal care* (4th ed.). Elk Grove Village, IL: Authors.

American College of Obstetricians and Gynecologists (ACOG). (1999). *Antepartal fetal surveillance.* Practice Bulletin No. 9. Washington, DC: Author.

Association of Women's Health, Obstetric and Neonatal Nurses (AWHONN). (1998). *Standards and guidelines for professional nursing practice in the care of women and newborns* (5th ed.). Washington: DC: Author.

Dildy, G. A. (1999). The physiologic and medical rationale for intrapartum fetal monitoring. *Biomedical Instrumentation and Technology, 33,* 143–151.

Dunster, R. K. (1999, December). Physiologic variability in the perinatal period: Origins measurement and applications. *Clinics in Perinatology, 26*(4), 801–809.

Huddleston, J. F. (1999, September). Intrapartum fetal assessment: A review. *Clinics in Perinatology, 26*(3), 549–568.

Ikeda, T., Murata, Y., Quilligan, E., Parer, J., Murayama, T., & Koono, M. (2000). Histologic and biochemical study of the brain, heart, kidney and liver in asphyxia caused by occlusion of the umbilical cord in near term fetal lambs. *American Journal of Obstetrics and Gynecology, 182*(2), 449–457.

Lindsay, M. K. (1999, September). Intrauterine resuscitation of the compromised fetus. *Clinics in Perinatology, 26*(3), 569–584.

Lowe, J. A., Victory, R., & Derrick, E. J. (1999). Predictive value of electronic fetal monitoring for intrapartum fetal asphyxia with metabolic acidosis. *Obstetrics and Gynecology, 93,* 285–291.

Schrifrin, B., & Harwal, R. (1999). FHR terminology. [Letter]. *Journal of Obstetric, Gynecologic, and Neonatal Nursing, 18*(2), 123.

Schuiling, K. D., & Sampselle, C. M. (1999). Clinical scholarship. Comfort in labor and midwifery art. *Image, 31*(1), 77–81.

Simpson, J., & Sharland, G. (1998). Fetal tachycardias: Management and outcome of 127 consecutive cases. *Heart, 79,* 576–581.

Vintzileos, A. M., Nochimson, D. J., Antsaklis, A., Varvarigos, I., Guzman, E. R., & Knuppel, R. A. (1995). Comparison of electronic fetal monitoring versus intermittent auscultation: A meta-analysis. *Obstetrics and Gynecology, 85,* 149–155.

MODULE 7

Induction and Augmentation of Labor

MARCELLA T. HICKEY

Oxytocin Labor Induction/Augmentation

OBJECTIVES

As you complete this module, you will learn:

1. Indications for labor induction/augmentation
2. A role for oxytocin in the active management of labor
3. Contraindications for labor induction/augmentation
4. Conditions necessary for the safe administration of oxytocin
5. Preinduction preparation of an "unfavorable" cervix using prostaglandins
6. To anticipate potential problems associated with the use of prostaglandins
7. The recommended method of oxytocin administration
8. To anticipate potential problems of oxytocin administration
9. The recommended nursing interventions when problems arise with the use of oxytocin or prostaglandins
10. The safe method of administering oxytocin for inducing/augmenting labor

KEY TERMS

When you have completed this module, you should be able to recall the meaning of the following terms. You should also be able to use the terms when consulting with other health professionals. The terms are defined in this module or in the glossary at the end of this book.

abruptio placentae
amniotomy
augmentation
biparietal diameter (BPD)
cephalopelvic disproportion (CPD)
chorioamnionitis
embolism
hydramnios

hyperbilirubinemia
hypertonic uterus
induction
multiple gestation
oxytocin
preinduction cervical ripening
prostaglandins
uterine dystocia

Induction and Augmentation of Labor

■ What is induction of labor?

Induction of labor is the deliberate starting of uterine contractions before they begin on their own. Several different ways of inducing labor are mentioned in this module.

■ What is augmentation of labor?

Occasionally, uterine contractions do not have the necessary power to cause cervical dilatation, effacement, or descent of the baby within a specific period of time. In this case, it is desirable to increase *(augment)* the contractions to help labor progress.

■ What is oxytocin?

Oxytocin is a hormone, normally released by the posterior pituitary gland, that causes the uterus to contract. Oxytocin can be administered to induce or augment uterine contractions in labor or postpartum. It can also stimulate the alveoli of the breast to contract, promoting milk "let down" in the postpartum period.

■ How does oxytocin function in labor?

Oxytocin increases free intracellular calcium, which is vital for smooth muscle activity. Within the uterine myometrium, the oxytocin receptors increase throughout pregnancy and labor. Gabbe reported the distribution of the receptor sites is greatest in the fundus and least in the cervix.[1] The increased number of sites is facilitated by an increase of estrogen as progesterone levels decrease. There is also an increase in prostaglandin. These processes contribute to the ripening of the cervix.[2]

■ What is the half-life of oxytocin?

The pharmacokinetic half-life of oxytocin is 10 to 15 minutes. *Three to five times the 10 to 15 minutes is needed to reach a steady-state concentration.* However, Poziac reports on several studies that demonstrate 40 minutes as the more realistic point for achieving a steady state.[2] **By delaying the increase from one level to the next, less hyperstimulation and fetal distress occur and an overall lower amount of oxytocin (Pitocin) is needed to achieve an active progressing labor.[2]**

■ How can labor be induced or augmented?

Common methods of inducing or augmenting labor include the following:

- **Amniotomy**—This is when the membranes are deliberately ruptured.

> Amniotomy is often done when the cervix is effaced and slightly dilated. The head of the fetus should be against the lower uterine segment and at least dipping into the pelvis. Rupturing membranes can cause the uterus to begin contracting, especially if the cervix is favorable.

- **Use of oxytocin infusion**—The intravenous (IV) administration of oxytocin will stimulate the smooth muscle of the myometrium of the uterus to contract. Because this often causes contractions that are more powerful than normal, the rate of oxytocin administration must be controlled carefully.
- **Nipple stimulation**—When the woman stimulates her nipples, oxytocin is released, causing the uterus to contract. Overstimulation of the uterus can result, however, so the contractions should be monitored closely.
- **Ambulation**—Mild or ineffective uterine contractions often can be stimulated by walking. In the upright position, pressure from the presenting part is maintained against the cervix and contractions become more efficient.
- **Prostaglandins**—In other countries, prostaglandin suppositories, gel, or tablets can be inserted into the cervix or vagina to induce labor. In the United States, prostaglandin E_2 (PGE_2) is commercially available and approved by the Food and Drug Administration (FDA) for use in the gel form and as vaginal inserts. PGE_2 gel (dinoprostone cervical gel) is marketed under the trade name of Prepidil Gel. PGE_2 vaginal insert (dinoprostone

vaginal insert) is marketed as Cervidil Vaginal Insert for placement in the posterior fornix of the vagina. Both are specifically approved for softening (to "ripen") the cervical tissue. This action makes the tissue more favorable for labor. It can also stimulate the muscles of the myometrium of the uterus, producing uterine contractions. Another form of prostaglandin—misoprostol, an E_1 analog—is being used as ripening agent. It is produced by Searle as Cytotec and is available in 100-μg tablets.[3] This use is not currently approved by the FDA.

The American College of Obstetricians and Gynecologists (ACOG) Committee on Obstetric Practice responded to Searle's warning about the use of misoprostol for cervical ripening. It recognizes that there are potential problems associated with the use of misoprostol in this manner. It also points to the published reports describing its safety and efficacy when used appropriately.[4]

Wing, in a review of published studies, noted that "most trials fail to demonstrate a significant change in the cesarean delivery rate with the use of this agent."[5] She notes that with the lower dosage of 25 μg every 4 hours, hyperstimulation is significantly decreased.

- **Stripping membranes and acupuncture**—These are other methods less commonly used to induce or augment labor.

Medical Indications for Induction/Augmentation of Labor

Indications for Induction/Augmentation of Labor

The following are situations in which induction or augmentation of labor might be necessary[6–8]:

- Vascular diseases that are life-threatening to the mother or her infant in second trimester or third trimester
- Preeclampsia (pregnancy-induced hypertension [PIH])
- Rh incompatibility
- Diabetes
- Premature rupture of membranes (PROM)
- Chorioamnionitis
- Postterm
- Biophysical profile less than 6 or oligohydramnios
- Intrauterine fetal death (induction of labor can also be accomplished by using prostaglandins)
- Uterine dystocia—usually described as poor-quality contractions that do not cause the proper cervical changes
- History of rapid labor
- The woman living a great distance from the hospital and possibly having psychosocial situations
- Prevention of prolonged labors (active management of labor)

> Initiating an induction for reasons of convenience may not be supported when evaluated in terms of risk versus benefit for maternal and neonatal outcomes. The woman needs this information to give an informed consent as recommended by the ACOG and JCAHO.[9]

■ What are the concerns for the health of the mother and fetus sometimes associated with induction/augmentation of labor?

Concerns for the mother include the following[8]:

- **Tetanic contractions**—These are powerful contractions with no rest period between contractions. Tetanic contractions can result in abruption of the placenta (abruptio placentae); rupture of the uterus; cervical tears; hypertension or stroke; postpartum hemorrhage; embolism (amniotic fluid); too-rapid birth; lacerations to the vagina, vulva, perineum, and rectum; and increased fear.

- **Water intoxication**—Oxytocin decreases the ability of the body to eliminate fluid, causing the mother to retain too much fluid (antidiuretic effect). Convulsions, coma, and death can result.

Concerns for the fetus include the following[8]:

- Fetal hypoxia (lack of oxygen)
- Fetal or newborn bradycardia (slow heartbeat)
- Injury or birth trauma
- Increased bilirubinemia *(hyperbilirubinemia)*—sometimes associated with oxytocin use

■ Can every woman be safely induced/augmented?

NO. With increased use of special monitoring equipment, safer preparation of drugs, and improved physician and nursing education, it has become a safer procedure for both mothers and babies. *However, there are many reasons why some women should NOT be induced.*

Contraindications for Induction/Augmentation of Labor

The following are examples of situations in which induction/augmentation should NEVER be done (absolute contraindications) (Display 7.1).[6,10]

DISPLAY 7.1   Contraindications to Induction/Augmentation[6]

CPD
Previous uterine surgery
Severe fetal distress
Soft tissue masses
Lack of patient willingness
Central or total placenta previa
Active genital herpes

- **Cephalopelvic disproportion (CPD)**—CPD is a condition in which the mother's pelvis is too small for the baby to pass through. The powerful labor contractions caused by induction could rupture the uterus or cause severe fetal distress.
- **Previous uterine surgery (e.g., removal of certain tumors)**—Contractions induced or augmented might be too powerful and may rupture the scar.
- **Severe fetal distress**—With each contraction of the uterus, there is a normal decrease in blood circulation and oxygen supply to the placenta and baby. Because oxytocin increases the intensity of the contractions, there can be an even greater loss of oxygen to the baby. If the fetus already shows signs of distress, it might not be able to survive the additional intensity of induced/augmented contractions.
- **Soft tissue masses (e.g., tumors, large ovarian cysts, pelvic kidneys)**—These masses might be large enough to prevent vaginal deliveries. Even though the pelvis is large enough under normal circumstances to birth the baby vaginally, labor should not be induced.
- **Lack of the woman's willingness**—In a conscious, mentally clear woman, labor should not be induced without full informed consent. Severe anxiety and tension will sometimes stop or prolong labor.
- **Central or total placenta previa**—The cervical os is completely covered by the placenta. This can be a life-threatening condition. Labor should be avoided and the fetus delivered by cesarean birth.
- **Active genital herpes infection**—In the presence of an active genital herpetic lesion, a cesarean birth is recommended to prevent neonatal herpes.

Relative Contraindications for Induction/Augmentation of Labor?

There are some situations in which induction/augmentation of labor might or might not present severe problems for mother and child (Display 7.2). These situations are known as *relative contraindications.*[6]

DISPLAY 7.2   Relative Contraindications to Induction/Augmentation[6]

Unfavorable cervix
Presenting part not engaged in pelvis
Abnormal presentation
Grandmultiparity
Multiple gestation
Hydramnios
Hypertonic or incoordinated uterus
Maternal exhaustion
Previous classic uterine incision

- **Unfavorable cervix**—Inductions are more successful when the cervix is favorable (i.e., soft, effaced greater than 50%, and dilated more than 2 cm). If the cervix is not favorable, the success rate for induction decreases. Preinduction use of prostaglandins can make the cervix more favorable for induction.
- **Presenting part not engaged in pelvis**—In this situation there is space between the presenting part and the bony pelvis. With forceful contractions, the bag of waters can rupture and the umbilical cord has room to prolapse. Also, if the presenting part is not engaged, it might indicate that the fetus is too large for the pelvis.
- **Abnormal presentation (breech, face, cord, or transverse lie)**—These presentations often indicate a small pelvis. A transverse lie presentation cannot be delivered vaginally.
- **Grandmultiparity**—In a woman who has had several children (five or more), the uterus is more likely to rupture with the powerful contractions caused by the induction/augmentation of labor.
- **Multiple gestation (e.g., twins, triplets)**—Caution must be taken to prevent overstimulation of a uterus already overly distended.
- **Hydramnios**—The uterus is overly distended and might not respond well. The possibility of an amniotic fluid embolus is increased.
- **Hypertonic or incoordinate uterus**—The uterus is contracting with too much power or does not rest between contractions (increased resting tone). The muscles of the uterus sometimes contract in an uneven rhythm. Induction/augmentation can worsen the situation.
- **Maternal exhaustion**—A relative contraindication to induction is extreme maternal fatigue. The mother should be given rest and fluids.
- **Previous cesarean delivery through a classic uterine incision**—Contractions induced or augmented might be too powerful, with subsequent rupturing of the uterine scar.

■ What is active management of labor?

Active management of labor is an augmentation protocol instituted by many institutions as a strategy to decrease cesarean births for dystocia. Its goal is to establish effective labor and delivery within 12 hours of admission. Although active management does not necessarily mean the routine use of oxytocin to augment labor progress, oxytocin is commonly used.

The term *active management of labor* is interpreted differently from one institution to another. Many of the protocols are based on the belief that **once labor had been diagnosed, the rate of cervical dilatation should be 1 cm per hour.** This rate of labor progress is actively supported by performing an amniotomy and using oxytocin, when necessary.[11]

The original protocol was developed in Dublin, Ireland, to shorten labor and conserve resources in maternity hospitals. All aspects of their protocol are not included in many U.S. hospitals. The following criteria are generally included[8]:

- Nulliparity
- More than 37 weeks' gestation
- Single fetus in no distress
- Spontaneous labor

Prerequisites for Induction/Augmentation of Labor

■ **What are some prerequisites for an induction/augmentation using oxytocin to be safe and effective?**

The woman should not have any of the contraindications for induction/augmentation.

The age (weeks of gestation) of the fetus should be accurately determined. This makes it possible to correctly anticipate the needs and management of the neonate. Methods of assessing gestational age or maturity are as follows:

- The last normal menstrual period (LNMP) and estimated date of confinement (EDC) recorded early in pregnancy.
- Initial examination before the fourteenth week reveals that there was agreement between estimated gestational age and uterine size at the time.
- Pregnancy established by successful infertility treatment.
- Establishing "quickening" (the first fetal movement perceived by the woman). It is predictable by 19 weeks' gestation in the primigravida and by approximately 17 weeks' gestation in the multipara.
- Auscultation of fetal heart tones. Sounds should be audible with the fetoscope between 16 and 18 weeks' gestation. With the electronic Doppler, sounds are audible between 12 and 14 weeks' gestation.[7]
- Ultrasound studies provide different dating information (Table 7.1).

TABLE 7.1	Ultrasound Dating Criteria
FETAL AGE	**FINDINGS**
5–7 weeks	Gestational sac volume is determined at 4 weeks; embryo seen at 4.5 weeks; fetal cardiac activity noted at 5 weeks.
6–12 weeks	Crown rump measurements—estimate error of ±3 days; biparietal diameter measurement (BPD) can be obtained at 10 weeks.
12–20 weeks	Using BPD as of 10 weeks, coupled with femur length and abdominal circumference (obtained as of 14 weeks), provides dating with a week's error for EDC.
20–32 weeks	Using BPD femur length and abdominal circumference provides dating with 1 to 1.5 weeks' possible error.
32 weeks and beyond	Using BPD, femur length, and abdominal circumference provides dating with 2.5 weeks' possible error

Data from Manning, F. A. (1999). General principles and application of ultrasound. In R. K. Creasy & R. Resnik (Eds.), *Maternal-fetal medicine* (4th ed., pp 169–202). Philadelphia: WB Saunders.

Evaluation of fetal growth pattern can be done to rule out a large-for-gestational-age (LGA) fetus, small-for-gestational-age (SGA) fetus, multiple gestation (e.g., twins, triplets), and hydramnios. Amniotic fluid studies can be done to determine the lecithin:sphingomyelin ratio and creatinine level.[6]

- The woman's health care provider must supervise the induction/augmentation and also needs to do the following:
- Have the woman examined before oxytocin is started and obtain informed consent from the woman.
- Be present when the infusion is started or ensure that a physician who has privileges to perform a cesarean section is readily available.
- Evaluate the woman and the fetal heart tones throughout the first few contractions and then regulate the infusion rate.
- Be at or near the labor unit when oxytocin is being administered.

It is the responsibility of the woman's health care provider to provide the woman with information about the procedure, answer her questions, and obtain an informed consent. In most instances, the informed consent can be expressed by oral or written words. Some hospitals have policies permitting nurses to obtain consents. See Module 16 for criteria that must be included in policies delegating this responsibility to nursing. Many hospital nurses have been prepared to assess cervical dilatation and effacement, and some hospitals have policies and guidelines enabling nurses to assume this responsibility.

■ What is a Bishop's score?

A Bishop's score is a method of evaluating how favorable or "ripe" the cervix is. A pelvic examination is done to evaluate cervical *dilatation, effacement, consistency* (i.e., softness or firmness), *and cervical position,* as well as *station* of the presenting part. The findings are scored on a scale that was developed based on studies of many women undergoing labor induction (Table 7.2). Successful inductions are more likely to occur when a woman's cervix has undergone certain changes. Based on the findings and using a scoring system for these changes, it is possible to predict which women are good candidates for labor induction.

TABLE 7.2 Bishop's Score

	SCORE[a]				
	0	**1**	**2**	**3**	**SUBTOTALS**
Dilatation (cm)	0	1–2	3–4	5–6	
Effacement (%)	0–30	40–50	60–70	80	
Station (cm)	−3	−2	−1	+1	
Cervical consistency	Firm	Medium	Soft		
Cervical position	Posterior	Midline	Anterior		
				Total	_____

[a]A multiparous woman (one who has delivered a child previously) can best be induced at a score of 5 or more. A nulliparous woman (one who has *not* delivered a child previously) can best be induced at a score of 7 or more.

Bishop developed this score based on observations of multiparous women. Over time it was applied to nulliparous women. Best outcomes for multiparous are seen with a score of 5 or more. The nulliparous woman has the best response with a score of 7 or greater.[8]

Use of Prostaglandins for Cervical Ripening

■ If the cervix is not favorable but a woman otherwise meets the criteria for induction, can PGE₂ be used to ripen the cervix?

PGE_2 (Prepidil Gel or Cervidil Vaginal Insert) is indicated for ripening (effacement, dilatation, and softening) the unfavorable cervix, at or near term, when there is a medical need for labor induction.

■ What are the potential concerns for the health of the mother and fetus when preinduction cervical ripening is achieved with PGE₂?

Concerns for the mother include the following:

- Tetanic contractions
- Gastrointestinal upset (e.g., nausea, vomiting, diarrhea)
- Fever
- Back pain
- Amnionitis
- PROM

Concerns for the fetus include the following:

- Fetal hypoxia
- Fetal heart rate abnormality (e.g., bradycardia, decelerations)
- Fetal sepsis

Contraindications for Preinduction Cervical Ripening With PGE$_2$

PGE$_2$ is not recommended in the following situations:

- Oxytocin is not recommended for the woman.
- The presentation is abnormal.
- Uterine patterns are hyperactive or hypertonic.
- Membranes are ruptured (**gel** contraindicated; **insert** may be placed).
- The woman is hypersensitive to prostaglandin or the gel ingredients.
- Placenta previa or unexplained vaginal bleeding occurred during this pregnancy.
- A vaginal delivery is not indicated (e.g., vasa previa or active herpes genitalia).
- There is definite evidence of fetal distress.

Special consideration must be given to administering PGE$_2$ to women with the following conditions[2]

- Asthma or a history of asthma
- Glaucoma or increased intraocular pressure
- Renal disease
- Hepatic disorders
- Previous delivery of six or more term pregnancies

Administration of PGE$_2$

> ■ **What precautions should be taken to provide safe administration of PGE$_2$ using endocervical or vaginal routes?**

To ensure the greatest safety for mother and fetus, it is recommended that[9]:

- Fetal heart tones and uterine activity be monitored electronically for a 20- to 30-minute baseline assessment before administration.
- After endocervical instillation, the mother should assume a side-lying position for 1 to 2 hours to help prevent leaking of the gel from the endocervix. (Some institutions recommend a modified Trendelenburg's position in their protocols.)
- Fetal heart tones and uterine activity be electronically monitored for at least 2 hours after instillation. In some cases, after this period of post–gel instillation observation, the woman is sent home and scheduled for reevaluation for induction the following day.
- After placement for a vaginal insert, the mother remain supine for 2 hours and then may ambulate.
- The vaginal insert be removed with onset of active labor or 12 hours after placement.
- Maternal blood pressure, pulse rate, and temperature be monitored every 15 to 30 minutes for the first hour, then every 4 hours.

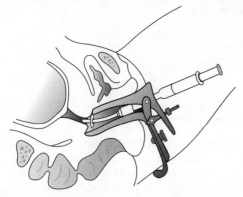

FIGURE 7.1 Prepidil Gel syringe and catheter. Application of gel for preinduction cervical ripening at or near term.

GEL PLACEMENT. Proper placement of the gel **in the endocervical canal** just below the internal os (**away from the membranes**) decreases complications. It is placed by a physician or nurse-midwife in the hospital. The appropriate-sized shielded endocervical catheter (10 or 20 mm) is selected and is attached to the prefilled, room temperature Prepidil (dinoprostone 0.5 mg) prostaglandin E$_2$ syringe. Air is expelled from the syringe. With the use of a sterile speculum, the cervix is visualized and the selected catheter is inserted through the external os *into the endocervix* (Fig. 7.1). It is critical to avoid intrauterine placement or placement against the amniotic membranes. Prepidil Gel is contraindicated for use with ruptured membranes.[12]

CERVICAL VAGINAL INSERT. Proper placement of the insert (dinoprostone 10 mg, released at 0.3 mg per hour over 12 hours) does not require visualization of the cervix or warming. Remove the insert from the foil package using sterile gloves and a very small amount of K-Y Jelly. Place the insert is transversely in the posterior fornix (not in the endocervical canal). Tuck the end of the retrieval system into lower vaginal space. This may be used with ruptured membranes.[13]

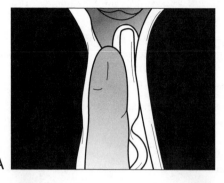

The Cervidil Vaginal Insert system is inserted into the vagina, up to the posterior fornix (Fig. 7.2A).

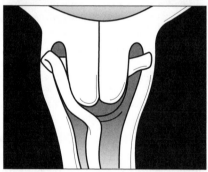

The system is left in place, transverse to the posterior surface of the cervix (Fig. 7.2B).

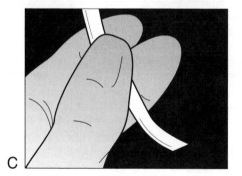

The Cervidil Vaginal Insert system can be easily grasped for gentle removal and discontinuation of drug administration (Fig. 7.2C).

FIGURE 7.2 Cervidil vaginal insert.

■ **If uterine hyperstimulation, fetal bradycardia, or decelerations in fetal heart rate occur, what actions should the nurse take?**

The woman should be placed on her left side, oxygen administered, uterine and fetal heart rate monitoring continued, and the woman's health care provider notified if no immediate improvement is observed. *If the Cervidil Vaginal Insert is in place, it must be removed.* IV fluids, tocolytic therapy, and cesarean section might be indicated. Specific protocols regarding nursing management of prostaglandin-related emergencies should be developed by each hospital using PGE$_2$ endocervical gel or vaginal inserts.[8]

■ **Can more than one dose of Prepidil Gel be administered if inadequate ripening occurs?**

A repeated dose of Prepidil Gel 0.5 mg can be administered after 6 hours. The maximum cumulative dose in a 24-hour period is 1.5 mg.[12]

■ **Can more than one dose of Cervidil Vaginal Insert be administered if inadequate ripening occurs?**

NO. The manufacturer does not currently recommend more than one application of the Cervidil because adequate studies have not been conducted on repeated dosing. Maximum overall time of administration is 12 hours.[13]

■ **With adequate cervical ripening and no labor, how soon after prostaglandin administration can oxytocin be administered for labor induction?**

It is recommended that 6 to 12 hours lapse between the last dose of Prepidil Gel and starting the IV oxytocin. It is recommended that Cervidil Vaginal Insert be removed at least 30 minutes before IV oxytocin is started.

Use of Misoprostol for Cervical Ripening* (see page 319)

Although not FDA approved for this indication, misoprostol is currently in use in many settings. Wilson presented considerations for developing a protocol for cervical ripening with misoprostol.[3] Misoprostol has been administered intravaginally in the posterior fornix using 50 μg every 6 hours and 25 μg every 3 hours. The higher dosage was associated with higher incidences of meconium uterine hyperstimulation and nonreassuring fetal heart patterns. The oral administration of 50 to 200 μg was repeated every 6 hours for a maximum of three doses. The higher dosage was associated with shortened labor but more hyperstimulation. In discussing the bioavailability of misoprostol, Wilson notes that "gastrointestinal or hepatic metabolism that occurs with oral routes makes them less effective."[3] The ACOG Committee on Obstetric Practice recommends 25 μg intravaginally as the initial dose.[14] After review of multiple studies, the committee concludes that 25 μg intravaginally every 4 hours achieves the best outcomes.

■ **Are there additional restrictions or concerns for the use of misoprostol?**

It is recommended that the woman be admitted to a hospital where continuous electronic monitoring is available. Women with a compromised cardiac status need careful evaluation. Careful observation is needed if chorioamnionitis is present. Women with a history of uterine surgery, including a low transverse cesarean section, should not receive the drug. Misoprostol also should not be used when fetal weight is less than 1800 g or greater than 4500 g, if there is any question of CPD, or in the presence of more than 12 contractions per hour.

Although the Food, Drug, and Cosmetic Act of 1938 was amended in 1962 to allow off-label use of approved drugs by physicians, the Association of Women's Health, Obstetric, and Neonatal Nurses (AWHONN) recommends that nurses check their state nurse practice act.[3,15] Protocols for the use of misoprostol should include data collection to document outcomes.

Recommendations for Safe Use of Misoprostol

To ensure the greatest safety for mother and fetus, it is recommended that *the following be true before administering misoprostol*[3,14]:

- The Bishop's score is less than 6.
- The woman is experiencing fewer than 12 contractions in an hour.
- The fetus has a reactive nonstress test (RNST) before the drug is placed.
- There is no history of uterine surgery.
- There is no concern for CPD.
- The pharmacist uses a 100-μg tablet and quarters it using a pill cutter to obtain a consistent dose of 25 μg.
- Terbutaline or magnesium sulfate is available if needed to treat hyperstimulation.
- IV access is in place.
- Electronic monitoring is done for 2 hours after each dose is inserted in the vagina.

- If membranes rupture after placement of misoprostol, the labor pattern and fetal response are observed for 2 hours before an additional dose is placed.
- Oral intake is restricted for 2 hours before and after placement.
- The facility has the capability of offering urgent/emergency cesarean delivery.
- Protocols are developed by the department and include guidelines for misoprostol use, evaluation of outcomes, and documentation of adherence to guidelines

---

MISOPROSTOL DOSAGE. The ACOG recommends starting with 25 μg in the posterior fornix.[15] Wing and Paul recommend 25 μg every 4 hours for a total of six doses in 24 hours.[14] Wilson offers a range of dosages: for induction of labor beyond 28 weeks, place 25 to 50 μg intravaginally every 4 to 6 hours or administer 50 to 100 μg by mouth every 4 to 6 hours.[3]

In the case of a fetal demise beyond 28 weeks, place 50 to 100 μg intravaginally every 4 to 6 hours **or** administer 100 to 200 μg by mouth every 4 hours.[3]

VAGINAL PLACEMENT. The tablet is placed in the posterior vaginal fornix with a minimum of lubricant. The patient voids before placement. The patient rests in bed for 30 minutes after placement. Before additional doses are placed, the following are done:

- Repeat the Bishop's score; withhold additional dose if score is 8 or more or cervical effacement is at 80% and dilatation is at 3 cm.
- Evaluate fetal heart pattern to determine level of fetal well-being.
- Evaluate uterine contraction pattern. Dose is withheld if contractions are every 5 minutes.[3,6,15]

OXYTOCIN ADMINISTRATION. If active labor is not established in 24 hours, oxytocin augmentation is indicated. Oxytocin may be started 2 hours after the last misoprostol dose.[15]

Administration of Oxytocin

■ **What is the recommended method of oxytocin administration?**

Oxytocin can be a dangerous drug if used improperly. Oxytocin should always be administered using the two-bottle system (one of which contains no oxytocin) "piggybacked," flexible IV catheters, and an infusion control pump. This method of administration:

- Ensures uniform control of dosage
- Prevents backup and clotting of blood
- Prevents air embolism and circulatory overload

INFUSION CONTROL PUMPS. Pumps provide a very carefully controlled flow of fluids. Several models are available on the market. It is critical to be aware of the manufacturer's guidelines for operation.

Every hospital should have a written and observed procedure for oxytocin use that includes the following[2,6]:

- Evaluation of the patient by a physician or a nurse qualified to assess the woman before administration of oxytocin

- Immediate availability, during oxytocin administration, of a physician qualified to perform a cesarean delivery should problems arise
- Use of an IV catheter, infusion pump, two-bottle system (one without oxytocin)
- Documentation of fetal heart rate, resting uterine tone, frequency and characteristics of contractions, flow rate, and blood pressure taken and recorded every 30 to 40 minutes (Continuous electronic fetal monitoring is recommended.)
- Guidelines for maximum concentration of solution and maximum rate of administration for both induction and augmentation

PRACTICE/REVIEW QUESTIONS *deliberate*

After reviewing this module, answer the following questions.

1. Define *induction of labor.* Starting of uterine ctx before the begin on their own

2. Define *augmentation of labor.* ↑ Contractions to help labor progress

3. What are four common ways to induce or augment labor?
   a. Amniotomy
   b. Pitocin
   c. Cervidil
   d. Ambulation / nipple stimulation

4. Oxytocin is a hormone secreted by the pituitary gland. Oxytocin causes the uterus to contract

5. Using commercially prepared FDA-approved products, how is PGE$_2$ administered?
   Vaginally - up by the cervix

6. Why is it necessary to carefully control the rate of oxytocin administration?
   Because you can cause more powerful/frequent contractions

7. Describe the best way to administer oxytocin so that the rate of administration is controlled.
   Infusion pump

8. List at least five medical indications for the induction or augmentation of labor.
   a. Preeclampsia / Biophysical profile ↓ 6
   b. Diabetes / Intrauterine fetal death
   c. PROM / uterine dystocia
   d. Post dates / H/O Rapid labor
   e. Macrosomia / living far away

9. What should be considered when a woman requests an induction for reasons of convenience?
   Well being of the fetus

10. Why are some institutions implementing active labor management protocols?
    To ↓ the chances of c/s d/t dystocia

11. List four criteria used to select women who might benefit from active labor management.

    a. *Nulliparity*

    b. *> 37 wks*

    c. *Single fetus in no distress*

    d. *Spontaneous labor*

12. Tetanic contractions resulting from induced labor can result in:

    a. *Abruption*

    b. *Rupture of uterus*

    c. *Cervical tears*

13. List at least five additional concerns of adverse effects for the mother who is experiencing induction/augmentation of labor.

    a. *Hypertension or stroke / water intoxication*

    b. *Postpartum hemorrhage / ↑ fear*

    c. *Embolism*

    d. *too rapid birth*

    e. *Lacerations to vagina, uterus, perineum + rectum*

14. List at least three concerns of adverse effects for the fetus during induction/augmentation.

    a. *Hypoxia*   *Bilirubinemia*

    b. *Bradycardia*

    c. *↑ trauma*

15. Match the definitions in Column B with the items in Column A. Choices may be used more than once.

    Column A

    d 1. Fetal distress

    a 2. Cephalopelvic disproportion

    c 3. Soft tissue masses

    b 4. Surgery for tumors on the uterus

    f / e 5. Active management of labor

    Column B

    a. Baby's head is too large for the woman's pelvis

    b. Potential for rupture of the scar with overstimulation of the uterus

    c. Tumors, large ovarian cysts

    d. Results from decreased oxygen to the placenta as a result of uterine contractions

    e. Often includes use of oxytocin to augment labor

    f. Deliberately rupturing the membranes

16. List six situation that are absolute contraindications for induction of labor. (Practice until you can do this without referring to the text.)

    a. *CPD*

    b. *Previous uterine surgical procedure*

    c. *Severe fetal distress*

    d. *Soft tissue mass*

    e. *Lack of willingness*

    f. *Placenta previa*

17. Match the definitions in Column B with the items in Column A. Choices may be used more than once.

Column A

g 1. Hydramnios
b 2. Favorable cervix
c 3. Grandmultipara
d 4. Primigravida
e 5. Abnormal presentation
a 6. Multiple gestation
f 7. Hypertonic uterus

Column B

a. When more than one embryo develops in the uterus at the same time

b. Must be effaced more than 50%, soft, and dilated more than 2 cm

c. A woman who has had five or more children

d. A woman who has never delivered a fetus before

e. The woman's pelvis is too small for the baby's head

f. Increased uterine resting tone

g. Excessive amounts of amniotic fluid

18. What are relative contraindications?

Conditions that May or May not present problems for Mother/Baby

19. List nine relative contraindications to the induction/augmentation of labor. (Practice until you can do this without referring to the text.)

a. *Unfavorable Cervix*
b. *Presenting part not engaged in the pelvis*
c. *Abnormal presentation*
d. *Grandmultiparity*
e. *Multiple gestation*
f. *Hydramnios*
g. *Hypertonic or incoordinate uterus*
h. *Maternal exhaustion*
i. *previous Classical Uterine incision*

20. For the following conditions, indicate whether they are contraindications (C) or relative contraindications (RC) to oxytocin induction/augmentation.

C a. Large soft tissue masses
RC b. Breech lie
C c. Cephalopelvic disproportion
RC d. Maternal exhaustion
RC e. Unfavorable cervix
C f. Severe fetal distress
RC g. Hydramnios
RC h. Twins
RC i. Hypertonic uterus
RC j. Woman's unwillingness
RC k. Presenting part not engaged in pelvis

21. Match the definitions in Column B with the items in Column A. Choices may be used more than once.

Column A

f 1. Premature rupture of membranes

g 2. Preeclampsia

l 3. Tetanic contractions

k 4. Amniotic fluid embolism

h 5. Rh incompatibility

e 6. Uterine dystocia

c 7. Hypoxia

j 8. Postterm

b 9. Abruptio placentae

d 10. Pitocin

a 11. Water intoxication

i 12. PGE$_2$

Column B

a. Decreased ability of the woman to eliminate fluid, leading to excessive fluid retention

b. Premature separation of a normally implanted placenta

c. Lack of oxygen

d. Trade name of oxytocin

e. Poor-quality contractions that fail to result in desirable cervical changes

f. Leaking of amniotic fluid through the cervix before the onset of labor

g. Hypertension with proteinuria and/or edema induced by pregnancy after the twentieth week of gestation

h. Contamination of the baby's red blood cells by maternal blood antibodies

i. Preinduction cervical ripening

j. Pregnancy that persists more than 42 weeks from the onset of the last normal menstrual period

k. Life-threatening conditions that can result in severe respiratory distress and circulatory collapse in the woman

l. Extremely powerful contractions with no rest periods

m. Effective method of regulating the flow of IV fluids

22. List at least three prerequisites for a safe and effective induction/augmentation.

a. *No Contraindications*

b. *Accurate EDC (Gestational Age)*

c. *health care provider must supervise*

23. State seven ways of assessing fetal gestation or maturity.

a. *Early + Accurate records of LMP + EDC*

b. *Establishment of quickening date*

c. *Auscultation of fetal ♡ tones*

d. *Early U/S by 20 wks*

e. *Serial U/S*

f. *evaluation of fetal growth pattern*

g. *amniotic fluid studies*

24. What is Bishop's score used to determine? *Whether the cervix is favorable for induction*

25. Mrs. J. is being assessed for induction of labor. Her cervix is dilated 1.5 cm and is 60% effaced. The vertex is at −1 station, cervical consistency is medium, and cervical position is midline. What is her Bishop's score? *7*

26. Match the definitions in Column B with the items in Column A.

Column A

d 1. Labor

c 2. Complete placenta previa

e 3. Hypertonic uterus

b 4. Premature rupture of membranes

a 5. Used to evaluate cervical status

Column B

a. Bishop's score

b. Indication for induction

c. Contraindications to induction/augmentation

d. Uterine contractions causing desired changes to cervix

e. Relative contraindications to induction/augmentation

f. Too-rapid birth

27. Oxytocin should always be administered using:

a. *Pump for infusion*

b. *two bottle system*

c. *flexible Catheter*

28. What evaluative technique is strongly recommended when using oxytocin?

Fetal / Uterine monitoring

29. Give at least two specific reasons why the two-bottle system, IV catheter, infusion control pump, and fetal monitoring should be used when giving oxytocin.

a. *Uniform control of dose*

b. *Allows close supervision of fetus / mother*

30. What should be included in the written procedures for oxytocin administration?

a. *Evaluation of Cervix*

b. *physician needs to be immediately available*

c. *Use of IV infusion pump*

d. *Maximum Concentrations of solution + rate of Administration*

e. *Monitor ctx, flow rate, BP q 30min*

31. List at least five concerns of effects for the mother who is receiving PGE$_2$ for preinduction cervical ripening.

a. *tetanic Contractions*

b. *Nausea / vomiting*

c. *fever*

d. *Back pain*

e. *Amnionitis and PROM*

32. List at least two concerns of effects for the fetus during preinduction cervical ripening.

a. *Hypoxia*

b. *♡ rate abnormality*

33. Prepidil Gel is not recommended in the following situations. (Practice until you can do this without referring to the text.)

    a. *oxytocin is not recommended*
    b. *presentation is abnormal*
    c. *uterine patterns are hyperactive, or* *hypertonic*
    d. *ROM*
    e. *hypersensitivity to prostglandin*
    f. *placenta previa or undiagnosed bleeding*
    g. *Vag delivery is not indicated*
    h. *definate evidence of fetal distress*

34. What are the relative contraindications for PGE$_2$?

    a. *Asthma or H/O*
    b. *Glaucoma or ↑ intraocular pressure*
    c. *Renal Disease*
    d. *Hepatic disorder)*
    e. *previous delivery of 6 or more* *term pregnancies*

35. Which one of the following dosages of misoprostol is recommended in the ACOG Committee Opinion?

    A. 50 μg every 6 hours in the posterior vaginal fornix
    B. An initial dose of 25 μg in the posterior vaginal fornix
    C. 50 μg every 6 hours by mouth
    D. 25 μg every 3 hours in the posterior vaginal fornix

36. The ACOG Committee Opinion on the use of misoprostol indicates that it is not recommended for women with a history of a low transverse cesarean section.

    A. True
    B. False

PRACTICE/REVIEW ANSWER KEY

1. Deliberately starting uterine contractions before they begin on their own

2. The act of helping increase contractions that have already started on their own

3. a. Amniotomy
   b. Use of oxytocin
   c. Ambulation
   d. Nipple stimulation

4. Hormone; posterior pituitary; contract

5. Instilled into the endocervical canal or placed in the posterior fornix of the vagina

6. Because it causes more powerful and frequent contractions than normal

7. Using an IV catheter in the arm, with a two-bottle system and the fluid flow rate controlled by an infusion control pump

8. Any five of the following:
   a. Life-threatening vascular disease
   b. Preeclampsia
   c. Rh incompatibility
   d. Diabetes
   e. Premature rupture of membranes
   f. Chorioamnionitis
   g. Postterm
   h. Intrauterine fetal death
   i. Uterine dystocia
   j. History of rapid labor
   k. Living a great distance from hospital or having psychosocial problems
   l. Prevention of prolonged labor
   m. Biophysical profile less than 6 or oligohydramnios

9. An induction for convenience may not be supported when evaluated in terms of maternal and/or fetal risk.

10. In an attempt to decrease the rate of cesarean deliveries for dystocia

11. a. Nulliparity
    b. More than 37 weeks' gestation
    c. Single fetus in no distress
    d. Spontaneous labor

12. a. Abruptio placentae
    b. Rupture of the uterus
    c. Cervical tears

13. Any five of the following:
    a. Hypertension or stroke
    b. Postpartum hemorrhage
    c. Embolism (amniotic fluid embolism)
    d. Too-rapid birth
    e. Lacerations to vagina, vulva, perineum, and rectum
    f. Water intoxication
    g. Increased fear

14. Any three of the following:
    a. Hypoxia
    b. Bradycardia
    c. Increased trauma
    d. Bilirubinemia

15. 1. d
    2. a
    3. c
    4. b
    5. e and f

16. a. Cephalopelvic disproportion
    b. Some previous uterine surgical procedures
    c. Severe fetal distress
    d. Soft tissue masses
    e. Lack of willingness
    f. Central or total placenta previa

17. 1. g
    2. b
    3. c
    4. d
    5. e
    6. a
    7. f

18. Conditions which *might* or *might not* present severe problems for mother and baby

19. a. Unfavorable cervix
    b. Presenting part not engaged in pelvis
    c. Abnormal presentation
    d. Grandmultiparity
    e. Multiple gestation
    f. Hydramnios
    g. Hypertonic or incoordinate uterus
    h. Maternal exhaustion
    i. Previous classical uterine incision

20. a. C
    b. RC
    c. C
    d. RC
    e. RC
    f. C
    g. RC
    h. RC
    i. RC
    j. C
    k. RC

21. 1. f
    2. g
    3. l
    4. k
    5. h
    6. e
    7. c
    8. j
    9. b
    10. d
    11. a
    12. i

22. a. The woman should not have any of the contraindications for induction/augmentation.
    b. Gestational age of the fetus should be accurate.
    c. The woman's health care provider should supervise the procedure.

23. a. Early and accurate records of LNMP and EDC
    b. Establishment of "quickening" date
    c. Auscultation of fetal heart tones with fetoscope at 16 to 18 weeks or with electronic Doppler at 12 to 14 weeks
    d. Early ultrasound by 20 weeks
    e. Serial ultrasounds
    f. Evaluation of fetal growth pattern
    g. Amniotic fluid studies

24. Whether the cervix is "favorable" for induction

25. 7

26. 1. d
    2. c
    3. e
    4. b
    5. a

27. a. Two-bottle system
    b. Flexible IV catheters
    c. An infusion control pump

28. Fetal/uterine monitoring

29. Any two of the following:
    a. Ensures uniform control of dosage
    b. Prevents backing up and clotting of blood
    c. Helps prevent an air embolism and circulatory overload
    d. Allows close observation of mother and fetus

30. a. Evaluation of cervical effacement and dilatation before administration
    b. Immediate availability, during administration, of a physician who has privileges to perform cesarean surgery
    c. Use of an IV catheter, infusion pump, two-bottle system
    d. Maximum concentration of solution and maximum rate of administration
    e. Monitoring of contractions, flow rate, and blood pressure at least every 30 minutes

31. a. Tetanic contraction
    b. Nausea and vomiting
    c. Fever
    d. Back pain
    e. Amnionitis and PROM

32. Any two of the following:
    a. Hypoxia
    b. Heart rate abnormality
    c. Sepsis

33. a. Oxytocin is not recommended for the woman.
    b. The presentation is abnormal.
    c. Uterine patterns are hyperactive or hypertonic.
    d. Membranes are ruptured.
    e. The woman is hypersensitive to prostaglandin or its gel.
    f. Placenta previa or undiagnosed vaginal bleeding occurred during the pregnancy.
    g. A vaginal delivery is not indicated.
    h. There is definite evidence of fetal distress.

34. a. Asthma or a history of asthma
    b. Glaucoma or increased intraocular pressure
    c. Renal disease
    d. Hepatic disorder
    e. Previous delivery of six or more term pregnancies

35. B

36. A

Oxytocin Labor Induction/Augmentation
SKILL UNIT 1

This skill unit instructs you on how to set up for an induction/augmentation of labor with oxytocin, how to identify equipment needed, and how to administer the drug.

Remember, induction or augmentation with oxytocin is a procedure that stimulates regular uterine contractions. The procedure must *always* be ordered by the health care provider managing the woman's labor. It is always performed for medical reasons. There must be no absolute contraindications present for the procedure implemented.

After you study this section, your preceptor should demonstrate the procedure and then give you an opportunity to demonstrate your skill.

Please remember, the types of equipment and supplies may vary from hospital to hospital, depending on the manufacturer and surgical supply houses used.

ALTERNATIVE PROCEDURES FOR OXYTOCIN ADMINISTRATION FOR INDUCTION, AUGMENTATION, OR ACTIVE MANAGEMENT OF LABOR MAKE IT CRITICAL FOR NURSES TO HAVE SPECIFIC PROTOCOLS AND GUIDELINES ESTABLISHED BY THE INSTITUTION.

COMPREHEHSIVE PROTOCOLS THAT ADDRESS NURSING RESPONSIBILITY IN OXYTOCIN ADMINISTRATION SHOULD INCLUDE CRITERIA FOR PATIENT SELECTION, RESPONSIBILITY FOR AND INFORMATION TO BE COVERED IN THE INFORMED CONSENT, DRUG PREPARATION AND ADMINISTRATION, PATIENT MONITORING, POTENTIAL SIDE EFFECTS, AND THERAPEUTIC GOALS.

ACTIONS	REMARKS
Assemble the Equipment	
Two-bottle IV	Piggyback setups vary from hospital to hospital, depending on IV products used. Refer to your hospital procedure manual for piggyback administration of drugs procedure.
IV fluid	Solution can be a balanced solution (lactated Ringer's or 0.9% sodium chloride).
1,000 mL of aqueous solution without medication	To decrease the possibility of water intoxication, avoid excessive use of D_5W.
10 units of Pitocin in 1,000 mL solution 20 units of Pitocin in 1,000 mL solution 15 units of Pitocin in 250 mL solution	The labor unit protocols need to specifically state which dilution is to be used.
Filter needle	If the pharmacy does not supply prefiltered unit dose packaging of drugs for IV use, oxytocin must be withdrawn from the ampule using a filter needle. The filter needle is then exchanged for another regular needle to add oxytocin to the IV solution.

ACTIONS	**REMARKS**
Flexible venous 18- to 20-gauge catheter	Most hospitals supply angiocaths, intracaths, or plastic needles.
Infusion control pump (Fig. 7.3)	Need to be familiar with the operation of the infusion control pump (Table 7.3).

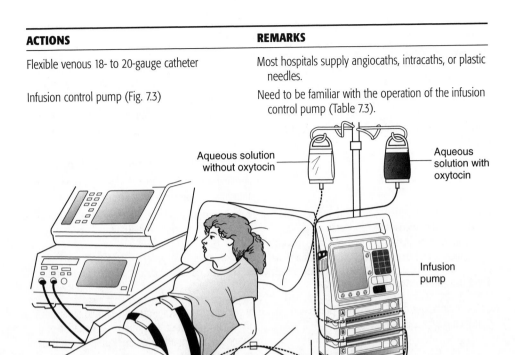

Aqueous solution without oxytocin

Aqueous solution with oxytocin

Infusion pump

FIGURE 7.3 Infusion control pump: setup for exytocin administration.

TABLE 7.3	Oxytocin Conversions		
	SOLUTION CONCENTRATION		
Rate (mU/min)	**10 U oxytocin/1,000 mL (10 mU/mL) (mL/hr)**	**20 U oxytocin/1,000 mL (0 mU/mL) (mL/hr)**	**15 U oxytocin/250 mL (60 mU/mL) (mL/hr)**
0.5	3	1.5	0.5
1	6	3	1
2	12	6	2
3	18	9	3
4	24	12	4
5	30	15	5
6	36	18	6
7	42	21	7
8	48	24	8
9	54	27	9
10	60	30	10
11	66	33	11
12	72	36	12
13	78	39	13
14	84	42	14
15	90	45	15
16	96	48	16
17	102	51	17
18	108	54	18
19	114	57	19
20	120	60	20

Adapted with permission from Poziac, S. (1999). Induction and augmentation of labor. In L. K. Mandeville, & N. H. Troiano (Eds.), *High-risk and critical care intrapartum nursing* (2nd ed.), pp. 139–158). Philadelphia: Lippincott.

ACTIONS	REMARKS
Prepare for IV Administration	
Obtain informed consent.	The woman must give permission with full awareness of the effects and side effects to herself and her baby. She needs your support and encouragement.
Start IV infusion. Use aqueous solution without oxytocin.	The woman must be evaluated before drug administration.
Set flow rate at 125 mL/hr.	This will provide the woman with adequate hydration.
Apply fetal and uterine monitor.	The monitor can be external or internal. Do not start Pitocin in the presence of a nonreassuring strip.
Record baseline information for 20 minutes before administration of medication: temperature, pulse, respirations, blood pressure, fetal heart rate, monitor frequency, and characteristics of any contraction.	Recordings must also be made at least every 30 minutes after medication administration begins.
Start the Administration of Oxytocin	
Connect the oxytocin infusion to the pump and start the piggyback infusion.	The woman's health care provider should order the initial flow rate dose. Maximum concentration and maximum rate of administration should be noted by hospital policy.
Adjust the flow rate until satisfactory contractions are established.	**To evaluate uterine and fetal response, the flow rate should not be increased any faster than every 30 minutes initially.** As the cervix starts to dilate, the flow rate might need to be reevaluated. See Display 7.3 for additional information. Some protocols will keep the rate stable, whereas others may gradually reduce or discontinue it.

DISPLAY 7.3 Adjusting the Oxytocin Flow Rate

For induction of labor:

1. Start infusion at 1 to 2 mU/min.
2. Increase dose every 15 minutes at rate of 1 mU per minute once uterine and fetal responses are known.
3. Once a regular pattern of uterine contractions is established, maintain infusion at current rate.

For augmentation of labor:

1. Start infusion at 0.5 to 1 mU/min.
2. Increase dose every 40 to 60 minutes at rate of 1 mU per minute. The time frame for changing the rate may be shortened if the expected response is not obtained.
3. Once a regular pattern of uterine contractions is established, maintain infusion at current rate.

From Mandeville, L. K., & Troiano, N. H. (1999). *High-risk and critical care intrapartum nursing* (2nd ed.). Philadelphia: Lippincott.

Discontinue flow	
Discontinue oxytocin administration during active labor, second stage, or postpartum, as ordered.	Opinions vary as to preferred time for oxytocin termination. Check the written order.
Discontinue oxytocin in the presence of a nonreas-	Fetal heart rate should remain stable with contractions of 40 to 60 seconds' duration and not exceeding 60 to 70 mm Hg. Contraction rate should not exceed five contractions in 10 minutes. Resting zone should be below 20 mm Hg.

suring fetal heart rate pattern or hyperstimulation.

ACTIONS	REMARKS

Record the Procedure

> Although some health care providers may order oxytocin via a bolus to manage postpartum hemorrhage, literature from pharmaceutical sources does not support or condone this route. Because bolus injections of oxytocin cause a significant and rapid drop in blood pressure in most women and could lead to circulatory collapse, bolus administration could prove dangerous to many women and should be avoided.

Observations and notes that must be recorded (in record and on monitor strip):

–date and time for each entry

–vital signs

–fetal heart rate

–resting uterine tone

–frequency, duration, and intensity of contractions and response to contractions

–vaginal findings: dilatation, effacement, station

–oxytocin infusion rate

–IV count

–fluid intake and output

–nurses' notes and signature

What Can Go Wrong?

The fetus might not get enough oxygen (hypoxia).	Monitor fetal heart rate continuously for bradycardia, sustained tachycardia, or loss of variability. If noted, discontinue oxytocin, place the woman on her left side, and administer oxygen.
The baby can be born too quickly and forcefully. This can cause trauma to the woman and the baby.	Assist with the birth. Support the woman and family. Observe and record the following: –indications of fetal distress (bradycardia, tachycardia, loss of variability) –maternal lacerations and uterine bleeding –birth injuries to the baby
The woman can retain too much fluid, causing water intoxication.	Closely regulate IV fluid intake and oxytocin dosage and measure urinary output. Administer oxytocin in aqueous solution according to the protocol, but limit D_5W to 2500 mL/24 hr. Observe the woman for confusion, amnesia, lethargy, vomiting, convulsion, or coma.
The woman's blood pressure can decrease, causing decreased oxygen supply to the baby.	Take vital signs at least every 30 minutes; position the woman on her side, preferably her left side. The frequency of assessing vital signs will depend on overall patient status and cervical changes.

> REMEMBER: The appropriately credentialed health care provider must order and supervise the regulation and administration of oxytocin.

ACTIONS	REMARKS
Good-quality contractions might not be achieved.	Most induction protocols recommend increasing the flow rate 1 mU/min. At this point, if further increases in the flow rate are needed, maintain each 1-mU/min increase for 1 hour.
	A good-quality pattern is usually considered three contractions in 10 minutes, resting tone 12 to 15 mm Hg (must be less than 20 mm Hg), and fetal heart rate 120 to 160 bpm with good variability in the baseline.
Contractions can be too strong and forceful.	If the length of contractions is more than 90 seconds, oxytocin should be discontinued. Support and evaluate the mother and evaluate fetal status. Administer oxygen and position the woman on her left side.
The cervix can dilate too rapidly.	Evaluate cervical dilatation after labor is established, before increasing the rate of infusion. If the cervix responds to contractions by pulling or stretching, as felt during a vaginal examination, do not increase rate.
Induction or augmentation with oxytocin might not produce the desired results (birth of the baby).	Support the woman and her family.

You will need to attend a skill session(s) to practice this skill with the help of your preceptor. Mastery of the skill is achieved when you can do the following:

- Assemble all of the necessary equipment
- Prepare the two-bottle IV solution administration setup
- Prepare the solution administration pump
- Apply the fetal and uterine monitor
- Use the fluid administration pump to increase the dosage of oxytocin
- Record observations on an appropriate flow sheet

R E F E R E N C E S

1. Fuchs, A. R., & Fuchs, F. (1996). Physiology and endocrinology of parturition. In S. G. Gabbe, J. R. Niebyl, & J. L. Simpson (Eds.), *Obstetrics: Normal & problem pregnancies* (3rd ed., pp. 111–136). New York: Churchill Livingstone.
2. Poziac, S. (1999). Induction and augmentation of labor. In L. K. Mandeville & N. H. Troiano (Eds.), *High-risk and critical care intrapartum nursing* (2nd ed., pp. 139–158). Philadelphia: Lippincott.
3. Wilson, C. (2000). The nurse's role in misoprostol induction: A proposed protocol. *Journal of Obstetric, Gynecologic, and Neonatal Nursing, 29*(6), 574–583.
4. ACOG. (2000). Committee Opinion Response to Searle's Drug Warning on Misoprostol #248. Washington, DC: Author.
5. Wing, D. A. (1999). Labor induction with misoprostol. *American Journal of Obstetrics and Gynecology, 181*(2), 339–345.
6. ACOG. (1999). Practice Bulletin Induction of Labor #10. Washington, DC: Author.
7. Bowes, W. A. (1999). Clinical aspects of normal and abnormal labor. In R. K. Creasy & R. Resnik (Eds.), *Maternal-fetal medicine* (4th ed., pp. 541–568.) Philadelphia: WB Saunders.
8. Simpson, K. R., & Poole, J. H. (1998). *Cervical ripening and induction and augmentation of labor.* Washington DC: AWHONN.
9. Kendrick, J. M., & Simpson, K. R. (2001). Labor and birth. In K. R. Simpson & P. A. Creehan (Eds.), *Perinatal nursing* (2nd ed., pp. 298–377). Philadelphia: Lippincot Williams & Wilkins.
10. Gibbs, R. S., & Sweet, R. L. (1999). Maternal and fetal infection disorders. In R. K. Creasy & R. Resnik (Eds.), *Maternal-fetal medicine* (4th ed., pp. 659–724) Philadelphia: WB Saunders.
11. Socol, M. L., & Peaceman, A. M. (1999). Controversies in labor management: Active Management of Labor. *Obstetrics and Gynecology Clinics, 26*(2), 287–294.
12. Upjohn. (1987). Prepidil Gel. Kalamazoo, MI: Upjohn Company.
13. Forest Pharmaceuticals. (1995). Cervidil. St. Louis: Forest Pharmaceuticals.
14. Wing, D. A., & Paul, R. H. (1999). Misoprostol for cervical ripening and labor induction: The clinician's perspective and guide to success. *Contemporary OB/GYN, 44*(4), 46–61.
15. ACOG. (1999). Committee Opinion Induction of Labor with Misoprostol #228. Washington, DC:

14. ACOG. (1999). Committee Opinion Induction of Labor with Misoprostol #228. Washington, DC: Author.
15. Wing, D. A., & Paul, R. H. (1999). Misoprostol for cervical ripening and labor induction: The clinician's perspective and guide to success. *Contemporary OB/GYN, 44*(4), 46–61.

*G. D. Searle & Co. submitted a supplemental new drug application to the FDA in 2000 for changes in the information listed under labor and delivery in the labeling of Cytotec (misoprostal). In April 2002 providers received copies of the new labeling information. They recognize the drug can induce or augment uterine contractions. The information goes on to state that the medication is used for cervical ripening, induction of labor and treatment of postpartum hemorrhage. They include cautions regarding uterine hyperstimulation, fetal bradycardia and uterine rupture particularly in the presence past uterine surgery (G. D. Searle & Co. (2002) Cytotec.)

SUGGESTED READINGS

Chyu, J. K., & Strasser, H. T. (1997). Prostaglandin E2 for cervical ripening: A randomized comparison of Cervidil versus Prepidil. *American Journal of Obstetrics and Gynecology, 177*(3), 606–611.

Impey, L., Hobson, J., & O'Herlihy, C. (2000). Graphic analysis of actively managed labor: Prospective computation of labor progress in 500 consecutive nulliparous women in spontaneous labor at term. *American Journal of Obstetrics and Gynecology, 183*(2), 438–443.

Jobe, A. H. (1999). Fetal lung development, tests for maturation, induction of maturation and treatment. In R. K. Creasy & R. Resnik (Eds.), *Maternal-fetal medicine* (4th ed., pp. 404–422). Philadelphia: WB Saunders.

Kramer, R. L., Gilson, G. J., Morrison, D. S., Martin, D., Gonzales, J. L., & Qualls, C. R. (1997). A randomized trial of misoprostol and oxytocin for induction of labor: Safety and Efficacy. *Obstetrics & Gynecology, 89*(3), 387–391.

O'Driscoll, K., & Stronge, J. M. (1975). The active management of labour. *Clinics in Obstetrics and Gynecology, 2*(1), 3–17.

Ruiz, R. J. (1998). Mechanisms of full-term and preterm labor: Factors influencing uterine activity. *Journal of Obstetric, Gynecologic, and Neonatal Nursing, 27*(6), 652–660.

Sanchez-Ramos, L., Chen, A. H., Kaunitz, A. M., Gavdier, F. L., & Delke, I. (1997). Labor induction with intravaginal misoprostol in term premature rupture of membranes: Randomized study. *Obstetrics & Gynecology, 89*(6), 909–912.

Searing, K. A. (2001). Induction vs. post-date pregnancies exploring the controversy of who's really at risk. *Lifelines, 5*(2), 44–48.

MODULE 8

Caring for the Woman at Risk for Preterm Labor or With Premature Rupture of Membranes

NANCY WEBSTER SMITH

As you complete this module, you will learn:

1. The definition of *preterm labor*
2. Strategies to identify women at risk for preterm labor
3. The limitations of risk appraisal
4. How to recognize and treat early symptoms of preterm labor
5. Care-seeking behaviors of expectant women
6. Management of preterm labor, including the following:
   a. Indications
   b. Contraindications
   c. Pharmacologic agents
   d. Nursing implications
   e. Controversies
7. The side effects of tocolytic agents and initiation of appropriate supportive measures
8. Appropriate education and counseling for women at risk for preterm labor to enhance their chances of delivering a mature infant
9. Decision making in telephone triage
10. The definition of *premature rupture of membranes*
11. Risks to the mother and fetus associated with premature rupture of membranes
12. Management methods when premature rupture of membranes occurs in a term pregnancy
13. Management methods when premature rupture of membranes occurs in a preterm pregnancy, including the following:
    a. How chorioamnionitis is diagnosed
    b. The role of amniocentesis in the management of premature rupture of membranes
    c. The relationship between premature rupture of membranes and the incidence of respiratory distress syndrome in the newborn
    d. The role of steroid therapy in the prevention of postdelivery complications in the newborn
14. Priorities for nursing interventions in caring for the woman with premature rupture of membranes

When you have completed this module, you should be able to recall the meanings of the following terms. You should also be able to use the terms when consulting with other health professionals. The terms are defined in this module or in the glossary at the end of this book.

amniocentesis
β-adrenergic agonist
β-adrenergic receptor
corticosteroid
corticotropin-releasing hormone
fetal fibronectin (fFN)
home uterine activity monitoring

phosphatidylglycerol (PG)
premature rupture of membrane (PROM)
preterm premature rupture of membranes (pPROM)
respiratory distress syndrome
salivary estriol
tocolysis

This module reviews current information regarding preterm labor and premature rupture of membranes. Continuing research is constantly changing our understanding of the process leading to these events. There is very little evidence that any of the medical strategies or behavioral interventions that have been widely used in the past 20 years have had any significant impact on the prevention of preterm labor or reduction in preterm births. The clinician must stay informed of the current evidence so that he or she can base practice decisions on proven strategies, better utilize resources, and avoid potentially harmful interventions.

Epidemiology of Preterm Labor

Despite the efforts of many different types of preterm birth prevention programs and millions of dollars in research focused on the prevention of preterm birth in the past 20 years, the incidence of preterm birth has actually risen. The incidence of preterm birth was 9.4% in 1981 and had risen to 11.4% by 1997. When further broken down by race, major differences exist: 8.8% of White births and 18.9% of African American births occur before 37 weeks' gestation. Nearly 70% of all infant mortality and about one third of all handicapping conditions come from low-birth-weight infants, especially infants born before 32 weeks. This is estimated to cost approximately $5 billion per year in the United States.[1]

■ How is preterm labor defined?

Preterm labor is usually defined as regular uterine contractions occurring between 20 and 37 weeks' gestation and accompanied by one or more of the following:

- Progressive cervical change (cervical dilatation or effacement detected by serial examination)
- Cervical dilatation of 2 cm or more
- Cervical effacement of 80% or more
- Rupture of membranes

Another definition sometimes used for research purposes is contractions occurring between 20 and 36 weeks' gestation at a rate of four in 20 minutes or eight in an hour, with at least one of the following:

- Cervical change over time
- Dilatation of 2 cm or more

> Standard criteria for diagnosing preterm labor often are not used. Without definitive diagnostic criteria and with a lack of consensus as to what constitutes successful treatment for preterm labor, evaluation of interventions is difficult.

Many women are inaccurately diagnosed with preterm labor. In recent years, efforts have been made to develop a diagnostic test to reliably differentiate between "true" and "false" labor. If, using standardized criteria, clinicians could more accurately identify those women truly at risk for having a preterm delivery, it would significantly reduce unnecessary hospitalizations, medical treatments, and the stress and risks related to these interventions.

Risk Assessment for Preterm Labor

The physiology of the onset of labor in humans at term or preterm is not fully understood. Even though there is no mechanism to accurately identify women who will experience preterm labor, certain factors appear to increase the risk for its occurrence. Most preterm birth prevention programs have been based on risk assessment tools designed to identify women at risk for preterm labor, with specific interventions aimed at reducing identified risk factors. Most of these programs have proven ineffective at reducing the rate of preterm birth. Risk assessment tools have had low detection rates, especially for primigravid women, and also appear to be population specific. Until the cause of preterm birth is better understood, it will be difficult to improve the detection rate of risk assessment tools.

> In most cases, the cause of preterm labor is probably related to an interplay of various factors related to socioeconomic status, clinical history, and behavioral and biologic factors.

Some of the conditions that seem to predispose to preterm labor and low birth weight are outlined in Display 8.1.[1]

DISPLAY 8.1 Risk Factors Associated With Preterm Labor

DEMOGRAPHIC RISKS

Maternal age ≤ 18 or ≥ 35 years
Non-Caucasian race
Low socioeconomic status
Unmarried
Low level of education

MEDICAL RISKS IN CURRENT PREGNANCY

Multiple gestation
Poor weight gain
Short interpregnancy interval
Infection
First or second trimester bleeding
Placental problems, such as previa or abruption
Hyperemesis
Hypertension: chronic or pregnancy induced
Hydramnios or oligohydramnios
Abnormal hemoglobin
Fetal anomalies
Incompetent cervix
Premature rupture of membranes

MEDICAL RISKS PREDATING PREGNANCY

Previous preterm birth
Multiparity ≥ 5
Low prepregnant weight for height
Uterine or cervical abnormalities or surgery
Nonimmune status for certain infections
Previous second trimester abortion
Diethylstilbestrol (DES) exposure
Maternal genetic factors
Chronic medical conditions, such as diabetes, hypertension, or heart disease

ENVIRONMENTAL/BEHAVIORAL/ PSYCHOSOCIAL RISKS

Smoking, especially ≥ 11 cigarettes per day
Alcohol or other substance abuse
Poor nutritional status
High altitude
Domestic abuse
Strenuous job activity
High stress
Lack of or inadequate prenatal care

> THE SINGLE GREATEST RISK FACTOR FOR PRETERM LABOR IS A PREVIOUS HISTORY OF PRETERM LABOR.

Screening for Preterm Labor Risk

■ **What other methods are used to identify women at risk for preterm delivery?**

Other methods used to identify woman at risk for preterm delivery include cervical assessment, transvaginal ultrasound, studies of biochemical markers, and home uterine activity monitoring.

Cervical Assessment

Routine digital assessment of dilatation of the cervix by itself is probably not an effective screening tool to detect women at high risk for preterm delivery. However, using *all* components of the Bishop score helps one correlate this finding more closely with preterm delivery.[2]

Transvaginal Ultrasound

The normal cervical length in the midtrimester of pregnancy is approximately 4 cm. Several studies have shown that the shorter the cervix, the higher the risk of preterm birth. The presence of funneling, a wedge of membranes and fluid pushing through the internal os, is also associated with preterm birth. Measuring cervical length by transvaginal ultrasound may be a valuable tool when used in conjunction with other parameters to predict preterm labor.[2]

Biochemical Markers

Because approximately half of all women with preterm contractions will go on to deliver at term,[3] biochemical markers to accurately identify those truly at risk for preterm birth would offer supplemental information that would help clinicians avoid providing unnecessary and costly treatment to those who will have a term delivery. Some of the biochemical markers being studied include the following:

- **Fetal fibronectin (fFN)**—fFN is a glycoprotein found in the placental membranes and amniotic fluid. fFN assays have been approved by the U.S. Food and Drug Administration (FDA) for clinical use in identifying women at risk for preterm labor. The fFN immunoassay is a qualitative test for the detection of this protein *in cervicovaginal secretions.* fFN can be measured in cervicovaginal secretions early in pregnancy and at term *but is rarely detectable between 21 and 37 weeks in normal singleton pregnancies.* Sampling is usually performed no earlier than 24 weeks and before 35 weeks in women with symptoms of preterm labor. The presence of fFN in these women has been associated with an increased risk of preterm birth. Although a negative test appears to be useful in ruling out imminent preterm birth (within 2 weeks), the clinical implications of a positive result are not fully understood. For this reason, it is not recommended as a routine screening tool for asymptomatic women.[3]
- **Salivary estriol**—Estriol levels have been shown to rise 3 to 5 weeks before labor begins. Estriol plays a role in preparing the body for labor and possibly signaling the onset of labor. Estriol levels can be monitored in saliva. The FDA has approved a laboratory technique for measuring salivary estriol as a risk assessment marker of preterm labor and delivery between 22 and 36 weeks' gestation. Like cervicovaginal fFN, salivary estriol has excellent negative predictive value (i.e., if the test is negative, the chance of preterm birth within 72 hours is very low). Because it produces a high percentage of false-positive results and is even less reliable before 30 weeks' gestation, it is not recommended for routine screening. However, there may be a role for salivary estriol testing in high-risk populations to determine which women are *not* at risk for early delivery.[4]
- **Corticotropin-releasing hormone**—Corticotropin-releasing hormone, a possible hormonal response to stress, may play a role in determining length of gestation. Abnormal or early elevations of these hormone levels in maternal plasma have been documented in preterm labor, implicating it as a possible contributor to the processes affecting the timing of delivery. An abnormal rise of corticotropin-releasing hormone may occur in response to psychosocial stress or physiologic stressors rising in the mother, fetus, or placenta. Recent research indicates that corticotropin-releasing hormone levels may be a potential marker for identifying patients at risk for preterm birth.[5]

Home Uterine Activity Monitoring

The role of *home uterine activity monitoring* in preventing preterm birth has been controversial. It was hoped that the monitoring of uterine activity using a portable external fetal monitoring system and telephone modem to transfer data to a monitoring center would hold promise for reducing the rate of preterm birth. Although it has been demonstrated that women who eventually deliver at preterm gestation have more uterine activity than other women at the same gestational age who eventually deliver at term, the difference is not reliable enough to be used effectively in screening for high-risk women. *The research to date shows no proven maternal, fetal, or neonatal benefit from the use of home uterine activity monitoring.*[6]

Signs and Symptoms of Preterm Labor

■ What are the warning signs of preterm labor?

The early warning signs of preterm labor are often subtle and can be difficult to differentiate from discomforts of pregnancy and therefore go unrecognized until labor is advanced. The key to treating preterm labor and preventing preterm delivery is early recognition and treatment. *Pregnant women should be educated to recognize the following symptoms:*

- **Uterine contractions**—Frequent uterine contractions, occurring every 10 minutes or less (more than five in an hour), might indicate preterm labor. Irregular uterine contractions, called Braxton Hicks contractions, occur normally as pregnancy progresses; however, frequent or regular contractions should not be ignored. Preterm labor contractions are *often painless* and might be described as a tightening of the uterus or as "the baby balling up."

- **Menstrual-like cramps**—These cramps in the lower part of the abdomen or upper thighs can be intermittent or constant.
- **Low, dull backache**—Backaches during pregnancy are not uncommon, but low backaches that are not relieved by rest or changes in position should be investigated. It can be described as "toothachy" or throbbing below the waistline, which can be intermittent or constant, and can radiate to the front or the abdomen.
- **Pelvic pressure**—Many women describe this as a heaviness in the lower abdomen, pelvis, back, or thighs, which feels as if the baby is pushing down. This is often a rhythmical pelvic pressure not relived by rest.
- **Abdominal cramping**—Intestinal cramps with or without diarrhea, sometimes described as "gas pains," can be associated with preterm labor.
- **Increase or change in vaginal discharge**—A milky white discharge is normal during pregnancy. However, a sudden increase or *change* in discharge, whether mucousy, watery, or tinged with blood, can be associated with preterm labor.

> A woman in preterm labor can have only one or all of these signs. The woman experiencing one or more of the signs of preterm labor must be examined and evaluated promptly. Early recognition is essential for optimal response to treatment of preterm labor.

In addition to educating women and their families, all personnel who might have contact with pregnant women should be knowledgeable about the early symptoms of preterm labor and the appropriate response. It is important to ensure that the expectant woman understands the terms used and can describe her symptoms. The importance of prompt reporting of these symptoms should be emphasized. The risks of delaying evaluation and treatment should be made clear, and women should be made to feel comfortable reporting symptoms even when they are found not to be in labor.

Management of the Woman at Risk for Preterm Labor

> ■ **What is the appropriate response to telephone calls from women with symptoms of preterm labor?**

If symptoms of preterm labor have been present for more than 1 hour or if the description of symptoms is vague, further investigation is needed.

If symptoms began while the woman was physically active and have been present for less than 1 hour, she should be instructed to do the following:

- Empty her bladder
- Rest on her side
- Drink fluids (2 to 3 glasses of water or juice)
- Palpate for uterine contractions
- Call back in 1 hour if symptoms persist or if symptoms recur with resumption of normal activities
- Report the following symptoms immediately:
  –Ruptured or leaking membranes
  –Frequent, strong contractions (every 10 minutes or less)
  –Changes in vaginal discharge
  –Vaginal bleeding

All personnel in hospital clinics or private practice offices who have contact with pregnant women need to be well sensitized to the dilemmas and subtleties of preterm labor. Secretaries are often the first contact when an inquiry is made by a pregnant woman confused by what she is experiencing. The woman needs to know from the person on the other end of the line that her call is welcomed and important. Pregnant women delay seeking care because they do not interpret what they feel as anything abnormal. They also delay because they fear subtle "putdowns" or being stereotyped as fearful or overanxious.

Before giving instructions, the woman's knowledge level of preterm labor, her pregnancy history, and distance from the hospital should be ascertained.

■ **What are important considerations for the woman at risk for preterm labor, and what other measures can be recommended to help prolong pregnancy?**

- Information about the signs and symptoms of preterm labor and the importance of seeking obstetric care immediately when they occur.
- Self-palpation and awareness of uterine contractions. Monitoring by palpation for contractions twice per day and any time symptoms occur.
- Maintaining a schedule of regular (weekly or bimonthly) prenatal visits to allow ongoing assessment of cervical status and uterine activity.
- Curtailing work or other physical activities and maintaining bed rest may not always be necessary. Activities may need to be modified depending on the type of employment, the occurrence of symptoms of preterm labor, and cervical status.
- Restricting travel.
- Maintaining adequate diet and hydration, prenatal vitamins and iron, and good hygiene.
- Avoiding smoking and other substance abuse.
- Avoiding stressful situations when possible. Stress and anxiety can contribute to preterm labor.

Considerations About Care-Seeking Behaviors of Pregnant Women[7,8]

Keep in mind as you review this section that risk appraisal fails to identify 50% of women who enter preterm labor.

- Preterm labor is usually not in the thinking of most expectant women.
- Women have difficulty bringing a meaningful interpretation to a symptom because pregnancy itself brings unexpected similar physical discomforts.
- The focus of women's advocacy groups and society in general is on the normalcy of pregnancy.
- Low-risk women often do not receive education about recognizing symptoms of preterm labor.
- The expectant woman attempts to make sense out of what she is feeling by taking several different steps.
  - She gathers data and seeks information by comparing with her own expectations and here she will often attempt to "normalize" her symptoms. She has no prior experiences to relate to if this is her first pregnancy.
  - She compares what she is feeling with the experiences of others (e.g., her mother, sister, friend).
  - She self-manages her symptoms as long as she can. Women rarely interpret sensations for preterm labor, but they think they "worked too hard," "got extra tired," "are coming down with the flu," or "strained their back."

NOTE: Care-seeking behaviors of people experiencing a myocardial infarction are not all that different than what has just been described.[7,8] Clinical studies reveal the following:

- *Prodromal symptoms*
- *Initial denial*
- *Self-evaluation*
- *Subsequent seeking of lay evaluation*
- *Finally medical evaluation*
- *Hospital travel*
- *Hospital evaluation*

- Having previous experience with contractions (a previous labor and delivery) does not always ensure that the present symptoms will be recognized as contractions.
- Some women have a high tolerance for discomfort and avoid seeking assistance for a prolonged time.

In seeking to understand why the expectant woman delays obtaining medical assistance until it is often too late to stop labor, you need to reflect on what has just been outlined. Care-seeking behaviors that are preceded by denial and/or normalizing are not at all unusual in many primary and acute care settings. Recognition of this is critical to how phone calls are handled and education of the expectant woman and her family is facilitated.

Finally, in offering reassurance of normal findings (often from a gentle cervical examination to rule out preterm labor), remind the woman to continue her vigilance of symptoms and to feel welcome to return for reassessments in the future. Avoid giving the impressions that the risk in no longer a possibility. Inadvertently at times, negative findings are incorrectly interpreted as meaning all is well now and for the next few hours, days, or weeks. *The onset of prodromal symptoms of preterm labor that night or the next day can be missed.*

Guidelines for Assessment and Intervention

■ **What might be included in the initial assessment and intervention for preterm labor?**

- Health history
- Reproductive history
- Prenatal course of this pregnancy—obtain records if possible
- Determination of precise fetal age, based on last menstrual period (LMP), early sonograms, fundal height measurements, date of quickening, first date of audible fetal heart tones
- Routine obstetric clinical parameters
- Assessment of signs/symptoms of preterm labor

> Document the occurrence of symptoms, onset, duration, and severity. Ask what activities preceded their onset and what relief measures have been tried.

- Bed rest—left lateral position for maximum placental perfusion; right lateral positions are certainly acceptable
- Hydration—oral or intravenous

> Preterm labor contractions will often stop with rest and hydration.

- Urine and cervical cultures

> Infection of the upper genital tract is a significant risk factor for preterm labor.[1,13]

- External monitoring—fetal and uterine
- Baseline cervical examination—should be done gently with minimal manipulation of the cervix

Serial gentle cervical examinations (without entry into the internal os) should be done by the same examiner, when possible, to improve reliability of assessing early or subtle cervical change. Evaluate and record the following:

- Position of the cervix
- Consistency
- Effacement (estimated length in centimeters)
- Dilatation
- Station of the presenting part

NOTE: *If there is suspicion of amniotic membrane rupture or leakage, a sterile speculum examination should be done. (See Module 3.)*

- Psychological and emotional status—maternal and family reaction

Preterm labor can be an extreme crisis for a family. Common responses might be guilt, fear, and/or anger. It is important to provide reassurance and support in an atmosphere that encourages expression of feelings.

■ **What are the nursing responsibilities in caring for the woman in preterm labor?**

- Monitor uterine status. External electronic fetal monitoring is usually done to document the frequency and quality of uterine contractions. Intensity of contractions should be assessed by palpation.

Instruct the woman to report continuation or change in symptoms of preterm labor, even in the absence of documentation of uterine contractions on the external monitor. *Do not depend on the monitor alone in assessing uterine contractility.*

- Reevaluate symptoms of preterm labor.
- Monitor fetal status. Electronic fetal monitoring is recommended.
- Monitor maternal vital signs (refer to Module 5).
- Monitor intake and output, especially during tocolytic therapy.
- Provide comfort measures and emotional support.
- Observe closely for side effects of tocolytic therapy: tremors, maternal and fetal tachycardia, headache, palpitations, anxiety, nausea, vomiting, hypotension, or widening pulse pressure.
- Educate the woman and her family about potential side effects of tocolytic therapy.
- Prepare for the possibility of the following:
  –Ultrasound
  –Amniocentesis
  –Tocolytic drug therapy
  –Steroid therapy
  –Baseline blood chemistry—serum potassium, glucose, complete blood count (CBC)
  –Baseline electrocardiogram (ECG)

Ultrasound and amniocentesis may be ordered to verify gestational age and fetal lung maturity.

Information to Consider Regarding Bed Rest

Bed rest has commonly been prescribed for the treatment or prevention of preterm labor even though there is evidence questioning its effectiveness. The assumption that bed rest is effective in preventing adverse pregnancy outcomes and is safe for the woman and her fetus is now being challenged. Clinical studies suggest that there are negative physical and emotional effects from immobilization during pregnancy. Bed rest in pregnancy may be associated with an increased risk for thromboembolic disease, muscle atrophy, bone loss, weight loss, insulin resistance, and calcium depletion. These effects appear to remain for a prolonged period after delivery also. The severity of adverse effects while on bed rest appears to be related to the amount of activity restriction and may be reduced by exercise. The severe emotional and economic effects of pregnancy bed rest on women and their families also needs to be taken into consideration. There are no guidelines for prescribing bed rest in pregnancy, and the amount and degree of activity restriction appear to vary greatly among practitioners. Still, nearly 20% of women end up on bed rest during pregnancy.[9]

The following areas need to be taken into consideration before bed rest is prescribed during pregnancy:

- Balancing maternal and fetal risks and benefits
- Involving the woman in decision making and planning regarding activity levels
- Discussing potential stressors for the whole family
- Including exercise in the plan of care while on bed rest

Information to Consider Regarding Smoking During Pregnancy

Smoking during pregnancy is associated with preterm birth. Smoking is also related to placenta previa, placental abruption, premature rupture of membranes, spontaneous abortion, and decreased birth weight and infant stature. Tobacco smoke contains more than 2,000 chemicals, most of which easily cross the placenta. Nicotine and carbon monoxide are two of the main chemicals thought to be responsible for poor fetal outcomes as the result of decreased oxygenation to the mother and fetus.

In the United States, 13% to 25% of pregnant women smoke. Approximately 6% to 7% of these women will stop smoking if they receive a formal smoking cessation program, but then 25% of these women will relapse and begin smoking again during pregnancy. The risk of preterm birth rises with the amount smoked. However, women who stop smoking by the sixteenth week of pregnancy decrease their risk to that of nonsmokers.

Because of the difficulty with stopping smoking and the high rate of relapse, tobacco dependence should be viewed as a chronic condition requiring repeated intervention. Smokers often view smoking as a stress reducer or coping tool in their lives, so interventions to encourage cessation should address this aspect as well as the impact that stopping smoking will have on the woman and her family. The most successful smoking cessation programs for pregnant women have addressed five important areas of concern[10]:

1. Risk of smoking
2. Benefits of quitting
3. Recommendation to quit
4. Feedback about fetal status
5. Teaching cognitive-behavioral strategies for quitting

Management of Preterm Labor

Past treatment methods for preterm labor have included bed rest, hydration, and the use of drugs such as progesterone, ethanol, narcotics, and sedatives to inhibit uterine contractions. None of these were effective in reducing the incidence of preterm birth. More recently, drugs that have a quieting or depressant effect on the myometrium of the uterus have been used. The depressant effect on the myometrium is called a *tocolytic effect*. The process of administering a drug for the purpose of inhibiting uterine contractions is called *tocolytic therapy*. It should be noted that the widespread use of tocolytics has not reduced the incidence of preterm deliveries. However, clinical studies indicate that tocolytics may prolong gestation for 24 to 48 hours. This can be beneficial to allow time for administration of corticosteroids to facilitate fetal lung maturity and to delay delivery until the pregnant woman can be transferred to a hospital where appropriate neonatal care is available.

■ **What are the indications for tocolytic therapy?**

Labor inhibition is generally indicated when:

- The diagnosis of preterm labor is made

- Gestation is beyond 20 weeks but prior to 35 weeks
- There is a live fetus without signs of severe distress or congenital anomalies incompatible with life

> Aggressive obstetric and neonatal interventions have a minimal effect on the survival of infants at 22 to 23 weeks or before. Always involve the woman and her family in the decision to start or stop tocolytic therapy.

ANTENENATAL CORTICOSTEROIDS SHOULD ALWAYS BE ADMINISTERED WHEN TOCOLYTIC THERAPY IS INITIATED.

■ **What are the contraindications to tocolytic therapy?**

Factors that threaten maternal and fetal status are contraindications to labor suppression (Display 8.2).

DISPLAY 8.2 Contraindications to Tocolysis for Treatment of Preterm Labor[a]

GENERAL CONTRAINDICATIONS	CONTRAINDICATIONS FOR SPECIFIC TOCOLYTIC AGENTS

Acute fetal distress (except intrauterine resuscitation)
Chorioamnionitis
Eclampsia or severe preeclampsia
Fetal demise (singleton)
Fetal maturity
Maternal hemodynamic instability
	β-Mimetic agents
	  Maternal cardiac rhythm disturbance or other cardiac disease
	  Poorly controlled diabetes, thyrotoxicosis or hypertension
	Magnesium sulfate
	  Hypocalcemia
	  Myasthenia gravis
	  Renal failure
	Indomethacin (Indocin)
	  Asthma
	  Coronary artery disease
	  Gastrointestinal bleeding (active or past history)
	  Oligohydramnios
	  Renal failure
	  Suspected fetal cardiac or renal anomaly
	Nifedipine (Adalat, Procardia)
	  Maternal liver disease

[a]Relative and absolute contraindications to tocolysis based on clinical circumstances should take into account the risks of continuing the pregnancy versus those of delivery.

American College of Obstetricians and Gynecologists. (1995).Preterm labor. Technical bulletin no. 206. Washington, DC: ACOG.

Drugs Currently Used for Tocolysis

Four classes of tocolytic agents are in use or under study (Table 8.1):

1. β-Mimetics
2. Magnesium sulfate
3. Calcium channel blockers
4. Nonsteroidal anti-inflammatory drugs (NSAIDs)

β-Mimetics or β-Adrenergic Agonists

There are two types of β-adrenergic receptors in humans:

1. β_1-Adrenergic receptors are found in the heart, liver, pancreas, kidney, small intestine, and adipose tissue.

TABLE 8.1. Drugs Most Commonly Used in the Treatment of Preterm Labor

DRUG	ACTION	DOSAGE/ROUTE	MATERNAL SIDE EFFECTS	FETAL SIDE EFFECTS	NURSING IMPLICATIONS
Magnesium sulfate	Central nervous system depressant	IV: 4-g loading dose diluted and infused over 20–30 min, then 1 g/hr maintenance dose until contractions stop Maintenance dose is based on serum magnesium level, reflex response, and patient response (serum therapeutic range is 4–7.5 mEq/L) Oral: Magnesium gluconate 1–2 g every 4 hr	Drowsiness, lethargy, slurred speech, blurred vision, ptosis, flushing, decreased gastrointestinal motility, headache, nausea, vomiting, muscular weakness, urinary retention, shortness of breath, diarrhea (pulmonary edema has been reported)	Decreased FHR variability, neonatal hypotonia, and drowsiness; possible bone abnormalities and congenital rickets have been associated with prolonged exposure	Closely monitor maternal vital signs and FHR; obtain serum magnesium levels as ordered Monitor intake and output; maintain fluid restriction as ordered Observe for signs of toxicity: increasing lethargy, hypotonia, extreme thirst Administration contraindicated if maternal respirations ≤12 breaths/min, urinary output ≤25 mL/hr, and patellar reflexes absent Have antidote (10% calcium gluconate) and resuscitation equipment immediately available
Terbutaline	β-Adrenergic agonist	IV: 1 mg/min initially; increase by 0.5 mg/min every 10 min to maximum of 8 mg/min until contractions stop Oral: 2.5–5 mg every 4 to 6 hr Subcutaneous: 0.25 mg every 1–6 hr The FDA has issued an alert regarding the potential dangers associated with terbutaline pump therapy and the lack of evidence supporting the efficacy of this treatment	Similar to ritodrine	Similar to ritodrine	See ritodrine

Drug	Classification	Dose	Maternal side effects	Fetal/neonatal effects	Nursing considerations
Ritodrine hydrochloride	β-Adrenergic agonist	IV: 0.05–0.1 mg/min; may be increased every 10 min to maximum of 0.35 mg/min until contractions stop Oral: 10 mg every 2 hr up to maximum of 120 mg/24 hr (first dose administered 30 min before IV infusion discontinued)	Palpitations, nervousness, tremors, tachycardia, sweating, headache, nausea, vomiting, thirst, chest pain ECG changes and cardiac dysrhythmia Hyperglycemia Hypocalcemia Pulmonary edema (increased risk with multiple gestation or concomitant use of corticosteroids) ↑ Serum insulin, glucose, and free fatty acids ↓ Serum potassium	Tachycardia, neonatal hypoglycemia	Closely monitor blood pressure and maternal and fetal heart rates; maternal heart rate should not exceed 120–130 bpm Note breath sounds and observe for signs of pulmonary edema (dyspnea, coughing, wheezing, rales) Monitor intake and output; maintain fluid restriction as ordered Before initiating IV therapy: Serum potassium Serum glucose Baseline ECG
Nifedipine	Calcium channel blocker	5–10 mg sublingual every 15–20 min (up to 4 times), then 10–20 mg orally every 4–6 hr	Transient hypotension, heartburn, headache, dizziness, cutaneous flushing, nausea	Intrauterine growth restriction	Closely monitor blood pressure; serial ultrasounds may be ordered to monitor fetal growth Avoid in diabetes; avoid concomitant use of magnesium sulfate
Indomethacin	Prostaglandin inhibitor	50–100 mg rectal suppository, then 25–50 mg orally every 6 hr × 24 hr May repeat for an additional 24 hr maximum	Headache, peptic ulcer, gastrointestinal upset, fluid retention, prolonged bleeding time, nausea or vomiting, pruritus, bowel changes, renal failure, hepatitis, gastrointestinal bleeding	Oligohydramnios Transient constriction of ductus arteriosus	Review history for contraindications: peptic ulcer disease, aspirin sensitivity, renal disease, coagulopathy, pregnancy beyond 30–32 weeks' gestation Amniotic fluid levels should be monitored in therapy continued ≥ 3 days Do not combine with magnesium sulfate use

2. β_2-Adrenergic receptors are found in smooth muscle of the uterus, blood vessels diaphragm, and bronchioles.

By binding to these receptor sites, β-mimetics initiate a series of reactions resulting in reduced levels of calcium and reduced sensitivity of the myosis-active contractile unit to calcium. This prevents the chemical interaction necessary for smooth muscle contraction. However, continued exposure to β-mimetics can lead to desensitization as the number of β-adrenergic receptors decrease. This reduces the efficacy of the drug and is called *down-regulation.*

Because β-adrenergic receptors are present in multiple sites, effects (side effects) can be seen on various organ systems and the probability of maternal risk is higher than with some of the other tocolytics. Some of these effects are as follows:

Cardiovascular	–Increases heart rate, systolic blood pressure, pulse pressure, stroke volume, and cardiac output.
	–Decreases diastolic pressure and peripheral vascular resistance.
	–Cardiac dysrhythmias have been reported.
	–Increased heart rate and myocardial contractility can predispose patients to myocardial ischemia.
Pulmonary	–Increases plasma renin and arginine vasopressin, which is associated with sodium and water retention. This predisposes patients to pulmonary edema, especially in multiple gestations. Excessive intravenous fluids combined with the antidiuretic effect of high dosages of β-mimetics can result in fluid overload.
Metabolic	–Increases maternal blood glucose levels and insulin levels. This effect is enhanced by concomitant administration of corticosteroids. Lipolysis can also be included, which can lead to severe metabolic acidosis in diabetic women.

Magnesium Sulfate (MgSO₄)

Magnesium sulfate is an inexpensive alternative to β-mimetic therapy. The side effects of parenteral magnesium for the treatment of preterm labor appear to be less severe and less frequent than those of β-mimetic therapy. $MgSO_4$ is also safer to use with insulin-dependent diabetic patients because it decreases the risk of uncontrolled hyperglycemia, which can occur with β-mimetics. The mechanism by which $MgSO_4$ inhibits uterine contractions is unknown but is thought to be related to its ability to block calcium uptake, binding, and distribution in smooth muscle cells.

Calcium Channel Blockers

Calcium channel blockers have shown some promise in inhibiting smooth muscle contractions. They produce vasodilatation and decreased peripheral vascular resistance, resulting in flushing of the skin and a transient increase in maternal and fetal heart rate. Postural hypotension can occur with sudden position changes.

Nonsteroidal Anti-inflammatory Drugs

NSAIDs, such as indomethacin, decrease the synthesis of prostaglandin, which stimulates uterine contractions.

Comprehensive protocols that address nursing responsibility in administering tocolytic therapy should be developed at each institution. These protocols need to include the following:

- Criteria for patient selection
- Responsibility for and information to be covered in the informed consent
- Drug preparation and administration
- Patient monitoring
- Potential side effects
- Therapeutic goals

■ How effective are tocolytics for the treatment of preterm labor?

Tocolytic drugs have not been shown to reduce the number of preterm deliveries, but they may prolong pregnancy for up to 48 hours. Postponing delivery may allow the administration of corticosteroids to enhance pulmonary maturity and reduce the incidence and severity of respiratory distress syndrome. It also allows time for transfer to a hospital where appropriate neonatal care is available. *(The use of tocolytics in a maintenance capacity following an episode of acute tocolysis has not been shown to the effective.)*

The efficacy of tocolytic drugs decreases if the cervix is 80% or more effaced or 3 to 4 cm or more dilated when therapy is initiated. If the cervix is dilated 5 cm or more, the chance of achieving inhibition of labor is minimal.

> THERE IS NO EVIDENCE THAT OUTPATIENT USE OF TOCOLYTICS PROLONGS GESTATION.[13]

■ When preterm labor is advanced or is unresponsive to tocolysis, what preparations should be made for delivery?

- If possible, women who are at less than 34 weeks' gestation should be transported to a tertiary care center *before delivery* so that intensive care facilities will be immediately available for the infant.
- Assess the family's understanding of the rationale for starting or stopping tocolytic therapy and their expectations for the preterm infant's appearance, needs, and care.
- Provide contact information for the neonatal care unit to facilitate communication.

Definitions, Etiology, and Risk Factors for Premature Rupture of Membranes

■ What is premature rupture of membranes?

Premature rupture of membranes (PROM) is the spontaneous rupture of membranes *before the onset of labor, regardless of gestational age.* This occurs in 11% of all term pregnancies and in about one third of preterm labor cases.[16] PROM at term is generally followed by the onset of labor.

■ What is preterm premature rupture of membranes?

Preterm premature rupture of membranes (pPROM) is rupture of membranes *before term* (i.e., before the completion of 37 weeks' gestation), with or without the onset of labor. pPROM remains the major cause of preterm birth and perinatal death resulting from prematurity and neonatal infections. This occurs in 3% of all pregnancies and contributes to 30% to 40% of all preterm births.[16]

> Infection is the single most common identifiable cause of pPROM.[13]

■ What is the cause of PROM?

Although risk factors that appear to be related to PROM have been identified, the exact cause is unknown. Infection of the upper genital tract is believed to be a significant and treatable risk factor. However, PROM often occurs in women without recognized risk factors.

Risk factors related to PROM include the following[16]:
- Lower socioeconomic status
- Sexually transmitted infections
- Prior preterm delivery or PROM
- Vaginal bleeding
- Cervical conization
- Smoking

Diagnosis, Management, and Nursing Interventions With PROM

■ How is PROM diagnosed?

Symptoms suggestive of PROM should be evaluated. An accurate diagnosis is essential to the appropriate management of suspected PROM. Symptoms suggestive of ruptured or leaking membranes should be evaluated promptly. Usually, ruptured membranes can be diagnosed on the basis of the history and physical examination.

- Observation of amniotic fluid pooling in the posterior vaginal vault is the best method to confirm the diagnosis.
- If the diagnosis is still in question, Nitrazine paper can be used to test the pH of the fluid. The pH of vaginal secretions is usually 4.5 to 6.0. Amniotic fluid has a higher pH of 7.1 to 7.3 and will therefore turn Nitrazine paper blue—a positive result.
- Ferning is another test that can be done by swabbing fluid from the posterior vaginal vault onto a glass slide and allowing it to dry. Under microscopic examination, the presence of a ferning pattern is suggestive of amniotic fluid in the vagina.
- Ultrasound may also be of value to confirm the diagnosis and to assess fetal presentation.
- Digital examination of the cervix may increase the risk of infection and *should be avoided* unless labor and imminent delivery are in process.
- A sterile speculum examination can usually verify the diagnosis of PROM and allows the clinician to inspect for cervicitis and umbilical cord prolapse, to do cervical cultures as indicated, and to assess cervical dilatation and effacement.

Blood, semen, and bacterial vaginosis are among the things that can cause a *false-positive result*. Vaginal discharge caused by urinary leakage, semen, cervicitis, vaginal douches or creams, or cervical dilatation can also be mistaken for ruptured membranes.

Risks Associated With PROM at Term

At term, maternal risks of ruptured membranes are low. Risks to the fetus from term PROM include fetal umbilical cord compression and ascending infection. *Maternal and fetal risks rise with the duration of time and with the number of digital vaginal examinations.*

Risks Associated With pPROM

Risks associated with pPROM are as follows:

- Intrauterine infection (chorioamnionitis)

- Fetal malpresentation
- Umbilical cord accident
- Placental abruption
- Complications of prematurity

Infection is evident in 13% to 60% of women with pPROM. The incidence of infection rises as gestational age decreases. The incidence of infection also rises with the number of cervical examinations done. Most women with pPROM will deliver within 1 week regardless of management.

■ What is the role of bacterial vaginosis in preterm labor and PROM?

Bacterial vaginosis (BV), the most commonly diagnosed cause of vaginal infection in women of childbearing age, has been shown to have a strong relationship to preterm delivery, especially in African American women. As many as 80% of early preterm births (between 24 and 28 weeks' gestation) may be related to intrauterine infection, with BV frequently being associated.

The American College of Obstetricians and Gynecologists (ACOG) has the following guidelines for the screening and treatment of bacterial vaginosis after the first trimester.[11]

- Screen all women at high risk for preterm labor.
- Treat those women who have positive test results or symptoms of BV with oral metronidazole.

NOTE: Vaginal treatment is not as effective in preventing preterm labor.

Paige et al. believe that identification and treatment of asymptomatic and symptomatic women can have a substantial impact on the incidence of preterm birth.[12]

Neither the Centers for Disease Control and Prevention (CDC) nor the ACOG recommends offering testing and treatment universally to pregnant women. This may change with future research. Some clinicians are currently screening all pregnant women (see Appendix A for a more detailed discussion).

■ What nursing interventions should be taken when a woman is admitted with PROM?

- Confirm membrane status and document the time of rupture, the time of onset of labor, and the color and odor of amniotic fluid. A sample of amniotic fluid may be obtained to assess fetal lung maturity. Avoid a digital examination—wait for the primary care provider unless an emergent situation presents (e.g., falling fetal heart tones with a prolapsed cord suspected).
- Review dating criteria for the pregnancy. Review data on LMP, early assessment of uterine size, and early sonograms.
- Monitor fetal heart rate and assess fetal status.
- Evaluate uterine activity.
- Determine group B streptococcus status and the need for antibiotic prophylaxis.
- Observe for signs of infection.
- Determine the need for transport to a tertiary care center based on gestational age and fetal status. If at less than 34 weeks' gestation and not in active labor, the woman should be transferred to a facility capable of providing intensive neonatal care.
- Assess the woman's understanding of the implications of PROM and management options. Provide psychosocial support.
- PREPARE FOR A HIGH-RISK INFANT IF INDICATED.
  –Pediatrician should be notified and present for delivery.
  –Resuscitation equipment should be in working order and in the delivery area.
  –Nursery should be notified of possible high-risk status of infant.
  –If there was not time to test for infection before the delivery, obtain a culture from the amniotic fluid, from the infant's ear, or from aspiration of stomach contents at the time of delivery.

■ What is the management of PROM?

Numerous controversies exist regarding optimal management and treatment of PROM, whether preterm or at term. Management decisions should be based on the following:

- Gestational age

- Presence or absence of labor
- Presence or absence of maternal infection
- Stability of the fetal heart rate tracing
- Stability of fetal presentation
- Cervical examination
- Availability of neonatal intensive care

Women with pPROM who are at 32 weeks' gestation or more, who have a mature fetal lung profile, and who are hospitalized where neonatal intensive care is available may be best managed by prompt induction of labor. **Antibiotic prophylaxis should be considered for all women when delivery is predicted to occur before 37 weeks' gestation or rupture of membranes is 18 hours or more in duration.**[13] Women with term PROM may be induced upon admission to the hospital or managed expectantly for 24 to 72 hours. At term, it is likely that spontaneous onset of labor and delivery will occur within 28 hours of membrane rupture.[14]

■ What is expectant management of pPROM?

When the potential complications associated with prematurity outweigh the risk of maternal and neonatal complications, expectant management is recommended. Hospitalization is usually required after pPROM. Women with pPROM who are at less than 32 weeks' gestation or who have an immature fetal lung profile may be managed expectantly. If the woman is not in active labor, she should be transferred to a high-risk medical center. Prophylactic tocolysis after pPROM has been shown to be beneficial in delaying the onset of contractions for 24 to 48 hours, allowing time for the beneficial effects of corticosteroid therapy, antibiotic therapy, and appropriate transfer.

Expectant management protocols may include the following:

- Modified bed rest
- Pelvic rest (e.g., avoid intercourse, sexual stimulation)
- Assessment for infection (chorioamnionitis)
  - Maternal or fetal tachycardia
  - Temperature greater than 100.4°F
  - Uterine tenderness
  - Foul-smelling purulent amniotic fluid

> Maternal tachycardia usually precedes a rise in maternal temperature and subsequent fetal tachycardia.

> Elevated white blood cell counts are not a reliable indicator of infection in women with PROM, especially if corticosteroids have been administered. During labor, even in the absence of infection, white blood counts can become elevated to levels of 25,000/mm³ or more.

- Surveillance for fetal compromise
  - Nonstress test
  - Ultrasound
- Prophylactic antibiotics
- Administration of corticosteroids
- Limited course of tocolytics

> Digital cervical examinations should not be done on women with PROM who are not in labor and in whom immediate induction of labor is not planned.

Fetal lung maturity tests can be performed accurately by vaginal pool *phosphatidylglycerol* (PG) on amniotic fluid samples aspirated from the vagina. If fetal lung maturity is documented, induction of labor should be considered.

Recommendations for Antenatal Corticosteroids

The appropriate use of corticosteroids to accelerate maturation of the fetus is one of the most effective ways to improve the outcomes of preterm births. Evidence from clinical trials since the 1970s has proven that antenatal corticosteroid administration is effective in reducing infant mortality by 30% and neonatal respiratory distress by 50%. **All women at risk for preterm delivery between 24 and 34 weeks' gestation are candidates for corticosteroid therapy** (Display 8.3). Studies have shown a decrease in the risk and severity of respiratory distress syndrome, intraventricular hemorrhage, neonatal mortality, and the cost and duration of neonatal care. The optimal benefit of antenatal corticosteroid therapy lasts for 7 days and is greatest more than 24 hours after starting therapy. Treatment for less than 24 hours is still associated with significantly improved outcomes. At this time, there is insufficient evidence to support the routine use of repeat courses of this treatment.[15]

DISPLAY 8.3	Corticosteroid Treatment Regimens[15]

Betamethasone 12 mg intramuscularly every 24 hours for two doses

OR

Dexamethasone 6 mg intramuscularly every 12 hours for four doses

---

> Antenatal corticosteroid therapy is one of the most effective strategies in the prevention of mortality and disability in preterm infants. A single course of corticosteroids should be given to all pregnant women between 24 and 34 weeks' gestation if at risk for preterm delivery within 7 days.[14]

PRACTICE/REVIEW QUESTIONS

After reviewing this module, answer the following questions.

1. Preterm labor is labor occurring after __20__ and before __37__ completed weeks' gestation.

2. The diagnosis of preterm labor is made when contractions less than 10 minutes apart are accompanied by:
   a. *progressive change in cervix*
   b. *cervical dilation of 2 cm or more*
   c. *cervical effacement of 80% or more*

3. The majority of perinatal morbidity and mortality in the United States are the result of:
   preterm births.

4. Five *demographic* risk factors related to low birth weight and preterm labor are:
   a. *Under age 18 or over 35*
   b. *Race – non white*
   c. *low socioeconomic status*
   d. *Unmarried*
   e. *low level of education*

5. The single greatest risk factor for preterm labor is
   previous preterm birth.

6. Five *behavioral* risk factors related to low birth weight and preterm labor are:
   a. _Smoking_
   b. _ETOH + Drugs_
   c. _Poor nutritional status_
   d. _High Altitude_
   e. _Domestic Abuse_

7. The keys to treating preterm labor and preventing preterm birth are _Early Recognition_ and _treatment_

8. List six warning signs of preterm labor.
   a. _Uterine ctx > 5/hr_
   b. _Menstrual like Cramps_
   c. _low, dull back ache_
   d. _pelvic pressure_
   e. _Abdominal Cramping_
   f. _↑ or change in vaginal discharge_

9. List three things to consider before giving telephone instructions to women complaining of vague symptoms of preterm labor.
   a. _pts Knowledge_
   b. _pg History_
   c. _distance from the hospital_

10. A knowledgeable patient with an uncomplicated pregnancy who experiences symptoms of preterm labor with physical activity might be instructed to do the following:
    a. _Empty her bladder_
    b. _Rest on side_
    c. _Drink 2-3 glasses of juice/water_
    d. _palpate for contractions_
    e. _Call back in 1 hr if symptoms persist_

11. The ultimate diagnosis of true labor progress is _of recur c resumption of normal Activity & cervical change_.

12. List five parameters used to determine fetal age.
    a. _LMP_
    b. _Early Sonograms_
    c. _fund height_
    d. _Date of quickening_
    e. _first date of audible heart tones_

13. About half the time, preterm labor contractions will stop with _Bed Rest_ and _hydration_

14. List four physiologic alterations in *nonpregnant* patients placed on bed rest.
    a. _loss of total Body mass_
    b. _Musle atrophy_
    c. _↓ blood + plasma volume_
    d. _↓ Cardiac output_

15. The best resting position for the woman with preterm labor contractions to achieve maximum placental perfusion is the _left side_

16. Well-controlled studies confirm that bed rest is an effective therapy for preterm labor.

    A. True

    B. False ✓

17. List five clinical observations that should be noted when doing a cervical examination on a woman at risk for preterm labor.

    a. _Position_
    b. _Consistency_
    c. _Effacement_
    d. _Dilation_
    e. _Station_

18. Women often react to their preterm labor by feeling _anger_ and _guilt_.

19. List the nursing responsibilities in caring for the woman being treated for preterm labor.

    a. _Monitor Uterine Status_
    b. _Reevaluate symptoms_
    c. _Monitor fetal Status_
    d. _Monitor Maternal VS_
    e. _Monitor intake and output_
    f. _provide comfort measure + support_
    g. _Observe closely for side effects of tocolytic_
    h. _Educate pt about side effects of " " therapy_
    i. _Prepare for possibility of US, Amnio, Drug therapy_

20. Risk appraisal (does) (does not) identify approximately 90% of women who will eventually experience preterm labor.

21. The expectant woman usually appreciates that preterm labor is a risk for her.

    A. True

    B. False ✓

22. Drugs that have a depressant effect on the myometrium of the uterus are called _Tocolytic drugs_.

23. The process of administering a drug for the purpose of inhibiting uterine contractions is called _tocolysis_.

24. What are three indications for tocolytic therapy?

    a. _Dx of preterm labor_
    b. _Gestation Between 20 - 35 wks_
    c. _live fetus s s/s of severe distress or congenital anomalies incompatible c life_

25. List eight contraindications to tocolytic therapy.
   a. _Chorioamnionitis_
   b. _eclampsia / severe preeclapsia_
   c. _Severe renal or cardiovascular dz_
   d. _Acute hemmorage_
   e. _pulmonary hypertension_
   f. _maternal hyperthyroidism_
   g. _fetal demise or anomaly incompatib_
   h. _Severe fetal growth restriction c̄ life_

26. Two drugs that are commonly used for tocolysis are _terbutaline_ and _Mag sulfate_

27. List seven side effects of β-adrenergic drugs.
   a. _tremors_
   b. _maternal & fetal tachycardia_
   c. _HA_
   d. _palpitations_
   e. _Anxiety / nervousness_
   f. _Nausea / vomiting_
   g. _Hypotension_

28. During tocolytic therapy, the physician should be notified if the maternal pulse exceeds _120_ bpm or the fetal heart rate exceeds _180_ bpm.

29. Intake should be monitored and limited to prevent _~~Asphyxia,~~ Pulmonary edema_

30. The nurse should listen to the patient's breath sounds before tocolytic therapy begins and should monitor for signs of pulmonary edema, including _Dyspnea Wheezing Coughing_ or _rales_.

31. MgSO₄, a central nervous system depressant, should never be administered in the absence of _patellar reflexes_

32. Seven potential side effects of MgSO₄ administration are:
   a. _Drowsiness_
   b. _↓ Sensorium_
   c. _Slurred speech_
   d. _heavy eyelids_
   e. _flushing_
   f. _↓ gastrointestinal Motility_
   g. _Respiratory depression_

33. The efficacy of tocolytic drugs decreases if the cervix is more than _80%_ effaced or more than _3-4 cm_ dilated.

34. List six potential adverse effects from tocolytic drug therapy.

    a. Maternal tachycardia
    b. Severe hypotension
    c. ECG Δ's or myocardial ischemia
    d. pulmonary edema
    e. patient intolerence
    f. Severe respiratory depression

35. Define *premature rupture of membranes.*

    Spontaneous rupture of membranes before the onset of labor regardless of gestational age

36. A vaginal infection known to have a strong relationship to preterm delivery, especially in African American women, is called bacterial vaginosis.

37. List nine nursing interventions when a woman is admitted with PROM.

    a. Confirm membrane status
    b. review dating criteria
    c. Monitor fetal heart tones
    d. Evaluate uterine activity
    e. Determine GBS
    f. Observe for signs of infection
    g. determine the need for transport
    h. Assess womens understanding offer info + support
    i. Prepare for delivery of high risk infant

38. List three possible complications resulting from PROM.

    a. Intrauterine infection
    b. preterm labor
    c. prolapsed cord

39. Name four signs of chorioamnionitis.

    a. ↑ temp > 100.4
    b. Maternal + fetal tachycardia
    c. uterine tenderness
    d. foul smelling

40. The management of PROM is determined by the gestational age of the fetus and the presence or absence of labor, Chorioamnionitis, and fetal lung maturity fetal distress

41. If the fetus is less than 34 weeks and the mother is not in active labor, her care should take place at high risk medical center

42. Every fetus between 24 and 34 weeks' gestation at risk for preterm delivery should be considered a candidate for antenatal treatment with Corticosteroids

43. If chorioamnionitis develops or if there is evidence of fetal distress, *immediate delivery* is indicated.

44. The benefits of antenatal administration of corticosteroids to the fetus at risk of preterm delivery include a reduction in the risks of *respiratory distress syndrome* and *intraventricular hemmrage*

PRACTICE/REVIEW ANSWER KEY

1. 20; 37

2. a. Progressive change in the cervix
   b. Cervical dilatation of 2 cm or more
   c. Cervical effacement of 80% or more

3. Preterm births

4. a. Age ≤18 or ≥35
   b. Race—non-White
   c. Low socioeconomic status
   d. Unmarried
   e. Low level of education

5. Previous preterm birth

6. Any five of the following:
   a. Smoking
   b. Alcohol and other substance abuse
   c. Poor nutritional status
   d. High altitude
   e. Domestic abuse
   f. Strenuous job activity
   g. High stress
   h. Lack of prenatal care
   i. DES exposure and other toxic exposures

7. Early recognition; treatment

8. a. Uterine contractions—five or more in hour
   b. Menstrual-like cramps
   c. Low, dull backache
   d. Pelvic pressure
   e. Abdominal cramping
   f. Increase or change in vaginal discharge

9. a. The patient's knowledge level of preterm labor
   b. Her pregnancy history
   c. Distance from the hospital

10. a. Empty her bladder
    b. Rest on her side
    c. Drink 2 to 3 glasses of water or juice
    d. Palpate for contractions
    e. Call back in 1 hour if symptoms persist or if symptoms recur with resumption of normal activities

11. Cervical change

12. a. LMP
    b. Early sonograms
    c. Fundal height measurements
    d. Date of quickening
    e. First date of audible fetal heart tones

13. Bed rest; hydration

14. Any four of the following:
    a. Loss of total body mass
    b. Muscle atrophy
    c. Reduced blood and plasma volume
    d. Decreased cardiac output
    e. Glucose intolerance
    f. Insulin resistance
    g. Increased anxiety, depression, and somatic complaints

15. Left lateral position

16. B

17. a. Position
    b. Consistency
    c. Effacement
    d. Dilatation
    e. Station

18. Anger; guilt

19. a. Monitor uterine status.
    b. Reevaluate symptoms of preterm labor.
    c. Monitor fetal status.
    d. Monitor maternal vital signs.
    e. Monitor intake and output.
    f. Provide comfort measures and emotional support.
    g. Observe closely for side effects of tocolytic therapy.
    h. Educate the patient and her family about potential side effects of tocolytic therapy.
    i. Prepare for the possibility of ultrasound, amniocentesis, tocolytic drug therapy, steroid therapy, baseline blood chemistry (serum potassium, glucose, CBC), and baseline ECG.

20. Does not

21. B

22. Tocolytic drugs

23. Tocolysis

24. a. Diagnosis of preterm labor
    b. Gestation between 20 and 35 weeks
    c. Live fetus without signs of severe distress or congenital anomalies incompatible with life

25. a. Chorioamnionitis
    b. Eclampsia/severe preeclampsia
    c. Severe renal or cardiovascular disease
    d. Acute hemorrhage or active uterine/vaginal bleeding
    e. Pulmonary hypertension
    f. Maternal hyperthyroidism
    g. Fetal demise or anomaly incompatible with life
    h. Severe fetal growth restriction

26. Terbutaline; magnesium sulfate

27. a. Tremors
    b. Maternal and fetal tachycardia
    c. Headache
    d. Palpitations
    e. Anxiety/nervousness
    f. Nausea and/or vomiting
    g. Hypotension

28. 120; 180

29. Pulmonary edema

30. Dyspnea; wheezing; coughing; rales

31. Patellar reflexes

32. a. Drowsiness
    b. Decreased sensorium
    c. Slurred speech
    d. Heavy eyelids
    e. Flushing
    f. Decreased gastrointestinal motility
    g. Respiratory depression

33. 80%; 3 to 4 cm

34. a. Maternal tachycardia greater than 140 bpm (β-mimetics)
    b. Severe hypotension (systolic pressure 80 to 90 mm Hg)
    c. ECG changes indicative of myocardial ischemia
    d. Pulmonary edema
    e. Patient intolerance
    f. Severe respiratory depression ($MgSO_4$)

35. The spontaneous rupture of membranes before the onset of labor, regardless of gestational age

36. Bacterial vaginosis

37. a. Confirm membrane status.
    b. Review dating criteria.
    c. Monitor fetal heart tones.
    d. Evaluate uterine activity.
    e. Determine group B streptococcus status and the need for antibiotic prophylaxis.
    f. Observe for signs of infection.
    g. Determine the need for transport.
    h. Assess woman's understanding of the implications of PROM and provide support and education.
    i. Prepare for delivery of a high-risk infant.

38. a. Intrauterine infection (chorioamnionitis)
    b. Preterm labor
    c. Prolapsed umbilical cord

39. a. Maternal or fetal tachycardia
    b. Temperature greater than 100.4°F
    c. Uterine tenderness
    d. Foul-smelling purulent amniotic fluid

40. Labor; chorioamnionitis; fetal distress; fetal lung maturity

41. A high-risk regional medical center

42. Corticosteroids (betamethasone)

43. Immediate delivery

44. Respiratory distress syndrome; intraventricular hemorrhage

REFERENCES

1. Heaman, M., Sprague, A., & Stewart, P. (2001). Reducing the preterm birth rate: A population health strategy. *Journal of Obstetric, Gynecologic, and Neonatal Nursing, 30,* 20–29.
2. Sullivan, C. (1998). Sonographic evaluation of the uterine cervix. *Obstetrics and Gynecology Clinics of North America, 25,* 623–637.
3. Leitich, H., Egarter, C., Kaider, A., Hohlagschwandtner, M., Berghammer, P., & Husslein, P. (1999). Cervicovaginal fetal fibronectin as a marker for preterm delivery: A meta-analysis. *American Journal of Obstetrics and Gynecology, 180*(5), 1169–1176.
4. Heine, R. P. (1999). Accuracy of salivary estriol testing compared to traditional risk factor assessment in predicting preterm birth. *American Journal of Obstetrics and Gynecology, 180*(1 Pt 3), S214–S218.
5. Lockwood, C. (1999). Stress-associated preterm delivery: The role of corticotropin-releasing hormone. *American Journal of Obstetrics and Gynecology, 180*(1 Pt 3), S264–S266.
6. American College of Obstetricians and Gynecologists. (1999). Home uterine activity monitoring. ACOG Committee Opinion, No. 172. Washington, DC: Author.
7. Patterson, E. T., Douglas, A. B., Patterson, P. M., & Bradle, J. B. (1992). Symptoms of preterm labor and self-diagnostic confusion. *Nursing Research, 41*(6), 367–372.
8. Patterson, K. A. (1993). Experience of risk for pregnant black women. *Journal of Perinatology, 13*(4), 279–284.
9. Maloni, J., Cohen, A., & Kane, J. (1998). Prescription of activity restriction to treat high-risk pregnancies. *Journal of Women's Health, 7*(3), 351–358.
10. Lumley, J., Oliver, S., & Waters, E. (2001). Interventions for promoting smoking cessation during pregnancy. *Cochrane Database System Review,* (2), CD001055.
11. American College of Obstetricians and Gynecologists. (1998). Bacterial vaginosis screening for prevention of preterm delivery. ACOG Committee Opinion, No. 198. Washington, DC.
12. Paige, D., Augustyn, M., Adih, W., Witter, F., & Chang, J. (1998). Bacterial vaginosis and preterm birth: A comprehensive review of the literature. *Journal of Nurse-Midwifery, 43*(2), 83–88.
13. Goldenberg, R. (1998). Low birthweight in minority and high-risk women: Patient outcomes research team (PORT) final report. Agency for Healthcare Policy and Research. Washington, DC.
14. American Academy of Pediatrics, Committee on Infectious Diseases and Committee on Fetus and Newborn. (1997). Revised guidelines for early onset group B streptococcal infection. *Pediatrics, 99*(3), 489–496.
15. National Institutes of Health Consensus Developement Panel. (2000). Antenatal corticosteroids revisited. *National Institutes of Health Consensus Development Conference Statement,* August 17–18.
16. American College of Obstetricians and Gynecologists. (1998). Premature rupture of membranes: Clinical management guidelines for obstetrician-gynecologists. ACOG Practice Bulletin, No. 1. Washington, DC: Author.

SUGGESTED READINGS

American College of Nurse-Midwives. (1998). Bacterial vaginosis in pregnancy. ACNM Clinical Bulletin, No. 4. Washington, DC: Author.

American College of Obstetricians and Gynecologists. (1995). Preterm labor. ACOG Technical Bulletin, No. 206, Washington, DC: Author.

Antenatal corticosteroids revisited: Repeat courses. NIH Consensus Statement 2000, 17(2), 1–10.

Brocklehurst, P., Hannah, M., & McDonald, H. (2000). Interventions for treating bacterial vaginosis in pregnancy. *Cochrane Database System Review,* (2), CD000262.

Crowley, P. (2000). Prophylactic corticosteroids for preterm birth. *Cochrane Database System Review,* (2), CD000065.

King, J., & Flenady, V. (2000). Antibiotics for preterm labor with intact membranes. *Cochrane Database System Review,* (2), CD000246.

Kovacevich, G. J., Gaich, S. A., Lavin, J. P., Hopkins, M. P., Crane, S. S., Stewart, J., Nelson, D., & Lavin, L. M. (2000). The prevalence of thromboembolic events among women with extended bed rest prescribed as part of the treatment for premature labor or preterm premature rupture of membranes. *American Journal Obstetrics and Gynecology, 182*(5), 1089–1092.

Majzorib, J., McGregor, J., Lockwood, C., Smith, R., Taggart, M. S., & Schulkin, J. (1999). A central theory of preterm and term labor: Putative role for corticotropin-releasing hormone. *American Journal of Obstetrics and Gynecology, 180*(1), S232–S241.

Maloni, J. (2001). Preventing low birth weight: How smoking cessation counseling can help. *AWHONN Lifelines, 5*(1), 32–35.

Maloni, J. (2000). Preventing preterm birth: Evidence-based interventions shift toward prevention. *AWHONN Lifelines, 4*(4), 26–33.

Maloni, J. (2000). *The prevention of preterm birth: Research-based practice, nursing interventions, and practice scenarios.* Washington, DC: Association of Women's Health, Obstetric and Neonatal Nurses.

Maloni, J., Brezinski-Tomasi, J., & Johnson, L. (2001). Antepartum bed rest: Effect upon the family. *Journal of Obstetric, Gynecologic, and Neonatal Nursing, 30*, 165–173.

Management of Preterm Labor. Summary, Evidence Report/Technology Assessment: No. 18. AHRQ Publication No. 01-E020, October, 2000. Agency for Healthcare Research and Quality, Rockville, MD.

Mercer, B. (1998). Antibiotic therapy for preterm premature rupture of membranes. *Clinical Obstetrics and Gynecology, 41*(2), 461–468.

Mercer, B. M., Goldenberg, R. L., Meis, P. J., Moawad, A. H., Shellhaas, C., Das, A., Menard, M. K., Caritis, S. N., Thurnau, G. R., Dombrowski, M. P., Miodovnik, M., Roberts, J. M., & McNellis, D. (2000). The Preterm Prediction Study: Prediction of preterm premature rupture of membranes through clinical findings and ancillary testing. The National Institute of Child Health and Human Development Maternal-Fetal Medicine Units Network. *American Journal of Obstetrics and Gynecology, 183*(3), 738–745.

Rini, C., Wadhwa, P., & Sandman, C. (1999). Psychological adaptation and birth outcomes: The role of personal resources, stress, and sociocultural context in pregnancy. *Health Psychology, 18*(4), 333–345.

Schroeder, C. (1998). Bed rest in complicated pregnancy: A critical analysis. *American Journal of Maternal Child Nursing, 23*, 45–49.

Tan, B. P., & Hannah, M. E. (2000). Oxytocin for prelabour rupture of membranes at or near term. *Cochrane Database System Review, (2)*, CD000157.

Wasser, S. (1999). Stress and reproductive failure: An evolutionary approach with applications to premature labor. *American Journal of Obstetrics and Gynecology, 180*(1), S272–S274.

M O D U L E   9

Caring for the Laboring Woman With Hypertensive Disorders Complicating Pregnancy

E. JEAN MARTIN

As you complete this module, you will learn:

1. The epidemiology of hypertensive disorders in pregnancy
2. The role of screening and diagnostic criteria in the assessment of women at risk for hypertensive disorders
3. Current terminology and a current classification system recommended for hypertensive disorders complicating pregnancy
4. The definition and characteristics of each hypertensive disorder associated with pregnancy
5. Factors that predispose a woman to chronic hypertension and pregnancy outcomes in women with chronic hypertension
6. Factors that predispose a woman to preeclampsia/eclampsia and pregnancy outcomes in women with the preeclampsia/eclampsia
7. Current theoretical and known pathophysiologic alterations that occur in women with preeclampsia
8. The significance of signs and symptoms that correlate with pathophysiologic changes in body systems in hypertensive disorders during pregnancy
9. Diagnostic criteria (including laboratory tests) considered valid and reliable for screening and monitoring women at risk for pregnancy-related hypertension
10. What to look for when reviewing the prenatal record during the admission process
11. Aspects of the physical examination that must be carried out in screening for hypertensive disorders
12. Priorities for treatment and nursing care
13. Issues of intrapartum pain management
14. Recommended anticonvulsant treatment regimens for administering magnesium sulfate ($MgSO_4 \cdot 7H_2O$) to the preeclamptic woman
15. Monitoring techniques and the therapeutic blood level range appropriate for the woman receiving magnesium sulfate
16. Signs of toxicity in magnesium sulfate overdose and treatment
17. Indications and nursing interventions for acute antihypertensive therapy in hypertensive emergencies in pregnancy
18. Guidelines for using antihypertensive therapy
19. Indications for maternal transport of a preeclamptic woman to a high-risk regional center
20. Special preparations for delivery of a potentially high-risk infant
21. Indications for postpartum care and education

When you have completed this module, you should be able to recall the meaning of the following terms. You should also be able to use the terms when consulting with other health professionals. Terms are defined in this module or in the glossary at the end of this book.

antiphospholipid antibodies
clonus

disseminated intravascular coagulation
endothelin-derived releasing factor (EDRF)

endothelium (endothelial lining)
epigastric pain
gestational hypertension
hydatidiform mole
hydralazine (Apresoline)
hydrops
iatrogenic
microangiopathy

oliguria
prostacyclin (PGI$_2$)
proteinuria
scotomata
thrombocytopenia
thromboxane
vasopressor

Introduction[1-3]

Hypertension associated with pregnancy complicates 6% to 8% of all pregnancies. The incidence of this serious disorder can vary greatly among racial and ethnic groups and is influenced by age and parity. Hypertension is the most common medical risk factor for pregnant women.

Among the four leading causes of maternal mortality in the United States—thromboembolic disease, hypertension, hemorrhage, and infection—hypertension during pregnancy is second only to thromboembolic disease. Current estimates attribute 12% to 18% of all pregnancy-related maternal deaths to hypertension disorders (i.e., approximately 70 maternal deaths in the United States and 50,000 maternal deaths worldwide occur each year). Because the fetus is exposed to maternal pathophysiologic alterations underlying a hypertensive disorder, pregnancy outcomes include stillbirths and neonatal morbidity and mortality.

Although the etiology and pathophysiology of hypertension in pregnancy have been intensively researched over the years, a great deal is still unknown. This module presents what is currently reflected in the literature as well as guidelines from the National High Blood Pressure Education Program Working Group Report on High Blood Pressure in Pregnancy.[2] The Working Group uses evidence-based findings and consensus in providing guidelines for management to clinicians.

Studying this module will perhaps involve repeated reading and a "letting go" of previous concepts and understanding. Diagnostic criteria have changed. For the nurse, nurse-midwife, and physician, astute and early assessments are critical to appropriate diagnosis and early intervention.

Terminology and Classification

Many classification schemes and terminology have been proposed by various authors, agencies, and even countries, resulting in confusing and nonstandardized diagnostic categories. A concise and clinically useful classification is needed.[4]

The most important issue in the classification of disorders of blood pressure (BP) in pregnancy is differentiating those hypertensive disorders occurring before pregnancy from those occurring during pregnancy with potentially serious consequences, specifically preeclampsia. Preeclampsia is peculiar to pregnancy and comprises a specific syndrome of the following:

- Reduced organ perfusion (brain, kidney, and liver), which is caused by the following:
- Vasospasm of tiny arteries (arterioles) occurring at the organ(s) site and elsewhere in the body's vasculature
- Activation of a coagulation process leading to abnormal fibrin deposition and platelet consumption (i.e., platelets are "used up")[2]

These pathophysiologic processes result in signs and symptoms in the pregnant woman that have degrees of significance and importance. Issues in making a diagnosis of a hypertensive disorder as complicating pregnancy have to do with the importance attached to the:

- Timing of the hypertensive disorder in relation to gestational age
- Timing of signs and symptoms in relation to gestational age
- Reliability of the sign or symptom (diagnostic criteria)

Diagnostic criteria or **diagnostic markers** are used in developing classification systems. A great deal of research has been done on behalf of substantiating the authenticity (reliability, reproducibility, and degree of predictability) of the diagnostic criteria used in the classification system presented by the Working Group.[2] The classification system is based on terminology and definitions similar to those developed by the American College of Obstetricians and Gynecologists (ACOG) in 1972 and modified by the ACOG in 1986 and 1994.

Clarification of Terms

Pregnancy-Induced Hypertension

A number of authors have used the term *pregnancy-induced hypertension* (PIH) broadly to describe all new onsets of hypertension in pregnancy, including hypertension not accompanied by proteinuria as well as hypertension with proteinuria (i.e., preeclampsia). Currently, key obstetric textbooks and journal articles are dropping the term; *pregnancy-induced hypertension* is no longer being used.[1,3–5] The Working Group Report on Hypertensive Disorders of Pregnancy has proposed a simplified classification system and defined terminology that might serve as a standard guideline. This module incorporates this new classification system.

Gestational and Transient Hypertension

The term *gestational hypertension* has been used to signify hypertension (BP of 140/90 mm Hg or greater) occurring after the twentieth week of gestation without proteinuria or edema. *If the elevated BP resolves rather quickly after delivery, it is diagnosed and termed as such retrospectively.*

NOTE: Gestational and transient hypertension previously fell under the broad category of PIH. The new classification system arranges these terms for the purpose of diagnosis somewhat differently.

Classification of Hypertensive Disorders Complicating Pregnancy

Each hypertensive disorder complicating pregnancy has distinguishing characteristics, diagnostic criteria, and risks of perinatal morbidity and mortality. Discussion will follow the Working Group Classification System:

1. Gestational hypertension
2. Preeclampsia/eclampsia

NOTE: HELLP syndrome—a serious extension of preeclampsia—is discussed within this category.

3. Preeclampsia superimposed upon chronic hypertension
4. Chronic hypertension

Important observations that reflect current understanding of the hypertensive disorders in pregnancy include the following:

- Pregnancy can induce hypertension in normotensive women *or* aggravate existing hypertension.
- Hypertensive states are classified according to certain signs or symptoms and time of occurrence in relation to the pregnancy.
- The term *pregnancy-induced hypertension* has sometimes been used to designate women with elevated BP but no proteinuria or edema. It is not a diagnostic category in the classification system presented by the Working Group Report.[2]
- The presence of hypertension before or very early in pregnancy increases the incidence of complications for both the mother and fetus, with a 10-fold higher risk of fetal loss.[2]
- When hypertension is documented before conception or before 20 weeks' gestation, it is much more likely to be chronic hypertension that is either essential hypertension from unknown causes or secondary hypertension with an identified cause (e.g., renal disease).[2]
- Elevated BP seen at midpregnancy (20 to 28 weeks) may be due to either early preeclampsia, which is rarely seen before 24 weeks; transient hypertension, which will resolve quickly after delivery; or chronic hypertension that has not been recognized in the woman and will remain beyond 12 weeks postpartum.[2]

- HELLP syndrome does not appear in the classification system because it is considered an extension of the pathophysiologic process of preeclampsia. HELLP syndrome is addressed later in this module.
- Fetal risks in a pregnancy complicated by hypertension include growth restriction, abruptio placentae, fetal distress, preterm birth, and low birth weight with subsequent perinatal morbidity and mortality.[6]
- The perinatal mortality rate increases as maternal BP and proteinuria increase.[6]
- Chronic hypertension and preeclampsia **do not** have the same etiology or pathophysiology and must be carefully differentiated.

Gestational Hypertension

- Formerly called PIH or transient hypertension
- Occurrence of BP elevation after 20 weeks' gestation to 140/90 mm Hg for the first time during pregnancy but without accompanying proteinuria
- Can progress to preeclampsia with development of proteinuria and other diagnostic indicators
- Is referred to as **transient hypertension of pregnancy** *if preeclampsia is not present at delivery and BP returns to normal by 12 weeks postpartum*

OR

- Is diagnosed as **chronic hypertension** *if BP elevation persists to beyond 12 weeks postpartum*

NOTE: *The diagnosis of gestational hypertension is used during pregnancy only until criteria (signs and symptoms) arise that define a more specific diagnosis.*

Preeclampsia/Eclampsia

- A pregnancy-specific syndrome usually occurring after 20 weeks' gestation

OR

- Occurring earlier in hydatidiform mole or hydrops (diseases of the trophoblast placenta)
- Determined by increased BP and proteinuria
- **Eclampsia**—the occurrence in a woman with preeclampsia of seizures that cannot be attributed to other causes

Preeclampsia Superimposed Upon Chronic Hypertension (Superimposed Preeclampsia)

- Occurrence of preeclampsia in a woman who enters pregnancy already in a hypertensive state

Chronic Hypertension

- Hypertension that is present and observable before pregnancy

OR

- Hypertension that is diagnosed before 20 weeks' gestation

Diagnosis

■ **How are the various hypertensive disorders diagnosed?**

Screening Criteria

In the past, noninvasive screening procedures were used to predict a woman's risk of developing hypertension or preeclampsia. The tests are mentioned here because their use needs to be put to rest once and for all. The three most commonly used tests were the following:

- Calculating the second trimester mean arterial pressure (MAP) to predict risks and associated perinatal morbidity and mortality
- Noting the absence of a decline in late second trimester BP, which might be interpreted as a pathophysiologic response predicting maternal or fetal risk
- Using the roll-over test (supine pressure test)—performed at 28 to 32 weeks' gestation to detect a woman's unique sensitivity to vasopressor substances in her circulatory system by assessing BP on her side and then on her back

These screening tests do not contain consistently predictable, reproducible, and reliable results and should not be used in screening women to predict a risk for preeclampsia.

Because reliable screening criteria are unavailable, the emphasis in clinical practice should be on timely and accurate assessment of *diagnostic criteria.*

Diagnostic Criteria

Using evidence-based medicine, the Working Group Report on High Blood Pressure in Pregnancy and others[2,6] identify reliable *diagnostic criteria* and guidelines to be used in the evaluation of hypertensive states in pregnancy. Display 9.1 illustrates the diagnostic criteria for each.

DISPLAY 9.1 Diagnostic Criteria Use in the Diagnosis of Hypertensive Disorders Complicating Pregnancy

Gestational Hypertension

BP ≥140/90 mm Hg for the first time during pregnancy

No proteinuria

BP returns to normal <12 weeks postpartum

Final diagnosis made only postpartum

May have other signs of preeclampsia, for example, epigastic discomfort or thrombocytopenia

Preeclampsia

Minimum Criteria:

BP ≥160/110 mm Hg

Proteinuria ≥300 mg per 24 hours or ≥1+ dipstick

Increased Certainty of Preeclampsia:

BP ≥160/110 mm Hg

Proteinuria 2 g per 24 hours or ≥2+ dipstick

Serum creatinine >1.2 mg/dL unless known to be previously elevated

Platelets <100,000/mm³

Microangiopathic hemolysis (increased LDH)

Elevated ALT or AST

Persistent headache or other cerebral or visual disturbance

Persistent epigastric pain

Eclampsia

Seizures that cannot be attributed to other causes in a woman with preeclampsia

Superimposed Preeclampsia (on Chronic Hypertension)

New-onset proteinuria >300 mg per 24 hours in hypertensive women but no proteinuria before 20 weeks' gestation

A sudden increase in proteinuria or blood pressure or platelet count <100,000/mm³ in women with hypertension and proteinuria before 20 weeks' gestation

Chronic Hypertension

BP >140/90 mm Hg before pregnancy or diagnosed before 20 weeks' gestation

OR

Hypertension first diagnosed after 20 weeks' gestation and persistent after 12 weeks postpartum

ALT, alanine aminotransferase; AST, aspartate aminotransferase; BP, blood pressure; LDH, lactate dehydrogenase; Adapted from National Blood Pressure Education Program. (2000). *Working Group report on high blood pressure in pregnancy.* Bethesda, MD: National Heart, Lung, and Blood Institute. Reprinted with permission from Cunningham, N. F. Gant, K. J. Leveno, L. C. Gilstrap, J. C. Hauth, & K. D. Wenstrom, K. D. (Eds.), (2001) *Williams' obstetrics* (21st ed., p. 569). New York: McGraw-Hill.

Gestational Hypertension

- Gestational hypertension is hypertension only, without proteinuria, with normal laboratory test results, and in the absence of symptoms.
- It has been defined and explained in terms of *criteria* and *timing* under the classification listing on the previous page.
- This classification no doubt includes women with hypertension of different etiologies. Some women may develop essential hypertension later in life.

- A rise of BP in the latter half of pregnancy should always be watched carefully. Both the mother and fetus could be in danger. Cunningham[1] cautions that treatment should not wait on the appearance of proteinuria because seizures can occur without proteinuria. Overdiagnosing preeclampsia is preferable to missing the diagnosis until the disease process has worsened.[1]
- Transient hypertension:
  - –Occurs in the absence of proteinuria or pathologic edema (generalized)
  - –Is considered a fairly benign disease that can recur in subsequent pregnancies (It may signal the possibility of future chronic hypertension as the woman ages.)
  - –*Is diagnosed in retrospect (when BP elevation resolves with no adverse sequelae)*
  - –Is not accompanied by poor birth outcomes
  - –Is sometimes seen in normotensive mothers within the first few hours after delivery, with subsequent return to baseline BP levels within 24 hours

Preeclampsia

Preeclampsia is the occurrence of gestational BP elevation accompanied by proteinuria.

Gestational BP elevation is defined as BP 140 mm Hg or greater systole or 90 mm Hg or greater diastole in a woman who has been normotensive before 20 weeks' gestation.

Remember, when distinguishing gestational hypertension from preeclampsia, *preeclampsia is more than hypertension—it is a syndrome.*

NOTE: *Preeclampsia is actually a syndrome that occurs only in the presence of pregnancy (the placenta plays a key role). Preeclampsia is caused by reduced perfusion of one or more organs, which results from vasospasm of arterioles and damage to the lining (endothelium) of the arterioles. It resolves with delivery of the fetus and placenta.*

While acknowledging that the cause of this disorder is unknown and most likely has no one single cause, Norwitz and Repke[3] state that preeclampsia is a multisystem disorder specific to the placenta. They cite the primary pathology as being a defect in placental development. The normal physiologic process involves embryo/fetal-derived cells of the trophoblast, which invade the uterine lining (decidua) and its vasculature, specifically the arteriole walls of uterine blood vessels. This invasion appears to play a critical role in the progressive and marked enlargement of the spiral arterioles in the endometrial lining. "The fetus is anchored to the mother." *The result ensures an adequate blood supply to the growing placenta and fetus.* Preeclampsia is characterized by a restriction of this process in which 30% to 50% of the placenta's spiral arteries show no evidence of trophoblastic invasion.[3]

According to Norwitz and Repke, "the end result in preeclampsia is an inability of the uterine vasculature to accommodate the necessary increase in blood flow with increasing gestational age . . . clinical manifestations of the disorder become apparent when the fetal placental unit outgrows its blood supply."[3] Underperfusion of the placenta is believed to produce chemical factors that enter the maternal circulation and eventually affect the vascular endothelium (the endothelial lining of the body's widespread arteriolar system). More of the pathophysiology is discussed later in this module.

Other important facts related to preeclampsia include the following:

- Preeclampsia can occur before the twentieth gestational week, when there are pathologic changes in the placenta, with the development of a hydatidiform molar pregnancy. In the United States and Europe, molar pregnancies occur in 1 per 1,000 expectant women and are typically characterized by the following[1]:
  - –Severe nausea and vomiting
  - –Elevated BP
  - –Elevated human chorionic gonadotropin (hCG) levels
  - –Absence of fetal movement or fetal heartbeat

Preeclampsia before 24 weeks' gestation necessitates evaluation to rule out a complete or partial molar pregnancy.

355

–Uterine size larger than dates by last menstrual period
–Vaginal bleeding
–Passage of grapelike clustered vesicles

- Preeclampsia occurs in approximately 5% of pregnant women, but this incidence is highly variable,[1] with a higher incidence in women younger than 20 or older than 35 years of age, in nulliparous women, and in women with multiple fetuses.
- Preeclampsia complicates approximately 20% of teenage pregnancies (younger than 20 years of age).
- It exists as a disease for weeks or even months before signs or symptoms are evident.
- It is often not accompanied by proteinuria until late in the disease (late third trimester or intrapartum period).
- Significant proteinuria means:
  –300 mg/L in a 24-hour specimen

  OR

  –2+ or greater on dipstick (tested twice 4 hours apart) in the absence of a urinary tract infection

---

Bacterial invasion of the vaginal or urinary tract mucosal lining causes tissue breakdown, releasing protein metabolites. Thus, protein found in the urine of a woman with a urinary tract or vaginal infection does not necessarily indicate kidney malfunction.

CLINICAL SIGNS OF PREECLAMPSIA CAN OCCUR SUDDENLY. NEVER UNDER-ESTIMATE THE IMPORTANCE OF EVEN MILD BP ELEVATIONS COMPLICATING A PREGNANCY.

Preeclampsia is usually categorized as mild or severe, based primarily on the degree of hypertension or proteinuria and whether other organ systems are involved.[4]

Mild preeclampsia occurs when the following are found:

- BP has reached 140/90 mm Hg or greater but is less than 160/110 mm Hg on two different occasions 4 hours apart. A rise in BP of 30 mm Hg systole or 15 mm Hg diastole is an important observation and warrants careful surveillance for other signs and symptoms.

A rise in the diastolic reading may be a more reliable indication of preeclampsia.

- Proteinuria, trace to +1 or about 300 mg in a 24-hour urine specimen, is noted.
- Signs that preeclampsia may be present are as follows:
  –Weight gain of more than 5 pounds per week during the second trimester or more than 2 pounds per week during the third trimester
  –Slight edema throughout the body

Severe preeclampsia occurs when the following are found:

- BP rises to 160/110 mm Hg or greater (some experts say 170/110 mm Hg or greater) on two different occasions 4 hours apart.
- Proteinuria is persistent 2+ or more (500 mg or greater per 24 hours).
- Urine output decreases to less than 500 mL in 24 hours (i.e., less than 30 mL per hour).

NOTE: Differentiating between mild and severe preeclampsia is not always clinically helpful because mild disease can rapidly progress to severe illness.[1]

In severe preeclampsia, the kidneys can go into failure with little output. This is a serious situation that can lead to permanent renal injury.

Symptoms of severe disease include:

Severe headaches
Visual problems (scotoma or blurring)
Epigastric pain
Nausea or vomiting
Thrombocytopenia
Irritability, restlessness, or apprehension
Pulmonary edema with respiratory
  distress

Signs of severe disease include[2-4]:

Severe proteinuria (3+ dipstick or greater)
Oliguria (less than 500 mL per 24 hours)
Low platelet count (less than 100,000/mm³)
Elevated hepatic enzymes (alanine amino-
  transferase [ALT] or aspartate aminotrans-
  ferase [AST])
Increased serum creatinine (greater than
  1.2 mg/dL unless known to be previously
  elevated)
Fetal intrauterine growth restriction
Coagulation abnormalities

> Early identification of worsening preeclampsia in a patient at a Level I or II hospital is critical. Transport to a high-risk regional center should be done while the patient is stable and before a critical state is reached. Both the mother and fetus are at risk.

When severe preeclampsia occurs before 32 weeks' gestation, the incidence of serious complications in the mother is high and fetal outcome is poor, often as a result of growth restriction and/or asphyxia at birth.

WATCH FOR SIGNS OF THE FOLLOWING:

- Abruptio placentae
- HELLP syndrome
- Eclampsia
- Disseminated intravascular coagulation (DIC)
- Acute renal failure

■ **Are certain pregnant women at risk for developing preeclampsia?**

Predisposing factors to preeclampsia exist in women:[1,2,4]

- Who are young and pregnant for the first time
- Who are young and experiencing a second pregnancy but with a new father
- With a partner who has fathered a preeclamptic pregnancy in another woman
- With a history of chronic hypertension or renal disease (renal vascular hypertension, nephrotic syndrome, adult polycystic kidney disease)
- With a twin pregnancy
- With diabetes
- With a history of preeclampsia
- Who are Black and older than 35 years of age
- With collagen vascular disease (i.e., lupus or antiphospholipid antibody syndrome)

> Pregnancies in which placental size is increased (e.g., multiple fetuses, diabetes, syphilis, isoimmunized pregnancies, hydatidiform moles) carry a higher risk because the placenta plays an important role in pathophysiologic processes.

> Race is not considered a significant risk factor by some. Hydramnios unaccompanied by fetal hydrops or diabetes is not a risk factor, nor is social class in general. The risk rises modestly in unmarried women.

Careful assessment should be done on women identified as at risk:

- Teenagers
- Black and other minority women 35 years of age and older

- Women with a multiple gestation
- Women with a history of chronic hypertension
- Women who were hypertensive during a previous pregnancy

HELLP Syndrome[5,7,9]

- HELLP syndrome is a hypertensive state in pregnancy that occurs in a small number of severely preeclamptic women who exhibit a certain set of symptoms *in addition to the criteria for severe preeclampsia.*
- It is named for its primary laboratory abnormalities—**H**emolysis, **E**levated **L**iver enzymes, and **L**ow **P**latelets (HELLP)
- Experts agree that hemolysis, liver dysfunction, and thrombocytopenia must be present for the diagnosis, but no agreement has been reached regarding specific criteria.
- HELLP syndrome involves a group of clinical/pathologic manifestations resulting from arteriolar vasospasm, which leads to the development of microangiopathic hemolytic anemia. Microvascular endothelial damage and intravascular platelet activation can be documented with laboratory studies. No one precipitating cause of this syndrome has been found.[5,7]
- The incidence of HELLP syndrome in preeclamptic women is reported to be 2% to 12%. An accurate rate of occurrence is unknown because of difficulties with agreement on diagnostic criteria.[5]
- HELLP syndrome occurs before term (late second or early third trimester) in more than 80% of women, with 11% of the cases occurring before 27 weeks; approximately one third of cases become evident during the postdelivery period.
- This syndrome occurs primarily with cesarean births and in multiparous women.
- A significant risk of maternal mortality, approaching 1.0% to 3.5%, is seen with HELLP syndrome.

NOTE: Women with HELLP syndrome often present with nonspecific symptoms or subtle signs. The woman is usually Caucasian and in her second or third trimester.

A common scenario is a woman complaining of "just not feeling good," "a flulike feeling," nausea, epigastric pain, or right upper quadrant pain. She may have no hypertension (15% of cases) or only mild hypertension (16% of cases). In addition, proteinuria may be absent or only 1+ on a urine dipstick. These women are very ill but are often misdiagnosed with the flu, gastroenteritis, appendicitis, viral hepatitis, gallbladder disease, or pyelonephritis.

- The *maternal* mortality rate approaches 1.0% to 3.5%.[9]
- Maternal mortality and morbidity are consequences of the following:
  - Spontaneous and postpartum hemorrhage
  - Development of superimposed DIC
  - Abruptio placentae
  - Renal failure
  - Pulmonary edema
  - Hepatic rupture
- The *perinatal* mortality rate ranges from 56 to 637 per 1,000 births.[9] Fetal death often occurs at gestational ages near the limit of viability because of the following:
  - Severe growth restriction
  - Abruptio placentae
- Many patients initially worsen after delivery and then begin to improve.

Eclampsia[1,2,8]

- Eclampsia is defined as the occurrence in a woman with preeclampsia of seizures and sometimes coma not caused by a neurologic disease (e.g., epilepsy).
- It represents a worsening of preeclampsia, with rapid deterioration of function in several organs and systems.
- The incidence is estimated at 1 in 3,250 for women in the United States.
- It is seen both in women without HELLP syndrome and in those with HELLP.
- Eclamptic women without HELLP syndrome usually have fewer adverse birth outcomes.[8]

- Eclamptic women with HELLP syndrome often experience the following:
  –Preterm labor
  –Earlier gestational ages
  –Lower birth weights
  –Lower Apgar scores
  –Greater perinatal morbidity and mortality

Maternal mortality is most often due to the following:

- Abruptio placentae
- Cerebral hemorrhage
- Acute renal or cardiac failure
- DIC

NOTE: Eclamptic convulsions can occur in women who have mildly elevated BP and mild proteinuria and in women who show few warning signs of a worsening condition.

Despite the rapid onset of convulsions characterizing eclampsia, ideally, no woman should experience eclampsia in a hospitalized setting. Signs, symptoms, and risk factors should indicate the woman's deterioration to medical and nursing personnel. However, a woman presenting to the labor unit with limited or no prenatal care can progress quickly to eclampsia.

■ What distinguishes eclampsia from preeclampsia?

The distinguishing characteristic of eclampsia is the presence of convulsions. Prior to convulsions, the BP often rises. The convulsive state involves the following:

- Initial twitching of facial muscles
- Fixed, protruding, and bloodshot eyes
- Alternating muscle contraction, with hands and teeth clenching and then relaxing
- Respirations that stop and then begin again with deep, heavy, and noisy breathing
- Coma, which can follow and last from 2 to 3 minutes to several hours

> This can signify pulmonary edema or pulmonary aspiration of gastric contents.

REMEMBER: Preeclampsia need not be severe to progress to eclampsia. Also, eclampsia can occur in the absence of proteinuria.

Preeclampsia Superimposed upon Chronic Hypertension[1,2,10]

- Preeclampsia superimposed upon chronic hypertension is defined as the occurrence of preeclampsia in women who are already hypertensive (i.e., who have chronic hypertension).
- *The prognosis for both the mother and fetus is much worse than with either chronic hypertension or preeclampsia alone.*
- The diagnosis is highly likely with the following findings[2]:
  –New-onset proteinuria (300 mg or greater or +1 or greater dipstick in 24 hours) in women at less than 20 weeks' gestation with hypertension but no proteinuria
  –Hypertension and proteinuria before 20 weeks' gestation
  –Sudden increase in proteinuria
  –Sudden increase in BP in a woman whose hypertension has previously been well controlled
  –Thrombocytopenia (platelet count less than 100,000 cells/mm³)
  –Increase in ALT or AST to abnormal levels
- The woman's history can include the following:
  –Multiparity
  –Hypertension with a previous pregnancy
  –History of essential hypertension
- The incidence of superimposed preeclampsia is about 25% in women with chronic hypertension.[1]

- The combination of hypertension and proteinuria in pregnancy significantly increases the risks of perinatal morbidity and mortality.
- The disease can progress to superimposed eclampsia.
- The risk of abruptio placentae is increased in these women.
- The fetus is at even greater risk of growth restriction than with preeclampsia or chronic hypertension alone.

Chronic Hypertension[1,2,10,11]

- Chronic hypertension is defined as hypertension that is present and observable before pregnancy or that is diagnosed before the twentieth week of gestation.

NOTE: *When hypertension is diagnosed for the first time during pregnancy and does not resolve by 12 weeks after delivery, it is diagnosed as chronic hypertension.*[2]

- Widespread variation and uncertainty exist regarding the best treatment for chronic hypertension in pregnancy. Studies to date reveal very few solid data to guide clinicians in the management of this disorder in pregnancy.[10]
- No universally accepted criteria exist for the diagnosis of hypertension in pregnancy. See Table 9.1 for a comparison of criteria.

TABLE 9.1 Definitions of Hypertension		
	BLOOD PRESSURE LEVELS	
	MILD HYPERTENSION	**SEVERE HYPERTENSION**
Working Group[2]	140–160/90–110 mm Hg	≥160/110 mm Hg
AHRQ[11]	140–169/90–109 mm Hg	≥170/110 mm Hg
ACOG[10]		≥180/110 mm Hg

- The prevalence of chronic hypertension in women of reproductive age varies according to age, race, ethnicity, and body mass index (Table 9.2).

TABLE 9.2 Prevalence of Hypertension in Women of Reproductive Age			
	18–29 YEARS	**30–39 Years**	**40–49 Years**
African American	2.0%	22.3%	30.5%
Caucasian	0.6%	4.6%	12.7%
Mexican American	1.0%	6.2%	10.6%

Data from AHRQ. (2000). *Management of chronic hypertension in pregnancy.* Evidence Report/Technology Assessment Number 14. (p. 12). Rockville, MD: U.S. Department of Health and Human Services.

- Women are experiencing pregnancies at a later age in the United States. Given the trend of childbearing at an older age, it is expected that the incidence of chronic hypertension in pregnancy will continue to rise.[11]
- Of all chronic hypertensive pregnant women, 90% have primary (or essential) hypertension (hypertension with no known cause).
- Many women have secondary hypertension, the cause of which lies in a pathologic process of an organ system (e.g., renal disease).
- Chronic hypertension occurs in 1% to 5% of pregnancies, depending on the population and diagnostic criteria used.[11]
- The prevalence of essential hypertension is two to three times greater in Black women than in White women.

- Pregnancies complicated by chronic hypertension are associated with increased rates of adverse outcomes such as fetal deaths, fetal growth restriction, small-for-gestational-age infants, premature delivery, and placental abruption. This is especially seen in women with superimposed preeclampsia, severe hypertension, and long-standing hypertension, as well as in women with preexisting cardiovascular renal disease.[11,12]
- Fortunately, most women with chronic hypertension do not go on to develop superimposed preeclampsia.
- When pregnant women experience mild, uncomplicated chronic hypertension, perinatal morbidity and mortality do not increase significantly.
- When renal disease is present, the woman has an increased risk of perinatal mortality and can experience reduced renal function during her pregnancy. She may require the following:
  –Sodium restriction
  –Weight reduction before, but not during, pregnancy
  –Pharmacologic treatment
  –Hospitalization
- During pregnancy, women with chronic hypertension but no complicating illnesses will require careful surveillance for high BP and other signs or symptoms of preeclampsia. Prenatal visits may be scheduled more frequently.

NOTE: Sodium restriction in pregnant women with mild or moderate chronic hypertension is not advocated because many of these women will have a lower plasma volume than normotensive women. Sodium restriction might lead to an even lower plasma volume.

Evidence-Based Findings on Clinical Management of Chronic Hypertension[9–11]

- Specific preconception BP management strategies to ascertain beneficial or adverse effects on conception or pregnancy outcomes *have not been studied in trials.*
- Data from randomized, controlled trials are too scant to either prove or disprove clinically significant benefits from treating mild to moderate hypertension during pregnancy.
- Treatment with antihypertensives or aspirin has not been proven to lower the increased risk of perinatal morbidity and mortality in pregnant women with mild to moderate chronic hypertension. There is insufficient evidence to prove or disprove moderate to large clinical effects of antihypertensive agents on perinatal outcomes. The quality of evidence addressing adverse effects of antihypertensive drugs is poor.
- Some evidence demonstrates an association between angiotensin-converting enzyme inhibitors use and fetal renal dysfunction. Also, some evidence suggests an association between alcohol use in early pregnancy and small-for-gestational-age infants.
- There is insufficient evidence to evaluate the effectiveness of a particular monitoring test or sequence of tests for women with chronic hypertension in pregnancy.
- No pertinent randomized, controlled trials were found that addressed nonpharmacologic treatment and outcomes (e.g., bed rest, diet, dietary supplements, smoking cessation, alternative medicine, biofeedback) in women with chronic hypertension in pregnancy. All trials involved either normotensive women or women with preeclampsia.

Management of the pregnant woman who has chronic hypertension remains unsubstantiated with evidence-based data. Rigorously designed research is needed to address the many unanswered questions on how best to treat and monitor the pregnant woman with chronic hypertension.

Major Theories Regarding the Etiology of Preeclampsia/Eclampsia

Epidemiologic evidence suggests that an immune maladaptive response is involved in the etiology of preeclampsia/eclampsia. Pregnancy normally involves degrees of maternal inflammatory responses. The presence of preeclampsia may be the result of an abnormal or exaggerated intravascular response to the presence of foreign genetic material (i.e., fetal and especially placental tissue).[1]

Paternity may also play a significant role in the pathogenesis of preeclampsia. Women conceiving with men from a different racial group have a higher incidence of preeclampsia. In addition, the multiparous woman appear to return to the nullipara's (first pregnancy) risk for developing preeclampsia when she conceives with a new partner. Immune mechanisms explaining these relationships have not been identified.[1,3,4]

Genetic disposition is thought to play a fairly strong role, and there is a significant amount of evidence supporting familial disposition to preeclampsia/eclampsia. Increased evidence is seen in the obstetric histories of mothers, daughters, and granddaughters. There may be maternal inheritance of single-gene recessive trait or a dominant gene with incomplete dominance.[1,3,4]

■ What are the major pathophysiologic and anatomic changes that occur during preeclampsia or eclampsia?

Many experts consider the placenta the pathogenic focus (primary origin point of pathology) for all manifestations of preeclampsia because delivery is the only definitive cure.[2] Understanding the pathophysiologic and anatomic changes that lead to preeclampsia and eclampsia can make medical management and nursing care for women far more insightful. The underlying disease process is one of widespread arteriolar vasospasm that probably results from abnormal sensitivity of a woman's vascular smooth muscle to vasoconstrictor substances produced in her body. The vasospastic episode leads to injury of the endothelial lining of blood vessels, with a subsequent platelet deposition and fibrin adherence to damaged cell walls. A damaged vascular endothelium results in capillary leakage of protein and fluid (referred to as *vascular permeability*). Intravascular fluid moves to the extravascular space.[13] The pathogenesis of preeclampsia remains incompletely understood, despite years of research. Hypertension is the primary clinical feature of the disease, but it is neither the cause nor the earliest symptom.[6]

Preeclampsia is a complex clinical syndrome that can involve one system or all organ systems. It is thought to develop early in pregnancy, perhaps as early as implantation, but is expressed late in the disease process as a vasospasm of arteriolar beds.

Remember that what seems to be involved here is a pathologic process that precedes the development of diagnostic signs by several weeks or months. Because vasospasms can occur within the placental bed, fetal circulation can be compromised long before warning signs are evident.

The rationale for nursing interventions and medical management is directly related to the pathophysiologic and anatomic changes that occur in preeclampsia.

■ Why do some pregnant women experience arteriolar vasospasm and hypertension?[1,2,5,14]

Women with pregnancy-induced hypertensive disorders fail to experience certain homeostatic, physical, and biochemical changes that are characteristic of normal pregnancy. Generally, homeostasis in humans is maintained between vasopressor (vasoconstriction) and vasodilator (vasodilatation) tendencies, resulting in "normal" BP. This finely tuned balance is mediated by complex chemical and neurogenic controls, many of which are not completely understood. The following are a few of the more widely accepted findings that explain pathophysiologic processes in pregnant woman that lead to increased sensitivity to circulating vasoconstricting substances.

Preeclamptic women have an imbalance in two potent vasoactive substances:

* **Prostacyclin (PGI$_2$)**
  – A hormone synthesized in the endothelial lining of blood vessels
  – A potent vasodilator
  – An inhibitor of platelet aggregation
  – Appropriate levels important for resisting circulating vasoconstrictors, such as angiotensin II and norepinephrine

* **Thromboxane**
  – Produced primarily by platelets
  – A potent vasoconstrictor
  – A stimulator of platelet aggregation

Studies indicate that, although the blood levels of both substances are increased in pregnancy, preeclamptic women demonstrate much higher levels of thromboxane.

Preeclamptic women have an increased sensitivity to a chemical substance called angiotensin II. This vasoconstrictor is produced by a complex conversion system that begins with renin production by the kidneys, ovaries, uterus, and placenta. Renin acts on the precursor angiotensinogen in the liver to convert it to an inactive chemical, angiotensin I. In turn, angiotensin I becomes biologically active angiotensin II, which effects smooth muscle contractions, stimulates aldosterone production and sodium retention, and enhances the reactivity of the smooth muscles of the vascular system to norepinephrine. In normal pregnancies, the vasoactive responses to angiotensin II are moderate and vascular tone is not unduly increased.

Recently, investigators have theorized that the vasoconstricting potential of some vasopressor substances such as angiotensin II and endothelin (produced in endothelial cells) is magnified in preeclampsia as a result of diminished nitric oxide synthase and endothelin-derived releasing factor (EDRF)—both substances playing a role in mediating delicate vasopressor/vasoconstrictor mechanisms.

Therefore, preeclamptic women appear to experience a deficiency of certain protective substances thought to be found in these prostaglandins. This deficiency predisposes the woman to increased vasopressor sensitivity, which leads to increased vascular tone and hypertension.

Preeclamptic women tend to have an abnormal placental implantation process, resulting in incomplete invasion of the uterine spiral arteries. Normally, as the developing placenta (called the trophoblast) implants in the uterine wall, it literally erodes into the spiral arteries found in the endometrium (the inner lining of the uterus). This process of erosion or migration into the spiral arteries converts small, narrow arteries to widened uteroplacental arteries that accommodate a generous blood supply that empties into the intervillous spaces of the placenta.

In preeclampsia, this process does not happen completely and is thought to lead to arterial vasoconstriction at the uteroplacental site.

Currently, many studies are underway to explore more completely the pathogenesis of this puzzling disorder. The etiology of the disease remains unknown.

The following are major areas affected by arteriolar vasoconstriction and vasospasm that give rise to symptoms.

- Kidney
- Cerebrum
- Uteroplacental unit
- Liver

■ How does the vasospastic process lead to pathophysiologic alterations?

Understanding the vasospastic process is critical for appreciating the diagnostic signs and symptoms in hypertensive disorders of pregnancy.

NOTE: *Microangiopathy is a disease of small blood vessels—as in diabetic microangiopathy, in which the basement membrane of capillaries thickens, or as in thrombotic microangiopathy, in which thrombi form in the arterioles and capillaries.*

An example using a visual life experience might aid in grasping the significance of microangiopathic changes in the vascular system.

Imagine a solid but flexible pipe, 4 inches in diameter. Fluids flow through it at a moderate pace. Because the pipe walls are intact, the volume of fluid flowing in and out remains unchanged.

Now imagine the pipe being subjected, for long periods, to great stress, such as severe vibrations or immense pressure on all sides. The pipe, initially whole and intact, begins deteriorating. The walls might begin to collapse, and/or small cracks or openings appear.

If the pipe narrows, the volume of fluid flowing through at a certain rate is reduced. If the pipe walls begin to crack, some of the fluid and its contents are lost through the tiny openings.

Now apply this imagery to a blood vessel—an arteriole or capillary. When subjected to intense vasopressor substances, the vessel might constrict and/or spasm. This stress can also cause the blood vessel to lose its integrity. Intense vasospasm causes injury to the endothelial cells, which make up the lining of the arterioles. Several changes can occur:

- Pressure within the arteriole is increased.
- Fluid or fluid components can seep out of the blood vessel. These components could be either protein substances (e.g., albumin), fluid, or both.

• Perfusion to the tissues that the arterioles supply is reduced not only in amount but possibly in content. Perfused components that could potentially be reduced are blood with its oxygen-carrying capacity and proteins.

When applying these activities to the blood supply of a body system such as the kidney, the overall result would be as follows:

• Hypertension within the kidney
• Reactive vasospasm in arterioles
• Breakdown in the endothelial lining of the arterioles
• Loss of blood and plasma content from the kidney vasculature
• Hemorrhage
• Change in oncotic pressures
• Poor perfusion leading to accumulation of extracellular fluid in kidney tissue and/or ischemia and necrosis

Imagine these alterations occurring at cerebral, hepatic, or uteroplacental sites. The result is poor perfusion to the site, as well as edema and the formation of hemorrhagic areas throughout the tissue of the particular target organ.

■ What about other pathophysiologic changes?

Arteriolar spasm leading to damage of the endothelial layer of small blood vessels remains the basis on which other changes occur.

1. The endothelial layer forms lesions (cracks in the pipe, so to speak), activating the body's immune system. Platelets accumulate at lesion sites and a fibrin network forms. Because blood continues to course through the damaged vessels, red blood cells are forced through the network under high pressure and are fragmented or "chopped up." This fragmentation of red blood cells results in hemolysis and is referred to as *microangiopathic hemolytic anemia*. It is a unique sign of the severest form of preeclampsia: HELLP syndrome.
2. Platelets are used up in this pathologic process, leading to thrombocytopenia.
3. As a consequence of vessel narrowing and changes in the coagulation process, microemboli form in the vasculature. The coagulation process leads to ischemia (diminished tissue perfusion) with subsequent tissue damage (e.g., the liver or kidney) and serious organ malfunction. When these pathologic alterations progress to the extreme, dire consequences that lead to maternal death occur from the following:

   –Abruptio placentae
   –Cerebral hemorrhage
   –Acute renal or cardiac failure
   –DIC

Figure 9.1 relates pathophysiologic alterations in severe hypertensive disease in pregnancy to their evolved signs and symptoms in the patient. Nursing and medical interventions make eminent sense when seen in this context.

Expert Clinical Assessment

Measuring Blood Pressure[15–17]

There is no substitute for BP appropriately measured using a calibrated mercury sphygmomanometer. This is noted despite the recent rise in the use of automated BP equipment, including the newer ambulatory BP monitoring devices.

Appropriate use of electronic devices requires periodic validation for accuracy in measurements. Electronic BP machines systematically underestimate diastolic pressures and overestimate systolic pressures. The main point is that the measurements should be taken using a consistent method that will track trends.

Recent consensus advises that diastolic BP be determined using the disappearance of auscultated sound.[2] Danforth suggests that in the 10% of women who demonstrate a large difference between the muffling (Korotkoff phase IV) and the disappearance of auscultated sound (phase V), it may be useful to record both sounds.[4]

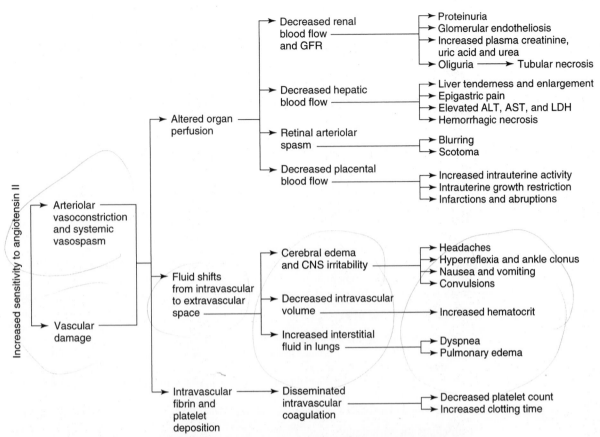

FIGURE 9.1 Pathophysiologic alterations occurring in severe hypertensive disease in pregnancy. ALT, serum alanine aminotransferase (formally known as SGPT); AST, aspartate aminotransferase (formally known as SGOT); GRF, glomerular filtration rate; LDH, lactose dehydrogenase. (Adapted with permission from Koniak-Griffen, D., & Dodgson, J. [1987]. Pathophysiologic alterations occurring in severe PIH. *Heart and Lung, 16*[6], 664.)

> Keep in mind that the clinical onset of preeclampsia can be insidious and might not be accompanied by overt symptoms.

When making an assessment of gestational hypertension, at least two BP readings taken 4 hours or more apart (but not more than 1 week apart) should be used. The woman should be in the same position, and the same arm and cuff size should be used. Checking BP should be delayed if the woman arrives at an office or hospital setting having been rushed or anxious. BP elevation is a systole of 140 mm Hg or greater OR a diastole of 90 mm Hg or greater.

Previous criteria of an increase of 30 mm Hg systole or 15 mm Hg diastole over baseline readings have limited diagnostic value. Recent studies have revealed that increases in systolic and diastolic BP can be either normal physiologic changes or signs of developing pathology. Some pregnant women develop preeclampsia with either systole or diastole elevations, but a certain percentage do not. For example[1,6]:

- From 67% to 73% of normotensive pregnant women experience a greater than 30 mm Hg systole increase or a greater than 15 mm Hg diastole increase. This is often a gradual increase during the second or third trimester.
- Women who develop preeclampsia might have higher baseline BP measurements in the first trimester than women who remain normotensive. Given the elevated first trimester BP, women with preeclampsia might never demonstrate any further significant increase in BP.

- Women with a diastolic BP of 85 mm Hg at 9 to 12 weeks' gestation have a 95% chance of remaining normotensive throughout pregnancy.

NOTE: Relative gradual increases in BP throughout a pregnancy should never be ignored or interpreted as "normal." Rather, they signify a need to remain alert to risk factors, to the possibility of an increase in the presence of existing hypertension, and to the development of additional signs and symptoms.

Evaluating Proteinuria

> Until recently, the diagnosis of preeclampsia required the presence of proteinuria or edema. Edema is no longer considered a reliable criterion.

The presence of protein in urine is key to the identification of preeclampsia and tends to develop late in the disease (or might not occur at all). Detection of protein in the hypertensive woman is considered a hallmark of the pathology occurring in the kidney.[18] When renal arteriolar pressures are severe, vasospasm in the arterioles results. Lesions of the endothelial lining develop, altering the glomerular filtration process. Protein normally retained within the renal artery is lost into the filtrate and appears in the urine in varying amounts.

Clinical Significance of Proteinuria

- Protein might be the most ominous sign of preeclampsia.
- When protein is 2+ or greater in the presence of hypertension, the perinatal mortality increases appreciably.
- In *mild preeclampsia,* the usual protein content in a 24-hour specimen is 300 mg to 2 g/L.
- Protein content reaching 5 g or greater in a 24-hour specimen serves as a standard criterion for a diagnosis of *severe preeclampsia.*

Guidelines for Technique[14]

Urinary dipstick analysis is only moderately reliable. Readings can be falsely positive or falsely negative based on the accuracy of the dipstick performance by the individual. In addition, a dipstick analysis of proteinuria on a urine specimen may not accurately represent protein excretion over a 24-hour period.[18]

- Interpretation when using a multiple reagent strip (dipstick) is as follows:
  Trace = 0.1 g/L
    1+ = 0.3 g/L
    2+ = 1.0 g/L
    3+ = 3.0 g/L
    4+ = 10.0 g/L

> Avoid "rounding up" of color assignments when reading the dipstick. This can lead to inaccurate readings.[18]

- "Significant" proteinuria should be based on either:
  −A 24-hour urine collection
           OR
  −A random clean-catch or catheter specimen
- Specimens showing 2+ proteinuria or 300 mg or greater are "significant."
- When obtaining a trace or more of proteinuria, do a repeated test of either a clean-catch or catheter specimen.
- Avoid using diluted urine because it can give false-negative results.
- Obtain clean urine samples.
- When using a multiple reagent strip, always test for specific gravity (SG) and pH.

NOTE: If SG is less than 1.010, beware of false-negative values resulting from diluted time. If SG is 1.030 or more, beware of false-positive values resulting from concentrated urine. When using sulfosalicylic acid (very alkaline) or when pH is 8.0 or higher, beware of false-negative tests.

- Vaginal and urinary tract infections can result in proteinuria because of the presence of bacterial activity. Exercise, posture, and urine contamination with blood can also influence proteinuria.[4]

A 24-hour urinary protein measurement is recommended for all pregnant women with hypertension.[18]

Pathologic Alterations and Assessment of Signs or Symptoms Reflecting Pathologic Alterations

- BP of 140/90 mm Hg or higher—BP elevation to this extent in a woman beyond 20 weeks' gestation on two occasions 4 hours or more apart may indicate early preeclampsia, transient hypertension, or chronic hypertension.

Look for the following:

- BP of 140/90 mm Hg or higher
- Significantly rising BP—should be watched carefully
- Development of other signs and symptoms—BP and laboratory values must be scrutinized

- Decreased oxygen and glucose delivery to all body tissues.
- Shift of fluids (especially blood plasma) from inside the circulatory system to the tissues of the body, resulting in decreased intravascular volume. Women with preeclampsia do not have the expanded blood volume normally experienced in pregnancy. This poses a great risk of hemorrhage at delivery. In addition, the intravascular space is contracted as a result of vasospasm. Therefore, the severe preeclamptic or eclamptic woman is sensitive to vigorous fluid therapy and even to normal blood loss at delivery.

Look for the following:

- Generalized edema (facial, digital, abdominal, sacral, and lower extremities)
- Large, sudden weight gain

NOTE: Plasma volume is lower than that of normal pregnancy, even in the presence of marked edema.
NOTE: Some of the most severe forms of preeclampsia occur in the absence of edema.

- Hemoconcentration within the circulatory system as the plasma content decreases.

Look for the following:

- Elevated or rising hematocrits

  OR

- Falling hematocrits if hemolysis is occurring

- Thrombocytopenia—The rates of change in platelet counts and lactate dehydrogenase (LDH) appear to correlate significantly with severity of the preeclampsia syndrome.[19]

Look for the following:

- Decreasing platelets; thrombocytopenia is present when platelets are[5]:
  Low = less than 100,000/mm^3
  Severe = less than 50,000/mm^3

NOTE: Currently, in hypertensive states, intracranial hemorrhage is one of the leading causes of maternal death. The presence of thrombocytopenia adds to this risk.[5]

- Proteinuria due to renal arteriolar vasospasm with resulting failure in the kidney's filtering process—Proteinuria usually develops late in the disease.

In normal pregnancies, renal blood flow increases by 25% and glomerular filtration by 50%. This leads to an *increase* in *urinary* creatinine and urea nitrogen levels with a concomitant *decrease* in *blood* values. *Serum* (or plasma) creatinine, blood urea nitrogen (BUN), and uric acid levels *decrease.*

With preeclampsia, renal perfusion and glomerular filtration are reduced. *Urinary levels of creatinine and urea nitrogen levels decrease, and plasma levels increase.* Plasma uric acid concentration tends to be high in women with severe disease. The pathologic plasma volume reduction seen in preeclampsia also contributes to plasma creatinine levels being elevated.

Look for the following:

- Proteinuria greater than 300 mg/L per 24 hours
- Elevated BUN
- Elevated uric acid
- Elevated plasma creatinine (in severe disease, plasma values can be up to several times nonpregnant values)[1]

NOTE: As urine BUN, uric acid, and creatinine levels fall, plasma levels rise.

- Spasm of the blood vessels and possibly edema in the brain or the optical vascular bed. Precise effects of preeclampsia and eclampsia on cerebral blood flow are unknown. Changes in cerebral perfusion and cerebral arterial wall damage may play a role in the development of headaches and altered consciousness. Cerebral hemorrhage can occur as a result of ruptured arteries in severe hypertension and is more common in older women with chronic hypertension.[1]

Look for the following:

- A complaint of visual disturbances, such as blurred vision, scotomata, and dizziness
- Persistent, sometimes severe headache

- Spasm of the blood vessels with subsequent hemorrhages in the liver capsule.

Look for the following:

- Changes in the liver enzymes with elevated AST or ALT more than two times the upper limit of normal
- A complaint of epigastric pain—pain in the upper right quadrant of the abdomen (This is a late and serious symptom of preeclampsia caused by hemorrhaging in the liver capsule, which leads to subcapsular hematoma and/or necrosis, or rupture, which is usually fatal.)
- Liver enlargement

- Irritation of the central nervous system.

Look for the following:

- The presence of hyperactive reflexes and/or clonus

- Decreased blood supply to the placental vascular bed, which reduces uteroplacental blood flow—Decreased blood supply can result in inadequate placental growth and function, thus compromising the fetus.

Look for the following:

- Signs of intrauterine growth restriction (IUGR), reflected in fundal height measurements below expected norms
- Ultrasonic verification of fetal size if IUGR is suspected from fundal height measurement
- Reduced amniotic fluid volume verified with ultrasonography

---

Look for the following:

- Signs of fetal hypoxia in electronic fetal monitoring tracings

NOTE: Nonstress testing (NST), ultrasound assessment of fetal activity, and amniotic fluid volume (BBP) are recommended antenatal fetal surveillance methods that may provide important fetal risk factors before admission.[2]

BE PREPARED FOR A HIGH-RISK BABY. When possible, stabilize the mother and transport her to a Level III hospital if severe preeclampsia or HELLP syndrome is suspected.

Detecting Preeclampsia While Admitting the Laboring Woman

- Look at all aspects of the laboring woman's record, as well as her present state.
- Review her past medical and obstetric history to note predisposing factors.
- Review her prenatal history during this pregnancy.

Assess the following:

- Baseline BP
  –Compare baseline BP with the BP ranges recorded throughout the woman's pregnancy. Ideally, a baseline BP is documented before the woman became pregnant.

BP readings taken within the first 8 weeks of pregnancy are often the only "baseline" BP readings obtainable. Keep in mind that in women predisposed to developing preeclampsia, BP can be somewhat elevated during the early weeks of gestation.

- Proteinuria at any time in the pregnancy (usually a late sign in preeclampsia)
- Weight gain
  –Note sudden, considerable weight gain or excessive overall weight gain.

SUDDEN, EXCESSIVE WEIGHT GAIN IS SOMETIMES THE FIRST SIGN OF IMPENDING PREECLAMPSIA. A weight gain of 5 pounds or more per week in the third trimester can precede signs of preeclampsia. This sudden weight gain is usually caused by fluid retention, regardless of whether it shows up as edema.

- A history of or current complaints of headache or blurred vision and/or severe edema of the hands, legs, feet, and face

Some edema of the hands, feet, and pretibial area is normal in pregnancy. The severity of edema in these areas, as well as facial, abdominal, and sacral edema, should alert you to the possibility of preeclampsia.

At the time of admission, assess the woman's status through questioning and physical examination.

- Take her BP.
- Check for edema in all body areas (including hands and feet) and especially facial, abdominal, and sacral areas.
- Check for hyperactive reflexes.
- Evaluate a clean-catch or catheterized urine specimen.
- Question her about recent:
  - –Headaches
  - –Blurred vision
  - –Loss of consciousness
  - –Nausea and vomiting
  - –Worsening of edema
  - –Epigastric pain
  - –General sick feeling

Detecting Severe Preeclampsia

Mild preeclampsia occurs when the following are found:

- BP has reached 140/90 to 160/110 mm Hg on two different occasions 4 hours apart. A rise of 30/15 mm Hg in BP is an important observation and warrants careful surveillance for other signs and symptoms.

An increase in the diastolic reading is a more reliable indication of preeclampsia.

- Proteinuria is 2+ or between 300 mg and 5 g in a 24-hour urine specimen.

Be alert when you see the following:

- Weight gain of more than 5 pounds per week during the second trimester or more than 2 pounds per week during the third trimester
- Slight edema throughout the body

Severe preeclampsia occurs when the following are found:

- BP rises to 160/110 mm Hg or higher on two different occasions 4 hours apart.
- Proteinuria is 5 g or higher in a 24-hour urine specimen.
- Urine output decreases to less than 400 mL in 24 hours (i.e., less than 30 mL per hour).

NOTE: *Clinical signs of preeclampsia can appear suddenly. Never underestimate the importance of even mild BP elevations complicating a pregnancy.*

In severe preeclampsia, the kidneys can go into failure with little output. This is a serious situation that can lead to permanent injury.

- *Symptoms develop and include the following:*
  - –Severe headaches
  - –Visual problems
  - –Epigastric pain
  - –Nausea or vomiting

–Thrombocytopenia
–Irritability, restlessness, or apprehension
–Pulmonary edema with respiratory distress

Early identification of worsening preeclampsia in a patient at a Level I or II hospital is critical.

When severe preeclampsia occurs before week 32 of gestation, the incidence of serious complications in the mother is high and the fetal outcome is poor, often as a result of growth restriction and/or asphyxia at birth.

Signs to watch for include the following:

- Abruptio placentae
- HELLP syndrome
- Eclampsia
- DIC
- Acute renal failure

Detecting HELLP Syndrome

Follow the same steps as described for detecting preeclampsia in the laboring woman. Particular care should be taken when obtaining the admission history.

Specifically question the woman about recent:	*The expectant mother might be assigned one of the following differential diagnoses:*
Nausea and vomiting	Viral hepatitis
General sick feeling	Gastroenteritis
Epigastric or right upper quadrant pain	Gallbladder disease
Worsening edema	Kidney stones
Diarrhea	Pyelonephritis
Hematuria	Peptic ulcer
Bleeding gums	Idiopathic thrombocytopenia
Abdominal, flank, or shoulder pain	Appendicitis
	Acute fatty liver of pregnancy
	Encephalopathy
	When in fact she has HELLP syndrome.

NOTE: Experts recommend that all pregnant women showing any of these signs or symptoms during the second half of pregnancy have a complete blood cell count with platelets, a peripheral blood smear, and determination of liver enzymes taken, irrespective of maternal BP level.[2,3,5]

These women are critically ill and must be rigorously and constantly assessed. Remember what is happening:

- Arteriolar vasospasms damage the endothelial layer of small blood vessels, forming lesions.
- Platelets accumulate at lesion sites, and a fibrin network forms.
- Red blood cells are forced through the fibrin network under high pressure, resulting in hemolysis with damaged erythrocytes (schistocytes, Burr cells).

Look for the following:	**H**—hemolysis as detected with the following:
- Falling hematocrit - Hyperbilirubinemia - Increased LDH - Jaundice inducing sclera	- Abnormal red blood cells on a peripheral smear - Bilirubin greater than 1.2 mg/dL

- Maternal liver failure results from microemboli in the hepatic vasculature, which causes ischemia and tissue damage within the liver.

Look for the following:

- Increased LDH
- Increased AST/ALT
- Feelings of malaise
- Viral-like syndrome
- Right upper quadrant pain

EL—elevated liver enzymes

- AST greater than 70 IU/L (also elevated ALT)
- LDH greater than 600 IU/L

- Thrombocytopenia occurs because of increased platelet consumption.

Look for the following:

- Falling platelet count
- Abnormal coagulation and fibrinolytic values

LP—low platelets

- Low   = less than 100,000/mm^3
- Severe = less than 50,000/mm^3

- Obstruction of hepatic blood flow and the continual deposit of fibrin causes hepatic distention.

Look for the following:

- Complaints of epigastric or right upper quadrant pain
- Complaints of nausea and vomiting
- Decreased blood glucose

IT IS IMPORTANT TO REMEMBER THAT THE PHYSICAL SYMPTOMS OF HELLP SYNDROME MIGHT NOT INITIALLY CORRELATE WITH PREECLAMPSIA. THE SYMPTOMS OF HELLP SYNDROME CORRELATE WITH ITS PATHOPHYSIOLOGY. THE CLASSIC TRIAD OF HYPERTENSION, PROTEINURIA, AND EDEMA NEED NOT BE PRESENT TO DIAGNOSE HELLP SYNDROME.

If appropriate for timing, distance, and her medical condition, a woman with HELLP syndrome needs to be referred to a tertiary care center for both maternal and fetal safety.

Priorities for Treatment and Nursing Management

Management of Preeclampsia

The primary goals in the management of the preeclamptic woman are as follows:

1. To prevent convulsions through the use of magnesium sulfate
2. To ensure adequate kidney function
3. To monitor fetal status continuously for signs of uteroplacental insufficiency
4. To stabilize the woman so that a vaginal or cesarean birth can be accomplished

The *definitive treatment* for preeclampsia is delivery.

In mild preeclampsia, clinical management usually involves a conservative approach, with office visits as frequent as twice a week, judiciously prescribed rest periods, and frequent laboratory and physical assessment. Fetal surveillance includes tests for fetal well-being, such as fetal movement counting, nonstress testing, contraction stress testing, and biophysical profiles. Hospitalization might be required for the woman who is uncooperative or whose condition does not improve. Along with bed rest, a regular diet with no salt restriction is promoted. A woman with preeclampsia might experience a reduced plasma volume; salt restriction can worsen the situation.

In severe preeclampsia, management is quite focused. Hospitalization facilitates the following:

- Intense maternal monitoring
- Administration of the anticonvulsant medication magnesium sulfate
- Administration of an antihypertensive medication, such as hydralazine or labetalol
- Delivery of the fetus by vaginal or cesarean birth depending on maternal and fetal conditions
- Electronic fetal monitoring

Nursing care for the laboring woman with severe preeclampsia includes the following[20–25]:

- Maintain a nurse:patient ratio of 1:1.[24]
- Assess vital signs every 15 to 30 minutes.
- Obtain standardized BP readings by practicing the following steps:
  –Use the same arm throughout. If pressure readings differ in each arm by more than 10 mm Hg, use the arm with the higher reading.
  –Keep the arm horizontal and at the level of the heart.
  –Fit a sphygmomanometer cuff appropriately sized for the woman's arm.
  –Ensure that BP readings are taken with the woman in the same posture each time.
  –Use the left lateral position consistently with the patient on bed rest.
  –Use the sitting position for the ambulatory patient.
  –To minimize compression of the inferior vena cava (and thus risk increasing BP), encourage a semirecumbent position at a 45-degree angle and on the same side as the arm used in measuring BP. A left or right side-lying position with a 15- to 30-degree tilt will give similar BP readings in pregnant women.[25] Consistent positioning minimizes false high or low readings. **Readings taken in different positions are not comparable.**

BP readings are:

- Highest when supine or standing
- Intermediate when sitting (recommended when possible)
- Lowest in the lateral recumbent position

  –Personnel on the unit should be consistent in the methods used for recording the diastolic reading. Consider the following:
  1. Using the fifth phase disappearance of the sound (i.e., the Korotkoff V sound) will place diastolic measurements abnormally low or even at the zero level in some women. Use of the fifth phase (Korotkoff V sound) was recommended for pregnant women in 1992 by the National Heart, Lung, and Blood Institute and in 2000 by the Working Group Report on High Blood Pressure in Pregnancy.
  2. The National Working Group Consensus Report encourages recording both the muffled sound (Korotkoff IV) and the disappearance sound (Korotkoff V).
  3. Some experts recommend that both phases be recorded and that the Korotkoff IV sound be used for diagnosis. This can result in an overdiagnosis of preeclampsia, but this "risk" is acceptable.

- Place the woman in a lateral recumbent or semirecumbent position. This avoids compression of the maternal vena cava and aorta; improves renal function by enhancing cardiac output, renal circulation, and urinary output; and can enhance uterine/placental perfusion, thus benefiting the fetus.

- Continuous fetal monitoring for uteroplacental insufficiency is done even after BP has been controlled because it is unclear whether the underlying pathologic condition has been controlled as well. Electronic fetal monitoring is recommended.
- Record hourly intake and output using a Foley catheter with a urometer. Careful assessment of fluid balance is critical in preventing a hydrostatic and oncotic pressure imbalance that could lead to pulmonary edema.

Oliguria (less than 30 mL per hour for 2 hours) can result from intravascular volume depletion, renal vasospasm, or cardiac failure. Oliguria is an ominous sign. Report a trend toward this immediately. Do not wait until fully evolved oliguria has occurred.

- Reduce stimulation from noise and light. Place the woman in the quietest room in the labor and delivery unit and dim the lights.
- Maintain the woman on strict bed rest. Side rails should be padded with a blanket for patients with severe preeclampsia or eclampsia.
- Give intravenous fluids to ensure adequate hydration and electrolyte balance and for drug administration.
  - Crystalloid solutions (e.g., 5% dextrose and water or lactated Ringer's solution) should be used.
  - Limit fluid administration to no more than 150 mL per hour. Some authorities suggest a more cautious use of 1 mL/kg per hour.[1]
  - Continuous monitoring is necessary to maintain adequate output.
- Obtain appropriate laboratory workup, which includes the following:
  - Complete blood count (CBC), type and crossmatch, and platelets
  - Liver studies
  - DIC profile
- Test the urine for protein every hour. *Use a fresh specimen* from the Foley catheter or urine collection bag.
- Assess every hour for hyperreflexia.
- Ask the woman to tell you if she develops a headache, blurred vision, dizziness, or epigastric pain, or if she feels uncomfortable or different.
- Observe the woman for restlessness or apprehension.
- HAVE EMERGENCY EQUIPMENT READY—SEIZURE PRECAUTIONS.
  - A padded tongue blade should be near the woman's head.
  - Oxygen and suctioning equipment must be immediately available. Check that the equipment is in operating order.
  - Keep an emergency cart nearby.
- Administer magnesium sulfate according to the physician's orders. Magnesium sulfate ($MgSO_4 \cdot 7H_2O$) is currently believed the safest and most effective anticonvulsant drug available. It can be given intramuscularly or intravenously.

Intravenous administration is recommended because it permits more precise control of serum magnesium blood levels in the woman. Also, the pain of an intramuscular injection is avoided.

The woman **with severe preeclampsia or eclampsia** needs intensive monitoring. She should never be left alone!

Management of HELLP syndrome

Management of the woman with HELLP syndrome is the same as that for the woman with severe preeclampsia.[1,5,8,20,26]

In addition:
- Monitor platelet count for changes indicating worsening thrombocytopenia.
- Assess for clinical signs and symptoms of bleeding:
  - –Petechiae
  - –Easy bruising
  - –Epistaxis
  - –Gingival bleeding
  - –Hematuria
  - –Gastrointestinal bleeding
  - –Conjunctival/retinal hemorrhage
  - –Oozing from the intravenous site
- Administer blood products per the physician's orders.
- Invasive hemodynamic monitoring may be used, but it is not always indicated.[1,22]
- Monitor serial liver function tests.
- Observe and report signs of the following:
  - –Malaise
  - –Anorexia
  - –Nausea and vomiting
  - –Right upper quadrant or epigastric pain
  - –Jaundice
  - –Hypoglycemia
- Keep 50% dextrose at the bedside.
- Avoid sedatives.

> **NOTE:** *Decreased blood glucose can occur as a result of hepatic congestion that is caused by microemboli in the small vessels of the liver.*

- Use internal fetal monitoring as soon as possible to assess for signs of fetal hypoxia.
- Deliver oxygen at 6 to 8 L per minute via face mask.

> **NOTE:** *Late decelerations and loss of short-term variability are nonreassuring signs associated with fetal hypoxia.*

Intrapartum Pain Management[1,2,8,27]

- Small intermittent doses (25 to 50 mg) of meperidine, used in the past, have been replaced by epidural anesthesia for many women.
- Local infiltration anesthesia can be used safely for all vaginal deliveries.
- Vaginal delivery is preferable to cesarean delivery, even with the presence of severe disease. Many authorities believe that epidural anesthesia is the preferred method for cesarean delivery in women with severe preeclampsia.[1,2,8]
- Regional anesthesia techniques are relatively contraindicated in preeclampsia accompanied by coagulopathy.[2]
- Given the current refinement of both general anesthesia and epidural anesthesia management for women with severe preeclampsia and eclampsia, both methods are viewed by many as equally acceptable for cesarean delivery.[27] A small percentage of women might develop pulmonary edema when given epidural anesthesia. This is thought to be due to intravenous fluid administration, required to circumvent epidural-induced hypotension.[27]
- Continuous epidural anesthesia for pain relief during labor in women with severe hypertensive disease does not appear to increase cesarean birth rates, maternal pulmonary edema, or acute renal failure.[27]

Anticonvulsant Therapy

> ■ **What is the current recommended treatment schedule for administering magnesium sulfate ($MgSO_4 \cdot 7H_2O$) to the preeclamptic woman?**[1,4,5,8,28]

> Magnesium sulfate is given for anticonvulsant therapy. **It is not given to treat hypertension.**

A number of sound clinical studies provide significant evidence that magnesium sulfate is the anticonvulsant drug of choice. Diazepam (Valium) and phenytoin (Dilantin) are no longer accepted anticonvulsant therapies for preeclampsia.

The following recommendations represent currently accepted therapeutic practices in the treatment of the preeclamptic woman with $MgSO_4 \cdot 7H_2O$. Respected authors vary in their recommendations. The regimen described here is according to Cunningham.[1]

- If a rapid therapeutic effect is desired, an initial loading dose of 4 to 6 g of magnesium sulfate in 100 mL of intravenous solution is administered intravenously over 15 to 20 minutes, followed by controlled, continuous infusion of 2 g per hour.
- Maintenance therapy is delivered at the rate of 2 g in 100 mL of solution per hour. Some women will require infusions of 3 g per hour to maintain effective plasma levels of magnesium.

NOTE: Administration of the loading dose at these rates is likely to induce vomiting. Do not speed up the loading dose infusion beyond the stated rate.

> The effect of magnesium sulfate is immediate when administered intravenously.

To make up a 4-g loading solution:

- Each 10-mL ampule of a 50% solution of $MgSO_4 \cdot 7H_2O$ contains 5 g of $MgSO_4 \cdot 7H_2O$.
- Add 40 g (8 ampules) to 1,000 mL of 5% dextrose and water or lactated Ringer's. Each 100 mL of solution will contain 4 g of $MgSO_4 \cdot 7H_2O$.
- To administer a 4-g loading dose in 25 minutes, run 100 mL of the solution at a rate of 4 mL per minute. This reduces the possibility of undesirable side effects (e.g., nausea, vomiting).

OR

To make up a 6-g loading solution:

- Use the aforementioned solution and run in 150 mL over 10 to 15 minutes, thus giving the woman 6 g of $MgSO_4 \cdot 7H_2O$ in 150 mL of solution.

OR

- Add 12 mL of 50% $MgSO_4 \cdot 7H_2O$ solution to 100 mL of 5% dextrose and water or lactated Ringer's and administer intravenously over 10 to 15 minutes, thus giving the patient 6 g of $MgSO_4 \cdot 7H_2O$ in 100 mL of solution.

At times, 4 g of $MgSO_4 \cdot 7H_2O$ can be given by intravenous push at a rate of 1 g per minute to stop a seizure.

> The physician should be present when $MgSO_4 \cdot 7H_2O$ is administered in a loading dose.

CHECK DRUG CONCENTRATIONS CAREFULLY BEFORE MAKING UP SOLUTIONS AND DOUBLE-CHECK YOUR CALCULATIONS BEFORE ADMINISTERING THESE SOLUTIONS.

The current treatment regimen recommends that the loading dose be followed by a smaller $MgSO_4 \cdot 7H_2O$ dose administered intravenously by infusion pump.

Loading doses of 4 to 6 g are usually followed by 1 to 2 g per hour.

Using the 4-g loading solution preparation outlined previously, various $MgSO_4 \cdot 7H_2O$ administration rates can be achieved (Table 9-3).

Magnesium sulfate is stable in both 5% dextrose and water and in lactated Ringer's solutions for extended periods. However, attention should be given to maintaining sterilization in a preparation administered over more than 24 hours. A new preparation of the solution is recommended.

TABLE 9.3	IV Administration Rates Using 40 g of MgSO$_4$/1,000 D$_5$W
IV RATE	**MgSO$_4$ DOSAGE PER HOUR**
25 mL/hr	1 g/hr
50 mL/hr	2 g/hr
75 mL/hr	3 g/hr
100 mL/hr	4 g/hr

CAUTION: Magnesium sulfate comes in ampules of 10%, 12.5%, and 50% solutions. Calculations for working with various concentrations must be done carefully.

Check each ampule when making up solutions or giving IM injections to be certain which percentage drug solution you are working with.

■ **What special monitoring of the patient is required during administration of magnesium sulfate?**

Magnesium is believed to exert a specific anticonvulsant action on the cerebral cortex. In therapeutic ranges, magnesium sulfate slows neuromuscular conduction and depresses central nervous system irritability. The purpose of giving the drug is to reduce muscle excitability and hyperreflexia, thus reducing the possibility of convulsions.

To monitor the woman during MgSO$_4$ • 7H$_2$O administration:

- Measure serum magnesium level every 4 to 6 hours and adjust the infusion to maintain levels between 4 and 7 mEq/L (4.8 and 8.4 mg/dL). Some experts recommend measuring the serum magnesium level 2 hours after the loading dose.
- Assess patellar reflexes. Absence of the reflex might mean the woman has received too much MgSO$_4$ • 7H$_2$O.
- Count respirations; they should not be less than 12 per minute and should be of normal depth. NO FURTHER DOSES OF MgSO$_4$ • 7H$_2$O SHOULD BE GIVEN IF RESPIRATIONS ARE BELOW 12 PER MINUTE. CONSULT THE PHYSICIAN IMMEDIATELY.
- Measure urinary output hourly. Use of a Foley catheter is imperative. Indications of impaired renal function as seen in laboratory tests (e.g., elevated plasma creatinine levels) or diminished urinary output (less than 30 mL per hour) necessitate a critical reevaluation of not only fluid therapy but also anticonvulsant therapy. **Because parenterally administered magnesium is cleared almost exclusively by renal excretion, notify the primary care provider immediately if you suspect any renal function compromise.**
- Assess the patient's state of consciousness.

The therapeutic range for MgSO$_4$ • 7H$_2$O administration is between 4 and 7 mEq/L (4.8 and 8.4 mg/dL) of serum magnesium. Concentrations greater than 7 mEq/L (8.4 mg/dL) result in signs of maternal toxicity, including the following:

- Nausea and vomiting
- Respiratory depression
- Disappearance of the patellar reflex
- Respiratory and cardiac arrest if toxicity is not remedied

Consider the following:

- Extensive experience indicates that intravenous doses of magnesium sulfate at dosages up to 2 g per hour are safe in the patient with normal renal function.

- If the dose is to be increased in a constant infusion, it could be done by increasing the concentration of solution and *not necessarily by increasing the volume of fluid.*
- Intramuscular administration of $MgSO_4 \cdot 7H_2O$ might be a safer route for treatment in the patient with abnormal kidney function. Constant nursing supervision is required, with a minimum of nurse:patient ratio of 1:2 for the woman receiving $MgSO_4 \cdot 7H_2O$ therapy.[20]
- In the event that the nursing staff is unable to adequately monitor the patient receiving the intravenous infusion of $MgSO_4 \cdot 7H_2O$, it may be necessary to consider intramuscular $MgSO_4 \cdot 7H_2O$.[20]
- Protocols for nursing supervision of patients with maternal disease, such as severe preeclampsia, should address a 1:1 nurse:patient ratio.[20,24]
- Magnesium sulfate is discontinued 24 hours after delivery.

TO AVOID TOXICITY:
Before giving each dose of $MgSO_4 \cdot 7H_2O$, make sure that the patient has excreted at least 100 mL of urine in the past 4 hours, that respirations are at least 12 per minute, and that patellar reflexes are not absent.

The most common causes of toxicity are:

1. Iatrogenic overdosage
2. Deteriorating renal function, which can be common with severe preeclampsia

---

■ How is a magnesium sulfate overdose managed?[1,2,8]

Calcium gluconate is the antidote to magnesium toxicity.

- Administer 1 g of calcium gluconate intravenously over 3 minutes; for example, use 10 mL of a 10% calcium gluconate solution (each milliliter contains 0.1 g of calcium gluconate). This administration can be repeated every hour, if needed, up to eight injections in a 24-hour period.
- Provide airway and ventilatory support as needed.

Calcium gluconate is commonly packaged in 1-g ampules containing 10 mL of a 10% solution. Read the label carefully when drawing up the solution. Keep a clearly labeled syringe of the solution at the bedside.

Antihypertensive Therapy: Current Recommendations[1,2,5,10,11,29]

Although controversy exists regarding how aggressively hypertension should be treated in pregnancy, there is a consensus that patients with diastolic BP measurements of 110 mm Hg or higher should be treated. In some situations, pressures lower than this might warrant antihypertensive treatment. For example, treatment of adolescents with a persistent diastolic pressure of 100 mm Hg might be considered if baseline pressures were 75 mm Hg or less. Maternal benefits from this therapy are the prevention of pulmonary edema and cerebral hemorrhage, two severe complications of preeclampsia.[1,5,10,11,29] The major concern in using antihypertensive drugs is that, while maternal BP is reduced, uteroplacental perfusion is also lowered, thus potentially compromising fetal oxygenation. Generally, therefore, treatment with these drugs is reserved for situations in which maternal BP is seriously elevated (higher than 105 to 110 mm Hg diastolic pressure). The goal of treatment is aimed at maintaining a diastolic pressure between 90 and 104 mm Hg, but not lower.[1,2]

A review of recent literature indicates a few selective drugs:

Hydralazine (Apresoline) (arteriolar dilator)	–A drug of choice for many in the treatment of severe hypertension near term or during labor –Administered intravenously and intramuscularly –See protocol that follows for specific directions

Labetalol (adrenergic blocker)

–Is used as a second-line drug of choice
–May be used in intravenous bolus injections beginning with 20 mg; if not effective within 20 minutes, give 40 mg, then 80 mg every 10 minutes, *but not to exceed 220 mg total dose*
–May be used as a continuous infusion of 1 mg/kg per hour as needed

NOTE: *The drug is premixed as a 20-mL vial containing a concentration of 5 mg labetalol per milliliter. Add 40-mL vial of labetalol to 160 mL of intravenous fluid; the resultant 200 mL contains 1 mg labetalol per milliliter.*

–Must watch for the delayed effect of sudden maternal hypotension (reactive hypotension); **stop the infusion immediately**
–Contraindicated in women with asthma and those with congestive heart failure

Nifedipine (calcium entry blocker)

–Used in preeclamptic hypertensive emergencies
–Start with 10-mg dose orally and repeat in 30 minutes if needed
–Short-acting nifedipine not approved by U.S. Food and Drug Administration for hypertension management

Guidelines for the Use of Hydralazine in Antihypertensive Therapy[1,2,5,30,31]

Hydralazine should be administered using plastic containers or syringes. A significant but unpredictable decrease in effectiveness has been observed when glass containers are used.[30]
NOTE: *The patient's response to vasodilators depends on the status of her intravascular blood volume. Severely preeclamptic patients have a depleted volume. WHEN ADMINISTERING HYDRALAZINE, WATCH FOR EARLY SIGNS OF HYPOTENSION. THESE PATIENTS CAN EXPERIENCE SUDDEN AND PROFOUND HYPOTENSION.[31]*

- A test dose of 1 mg is given intravenously over 1 minute. BP is checked to determine any idiosyncratic hypotension.
- Administer a 5-mg dose intravenously over 1 to 2 minutes, or give 10 mg intramuscularly.
- Check BP every 2 to 5 minutes thereafter.
- Subsequent doses are dictated by the patient's response to the initial dose. For example, another 5- to 10-mg dose may be given intravenously after 20 minutes if the diastolic BP remains greater than 110 mm Hg.
- Recheck BP every 5 minutes.

The pharmakinetics of hydralazine involve a peak and maximal effect in 20 minutes, with a 6- to 8-hour duration of action. This is why intermittent bolus injections are appropriate. However, because the time to maximum effect of any given dose can vary, DO NOT ADMINISTER THE 5-MG DOSES TOO CLOSE TOGETHER.[2]

- Once BP control is achieved, the dose is repeated as needed—usually about every 3 hours.
- Maintain a properly functioning IV line. Monitoring of input and output is critical to prevent hypotensive episodes or overload.
- Do not mix this medication with any other medications in the same intravenous bag.

NOTE: *A desired response to hydralazine therapy is defined as a decrease in the diastolic BP to 90 to 100 mm Hg, but not any lower because placental perfusion can be compromised. If,* *after giving 20 mg intravenously or 30 mg intramuscularly total dose, success has not be achieved, another drug should be considered.*

> COMPREHENSIVE PROTOCOLS THAT ADDRESS NURSING RESPONSIBILITIES FOR ANTICONVULSANT THERAPY OR ANTIHYPERTENSIVE THERAPY (e.g., HYDRALAZINE) SHOULD BE DEVELOPED AT EACH INSTITUTION. THESE PROTOCOLS SHOULD INCLUDE CRITERIA FOR PATIENT SELECTION, RESPONSIBILITY FOR INFORMATION TO BE COVERED IN THE INFORMED CONSENT, DRUG PREPARATION AND ADMINISTRATION, PATIENT MONITORING, POTENTIAL SIDE EFFECTS, AND THERAPEUTIC GOALS.

Special Delivery Preparations

- Maternal corticosteroid administration is strongly recommended to reduce the risk of newborn respiratory distress syndrome if a preterm birth is anticipated. A single course of corticosteroids should be given 24 hours before birth is anticipated. All pregnant women between 24 and 34 weeks' gestation should be considered candidates.[32] See Module 8 for treatment dose.
- If the preeclamptic woman is at a Level I or Level II hospital, is preterm, and does not respond to the conservative management of diet control and bed rest with a decrease in BP, disappearance of proteinuria, and lessening of edema, it is recommended that she be transferred to a high-risk regional center. She may need fetal maturity tests, electronic fetal monitoring, and induction of labor. **PREPARE FOR A HIGH-RISK INFANT.**
- If a preterm or term woman is admitted to the labor and delivery unit of a Level I or Level II hospital with severe preeclampsia, it is recommended that she be transferred to the high-risk regional center as soon as she is stabilized enough for the transfer.
- In the event that the preeclamptic woman delivers at the community hospital because there is no time for transfer to the regional center, **PREPARE FOR A HIGH-RISK INFANT.**
- *The preeclamptic woman maintained on therapeutic levels of $MgSO_4 \cdot 7H_2O$ is at risk for postpartum hemorrhage. This is of great concern because the woman with severe preeclampsia or eclampsia is unable to tolerate a large blood loss at delivery. She is already experiencing reduced blood volume and hemoconcentration. Be prepared for this. Oxytocic drugs and manual uterine stimulation usually will control uterine atony.*

> Recognize that any significant fall in BP soon after delivery in these women often reflects excessive blood loss and not the disappearance of vasospasm with return to a more normotensive state.[32]

> Oliguria soon after delivery may signify blood loss. Hematocrit should be evaluated frequently to detect this. Treatment with careful blood transfusion might be implemented.[33]

Cross matched blood should be available in the labor and delivery setting for these patients.

- **Whenever anticipating a possible HIGH-RISK INFANT** *have the appropriate personnel on hand—not on call.* Their presence at the birth can make a critical difference to the quality of life for the newborn.
- Epidural anesthesia is considered safe and is the anesthetic of choice in severe preeclampsia, if preceded by volume preloading, to prevent maternal hypotension.[27] Fluid management consists of crystalloid infusion of normal saline or lactated Ringer's solution at a rate of 100 to 125 mL per hour. Intravenous fluids can decrease colloidal osmotic pressure and also result in fluid accumulation in interstitial tissue. Be vigilant in monitoring for hypotension and pulmonary edema. Women who are experiencing severe preeclampsia or eclampsia and develop pulmonary edema most often do so in the postpartum period.

Postpartum Care and Education, Including Long-Term Prognosis[1,2,9,34]

- Delivery is the "cure" for preeclampsia.
- Magnesium sulfate should be continued in the severely preeclamptic and eclamptic woman for at least 24 hours after delivery and even longer if the woman complains of persistent headache, blurred vision, or scotomata.
- BP monitoring is continued after magnesium sulfate administration is discontinued.
- Approximately 25% to 30% of eclampsia cases occur within the first few days postpartum.
- Recovery, including resolution of abnormal laboratory values, is not always immediate in women with HELLP syndrome. These women are very ill.
  - –Thrombocytopenia worsens for 3 to 4 days after delivery.
  - –Patients may appear to worsen initially and then slowly begin to improve.
- Close monitoring within the first 48 hours is critical to detect the development of pulmonary edema, renal failure, or hypertension encephalopathy. Watch for the following:
  - –Hemoconcentration
  - –Oliguria
  - –Respiratory changes, such as pulmonary rales, tachypnea, and dyspnea; chest discomfort; and tachycardia
- Women who are especially at risk for postpartum complications are those with underlying cardiac disease, chronic renal disease, superimposed preeclampsia, placental abruption complicated with DIC, and hypertension that requires several antihypertensive medications.
- Breastfeeding is encouraged and can be done safely using selected antihypertensive drugs and reduced doses under careful BP supervision. Studies indicate that all antihypertensive agents are excreted into human breast milk. The breastfed infant requires close monitoring for any adverse effects.[2]
- At 3 months postpartum, BP is usually normal and proteinuria disappears. However, in some women hypertension may persist for as long as 3 months.

> The longer hypertension diagnosed during pregnancy persists postpartum, the greater the likelihood that the cause is underlying chronic hypertension.[9]

> The existence of normal BP in a pregnancy subsequent to a hypertension-complicated pregnancy has been found to be predictive of reduced risk for chronic hypertension in the future.[1]

- The sequelae of underlying renal disease are few.
- Approximately 3% to 19% of women with HELLP syndrome will experience the disorder in a subsequent pregnancy; 43% will experience preeclampsia.[1] When the syndrome does occur, it tends to develop later in the pregnancy and tends to be less severe after two episodes.[1]

NOTE: Preeclampsia does not cause chronic hypertension.[1]

- Oral contraceptives usually can be used safely under medical BP supervision.
- Women with HELLP syndrome should be screened for the presence of antiphospholipid antibodies (APLA testing), which may be indicative at specified levels of a syndrome associated with a variety of medical problems, including arterial and venous thrombosis, autoimmune cytopenia, and fetal loss.[34]

PRACTICE/REVIEW QUESTIONS

After reviewing this module, answer the following questions.

1. Hypertension complicates pregnancy in approximately ____6____ % to ____8____ % of women.

2. A general term that has been used to describe all new onsets of hypertension in pregnancy
is *Pregnancy induced hypertension* .

3. A general term identifying chronic hypertension worsened by pregnancy is
Pre Superimposed hypertension

4. A hypertensive state in pregnancy that occurs after the twentieth week and is characterized
by convulsions is *Eclampsia* .

5. Pregnancy complicated by hypertension and proteinuria is called *Preeclampsia*

6. Match the terms in Column B with the descriptions given in Column A.

Column A

b 1. Hypertension during the last 20 weeks of pregnancy or in the first 24 hours postpartum without other signs of preeclampsia

g *a* 2. A term sometimes used to designate expectant women who have elevated BP after 20 weeks but without accompanying proteinuria

e 3. A subset of preeclampsia

b 4. Sometimes seen in normotensive women within the first hours after delivery but with a subsequent return to baseline BP levels in 24 hours

a 5. The development of a BP of 140/90 mm Hg or higher after the twentieth gestational week and accompanied by proteinuria

a 6. Occurs before the twentieth week in the presence of pathologic changes in the placenta

a 7. A disorder that can begin with implantation but has no overt signs or symptoms for weeks or even months

a 8. Exists in a severe form when BP reaches 160/110 mm Hg or higher

f 9. Can occur in women who enter pregnancy with preexisting hypertension

e 10. Has as its underlying pathophysiology arterial vasospasm leading to microangiopathic hemolytic anemia

c 11. Is accompanied by convulsions not caused by neurologic disease

d 12. Is diagnosed with a history of persistent BP elevation of at least 140/90 mm Hg before the twentieth gestational week

c 13. Convulsions can occur in the presence of mildly elevated BP or mild proteinuria

d 14. The presence of this hypertensive disorder, together with diabetes, renal disease, or a cardiac condition, increases the mother's risk

Column B

a. Preeclampsia
b. Transient hypertension
c. Eclampsia
d. Chronic hypertension
e. HELLP syndrome
f. Superimposed preeclampsia
g. Gestational hypertension

7. The following statements elicit your understanding of the current thinking about hypertensive states in pregnancy.

   a. Perinatal mortality rates tend to increase as maternal BP increases.

   (A.) True

   B. False

   b. Chronic hypertension and preeclampsia have the same etiology.

   A. True

   (B.) False

   c. Several reliable screening tests can be used to identify women at risk for pregnancy-induced hypertensive disorders.

   A. True

   (B.) False

   d. Eclampsia can be mild or severe.

   A. True

   (B.) False

   e. A diagnostic criterion for hypertension is a BP of 140/90 mm Hg.

   (A.) True

   B. False

   f. Severe hypertension is diagnosed when the BP reaches 150/100 mm Hg.

   A. True

   (B.) False

   g. Gestational hypertension is the same thing as transitional hypertension.

   (A.) True

   B. False

   h. A BP of 146/100 mm Hg in a laboring woman with no previous hypertension history and with no proteinuria can indicate transient hypertension or preeclampsia.

   (A.) True

   B. False

   i. If the laboring woman mentioned above in "h" has transient hypertension, it can be diagnosed only in the postpartum period.

   (A.) True

   B. False

8. Name the two principal signs present in the hypertensive states of pregnancy.

   a. *Elevated BP 140/90*

   b. *Proteinuria*

9. Select the hypertensive state that fits the descriptions given in a through j.

   T = Transient hypertension

   P = Preeclampsia

   H = HELLP syndrome

   E = Eclampsia

I a. Is not accompanied by adverse fetal outcomes

P b. Complicates approximately 20% of teenage pregnancies

H c. Is characterized by microangiopathic hemolytic anemia, as diagnosed by abnormal red blood cells on a peripheral smear

H d. Accompanied by malaise, flulike symptoms, and nausea and vomiting

P e. A disorder that can begin with implantation

I f. A fairly benign disease that can, however, be predictive of possible future chronic hypertension with aging

P,E,H g. Proteinuria often a late sign

H h. Microvascular damage to the endothelial lining of blood vessels and platelet activation diagnosed in laboratory studies

E i. Convulsions that are sometimes not accompanied by dramatic warning signs

H j. Associated with poor maternal and perinatal outcomes and its presence is a risk factor for postpartum eclampsia

10. State at least five predisposing risk factors for developing preeclampsia.

a. *Young (pregnant for 1st time*

b. *H/O chronic hypertension*

c. *Twin pregnancy*

d. *Diabetes*

e. *H/O preeclampsia*

11. "Significant" proteinuria means:

A. 300 mg or more in 24 hours

B. 200 mg in 24 hours

C. 1+ on dipstick tested twice 4 hours apart

D. The presence of a urinary tract infection

12. When a pregnant woman presents with a BP of 144/96 mm Hg, how is a diagnosis of chronic hypertension versus preeclampsia made?
history of BP before 30th wk of pg

13. Mark with an "X" the statements that characterize what is known about chronic hypertension and pregnancy.

X a. Most chronic hypertensive pregnant women have primary or essential hypertension.

___ b. It occurs more often in White women than in Black women.

___ c. It is not associated with increased risk of intrauterine growth restriction.

___ d. Mild, uncomplicated chronic hypertension in pregnancy is associated with moderate maternal and fetal morbidity.

___ e. Preconceptional and antepartal antihypertensive medication are not advised in the moderately chronic hypertensive woman.

___ f. Sodium restriction is advocated to reduce the potential for edema.

14. Pregnancy-aggravated hypertension exists in two forms:
Superimposed eclampsia and *Superimposed preeclampsia*.

15. State at least five characteristics that are common to the woman presenting with HELLP syndrome.

    a. *Caucasion - in her 2nd or 3rd trimester*

    b. *C/O "Just not feeling good" flu-like symptoms*

    c. *nausea*

    d. *epigastric*

    e. *(R) upper quadrant pain*

16. The second leading cause of maternal death in the United States is:

    A. Hemorrhage

    B. Infection

    C. Thromboembolic disease

    D. Preeclampsia

17. The underlying disease process in preeclampsia is:

    A. Not known

    B. Thought to be strictly neurologic in origin

    C. Widespread vasospasms of the arterioles

    D. DIC

18. In preeclampsia, hypertension is the:

    A. Primary clinical feature

    B. Cause of the disease

    C. Earliest symptom

    D. Latest symptom

19. Preeclampsia:

    A. Can involve one or more organ systems

    B. Is thought to be inherited

    C. Begins late in pregnancy

    D. Never occurs in the older primigravida

20. Pathophysiologic processes related to preeclampsia involve all of the following except:

    A. A balance in two potent vasoactive substances

    B. Increased sensitivity to angiotensin II

    C. Incomplete invasion of the spiral arteries in the endometrium

    D. Microangiopathy

21. Match the terms in Column B with the descriptions given in Column A.

    Column A

    a 1. Stimulates platelet aggregation

    b 2. Synthesized in the endothelium of blood vessels

    b 3. A potent vasodilator

    b 4. Inhibits platelet aggregation

    a 5. A potent vasoconstrictor

    d 6. A precursor in the liver requiring the action of renin

    c 7. Affects smooth muscle contractions, stimulates aldosterone production, and sensitizes smooth muscles of the vasculature to norepinephrine

    Column B

    a. Thromboxane
    b. Prostacyclin
    c. Angiotensin II
    d. Angiotensinogen

22. Fill in the blanks from the following list of terms:

    Angiotensin I
    Angiotensin II
    Angiotensinogen
    Endothelin-derived releasing factor

    Prostacyclin
    Renin
    Thromboxane

    Preeclamptic women have increased sensitivity to a chemical substance called ___Angiotensin II___. In the liver, ___~~Anga~~ renin___ converts ___angitensinogen___ to an inactive substance called ___Angiotensin I___. In turn, this becomes biologically active ___Angiotensin II___. Normal pregnant women have a moderate vasoactive response to angiotensin II.

23. Define *microangiopathy*.

    A disease of small blood vessels in which the basement membrane of capillaries thickens, or thrombi. Microangiopathy in which thrombi form in arterioles of capillaries

24. List the changes that vasospasms can lead to in terms of the following:

    a. Pressure and blood flow through the arteriole

    Pressure is increased (hypertension) and blood flow is diminished

    b. Loss of fluid components

    lesions in the vessel wall result in fluid (plasma) loss leading to Δ's in oncotic pressures + extracellular fluid accumulation

    c. Blood supply to target organs

    Perfusion to target organ's is reduced leading to ischemia and necrosis.

25. Vasospasm leading to formation of endothelial lesions activates the body's ___immune___ system. ___Platelets___ accumulate at lesion sites, and a ___fibrin___ network forms. Blood continues to be forced through the damaged vessels, and consequently, ___RBC___ are forced through the fibrin network. The damage sustained by the fragmentation of these cells results in ___hemolysis___

26. The process described in question 25 results in a disorder called *Microangiopathic hemolytic anemia*. This is a unique sign of what disease state? *HELLP Syndrome*

27. Ongoing endothelial vessel damage continues to result in more lesions with increasing numbers of platelets used up in laying down fibrin networks. This platelet consumption results in *thrombocytopenia*.

28. Maternal death resulting from the extreme pathologic processes described in questions 23 through 27 is usually caused be one of four conditions:
    a. *abruptio placentae*
    b. *Cerebral hemorrhage*
    c. *Acute and renal or Cardiac failure*
    d. *DIC*

29. A significant elevation of BP requiring careful watching is a diastole of *90 15* mm Hg or a systole of *140 30* mm Hg.

30. A BP elevation to 140/90 mm Hg seen throughout a morning in a woman in the clinic who is beyond 20 weeks' gestation indicates *Gestational hypertension*

31. With preeclampsia, there is a shift of fluids within the circulatory system, resulting in decreased *Intravascular volume*. A sign of this can be either *edema* or *Weight gain*

32. This shift of fluid also results in hemoconcentration within the circulatory system. A sign of this can be seen in a rising *hematocrits*

33. Thrombocytopenia is diagnosed with platelets lower than *$100,000 mm^3$*. It is severe with a platelet count of less *$500,000 mm^3$*

34. Proteinuria:
    A. Usually develops early in the disease process
    (B.) Is a result of renal arteriolar vasospasm
    C. Generally indicates integrity of kidney tissue
    D. Is correlated with a mild disease process

35. Patient complaints of what four symptoms may indicate spasm of blood vessels and edema in the brain and/or optical?
    a. *Blurred vision*
    b. *Scotomata*
    c. *Dizziness*
    d. *Persistent Sometimes Severe HA*

36. Vascular spasms occurring in the liver capsule should be suspected when the patient complains of *(R) upper quadrant pain*

37. Irritation of the central nervous system is suspected in the presence of *hyperactive reflexes or clonus*.

38. Hypertension in pregnancy can compromise blood supply to the placenta and lead to *inadequate placental growth*

39. Increases in systolic and diastolic pressures are always pathologic.

    A. True
    B. (False)

40. In some women, even a 10-mm Hg elevation of BP can be pathologic.

    A. (True)
    B. False

41. Relative gradual increases in BP can be interpreted as "normal."

    A. True
    B. (False)

42. The diagnosis of preeclampsia requires the presence of proteinuria and edema.

    A. True
    B. (False)

43. Edema is not a valid diagnostic sign of preeclampsia.

    A. (True)
    B. False

44. Most pregnant women exhibit some edema.

    A. (True)
    B. False

45. A 19-year-old gravida 1 is at 37 weeks' gestation; her BP is 150/100 mm Hg, and she has no lower extremity edema. A 24-hour urine specimen collected is reported to have 5 g of protein. By definition the diagnosis is ___*Preeclampsia*___.

46. Significant proteinuria is based on:
    300mg/L or more protein in a 24hr specimen, or protein concentration of 2+ or higher on a least two random urine tests done 6 hrs apart.

47. A 17-year-old African American primigravida is admitted to labor and delivery in a Level I hospital at 27 weeks' gestation. Her BP is 170/114 mm Hg, and her urine output is 30 mL per hour. Stabilization and transport to a high-risk regional center is important because *she needs to be delivered + her baby will require level III nursery.*

48. List three diagnostic criteria for HELLP syndrome.

    a. *Hemolysis*
    b. *elevated liver enzymes*
    c. *low platelets*

49. Indicate whether the following statements are true (T) or false (F).

    _T_ a. Arteriolar vasospasm is the underlying factor in hemolytic anemia that occurs in HELLP syndrome.
    _F_ b. In HELLP syndrome, platelets accumulate in small blood vessels, causing those vessels to swell and rupture.
    _T_ c. The liver is the primary organ that is damaged as a result of HELLP syndrome.
    _T_ d. Hepatic distention can cause subjective symptoms of epigastric pain or right upper quadrant pain.

50. To diagnose the complication of HELLP syndrome, a pregnant woman must show clinical evidence of preeclampsia (i.e., hypertension, proteinuria, and edema).

    A. True

    B. False *(circled)*

51. List at least five areas that you need to address in admission history when screening a woman for HELLP syndrome.

    a. *Nausea/vomiting*

    b. *Right upper quadrant pain*

    c. *edema*

    d. *Bleeding gums*

    e. *just not feeling well*

52. State four primary nursing management goals in the care of a preeclamptic woman.

    a. *to prevent convulsions c̄ the use of Mag*

    b. *ensure adequate kidney function*

    c. *to monitor fetal status continuously for signs of Uteroplacental deficiency*

    d. *to stabalize the women so delivery can happen*

53. What four steps should be taken to ensure that BP readings on the preeclamptic woman are standardized?

    a. *Use the same arm*

    b. *Use the arm c̄ the higher readings*

    c. *Use the correct BP cuff size*

    d. *Take BP when women is in the same position each time.*

54. Match the correct responses. BP readings are:

    Column A   Column B

    c 1. Lowest   a. Supine, standing

    a 2. Highest   b. Sitting

    b 3. Intermediate   c. Laterally recumbent with a 15- to 30-degree tilt

55. In the severely preeclamptic patient, how often is assessment of the following recommended?

    a. BP: *every 15 → 30 minutes*

    b. Proteinuria: *every hour*

    c. Hyperreflexia: *every hour*

    d. Urinary output: *every hour*

56. An appropriate nurse:patient ratio with a severely preeclamptic woman is

    1:1 .

57. Appropriate laboratory workup for the preeclamptic woman includes:

    a. *CBC c̄ peripheral smear*

    b. *Type + cross match*

    c. *liver enzymes*

    d. *DIC profile*

    e. *serum creatinine*

58. State five precautions to be taken in caring for the severely preeclamptic woman.
    a. *Keep lights dim, noise level & visitors to a minimum*
    b. *Pad the sides of the bed*
    c. *place a tongue blade @ side of the bed*
    d. *have O₂ & suction available*
    e. *Emergency cart nearby*

59. State the initial steps you would take if an 18-year-old primigravida at 34 weeks' gestation presented in early labor at the labor unit of a Level I hospital and had signs and symptoms of severe preeclampsia.
    Notify the physician. Stabalize the pt and prepare her for transport to a high risk hospital.

60. The woman with HELLP syndrome is at risk for hemorrhage due to a severely low platelet count. Which of the following are clinical signs and symptoms of this condition? (Circle all that apply.)

    A. Hematuria   F. Epigastric pain
    B. Epistaxis   G. Easy bruising
    C. Proteinuria   H. Oozing from the IV site
    D. Petechiae   I. Bleeding gums
    E. Hypertension

61. When caring for the woman with HELLP syndrome, what two laboratory values should be monitored closely?
    a. *liver enzymes*
    b. *Platelets*

62. The recommended fetal monitoring approach for a woman with HELLP syndrome is intermittent, external fetal monitoring throughout her labor.
    A. True
    B. False

63. Epidural blocks can safely be used for pain management during labor and delivery and for anesthesia during cesarean delivery in the woman with HELLP syndrome.
    A. True
    B. False

64. All women with HELLP syndrome should have a cesarean delivery.
    A. True
    B. False

65. To give a woman a loading dose of MgSO₄ • 7H₂O means that:
    Must be infused over 20 Minutes in 100mL Bag

66. To administer 4 to 6 g of $MgSO_4 \cdot 7H_2O$ in loading doses, you must be able to perform certain calculations using known $MgSO_4 \cdot 7H_2O$ concentrations. One ampule (10 mL) of a 50% solution contains 5 g of $MgSO_4 \cdot 7H_2O$. This means that 1 g of $MgSO_4 \cdot 7H_2O$ is in ___*2 mL*___ mL of solution. To add 4 g of $MgSO_4 \cdot 7H_2O$ to any IV solution, you would draw up ___*8 mL*___ mL. To administer a 4-g loading dose using the 50% $MgSO_4 \cdot 7H_2O$ solution just described, you would add ___*8*___ ampules to 1,000 mL of 5% dextrose and water or lactated Ringer's solution run at ___*4*___ mL per minute over a 25-minute period. To give a 6-g loading dose using this same solution, you would administer ___*150*___ mL of solution over a set time (e.g., 10 to 15 minutes).

67. You have 10-mL ampules of 50% concentrate $MgSO_4 \cdot 7H_2O$ solution available. To prepare an IV solution to administer 2 g of $MgSO_4 \cdot 7H_2O$ over 1 hour, you add ___*40*___ g or ___*8*___ ampules to 1,000 mL of 5% dextrose and water or lactated Ringer's solution and run it at the rate of ___*50*___ mL per hour by infusion pump.

68. State three signs of magnesium sulfate overdose.
    a. ___*poor reflexes*___
    b. ___*Nausea / vomitting*___
    c. ___*Respiratory Depression*___
    late signs - Respiratory and Cardiac arrest

69. In treating the preeclamptic patient with $MgSO_4 \cdot 7H_2O$, the aim is to achieve a therapeutic blood level of ___*4-7*___ mg/dL of serum magnesium. This laboratory test is usually done every ___*4-6*___ hours.

70. The antidote to $MgSO_4 \cdot 7H_2O$ toxicity is the administration of ___*Calcium*___. This should be administered at an intravenous rate of ___*3 minutes*___. *Glucanate*

71. The initial dose of hydralazine (Apresoline) to the severely hypertensive patient is *the (5mg over 1-2min test dose (Initial)* ___*1*___ mg intravenously over ___*1*___ minutes. BP during hydralazine therapy should be checked every ___*2-5*___ minutes. Another ___*5*___ mg may be given intravenously after ___*20*___ minutes if the diastolic BP remains above 110 mm Hg.

72. Explain why it is critical to observe for any sign of hypotension when administering a vasodilator, such as hydralazine (Apresoline), to the severely hypertensive or eclamptic woman.
    ___*Because the pt can experience sudden and profound hypotension.*___

73. A significant drop in BP after delivery in a woman with a severe hypertensive disorder likely reflects ___*severe blood loss*___.

74. When a high-risk baby is anticipated at delivery, it is imperative to prepare by ___*have appropriate people a delivery not on call*___

75. The "cure" for preeclampsia is ___Delivery_____ .

76. Eclampsia occurs in almost ___25___ % to ___30___ % of cases during the _Postpartum_period.

77. Postpartum recovery from HELLP syndrome is:

   A. Gradual

   B. Preceded by worsening of laboratory values and illness

   C. Quite rapid

   D. Uneventful

78. State five signs and symptoms that indicate the development of pulmonary edema.

   a. _Chest discomfort_____

   b. _Tachycardia_____

   c. _pulmonary rales_____

   d. _Tachypnea_____

   e. _Dysphnea_____

79. Breastfeeding can be done safely in women taking selected antihypertensive drugs with carefully reduced dosages and BP supervision.

   A. True

   B. False

80. The longer hypertension occurring for the first time during pregnancy persists postpartum, the greater the likelihood that the underlying cause is chronic hypertension.

   A. True

   B. False

81. Most women experiencing HELLP syndrome for the first time have a high risk of reoccurrence in a subsequent pregnancy.

   A. True

   B. False

PRACTICE/REVIEW ANSWER KEY

1. 6; 8%

2. Pregnancy-induced hypertension

3. Superimposed hypertension

4. Eclampsia

5. Preeclampsia

6. 1. b
   2. g
   3. e
   4. b
   5. a
   6. a
   7. a
   8. a
   9. f
   10. e

11. c
12. d
13. c
14. d

7. a. A
   b. B
   c. B
   d. B
   e. A
   f. B
   g. A
   h. A
   i. A

8. a. Elevated BP: 140/90 mm Hg or higher
   b. Proteinuria

9. a. T
   b. P
   c. H
   d. H
   e. P
   f. T
   g. P, E, or H
   h. H
   i. E
   j. H

10. Any five of the following:
    a. Young and pregnant for the first time
    b. Young and experiencing a pregnancy with a new father
    c. History of chronic hypertension
    d. Twin pregnancy
    e. Has diabetes
    f. History of preeclampsia
    g. Black race and older than 35 years of age

11. A

12. A diagnosis of chronic hypertension preceding pregnancy is made based on a history of persistent BP elevation before the twentieth week of gestation. Preeclampsia is diagnosed with BP elevations after the twentieth week of gestation.

13. Mark an "X" by statement a.

14. Superimposed preeclampsia; superimposed eclampsia

15. Any five of the following:
    a. Is remote from term (less than 36 weeks' estimated gestational age)
    b. Is White, multiparous, and 25 years of age or older
    c. Demonstrates excessive weight gain with generalized edema
    d. Complains of epigastric or right upper quadrant pain and a history of malaise for a few days
    e. Complains of flulike symptoms and nausea and vomiting
    f. Complains of hematuria, bleeding gums, jaundice, or diarrhea

16. D

17. C

18. A

19. A and B

20. A

21. 1. a
    2. b
    3. b
    4. b
    5. a
    6. d
    7. c

22. Angiotensin II; renin; angiotensinogen; angiotensin I; angiotensin II

23. A disease of small blood vessels in which the basement membrane of capillaries thickens, or thrombi microangiopathy, in which thrombi form in arterioles or capillaries

24. a. Pressure is increased (hypertension) and blood flow is diminished
    b. Lesions in the vessel wall result in fluid (plasma) loss, leading to changes in oncotic pressures and extracellular fluid accumulation
    c. Perfusion to the target organs is reduced, leading to ischemia and necrosis

25. Immune; platelets; fibrin; red blood cells; hemolysis

26. Microangiopathic hemolytic; HELLP syndrome

27. Thrombocytopenia

28. a. Abruptio placentae
    b. Cerebral hemorrhage
    c. Acute renal or cardiac failure
    d. DIC

29. 30; 15

30. Gestational hypertension

31. Intravascular volume; edema; sudden weight gain

32. Hematocrit

33. 100,000 mm^3, 50,000 mm^3

34. B

35. a. Blurred vision
    b. Dizziness
    c. Scotomata
    d. Headache

36. Epigastric pain in the right upper quadrant of the abdomen

37. Hyperactive reflexes

38. Intrauterine growth restriction

39. B

40. A

41. B

42. B

43. A

44. A

45. Preeclampsia

46. 300 mg/L or more of protein in a 24-hour specimen or protein concentration of 2+ or higher on at least two random urine tests done 6 hours apart

47. She has severe preeclampsia. If delivery is required, a preterm, low-birth-weight infant will require neonatal intensive care.

48. a. Hemolysis
    b. Elevated liver enzymes
    c. Low platelets

49. a. T
    b. F
    c. T
    d. T

50. B

51. Any five of the following:
    a. Nausea and vomiting
    b. General sick feeling
    c. Epigastric or right upper quadrant pain
    d. Worsening edema
    e. Diarrhea
    f. Hematuria
    g. Bleeding gums
    h. Abdominal, flank, or shoulder pain

52. a. To prevent convulsions through the use of magnesium sulfate
    b. To ensure adequate kidney function
    c. To monitor fetal status continuously for signs of uteroplacental insufficiency
    d. To stabilize the woman so that a vaginal or cesarean birth can be accomplished

53. a. Use the same arm throughout.
    b. Use the arm with the higher reading if pressure readings differ in each arm by more than 10 mm Hg.
    c. Fit the appropriate size sphygmomanometer to the patient's arm.
    d. Perform BP readings with the woman in essentially the same position each time, preferably laterally recumbent and at a 15- to 30-degree tilt when on bed rest.

54. 1. c
    2. a
    3. b

55. a. Every 15 to 30 minutes
    b. Every hour
    c. Every hour
    d. Every hour

56. 1:1

57. a. CBC with peripheral smear
    b. Type and cross match
    c. Liver enzymes
    d. DIC profile
    e. Serum creatinine

58. a. Control the environment by keeping lights dim, noise level down, and visitors to a minimum.
    b. Pad the sides of the bed.
    c. Place a tongue blade at the bedside.
    d. Have oxygen and suctioning equipment available.
    e. Check that the equipment is in operating order and have the emergency cart nearby.

59. Notify the primary care provider immediately. Anticipate a maternal transport to a high-risk regional center after the patient is stabilized.

60. A, B, D, G, H, I

61. a. Platelet count
    b. Liver enzymes

62. B

63. B

64. B

65. The woman receives 4 to 6 g of $MgSO_4 \cdot 7H_2O$ in 100 mL of solution administered at a rate that ensures that the entire 4 to 6 g is received over a 15 to 20-minute period. This is done when a rapid therapeutic effect is desired. To reduce the risk of vomiting (the side effect of rapid $MgSO_4 \cdot 7H_2O$ administration), administer the dose over 25 to 30 minutes in nonemergency situations.

66. 2; 8; 8; 4; 150

67. 40; 8; 50

68. a. Absence of the patellar reflex
    b. Respirations that are shallow and fewer than 12 per minute
    c. Urinary output less than 25 mL per hour

69. 4.8 to 8.4; 2 to 6 (e.g., 2 hours after a loading dose, every 6 hours during maintenance therapy)

70. Calcium gluconate; using 10 mL of a 10% calcium gluconate solution (each milliliter contains 0.1 g of calcium gluconate), administer 1 g over 3 minutes

71. 5 mg; 1 to 2 minutes; 2 to 5 minutes; 5 to 10 mg; 20 minutes

72. Women who are severely hypertensive or eclamptic usually have reduced intravascular blood volume. Giving a potent vasodilator such as hydralazine causes blood vessels to dilate. This can result in poor blood return to vital organs in a patient with an abnormally low blood volume. The woman might experience sudden, severe hypotension.

73. Excessive blood loss

74. Having appropriate personnel present, not on call

75. Delivery

76. 25; 30; postpartum

77. B

78. a. Chest discomfort
    b. Tachycardia
    c. Pulmonary rales
    d. Tachypnea
    e. Dyspnea

79. A

80. A

81. B

REFERENCES

1. Cunningham, F. G., Gant, N. F., Leveno, K. J., Gilstrap, L. C., Hauth, J. C., & Wenstrom, K. D. (Eds.). (2001). Hypertensive disorders in pregnancy. In *Williams' obstetrics* (21st ed., pp. 567–618). New York: McGraw-Hill.
2. National High Blood Pressure Education Program. (2000). *Working Group report on high blood pressure in pregnancy.* Bethesda, MD: National Heart, Lung, and Blood Institute.
3. Norwitz, E. R., & Repke, J. T. (2000). Preeclampsia prevention and management. *Journal of the Society for Gynecologic Investigation, 7*(1), 21–36.
4. Branch, D. W., & Porter, T. F. (1999). Hypertension disorders in pregnancy. In J. R. Scott, P. J. DiSaia, C. B. Hammond, & W. N. Spellacy (Eds.), *Danforth's obstetrics and gynecology* (8th ed.). Philadelphia: Lippincott Williams & Wilkins.
5. Roberts, J. M. (1999). Pregnancy-related hypertension. In R. K. Creasy & R. Resnik (Eds.), *Maternal fetal medicine* (4th ed., pp. 833–872). Philadelphia: WB Saunders.
6. Roberts, J. (1994). Current perspectives on preeclampsia. *Journal of Nurse-Midwifery, 39*(2), 70–90.
7. Dekker, G. A. (1999). Risk factors for preeclampsia. *Clinical Obstetrics and Gynecology, 42*(3), 422–435.
8. Association of Obstetricians and Gynecologists. (1996). Hypertension in pregnancy. ACOG Technical Bulletin No. 219.
9. Saphier, C. J., & Repke, J. T. (1998). Hemolysis, elevated liver enzymes, and low platelets (HELLP) syndrome: A review of diagnosis and management. *Seminars in Perinatology, 22*(2), 118–133.
10. ACOG Practice Bulletin. (2001). Chronic hypertension in pregnancy. ACOG Committee on Practice Bulletins. *Obstetrics and Gynecology, 98*(1), 177–185.
11. Mulrow, C. D., Chiquette, E., Ferrer, R. L., Sibai, B. M., Stevens, K. R., Harris, M., Montgomery, K. A., & Stamm, K. (2000). *Management of chronic hypertension in pregnancy.* Evidence Report/Technology Assessment No. 14 (Prepared by the San Antonio Evidence-based Practice Center based at the University of Texas Health Science Center at San Antonio under Contract No. 290-97-0012). AHRQ Publication No. 00-E011. Rockville, MD: Agency for Healthcare Research and Quality.
12. Haddad, B., & Sibai, B. M. (1999). Chronic hypertension in pregnancy. *Annals of Medicine, 31*(4), 246–252.
13. Kelley, M. A. (1999). Triage and management of the pregnant hypertensive patient. *Journal of Nurse-Midwifery, 44*(6), 558–571.
14. Cowles, T., Saleh, A., & Cotton, D. B. (1994). Hypertension disorders of pregnancy. In D. K. James, P. J. Steer, C. P. Weiner, & B. Gonik (Eds.), *High risk pregnancy management options.* Philadelphia: WB Saunders.
15. Joint Committee on Prevention, Detection, Evaluation, and Treatment of High Blood Pressure. (1997). *The Sixth Report of the Joint Committee on Prevention, Detection, Evaluation, and Treatment of High Blood Pressure* (pp. 11–16). Bethesda, MD: National Institutes of Health.
16. Brown, M. A., & Whitworth, J. A. (1999). Management of hypertension in pregnancy. *Clinical and Experimental Hypertension, 21*(5 & 6), 907–916.
17. Shennan, A. H., & Halligan, A. W. F. (1999). Measuring blood pressure in normal and hypertensive pregnancy. *Bailliere's Clinical Obstetrics and Gynecology, 13*(1), 1–26.
18. Bell, S. C., Halligan, A. W. F., Martin, A., Ashmore, J., Shennan, A. H., Lambert, P. C., & Taylor, D. J. (1999). The role of observer error in antenatal dipstick proteinuria analysis. *British Journal of Obstetrics and Gynecology, 106,* 1177–1180.
19. Rinehart, B. K., Terrone, D. A., May, W. L., Magann, E. F., Isler, C. M., & Martin, J. N. (2001). Change in platelet count predicts eventual maternal outcome with syndrome of hemolysis, elevated liver enzymes and low platelet count. *Journal of Maternal-Fetal Medicine, 10*(1), 28–34.

20. Kruppel, R. A., & Drukker, J. E. (1993). Hypertension in pregnancy. In R. A. Knuppel & J. E. Drukker (Eds.), *High-risk pregnancy: A team approach* (2nd ed.). Philadelphia: WB Saunders.

21. Surrat, N. (1993). Severe preeclampsia: Implications for critical care obstetric nursing. *Journal of Obstetric, Gynecologic & Neonatal Nursing, 22*(6), 500–507.

22. Koenigseder, L. A., Crane, P. B., & Lucy, P. W. (1993). HELLP: A collaborative challenge for critical care and obstetric nurses. *American Journal of Critical Care, 2,* 385–394.

23. Leicht, T. G., & Harvey, C. J. (1999). Hypertensive disorders in pregnancy. In L. K. Mandeville & N. H. Troiano (Eds.), *AWHONN high-risk and critical care intrapartum nursing* (2nd ed., pp. 159–172). Philadelphia: Lippincott.

24. Association of Women's Health, Obstetric and Neonatal Nurses. (1993). *Didactic content and clinical skills verification for professional nurse providers of basic, high-risk, and critical care intrapartum nursing* (p. 29).Washington, DC: Author.

25. National High Blood Pressure Education Program. (1990). Working Group report on high blood pressure in pregnancy. *American Journal of Obstetrics and Gynecology, 163,* 1689–1712.

26. Sibai, B. H. (1990). Preeclampsia-eclampsia: valid treatment approaches. *Contemporary OB/GYN, 37*(8), 84–100.

27. Hogg, B., Hauth, J. C., Caritis, S. N., Sibai, B. M., Lindheimer, M., Van Dorsten, J. P., Klebanoff, M., MacPerson, C., Landon, M., Paul, R., Miodovnik M., Meis, P., Thurnau, G., Roberts, J., & McNellis, D., for the NICHD Maternal Fetal Medicine Units Network. (1999). Safety of labor epidural anesthesia for women with severe hypertensive disease. *American Journal of Obstetrics and Gynecology, 181*(5), 1096–1101.

28. Idamo, T. O., & Lindow, S. W. (1998). Magnesium sulfate: A review of clinical pharmacology applied to obstetrics. *British Journal of Obstetrics and Gynaecology, 105*(3), 260–268.

29. Ferris, T. F. (1995). Hypertension and preeclampsia. In G. N. Burrow & T. F. Ferris (Eds.), *Medical complications during pregnancy* (pp. 1–28). Philadelphia: WB Saunders.

30. Perkins, R. P. (1985). Toxemia. In N. Nelson (Ed.), *Current therapy in neonatal-perinatal medicine, 1985–1986* (p. 75). St. Louis: Mosby.

31. Dildy, G. A., Phelan, J. P., & Cotton, D. B. (1991). Complications of pregnancy-induced hypertension. In S. L Clark, D. B. Cotton, G. D. V. Hawkins, & J. P. Phelan (Eds.), *Critical care obstetrics* (pp. 257, 710). Boston: Blackwell Scientific Publications.

32. Antenatal corticosteroids revisited: Repeat courses. (2000). *NIH Consensus Statement, 17*(2), 1–18.

33. Levano, K. J., & Cunningham, F. G. (1999). Management of preeclampsia. In M. D. Lindheimer, J. M. Roberts, & F. G. Cunningham. *Chesley's hypertensive disorders* (p. 573). Stamford, CT: Appleton & Lange.

34. Silver, R. M., & Boanch, D. W. (1999). Immunologic disorders. In R. K. Creasy & R. Resnik (Eds.), *Maternal-fetal medicine* (4th ed., p. 465). Philadelphia: WB Saunders.

MODULE 10

Intrauterine Growth Restriction: Perinatal Issues and Management

JOAN G. ANDRES

As you complete this module, you will learn:

1. To differentiate between intrauterine growth restriction (IUGR) and small for gestational age (SGA) conditions
2. The problems encountered with the definition of IUGR
3. To recognize potential neonatal complications associated with IUGR and priorities for nursing care
4. To identify the intrauterine growth-restricted neonate by its physical characteristics
5. The three phases of normal cellular growth and the factors that influence these phases
6. The maternal, fetal, and placental factors contributing to IUGR
7. The difference between symmetric and asymmetric IUGR and the significance of each classification
8. How IUGR is diagnosed
9. To identify maternal risk factors for having a growth-restricted infant
10. The parameters of ultrasonic assessment for fetal size, growth, and well-being
11. Common fetal surveillance tests and criteria for interpretation
12. The general principles of management for the fetus suspected of having growth restriction
13. Criteria used to determine the timing and method of delivery
14. The antepartum plan of care for a woman having or suspected of having a growth-restricted fetus
15. Intrapartum nursing care for a woman with fetal growth restriction
16. The prognosis for an infant experiencing IUGR

When you have completed this module, you should be able to recall the meanings of the following terms. You should also be able to use the terms when consulting with other health professionals. Terms are defined in this module or in the glossary at the end of this book.

abdominal circumference (AC)
amniocentesis
amniotic fluid volume (AFV)
asymmetric IUGR
biophysical profile (BPP)
biparietal diameter (BPD)
circumvallate placenta
contraction stress test (CST)
cordocentesis
crown-rump length (CRL)
dizygotic
Doppler flow studies

head circumference:abdominal circumference ratio (HC/AC)
hyperplasia
hypertrophy
hypoglycemia
intrauterine growth restriction (IUGR)
monozygotic
nonstress test (NST)
oligohydramnios
placenta accreta
placenta previa
polycythemia

femur length (FL)
fetal karyotype
fundal height
head circumference (HC)

small for gestational age (SGA)
symmetric IUGR
vibroacoustic stimulation

Definitions and Incidence

Intrauterine growth restriction (IUGR), also called intrauterine growth retardation, fetal growth restriction, or fetal growth retardation, has several definitions. The most widely used definition is a fetus whose estimated weight is below the 10th percentile for its gestational age. The negative connotation of the word *retardation* has prompted the change of this term to *restriction.* Other definitions use birth weights below either the 15th, 5th, or 3rd percentile for gestational age.

> *Intrauterine growth restriction* is defined as a fetus whose estimated weight is below the 10th percentile for its gestational age.

Small for gestational age (SGA) is a neonatal diagnosis and describes an infant with a birth weight less than the 10th percentile for gestational age.[1] It may appear that these two definitions are the same and could be used interchangeably; however, they are two different entities. IUGR is the pathologic counterpart for SGA. With IUGR, the fetus has not reached its growth potential at a given gestational age as a result of one or more causative factors.[2] Growth-restricted fetuses are at increased risk for a poor outcome. SGA babies, on the other hand, are small but have reached their appropriate growth potential. These babies are simply small because of their genetic makeup and are otherwise normal.

> *IUGR* and *SGA* are not terms to be used interchangeably.

■ What problems exist with this definition?

Using this current definition of IUGR, two potential problems exist:

1. **The definition is based on the size of the fetus, not its growth potential.**[3,4] This could cause two potential problems. As already discussed, SGA babies are small but healthy babies. This sized-based definition would lead to many incorrectly diagnosed babies as having IUGR. On the other end of the spectrum, IUGR could be manifested as a weight above the 10th percentile for gestational age. A fetus may be initially well, within normal weight limits, and then exposed to an intrauterine stress that restricted its growth. Its birth weight, being above the 10th percentile, would incorrectly exclude it from being identified as a growth-restricted fetus.
2. **Variations in birth weight for gestational age standards exist.**[4,5] Not all growth standards use the same weights. Any factor contributing to the birth weight can affect the standards. The most influential factors include altitude, race, fetal sex, maternal parity, maternal height, paternal height, and socioeconomic status. Higher altitudes may impair maternal and fetal oxygenation and limit fetal growth. More and more specific based growth curves are being used. However, these become even more difficult in geographically mobile and ethnically heterogeneous populations. In addition, some standards round off gestational age to the nearest week, whereas others express weights by weeks completed.

Obviously, a better definition of IUGR is needed, specifically, one recognizing growth restriction as a pathologic process interfering with fetal growth and resulting in increased morbidity and mortality.

■ **What is the incidence of IUGR?**

Until a better definition is uniformly applied, it remains difficult to accurately assess the incidence, effectiveness of treatment, and outcomes of the truly growth-restricted fetus. By definition, the incidence of IUGR should be 10%. However, as already noted, not all fetuses with IUGR are identified, and others who are included really are not growth restricted. The reported incidence varies by author. Approximately 70% of fetuses with a birth weight below the 10th percentile for gestational age are constitutionally small; in the remaining 30%, the cause of IUGR is pathologic.[2,3]

Complications Associated With IUGR

IUGR is the second leading cause of perinatal morbidity and mortality, outranked only by prematurity.[5] Perinatal morbidity and mortality are significantly increased with weights below the 3rd percentile for gestational age.[2] Complications associated with IUGR are grouped under antepartal complications and neonatal complications (Display 10.1).

DISPLAY 10.1	Complications of IUGR
ANTEPARTUM	**NEONATAL**
Intrauterine fetal death	Meconium aspiration
Oligohydramnios	Hypoglycemia
Intrapartum hypoxia	Polycythemia
	Hyperbilirubinemia
	Hypothermia

Antepartum Complications

- **Intrauterine fetal death** can occur at any time during the pregnancy but is more common after 36 weeks' gestation and before the onset of labor.[4] According to Peleg, Kennedy, and Hunter[5] and Vandenbosche and Kirchner[4], the overall perinatal mortality for the growth-restricted infant in the United States is 6 to 10 times higher than that observed in normal pregnancies. One study found that 26% of all stillbirths had IUGR.[3] The risk of death is also affected by gestational age and the primary cause of the IUGR.
- **Oligohydramnios** is a reduction in amniotic fluid. It is diagnosed by ultrasonography and is addressed later in this module. Oligohydramnios occurs in approximately 77% to 85% of pregnancies with IUGR.[3,4] It results from chronic stress being placed on the fetus. Blood is redistributed from the fetal kidneys to the brain. This shunting process decreases renal perfusion, thus decreasing fetal urinary output. The final result is less-than-normal amniotic fluid. Severe oligohydramnios signifies prolonged stress and is considered an ominous sign with respect to fetal well-being.
- Up to 50% of growth-restricted fetuses develop **hypoxia during labor.**[1,3] This is evidenced by late decelerations, absent or decreased variability, and/or bradycardia (see Module 6). Incidence of low Apgar scores and cord blood acidemia (a blood pH of less than 7.20) increases significantly in IUGR neonates.

Neonatal Complications and Priorities for Nursing Care

Meconium aspiration is related to the fetus gasping in utero in response to asphyxia. With fetal hypoxia, there is a reflex relaxation of the anal sphincter and an increase in intestinal movement. This combination causes fetal release of meconium in utero. This is not usually seen before 34 weeks' gestation. Meconium aspiration used to be a major cause of mortality and morbidity; however, with the use of amnioinfusion during labor and the resuscitative techniques used at delivery, the incidence and severity have decreased. Amnioinfusion involves the installation of fluid, via an intrauterine pressure catheter, into the uterus to dilute the meconium (see Module 5). Careful suctioning of the nasopharynx and oropharynx on the perineum before delivery of the shoulders also helps reduce the incidence of aspiration.

> **BE PREPARED FOR A HIGH-RISK BABY.** Nursing responsibilities are to do the following:
>
> - Notify appropriate personnel to attend the delivery
> - Have functioning resuscitative equipment at the bedside
> - Know how to carefully suction the nasopharynx and oropharynx before delivery of the baby's shoulders, if called upon to do so

Further clearing of the airway after delivery can be accomplished by direct laryngoscopy and aspiration by an experienced provider.

Hypoglycemia is a blood glucose less than 40 mg/dL in a term infant and less than 25 mg/dL in a premature infant.[6] In preparation for extrauterine life, the fetus stores glucose in the form of glycogen in the liver and muscle. *With IUGR, these glycogen stores are inadequate.* Signs and symptoms of hypoglycemia include the following:

- Jitteriness
- Tremors
- Weak cry
- Lethargy
- Floppy posture
- Hypothermia
- Poor feeding
- Seizures (occasionally)

Nursing care consists of early oral feedings (either breast, bottle, or a dextrose solution). Intravenous (IV) solutions may be needed until the infant is able to suck vigorously enough to have sufficient feedings.

Polycythemia is a hemoglobin greater than 22 g/dL or a hematocrit greater than 65%. Polycythemia occurs three to four times more frequently among the growth-restricted population. The fetus attempts to compensate for hypoxia by increasing its red blood cell (RBC) production (i.e., polycythemia). Also, with asphyxia, there is a transfer of blood volume from the placental circulation to the fetal circulation. With polycythemia, there is an increase in RBC breakdown, which leads to an increase in bilirubin (i.e., **hyperbilirubinemia**).

Hypothermia, a body temperature less than normal, is another problem seen in growth-restricted newborns. One way neonates regulate heat is through nonshivering thermogenesis. This refers to the utilization of brown fat for heat production. Brown fat deposits are located in and around the upper spine, clavicles, sternum, kidneys, and major blood vessels. *The amount of brown fat depends on gestational age and is decreased in growth-restricted fetuses.* Clinical symptoms may be subtle and include tachypnea and tachycardia. Nursing care focuses on the maintenance of thermoneutrality to promote recovery from perinatal asphyxia. An external heat source may be necessary.

Other neonatal complications are related to the specific cause or causes of the growth restriction. They are discussed later in this module.

Physical Appearance of the Growth-Restricted Newborn

> ■ **What are the physical characteristics of the growth-restricted newborn?**

Physical characteristics of the growth-restricted newborn include the following[6]:

- The skull is normal size. However, with decreased dimensions of the rest of the body, it appears large. Scalp hair is sparse. The sutures are wide as a result of inadequate bone growth.
- The skin is loose, dry, and thin. It is possible to grasp large skin folds, particularly around the shoulders and upper back. This is because of a deficiency in subcutaneous, deep, and brown fat.
- Meconium staining of the skin and cord is often seen. The cord tends to be limp, dull, and dry. (A normal cord is gray, glistening, round, and moist.)

- The abdomen is scaphoid; the ribs protuberant; and the muscle mass of the arms, buttocks, and thighs decreased.
- There is an alert, wide-eyed appearance. This results from prolonged hypoxia.
- In most cases the head circumference is greater than the abdominal circumference.
- Most of the time the birth weight and placenta weight are less then the 10th percentile.

> **The appearance of the IUGR baby and the SGA baby will not be the same.**

When the physical appearance of the growth-restricted infant is compared with a constitutionally SGA infant, they both may have a birth weight less than the 10th percentile. However, the SGA baby has a symmetric development of the head and abdomen, adequate subcutaneous fat, normal muscle mass, and a normal cord.

Normal Fetal Growth

Before one can understand the etiology of growth restriction, it is necessary to understand the cellular phases of normal growth and the factors that influence these phases.

■ What are the three phases of normal cellular growth?

Fetal growth is viewed as having three consecutive cell growth dynamic phases. The first phase, **cellular hyperplasia,** occurs during the first 16 weeks of gestation. During this phase, a rapid increase in the cell number occurs. The second phase is known as the phase of **concomitant cellular hyperplasia and hypertrophy.** This phase occurs midgestation and involves both an increase in cell number and an increase in cell size. The last phase of cellular growth occurs after 32 weeks' gestation and is called **cellular hypertrophy.** There is a rapid increase in cell size during this phase. The corresponding fetal growth rates during these phases are from 5 g/day at 15 weeks, 15 to 20 g/day at 24 weeks, and 30 to 35 g/day at 34 weeks of gestation.[2]

Factors Influencing Fetal Growth

Along with the phases of normal growth, certain factors influence the fetus' ability to grow to its inherent growth potential.

- **Genetic factors**—The genetic makeup alone can influence the size of the fetus. This is why SGA babies can exist without experiencing growth restriction. Although both parents' genes affect childhood growth and final adult size, maternal genes mainly influence birth weight.[5]
- **Substrates**—The availability of certain substrates are needed for normal growth. The most important of these are oxygen, glucose, and amino acids. Oxygen crosses the placenta by simple diffusion. Glucose crosses via facilitated diffusion and is burned with oxygen to produce energy in the form of adenosine triphosphate. This energy is used to convert amino acids into protein, and the result is a growing intrauterine infant. In a steady state, the maternal and fetal blood glucose levels are similar, with the fetal level being about 80% of the maternal level. Amino acids are actively transported to the fetus and thus are in higher concentration in fetal than maternal blood.
- **Adequate vascular support**—An adequate vascular support is needed to transport the substrates. Transplacental transfer depends on uteroplacental blood flow (blood flow from the uterine artery to the placenta), fetoplacental blood flow (blood flow from the umbilical artery to the placenta), and the villous structure at the interface of fetal and maternal blood. A disruption in any of these can decrease the amount of substrates the fetus receives.

Etiology of Intrauterine Growth Restriction

■ What causes IUGR?

Insult to any of the three phases of cellular growth or to one or more of the growth determinants can lead to an inability of the fetus to reach its growth potential. Various schemes attempt to classify the etiologic factors of IUGR. Some classify these factors as intrinsic or extrinsic. Others classify by most to least common causes. Still others view the pathophysiologic basis as being maternal, fetal, or placental in origin, which is how it is discussed in this module (Display 10.2).

DISPLAY 10.2	Maternal, Fetal, and Placental Factors Affecting IUGR	
MATERNAL FACTORS	**FETAL FACTORS**	**PLACENTAL FACTORS**
Nutritional status	Chromosome abnormalities	Inadequate development or maintenance
Maternal age	Structural anomalies	of the placenta
Environmental/social factors	Multifetal gestation	Impaired umbilical blood exchange
Poor obstetric history	Premature infants	Elevated maternal serum α-fetoprotein (AFP)
Maternal disease	Intrauterine infections	level

Maternal Factors

■ **What maternal factors influence IUGR?**

Maternal prepregnancy weight and **weight gain during pregnancy** are considered strong predictors of birth weight. Low prepregnancy weight and low maternal weight gain have been positively associated with an increase in IUGR.[3] The current consensus is that a maternal weight gain of less than 10 kg (22 pounds) by 40 weeks' gestation is clearly a risk factor for IUGR.[4]

Extremes in maternal age (i.e., younger than 16 or older than 35 years of age) are also associated with IUGR.[3]

Maternal environmental/social factors can cause IUGR. These factors include cigarette smoking, alcohol consumption, illicit drug use, and medications.

- **Maternal smoking** may be the cause of 30% to 40% of IUGR cases occurring in the United States.[4] Of all pregnant women, 15% to 20% smoke cigarettes.[7] There is a direct relationship between the severity of fetal growth impairment and the quantity of cigarettes smoked per day, although the exact mechanism by which tobacco affects birth weight is unknown. Nicotine, a powerful vasoconstrictor, decreases uterine and placental blood flow, resulting in fetal hypoxia. Because placental blood flow is diminished, there may be a decrease in nutrients reaching the fetus, which adversely affects fetal growth. Carbon monoxide can damage cells and directly decrease fetal growth. It can also reduce the capacity of the RBCs to carry oxygen by combining with hemoglobin to produce carboxyhemoglobin. Cyanide, which is produced by cigarette smoking, is directly toxic to cells and fetal growth. Finally, women who smoke tend to consume fewer calories and gain less weight. All of these factors can contribute to the decrease in birth weight.[7]
- Early use of **alcohol** by the pregnant mother may lead to fetal alcohol syndrome, whereas use during the second or third trimester may result in growth restriction.[4] Alcohol causes relaxation of the smooth muscle of the umbilical vessels, causing them to collapse and impair blood flow. This results in hypoxia and acidosis. As little as one to two drinks per day has been shown to result in growth delay in a child.
- **Illicit drug use** may result in IUGR in a fetus by a direct toxic effect on its growth, as well as through the likely association of inadequate diet, lack of prenatal care, and other socioeconomic factors. Cocaine acts by preventing catecholamine (norepinephrine and epinephrine) reuptake at presynaptic nerve endings. The increase of catecholamine concentration at the synapses stimulates the peripheral and central nervous systems. These effects increase blood pressure and cause tachycardia and vasoconstriction.[8] Cocaine abuse in pregnancy is associated with delivery of a growth-restricted infant in 30% or more of cases.[3] The incidence of IUGR in mothers with heroin addiction is as high as 50%.[3]
- **Maternal ingestion of certain medications** is another recognizable cause of IUGR. The incidence and severity vary by substance, gestational age at exposure, duration of exposure, and dosage. Known medications associated with IUGR include anticonvulsants (e.g., trimethadione, phenytoin), folic acid antagonists (e.g., methotrexate), and warfarin.

Women who have previously given birth to an IUGR baby are at increased risk for this condition in subsequent pregnancies. These women have up to a twofold to fourfold increased risk of another similarly affected fetus.[5]

Maternal diseases that affect the microcirculation, thereby causing fetal hypoxemia, vasoconstriction, or a reduction in fetal perfusion, are also significantly associated with IUGR. These include asthma, cystic fibrosis, cyanotic heart disease, preeclampsia, chronic hypertension, diabetes, lupus, and sickle cell disease. Chronic hypertension is the most common cause of IUGR. Growth-restricted infants of hypertensive mothers have a threefold increase in perinatal mortality compared with growth-restricted infants born of normotensive mothers.[4]

Fetal Factors

■ **What fetal factors are associated with IUGR?**

From 15% to 20% of fetal growth restrictions may be caused by fetal factors.[2]

Chromosomal and structural anomalies are major causes of IUGR. The relative risk ranges from as high as 24.7 with anencephaly to as low as 1.2 with pyloric stenosis.[3] Chromosomal abnormalities may constitute up to 7% of all cases of IUGR.[2]

IUGR is a complication that occurs in **multifetal gestation.** It is more pronounced in higher-order multiple gestations than with twins.[3] Growth restriction occurs 10 times more frequently in twin pregnancies than in singleton pregnancies. The incidence of IUGR in twins is about 15% to 25%.[4] Reasons include a decrease in placental mass in relation to fetal mass, abnormal placentation, and twin-to-twin transfusion. Growth restriction can occur with dizygotic twin gestations (twin pregnancies resulting from two fertilized ova) but is more common and severe with monozygotic twins (resulting from one fertilized ovum that splits).[3]

Prematurity is another risk factor for IUGR. The incidence of preterm growth restriction is at least three times higher than that of term growth restrictions. Preterm IUGR babies have the worst prognosis among all IUGR babies.[2]

Intrauterine infections account for about 10% of all cases of IUGR.[4] These include the TORCH groups: *TO*xoplasmosis, *R*ubella, *C*ytomegalovirus, and *H*erpes simplex. About one third of TORCH-affected infants have restricted growth.[1]

Other infections causing IUGR are HIV, hepatitis A, hepatitis B, parvovirus B19, and *Treponema pallidum* (syphilis). Bacterial infections have not been shown to cause growth restriction.[3]

Placental Factors

■ **What placental factors affect IUGR?**

Placental insufficiency is a well-established cause of fetal growth restriction. The main cause is inadequate blood flow, either on the maternal side or on the fetal side of the placenta. The reduced blood flow is caused by **inadequate development or maintenance of the vascular beds.**[9] This leads to alterations in placental surface area. Because the placenta is the source of nutrition and respiratory support necessary to sustain fetal life, any absolute or relative alteration in placental surface area affects the quantity of substrate the fetus receives. The following are all associated with altered surface areas: placenta previa, circumvallate placenta, partial placenta abruption, placenta accreta, placental infarctions, and multiple gestations. An abnormal umbilical cord can cause IUGR. Velamentous insertion, a condition in which the blood vessels of the umbilical cord course through the membranes before attachment to the placenta, or a single umbilical artery can cause an **impaired umbilical blood exchange.** Once again, if the fetus does not have adequate blood exchange, hypoxia and acidosis result. An **unexplained elevated maternal serum α-fetoprotein (AFP) level** greater than two times the multiple of the mean (MOM) is associated with an increased risk of IUGR. This may result from an early (16 week) placental disruption that results in leakage of fetal AFP into the maternal blood. These breaks in the placenta may prevent the later development of a larger, normal-sized placenta, decreasing substrate transfer of oxygen and nutrients and affecting fetal growth.[1]

Classifications of Intrauterine Growth Restriction

■ **How is IUGR classified?**

Most IUGR articles contain a discussion of its classifications. The American College of Obstetricians and Gynecologists (ACOG) does not address this in its practice bulletin because it is unclear whether the distinction is important with respect to etiology or neonatal outcome.[3] It is discussed here.

The classification of IUGR is based on the relationship between the size of the fetal abdomen and the size of the fetal head. There are two types of IUGR: symmetric (type I) and asymmetric (type II) (Display 10.3).

DISPLAY 10.3	Classification of IUGR
SYMMETRIC (Type 1)	**ASYMMETRIC (Type II)**
20% to 30% incidence Fetal head and abdomen are decreased Associated with an earlier insult	70% to 80% incidence "Brain-sparing" Associated with a later insult

Symmetric IUGR

Symmetric IUGR is a growth pattern in which the growth of both the fetal head and abdomen are decreased equally; hence, the classification of symmetric IUGR. Occurrence rates for symmetric IUGR are 20% to 30%.[2] This type of growth restriction is associated with an earlier insult that impairs fetal hyperplasia on all organs and is assumed to result from long-term intrauterine growth impairment. Symmetric IUGR may be caused by a fetal chromosomal disorder or infection.

Asymmetric IUGR

Asymmetric IUGR is a disproportionate decrease in the size of the fetal abdomen with respect to the head. This is the more common type, occurring 70% to 80% of the time.[2] This insult is associated with a later insult that impairs cellular hypertrophy. The disproportionate decrease in fetal organ size seen with this type of IUGR is due to the capacity of the fetus to adapt and redistribute its cardiac output from the less vital organs (i.e., liver, muscle, and fat) to the brain. This type is also called "brain-sparing" IUGR.

It is now believed that most cases of IUGR are a continuum from asymmetry (early stages) to symmetry (late stages).

Diagnosing Intrauterine Growth Restriction

The main prerequisite for determining IUGR is precise dating of the pregnancy (see Module 4). Without accurate dating, there is not a correct gestational age to compare the estimated weight with. Once accurate dating has been established, two essential steps are involved in the antenatal recognition of growth restriction. The first step involves the **identification of maternal risk factors** associated with IUGR and **clinical assessment of uterine size** in relation to gestational age. The second step involves **ultrasonic assessment** of fetal size and growth, supplemented by invasive fetal testing for chromosomal abnormalities or viral infections in select cases.

Identification of Maternal Risk Factors

■ **What maternal risk factors should be assessed?**

Assessing risk factors should begin at the first prenatal visit and continue at each subsequent visit. This assessment should include past medical and obstetric history, medication use, recent infections, social/environmental history, and present pregnancy history.

Medical History
- Chronic hypertension
- Asthma
- Cystic fibrosis
- Cyanotic heart disease
- Diabetes
- Lupus
- Sickle cell disease

407

Obstetric History
- History of chromosomal/congenital defects
- Prior IUGR infant
- Prior stillborn after 20 weeks' gestation
- Three or more consecutive spontaneous abortions

Medication Use
- Anticonvulsants
- Folic acid antagonists
- Warfarin

Recent Infections or Exposures
- Toxoplasmosis
- Rubella
- Cytomegalovirus
- Herpes
- Parvovirus B19
- HIV
- Hepatitis A or hepatitis B
- Syphilis

Social/Environmental History
- Prepregnant weight
- Cigarette smoking
- Alcohol consumption
- Illicit drug use

Present Pregnancy History
- Placenta previa
- Preeclampsia
- Multiple gestation
- Elevated maternal serum AFP

Clinical Assessment of Uterine Size

Before the development of ultrasonography, delayed fetal growth was indicated by **low maternal weight gain, Leopold maneuvers** (see Module 4), and **lagging fundal height.** Currently, IUGR is still often suspected on the basis of fundal height measurements. Fundal height is the measurement from the uppermost border of the symphysis pubis to the uppermost border of the fundus in the center of the abdomen. To measure fundal height, the mother should have an empty bladder and should be in the same position on the same examination table each time she is measured. Ideally, the same practitioner should perform the measurement at each visit. A fundal height that lags by more than 3 cm or is increasing in disparity may be a signal of IUGR.[4,5] Fundal height techniques are prone to considerable inaccuracy and should be used for screening only, not as the sole indicator. Studies have shown that in using fundal height alone to make the diagnosis, IUGR will go undetected in about one third of the cases and will be incorrectly diagnosed approximately half of the time.[3]

Ultrasonic Assessment of Fetal Size, Growth, and Well-being

Once IUGR is suspected, the next and most important diagnostic test performed is an **ultrasound.** Accurate ultrasound measurement requires knowledge of the fetus' gestational age. The timing of ultrasonography varies depending on the primary reason for doing it. Reasons include the following: to determine gestational age, to identify fetal anomalies, to calculate amniotic fluid volume, to grade the placenta, to estimate fetal weight, to determine adequate fetal growth, and to assess fetal well-being.

When it is impossible to accurately date a pregnancy by patient history and clinical examination, the first ultrasound is usually done to confirm gestational age. Ideally, to increase accuracy, ultrasounds performed for the purpose of dating a pregnancy should be done early (8 to 13 weeks' gestation). Fetal anomalies can be detected by ultrasound at 18 to 20 weeks' gestation. Once IUGR is suspected (i.e., lagging fundal height), ultrasound is performed. Remember, IUGR is based on the inability of the fetus to grow. Fetal growth, as opposed to fetal size, is a dynamic process and requires more than one ultrasound for diagnosis. Ultrasounds are performed no more than every 2 to 4 weeks. Measurements at shorter intervals may overlap with measurement errors.[3]

To assess fetal size, growth, and well-being, several different ultrasonic parameters are obtained (Display 10.4). These parameters include crown-rump length, abdominal circumference, biparietal diameter, head circumference, femur length, head circumference:abdominal circumference ratio, estimated gestational age, estimated fetal weight, amniotic fluid volume, and placental grading.

DISPLAY 10.4 | Ultrasound Parameters

Crown-rump length (CRL)	HC/AC ratio
Abdominal circumference (AC)	Estimated gestational age (EGA)
Biparietal diameter (BPD)	Estimated fetal weight (EFW)
Head circumference (HC)	Amniotic fluid volume (AFV)
Femur length (FL)	Placental grading

Crown-Rump Length

Most authorities agree that the **crown-rump length (CRL)** is the most accurate ultrasonic pregnancy dating method currently available. The distance from the upper part of the fetal cephalic pole (crown) to the lower portion of the fetus (rump) is measured. Adding 6.5 to the centimeter measurement will give you a rough gestational age estimate. More than 90% of the time this is accurate within 5 to 6 days of the estimated date of confinement.[10]

Abdominal Circumference

The **abdominal circumference (AC)** measurement is the best single measurement. AC measurements can be used after 14 weeks' gestation. For detecting growth restriction, it is a more sensitive measurement than the estimated fetal weight.[11] In all growth-restricted fetuses, the abdominal circumference is the first measurement to change.

Biparietal Diameter

The **biparietal diameter (BPD)** was the first sonographic parameter used to determine gestational age and to assess fetal growth. Measurements are taken at the level of the thalamus. Although this method can be used any time after the twelfth week of pregnancy, it is most accurate before the twenty-eighth week and optimally before the twentieth week. BPD is no longer the primary method for identifying the IUGR fetus because of the following limitations: Changes in the BPD may represent normal alterations in head shape; late in the third trimester, the normal variability of this measurement is relatively large, making it less effective; and identification of fetuses with asymmetric growth restriction is difficult because of the redistribution of blood flow favoring the brain.

Head Circumference

The **head circumference (HC)** is more commonly used than the BPD for evaluating fetal growth or investigating evidence of fetal anomalies. Molding will affect the BPD but will not affect the HC.

Femur Length

Measurements of fetal long bones are often used for estimation of gestational age. **Femur length (FL)** is rarely affected by IUGR, except in severe cases, and therefore in and of itself is not diagnostic. It does assume greater importance when combined with other parameters in the assessment of gestational age and in estimating fetal weight. It is easy to obtain and is not affected by molding or abnormal fetal positions.

Head Circumference:Abdominal Circumference Ratio

Morphometric ratios are used in diagnosing IUGR. The most commonly used is the **head circumference:abdomen circumference (HC/AC) ratio.** With asymmetric IUGR, the size of the liver tends to be disproportionately small. This is reflected by an AC that is smaller than expected based on the head size or body length. The HC/AC ratio compares the most preserved organ (i.e., the brain) in the malnourished fetus with the most compromised (i.e., the liver). The HC/AC ratio is normally 1 at 32 to 34 weeks and falls below 1 after 34 weeks. A ratio of greater than 1 detects about 85% of growth-restricted fetuses.[4] The ratio is normal in symmetric IUGR.

Estimated Gestational Age

Ultrasound machines have a built-in computer that can determine the **estimated gestational age (EGA)** by averaging the routine fetal measurements discussed previously. If good clinical dating is present, the ultrasonic EGA is compared with the clinical EGA. The difference between the two gives the care provider a quantitative idea of the severity of the growth impairment.

Estimated Fetal Weight

Although the abdominal circumference is considered the one best measurement, the **estimated fetal weight (EFW)** is the most common screen. It is based on the measurements of HC, AC, and FL. These parameters are converted to fetal weight estimates using published formulas and tables. An estimated fetal weight of less than the 6th percentile strongly correlates with growth restriction, and an estimated fetal weight greater than the 20th percentile virtually rules out IUGR. An estimated fetal weight at or less than the 15th percentile, or a decreasing fetal weight as determined by serial ultrasound measurements, is suggestive of IUGR.[4] When IUGR is suspected, serial measurements of fetal parameters provide an estimated growth rate. This is important for diagnosing or ruling out IUGR, as well as for assessing the progression and severity of the growth restriction.

Amniotic Fluid Volume

The first radiographic sign of IUGR may be decreased **amniotic fluid volume.** Oligohydramnios is diagnosed ultrasonographically in approximately 77% to 85% of pregnancies with fetal growth restriction.[3,4] Fluid volume can be measured in two different ways. The first way assesses the largest pocket of fluid in two perpendicular planes. Amniotic fluid volume is termed *normal* if at least one pocket measuring at least 2 cm is identified, marginal if a 1- to 2-cm pocket is seen, and decreased if a pocket less than 1 cm is noted. A pocket less than 1 cm, regardless of gestational age, is found in about 39% of cases of IUGR.[4] Another way of assessing fluid volume is the four-quadrant method. This method consists of measuring the largest pocket of fluid found in each of the four quadrants of the uterus. The measurements are then added to obtain the amniotic fluid index (AFI). If the total is less than 10 cm, it is considered decreased. If it totals less than 5 cm, it is considered significantly decreased and the risk of IUGR is increased.[4] The amniotic fluid volume often is normal in a fetus with significant growth restriction; thus, the absence of oligohydramnios should not detract from the diagnosis of IUGR.

Placental Grading

Ultrasonic **placental grading** has been studied with respect to IUGR. Placental maturation is described in four stages, based on calcium deposits within the placental septa. With progression from the least mature, grade 0, to the most mature, grade 3. Normally, a grade 3 placenta is not detected before 36 weeks' gestation. The presence of this before 36 weeks, along with an estimated fetal weight of less than 2,700 grams (5 pounds, 14 ounces), carries a fourfold risk of IUGR.[4]

General Management Principles for IUGR

> ■ **What are the general principles of management for a fetus suspected of having growth restriction?**

According to the ACOG,[3] evidence from randomized, controlled trials find few interventions beneficial in preventing or treating IUGR.

Management of suspected IUGR pregnancies depends on the following general principles:

- Eliminate contributing factors.
- Increase uterine blood flow and improve fetal oxygenation.
- Perform fetal surveillance testing.
- Include treatment therapies.
- Deliver at the appropriate time and place.

Eliminate Contributing Factors

The first step in decreasing the incidence of IUGR pregnancies is to eliminate contributing factors, such as poor dietary intake, cigarette smoking, alcohol consumption, and illicit drug use. The mother should be counseled on the importance of **good nutrition and adequate weight gain.** Her diet should contain about 300 calories per day (i.e., 2,100 to 2,300 calories total) more than the nonpregnant woman. The appropriate weight gain in the underweight woman should be 28 to 40 pounds; in the normal-weight woman, 25 to 35 pounds; in the overweight woman, 15 to 25 pounds; and when carrying twins, 35 to 45 pounds. The patient should be encouraged to **stop smoking.** Women who stop smoking by the twentieth week of pregnancy have babies of approximately equal size and health as women who never smoked. Women who stop smoking by the thirtieth week of pregnancy still have significant increases in the birth weight of their babies, compared with women who do not stop at all.[7] The woman should be encouraged to **stop drinking and using illicit drugs.** Other identifiable causes should be corrected, if possible.

Increase Uterine Blood Flow and Improve Fetal Oxygenation

The second step in the management of IUGR is to increase uterine blood flow as much as possible. **Bed rest** in the left lateral position is advocated to increase uterine blood flow, although studies have not proven this.[1,3] Even though exercise and physical activity do not seem to present a problem in the normal infant, they are contraindicated in high-risk pregnancies. **IV hydration** is given to improve uteroplacental perfusion and increase amniotic fluid volume. Intensive oxygenation therapy given to the mother has been attempted. However, fetal growth pattern, gross body movements, and heart rate variability do not change. Studies have shown that short-term oxygen therapy may have some benefit in prolonging pregnancies while corticosteroids can be administered.[4,11]

Perform Fetal Surveillance Testing

The goal of fetal surveillance is to prevent fetal death. Techniques such as maternal perception of fetal movement, electronic fetal monitoring, and real-time ultrasonography can identify the fetus that is either suboptimally oxygenated or, with increasing degrees of placental dysfunction, acidemic. *Identification of suspected fetal compromise provides the opportunity to intervene before progressive metabolic acidosis can lead to fetal death.*[12] Before an intensive fetal surveillance program is begun, a fetal karyotype may be done if there is serious risk of chromosome abnormalities in the normally pregnant woman with severe symmetric IUGR. Fetal karyotype is a schematic arrangement of the chromosomal analysis of fetal cells. Fetal cells can be obtained through **cordocentesis** or **amniocentesis.** Cordocentesis involves the removal of 0.5 to 5 mL of fetal blood via the insertion of a needle transabdominally through the uterus into either the umbilical artery or umbilical vein. After completion, the needle is removed and the site is visualized by ultrasound to observe for blood leakage. Amniocentesis, the removal of amniotic fluid via needle aspiration, is done for fetal karyotyping and assessment of fetal lung maturity. If the patient is Rh negative, RhoGam is given after either procedure.

■ **What fetal surveillance tests are performed?**

Fetal Kick Counts

A decrease in the maternal perception of fetal movement often, but not invariably, precedes fetal death, in some cases by several days. This is the reason for instructing the patient on "kick counts" as a means of fetal surveillance.[12] The woman should be encouraged to assess fetal activity every day. Several different protocols (e.g., time used to count and number of minimal accepted movements) are used. Some protocols require a minimum of four movements in 1 hour, some require 10 movements in 2 hours, and still others have the patient count for 1 hour three times a week comparing the number of movements with previous counts (they should equal or exceed the previous count). No optimal number of movements or minimal duration for counting movements has been defined.

Nonstress Test

The **nonstress test (NST)** is the first fetal assessment test performed. It is based on the premise that the heart rate of a fetus that is not acidotic or neurologically depressed will temporarily accelerate with fetal movement. Steps for performing an NST are as follows:

1. The patient lies in the left lateral tilt position.
2. The fetal heart rate is monitored with an external transducer.
3. The tracing is observed for heart rate accelerations that increase by at least 15 beats per minute, above the baseline and last (from beginning to end) at least 15 seconds.

If two accelerations are noted in a 20-minute period, the NST is interpreted as reactive. It is nonreactive if there are not two accelerations. Because of normal fetal sleep–wake cycles, the test may need to continue for 40 minutes or longer. Using **vibroacoustic stimulation (VAS)** during the NST decreases the amount of time needed to complete the test and decreases the false-negative rate by 50%.[11] VAS uses an artificial larynx to deliver both vibratory and acoustic stimuli to the fetus, which responds with a startle and accelerations in the heart rate. To perform VAS, the artificial larynx is positioned on the maternal abdomen and a stimulus of 1 to 2 seconds is applied. This may be repeated up to three times for progressively longer durations of up to 3 seconds to elicit fetal heart rate accelerations.[12] A reactive fetal heart rate tracing should be seen by 32 weeks' gestation. From 28 to 32 weeks, 15% of NSTs will be nonreactive despite a normal fetus. *Fifty percent of NSTs will be nonreactive from 24 to 28 weeks' gestation.*[12] *For these earlier gestations, a 10-beat acceleration often is acceptable.*[11] A reactive NST correlates with fetal well-being. A nonreactive NST does not necessarily indicate fetal compromise. The presence of late decelerations correlates with fetal hypoxemia. Variable decelerations are associated with oligohydramnios and/or cord compression. Timing of NSTs varies from daily (with severe IUGR) to weekly or twice weekly depending on the source and the fetal condition. *An NST should always be ordered if the mother notes a decrease in fetal movement.* Because of the possibility of a false-positive result, if an NST is nonreactive, further evaluation is needed before a management plan is formed.

Contraction Stress Test

The next test performed is either a **contraction stress test (CST)** or a **biophysical profile (BPP).** CSTs can be done by nipple stimulation (causing endogenous release of oxytocin from the posterior pituitary gland) or by a continuous IV oxytocin drip (called an *oxytocin challenge test*). The goal is to obtain three contractions in 10 minutes. Once three contractions are obtained, the fetal heart rate is observed for the presence of decelerations. Interpretation of the CST results is categorized as follows[12]:

- Negative—No late or significant variable decelerations
- Positive—Late decelerations following 50% or more of contractions (even if the contraction frequency is less than three in 10 minutes)
- Equivocal-suspicious—Intermittent late decelerations or significant variable decelerations
- Equivocal-hyperstimulatory—Fetal heart rate decelerations that occur in the presence of contractions more frequent than every 2 minutes or lasting longer than 90 seconds
- Unsatisfactory—Fewer than three contractions in 10 minutes or an uninterpretable tracing

Relative contraindications to the CST generally include preterm labor (or those at risk for preterm labor), premature rupture of membranes, history of extensive uterine surgery or classical cesarean delivery, and known placenta previa.

EVERY PRACTICE/INSTITUTION CONDUCTING NSTs AND CSTs SHOULD HAVE A WRITTEN AND OBSERVED PROCEDURE FOR EACH TEST. INTERPRETATION OF WHAT CONSTITUTES NORMAL AND ABNORMAL RESULTS SHOULD BE CLEARLY STATED IN THE PROCEDURE.

Biophysical Profile

The BPP can be performed if the NST is nonreactive. It is often done weekly or biweekly once a diagnosis of IUGR has been made. Multiple-parameter biophysical testing was introduced in 1980 by Manning. The BPP consists of an NST combined with four observations made by ultrasound. These observations include fetal breathing movements, fetal movements, fetal tone, and qualitative amniotic fluid volume. Each parameter is scored as either 2 (normal) or 0 (abnormal). Refer to Display 10.5 for scoring criteria for each parameter.

DISPLAY 10.5 | Biophysical Profile Scoring[12]

NONSTRESS TEST (If all four components of the ultrasound are normal, the NST can be omitted without compromising the validity of the test results.)

2: Reactive
0: Nonreactive

FETAL BREATHING

2: One or more episodes of rhythmic fetal breathing movements of 30 seconds or longer occurring within 30 minutes
0: Less than 30 seconds or no fetal breathing movements within 30 minutes

FETAL MOVEMENT

2: Three or more discrete body or limb movements within 30 minutes
0: Less than three or no discrete movements within 30 minutes

FETAL TONE

2: One or more episodes of extension of a fetal extremity with return to flexion, or opening or closing of a hand, within 30 minutes
0: Fetal movement not followed by return to flexion, or no opening of hand, within 30 minutes

QUALITATIVE AMNIOTIC FLUID VOLUME

2: A single vertical pocket of amniotic fluid exceeding 2 cm
0: Less than a 2-cm vertical pocket of amniotic fluid

A cumulative score of 8 or higher has been associated with a good pregnancy outcome. A score of 6 is considered equivocal, and a score of 4 or less is abnormal. Regardless of the composite score, in the presence of oligohydramnios, further evaluation is needed.[12] The effects of fetal hypoxia and acidosis on the score depend on many factors: chronicity, frequency, duration, and degree of hypoxia. Acute insults abolish the biophysical activities in a predictable order. Chronic hypoxia may result in the redistribution of blood flow from nonvital organs. Oligohydramnios has traditionally been considered a chronic marker of the fetal condition because it is not influenced by acute hypoxic episodes. Biophysical activities that appear last during fetal neurodevelopment (fetal heart rate reactivity and fetal breathing movements) are the first to be abolished. Fetal movements and fetal tone are lost last in the process of fetal asphyxia.

Doppler Flow Studies

Doppler ultrasonography is a noninvasive technique used to assess the hemodynamic components of vascular impedance. This technique can differentiate between the IUGR fetus and the SGA fetus. Basically, the Doppler flow velocity waveforms are ultrasonically derived from movement of RBCs within the vessel lumen and reflect downstream resistance in a given circulatory bed. Waveforms in the umbilical artery reflect resistance in the placental circulation. The umbilical flow velocity waveform of a normally growing fetus is characterized by high-velocity diastolic flow, whereas with IUGR, there is diminution of umbilical artery diastolic flow. In some cases of extreme IUGR, flow is absent or even reversed. The perinatal mortality rate in these pregnancies is high.

Include Treatment Therapies

■ **What treatment therapies are available?**

Corticosteroids may be administered if the fetus is less than 34 weeks' gestation (see Module 7).

Administration of daily **low-dose aspirin** has been advocated for the treatment of placental insufficiency in pregnancies complicated by IUGR. Studies show mixed results. Therefore, aspirin therapy should be used only in experimental protocols.[3]

Deliver at the Appropriate Time and Place

Proper timing of delivery for the mother experiencing IUGR is critical. The risks of prematurity versus a deteriorating intrauterine environment must be weighed. If all surveillance tests are normal, the optimal time for delivery appears to be about the thirty-eighth week of pregnancy.[1] If surveillance tests become abnormal before that time, assessment of fetal lung maturity needs to be done via amniocentesis. Once lung maturity is documented, there is nothing to gain by postponing delivery. Remember, the majority of intrauterine demises occur after 36 weeks' gestation and before the onset of labor. If the NST is nonreactive, either a CST or BPP is done. It is recommended that the baby be delivered if one or more of the following conditions are true:

- The CST is positive.
- The BPP score is low. (Some authors just use the word *low;* some define *low* as less than 4 at 32 weeks' gestation.)
- There is "severe" oligohydramnios.
- There is complete cessation of fetal growth, assessed ultrasonographically over a 2- to 4-week interval.
- Umbilical Doppler flow studies demonstrate absent or reversed flow.

Location of delivery depends on the severity of the growth restriction and the fetal gestational age. The patient may need to be transferred to a tertiary center where appropriate neonatal care is available. If the cervix is favorable and antenatal testing is normal, vaginal delivery can be attempted. Approximately one third of pregnancies with IUGR require cesarean section.[11]

Intrapartum Care

Excluding congenital defects, intrapartum asphyxia is the major cause of perinatal morbidity and mortality. *IUGR fetuses are more susceptible to intrapartum asphyxia than normally grown fetuses.* With increasing contractions, blood flow within the intervillous space decreases, resulting in decreased fetal oxygenation. The fetus then becomes hypoxic, which is reflected in the fetal heart tracing. For this reason, **continuous electronic fetal monitoring** should be applied to all woman who are suspected of having a pregnancy complicated by IUGR (Display 10.6).

DISPLAY 10.6 | Intrapartum Nursing Care

Continuous electronic fetal monitoring
Left lateral position
IV hydration
Oxygen therapy
Epidural (for pain relief)
Adequate personnel at the delivery

Left lateral position will improve uteroplacental blood flow. **IV hydration** is instituted to increase maternal blood volume, thereby improving uteroplacental perfusion. Thick meconium or the presence of variable decelerations (secondary to oligohydramnios) warrants **amnioinfusion. Oxygen therapy** should be considered in the presence of any abnormal fetal tracing. The best choice for pain relief is **epidural anesthesia.** Care must be taken to prevent the development of hypotension. To do this, the nurse should give an IV bolus before the epidural catheter is placed. IV sedation is not recommended because of its effects on the fetus. At delivery, **someone capable of neonatal resuscitation** should be present. Depending on the institution, this may be a pediatrician, neonatologist, or nursery nurse. All **resuscitative equipment** should be at the bedside and checked before delivery.

Long-Term Prognosis

■ What is the prognosis for IUGR babies?

Because more and more babies are surviving the neonatal period, more attention is being focused on their long-term prognosis. In most cases, infants with IUGR ultimately have good outcomes, with a reported mortality rate of only 0.2% to 1%.[4] Long-term development depends, in part, on the cause of the growth restriction. In infants with chromosomal abnormalities or viral infections, the cause rather than the birth weight ultimately determines their outcome.[3] There are conflicting data on whether IUGR infants experience a "catch up" in growth. Most authorities believe that babies who experience IUGR because of placental insufficiency will experience normal catch-up growth between 3 months and 2 years of age, although this pattern may not be seen universally in severely affected infants. At least one third of infants who experienced IUGR never achieve normal height.[5] The lower the birth weight and the earlier the gestational age, the less the chance a child has of catching up.

Prognosis summary:

- Long-term development depends, in part, on the cause of the growth restriction.
- The lower the birth weight and the earlier the gestational age, the less the chance a child has of catching up.
- Decreased intrauterine growth may have a negative effect on brain growth and mental development potential.
- Overall, most IUGR babies have an excellent long-term prognosis

Decreased intrauterine growth may have a negative effect on brain growth and mental development potential. Fattal-Valevski, Leitner, Kutai, Tal-Posener, Tomer, Lieberman, Jaffa, Many, and Harel[13] found minor neurodevelopmental problems (e.g., the inability to cut paper, walk up stairs alone, or copy circles) in 3-year-olds who experienced IUGR. They did not find any significant differences in IQ scores. Zubrick, Kurinczuk, McDermott, McKelvey, Silburn, and Davies[14] studied children 4 to 13 years of age. They found poor fetal growth was related to an increased risk of clinically significant mental health problems. Children born with weights less than the 2nd percentile were more likely to be academically impaired. The research shows no consistent findings. Long-term studies have shown that IUGR babies are more prone to develop hypertension, cardiovascular complications, and type 2 diabetes as adults.[3,4] Overall, most infants with IUGR have an excellent long-term prognosis.

PRACTICE/REVIEW QUESTIONS

After reviewing this module, answer the following questions.

1. *IUGR* is defined as a fetus whose estimated weight is below the ___10th___ percentile for its gestational age.

2. The terms *IUGR* and *SGA* are correctly used interchangeably.

   A. True

   B. False

3. State your rationale for the answer to question 2.

   IUGR- fetus below the 10th percentile
   SGA - neonate below the 10th percentile

4. Discuss the two problems with the definition of IUGR.

Variations II

   a. The definition is based on the size of the fetus not its growth potential
   b. Differences in birth weight for gestational age standards exist

5. List seven factors that contribute to birth weight that can affect the growth standards.

   a. altitude
   b. fetal sex
   c. race
   d. maternal parity
   e. maternal height / paternal height
   f. maternal weight
   g. Socioeconomic Status

6. The incidence of IUGR is 10% as the definition implies.

   A. True
   (B) False

7. IUGR is the ___2nd___ leading contributor to the perinatal mortality rate, prematurity is the ___1st___.

8. List three antepartum complications that can occur from growth restriction.

   a. Intrauterine fetal death
   b. Oligohydramnios
   c. Intrapartum hypoxia

9. With IUGR, intrapartum fetal death can occur at any time during a pregnancy. However, it is most common after ___36___ weeks of gestation and before the onset of labor

10. Oligohydramnios is considered a(n) acute/(chronic)(please circle) insult and is caused by:
    Chronic stress being put on the fetus

11. Oligohydramnios occurs in approximately ___77___ % to ___85___ % of pregnancies with IUGR.

12. List three signs of fetal hypoxia as seen on a fetal monitor.

    a. late decelerations
    b. absent or decreased variability
    c. and bradycardia

13. List five neonatal complications seen with IUGR.

    a. Meconium aspiration
    b. hypoglycemia
    c. polycythemia
    d. Hyperbilirubinemia
    e. hypothermia

14. What causes the release of meconium from an IUGR fetus?

hypoxia in the fetus causes relaxation of the anal spincter

15. Meconium aspiration is a problem not usually seen before ___*34*___ weeks of gestation.

16. What two interventions help reduce the incidence of meconium aspiration?
    a. *IUPC (Amnioinfusion*
    b. *resucitative tecniques used @ delivery*

17. When meconium is present, nursing care includes what two things?
    a. *notify appropriate personnel to be @ delivery*
    b. *and have appropriate resucitative equipment @ the BS*

18. Hypoglycemia is a blood glucose level less than ___*40*___ mg/dL in a term infant and less than ___*25*___ mg/dL in premature infant. It is caused by:

19. List six signs/symptoms of hypoglycemia.
    a. *jitteriness*
    b. *tremors*
    c. *weak cry*
    d. *lethargy*
    e. *floppy posture*
    f. *hypothermia, poor feeding, Occasionally seizures*

20. Nursing care for the treatment of hypoglycemia consists of:
    Early oral feedings; IV may be needed until the infant is able to suck rigorousley enough to have sufficient feedings.

21. *Polycythemia* is defined as *hemogleobin > 25 g/dL or a crit > 65%*

22. Two causes of polycythemia in the growth-restricted infant are:
    a. *fetus tries to compensate for hypoxia by ↑ its RBC produ*
    b. *Also c asphyxia there is a transfer of blood volume from the placental circulation to the fetal circulation*

23. The increase in RBC breakdown associated with polycythemia can lead to *hyperbilirubinemia*

24. Why is the growth-restricted infant prone to hypothermia?
    The amount of brown fat depends is ↓ in growth restricted infants.

25. List two signs/symptoms of hypothermia.

    a. *tachypnea*

    b. *tachycardia*

26. A(n) *external heat source* may be necessary for maintaining thermoneutrality.

27. The appearance of the IUGR baby and the SGA baby are the same.

    A. True

    B. False

28. Provide your rationale for the answer to question 27.

    The SGA Baby has symetric development of of the head and abdomen

The following questions are related to the appearance of an IUGR newborn.

29. The skull is larger than normal.

    A. True

    B. False

30. The skin is *loose* , *dry* , and *thin* .

31. The cord tends to be glistening, round, and moist.

    A. True

    B. False

32. The abdomen is distended, the ribs protuberant, and the muscle mass decreased.

    A. True

    B. False

33. The eyes are alert and wide.

    A. True

    B. False

34. Circle the correct answer: Most of the time the head circumference is (greater than) (less than) (equal to) the abdominal circumference.

35. Name the three normal phases of cellular growth, define when each occurs, and state what happens during each phase.

    a. *Cellular hyperplasia - occurs during the 1st 16wks - rapid ↑ in cell # too.*

    b. *Concomitant cellular hyperplasia + hypertrophy occurs mid gestation + involves both an ↑ in cell # + size*

    c. *Cellular hypertrophy - occurs after 3 awks rapid ↑ in cell size*

36. Name three factors that influence fetal growth.

    a. _____

    b. _____

    c. _____

37. Maternal genetic factors have less of an influence of birth weight than paternal factors.

    A. True

    B. False

38. List the three substrates needed for a fetus to reach its growth potential.

    a. _____

    b. _____

    c. _____

39. Glucose is burned with oxygen to produce _____, which converts

    _____ into protein.

40. Fetal glucose levels are about _____% of the maternal levels.

41. Why is it important to have adequate vascular support for fetal growth?

    _____

42. The pathophysiologic basis for discussion of the etiology of IUGR are divided into

    _____ factors, _____ factors, and _____ factors.

43. Name the two strong predictors of birth weight.

    a. _____

    b. _____

44. A maternal weight gain of less than _____ kg or _____ pounds
    by 40 weeks' gestation is clearly a risk factor for IUGR.

45. What are the maternal ages associated with growth restriction?

    _____

    _____

46. List four environmental factors known to cause IUGR.

    a. _____

    b. _____

    c. _____

    d. _____

47. Maternal smoking may cause _____% to _____% of IUGR
    occurring in the United States.

48. There is no relationship between the severity of fetal growth impairment and the quantity
    of cigarettes smoked per day.

    A. True

    B. False

49. Vasoconstriction _____ uterine and placental blood flow.

    A. Increases

    B. Decreases

50. Alcohol consumption relaxes the umbilical vessels, causing them to collapse and impair blood flow to the fetus.

   A. True

   B. False

51. Early use of alcohol by the mother may cause _____, while second or third trimester use may result in _____.

52. Cocaine causes _____, which decreases blood flow to the fetus.

   A. Vasoconstriction

   B. Vasodilatation

53. Cocaine abuse in pregnancy is associated with a delivery of a growth-restricted infant in _____% or more of cases.

54. Name three medications that cause IUGR.

   a. _____

   b. _____

   c. _____

55. IUGR in previous pregnancies does not affect the risk of IUGR in future pregnancies.

   A. True

   B. False

56. List six maternal diseases that can cause IUGR.

   a. _____

   b. _____

   c. _____

   d. _____

   e. _____

   f. _____

57. _____ is the most common cause of IUGR.

58. From _____% to _____% of fetal growth restrictions may be due to fetal factors.

59. List five fetal causes of IUGR.

   a. _____

   b. _____

   c. _____

   d. _____

   e. _____

60. How are multifetal gestations associated with IUGR?

   _____

   _____

   _____

61. What is the incidence of IUGR in twin gestation? _____

62. Growth restriction is more common and severe in _____ twins.

    A. Monozygotic

    B. Dizygotic

63. The incidence of preterm growth restriction is at least _____ times higher than that of term growth restrictions.

64. Name the TORCH infections.

    a. _____

    b. _____

    c. _____

    d. _____

65. Bacterial infections have been shown to cause IUGR.

    A. True

    B. False

66. Why is the placental surface a factor in IUGR?

    _____

    _____

67. List four things that alter the placental surface area.

    a. _____

    b. _____

    c. _____

    d. _____

68. A low maternal serum α-fetoprotein is associated with IUGR.

    A. True

    B. False

69. What are the two types of IUGR?

    a. _____

    b. _____

70. What distinguishes the types?

    _____

    _____

71. Discuss the pathophysiology for the asymmetric growth-restricted fetus.

    _____

    _____

72. Indicate whether the following are characteristic of symmetric (S) or asymmetric (A) IGUR.

    A. _____ Usually occurs as a result of an early insult

    B. _____ Also called "brain-sparing"

    C. _____ Insult impairs cellular hypertrophy

    D. _____ Type I

    E. _____ The more common type

    F. _____ Fetal head and abdomen are proportionately decreased

73. _____ is the main prerequisite for precise and early detection of IUGR.

74. After accurate dating has been established, what are the next two essential steps involved in diagnosing intrauterine growth restriction?

    a. _____

    b. _____

75. Assessment of risk factors for growth restriction occurs during the first prenatal visit only.

    A. True

    B. False

76. To assess risk factors for IUGR, a complete patient history must be obtained. Name six components of the history.

    a. _____

    b. _____

    c. _____

    d. _____

    e. _____

    f. _____

77. List three factors from a prior pregnancy that increase the risk for IUGR in a current pregnancy.

    a. _____

    b. _____

    c. _____

78. List three social/environmental risk factors for IUGR.

    a. _____

    b. _____

    c. _____

79. Identify four things in a current pregnancy that increase the risk for IUGR.

    a. _____

    b. _____

    c. _____

    d. _____

80. Before the development of ultrasound, IUGR was often indicated by what three assessments?

    a. _____

    b. _____

    c. _____

81. _____ is the most common clinical method used for the initial suspicion of IUGR.

82. How is the fundal height measurement done?

    _____

    _____

    _____

83. What two deviations in fundal height should increase the practitioner's suspicion of the possibility of a growth-restricted fetus?

    a. _____

    b. _____

84. Once IUGR is suspected, the next and most important test performed is a(n)

    _____.

85. List five reasons an ultrasound may be done.

    a. _____

    b. _____

    c. _____

    d. _____

    e. _____

86. At what gestational age should an ultrasound ideally be done when attempting to date a pregnancy? _____

87. When can fetal anomalies be detected? _____

88. One ultrasound is not sufficient to diagnose IUGR.

    A. True

    B. False

89. State your rationale for the answer to question 88.

    _____

    _____

    _____

90. How often are ultrasounds performed to assess fetal growth? _____

91. Match the term in Column B with the correct definition in Column A.

    Column A

    1. _____ Molding will affect this

    2. _____ Is used more often than BPD for assessing the head

    3. _____ Most accurate measurement for dating

    4. _____ The best single measurement

    5. _____ Compares the most preserved organ with the most compromised

    6. _____ Reflects the size of the liver

    7. _____ Adding 6.5 to this measurement will yield the gestational age

    8. _____ The distance from the upper part of the fetal cephalic pole to the lower portion of the fetus.

    9. _____ The first measurement to be affected by IUGR

    10. _____ If normal, IUGR is practically ruled out

    11. _____ Most common long bone measurement

    Column B

    a. Crown-rump length

    b. Biparietal diameter

    c. Head circumference

    d. Abdominal circumference

    e. Femur length

    f. HC/AC ratio

92. What is the most common parameter for diagnosing IUGR?

    _____

93. The first radiographic sign of IUGR may be what? _____

94. Discuss the two methods used to assess amniotic fluid volume. Include the normal and abnormal values in your discussion.

    _____
    _____
    _____
    _____
    _____

95. Grade 2 placentas before 36 weeks' gestation increase the risk of IUGR.

    A. True

    B. False

96. List five general management principles for IUGR.

    a. _____
    b. _____
    c. _____
    d. _____
    e. _____

97. State the appropriate amount of weight each of the following pregnant patients should gain:

    a. Underweight: _____

    b. Normal weight: _____

    c. Overweight: _____

    d. Carrying twins: _____

98. Women who stop smoking by the twentieth week of pregnancy still have growth-restricted babies.

    A. True

    B. False

99. List two reasons IV hydration is given.

    a. _____

    b. _____

100. What is the goal of antepartum fetal surveillance?

    _____

101. If severe symmetric IUGR is suspected, what test is often done before an intensive fetal surveillance program is initiated? _____

102. Fetal karyotyping can be obtained through what two procedures?

    a. _____

    b. _____

103. Why are fetal kick counts important?

    _____

    _____

104. What is the first test done to evaluate fetal well-being? _____

105. Define *reactivity*.

    _____

    _____

106. At how many weeks should an NST be reactive? _____

107. Name two tests that can be ordered if the NST is nonreactive.

    a. _____

    b. _____

108. Name two ways a CST can be performed.

    a. _____

    b. _____

109. Differentiate between a negative and a positive CST.

    Negative: _____

    _____

    Positive: _____

    _____

110. List four relative contraindications for performing a CST.

a. _____

b. _____

c. _____

d. _____

111. List the five elements of a BPP.

a. _____

b. _____

c. _____

d. _____

e. _____

112. Discuss how fetal breathing is evaluated.

_____

_____

113. How many fetal movements must be present for a score of 2? _____

114. Discuss how fetal tone is evaluated.

_____

_____

115. Discuss how amniotic fluid volume is evaluated.

_____

_____

116. In a BPP, a score of _____ or more is associated with a good pregnancy outcome.

117. Which parameter has been traditionally considered a chronic marker of fetal condition?

_____

118. _____ and _____ will be the first biophysical elements to be abolished on a BPP.

119. Doppler flow studies cannot differentiate between the IUGR and SGA fetus.

A. True

B. False

120. Doppler flow velocity waveforms are derived from movement of _____ within the vessel and reflect _____ in a given circulatory bed. Waveforms in the umbilical artery reflect resistance in the _____.

121. In the growth-restricted fetus, Doppler evaluation shows _____ diastolic umbilical artery flow. In some extreme cases, flow may be _____ or _____.

122. _____ are given to mature fetal lungs.

123. Low-dose daily aspirin therapy is indicated for the treatment of IUGR.

    A. True

    B. False

124. What is the decision to deliver a growth-restricted fetus based on?

    _____

    _____

125. The baby should be delivered if:

    a. _____

    b. _____

    c. _____

    d. _____

    e. _____

    f. _____

    g. _____

126. As the nurse caring for this woman, what are some of the nursing interventions you can do to improve fetal outcome?

    _____

    _____

    _____

    _____

    _____

    _____

127. State two reasons why amnioinfusion is used.

    a. _____

    b. _____

128. Most authorities believe that babies who experience IUGR because of placental insufficiency do not experience a "catch up" in growth.

    A. True

    B. False

129. The lower the birth weight and the earlier the gestational age, the less the chance a child has of catching up.

    A. True

    B. False

130. Studies are inconsistent with regard to neurodevelopmental delays experienced by the IUGR infant.

    A. True

    B. False

131. IUGR babies are more prone to developing hypertension, cardiovascular complications, and type 2 diabetes as adults.

    A. True

    B. False

PRACTICE/REVIEW ANSWER KEY

1. 10th

2. B

3. IUGR is the pathologic counterpart for SGA. With IUGR, the fetus has not reached its growth potential because of one or more causative factors. They are at increased risk of poor outcomes. SGA babies are small but have reached their growth potential. They are not at risk for poor outcomes.

4. a. The definition is based on the size of the fetus not its growth potential.
   b. Variations in birth weight for gestational age standards exist.

5. a. Altitude
   b. Race
   c. Fetal sex
   d. Maternal parity
   e. Maternal height
   f. Paternal height
   g. Socioeconomic status

6. B

7. Second, first

8. a. Intrauterine fetal death
   b. Oligohydramnios
   c. Intrapartum fetal hypoxia

9. 36, the onset of labor

10. Chronic; chronic stress placed on the fetus. Blood is redistributed from the kidneys to the brain. This shunting process decreases renal perfusion, thus decreasing urinary output.

11. 77; 85

12. Any three of the following:
    a. Late decelerations
    b. Absent variability
    c. Decreased variability
    d. Bradycardia

13. a. Meconium aspiration
    b. Hypoglycemia
    c. Polycythemia
    d. Hyperbilirubinemia
    e. Hypothermia

14. With fetal hypoxia, there is a reflex relaxation of the anal sphincter and an increase in intestinal movement. This combination causes fetal release of meconium.

15. 34

16. a. Amnioinfusion
    b. Resuscitative techniques at delivery

17. a. Notifying appropriate personnel to attend delivery
    b. Having functioning resuscitative equipment at the bedside

18. 40; 25; inadequate glycogen stores in the liver and muscle

19. Any six of the following:
    a. Jitteriness
    b. Tremors
    c. Weak cry
    d. Lethargy
    e. Floppy posture
    f. Hypothermia
    g. Poor feeder
    h. Seizures (occasionally)

20. Early oral feedings (either breast, bottle, or a dextrose solution); IV feedings may be needed until the infant is able to suck vigorously enough to have sufficient feedings.

21. A hemoglobin greater than 22 g/dL or a hematocrit greater than 65%

22. a. The fetus attempts to compensate for hypoxia by increasing its RBC production.
    b. With asphyxia, there is an increase in blood volume from the placental circulation to the fetal circulation.

23. Hyperbilirubinemia

24. There is decreased brown fat in an IUGR infant. Brown fat is needed for heat production.

25. a. Tachypnea
    b. Tachycardia

26. External heat source

27. B

28. With an SGA baby, there is symmetric development of the head and abdomen. There is adequate subcutaneous fat, normal muscle mass, and a normal cord.

29. B

30. Loose; dry; thin

31. B

32. B

33. A

34. Greater than

35. a. Cellular hyperplasia (first 16 weeks of gestation); increase in the cell number
    b. Cellular hyperplasia and hypertrophy (midgestation); increase in cell number and size
    c. Cellular hypertrophy (after 32 weeks of gestation); increase in cell size

36. a. Genetic factors
    b. Substrates
    c. Adequate vascular support

37. B

38. a. Oxygen
    b. Glucose
    c. Amino acids

39. Energy; amino acids

40. 80

41. To transport the substrates

42. Maternal; fetal; placental

43. a. Maternal prepregnancy weight
    b. Weight gain during pregnancy

44. 10; 22

45. Less than 16 years of age; older than 35 years of age

46. a. Cigarette smoking
    b. Alcohol consumption
    c. Illicit drug use
    d. Medications

47. 30; 40

48. B

49. B

50. A

51. Fetal alcohol syndrome; IUGR

52. A

53. 30

54. a. Anticonvulsants (trimethadione, phenytoin)
    b. Folic acid antagonists (methotrexate)
    c. Warfarin

55. B

56. Any six of the following:
    a. Asthma
    b. Cystic fibrosis
    c. Cyanotic heart disease
    d. Preeclampsia
    e. Chronic hypertension
    f. Diabetes
    g. Lupus
    h. Sickle cell disease

57. Chronic hypertension

58. 15; 20

59. a. Chromosome abnormalities
    b. Structural anomalies
    c. Multifetal gestation
    d. Premature infants
    e. Intrauterine infections

60. Decrease in placental mass in relation to fetal mass; abnormal placentation; twin-to-twin transfusion

61. 15% to 25%

62. A

63. Three

64. a. Toxoplasmosis
    b. Rubella
    c. Cytomegalovirus
    d. Herpes simplex

65. B

66. The placenta is the source of nutrition and respiratory support necessary to sustain fetal life.

67. Any four of the following:
    a. Placenta previa
    b. Circumvallate placenta
    c. Partial placenta abruption
    d. Placenta accreta
    e. Placental infarctions
    f. Multiple gestation

68. B

69. a. Symmetric
    b. Asymmetric

70. The relationship between the size of the fetal head and the size of the abdomen

71. Blood is shifted from the less vital organs (i.e., liver, muscle, and fat) to the brain.

72. A. S
    B. A
    C. A
    D. S
    E. A
    F. S

73. Precise dating of the pregnancy

74. a. Identification of maternal risk factors and clinical assessment of uterine size
    b. Ultrasonic assessment

75. B

76. a. Medical history
    b. Obstetric history
    c. Medication use
    d. Recent infections or exposures
    e. Social/environmental history
    f. Present pregnancy history

77. Any three of the following:
    a. History of chromosomal/congenital defects
    b. Prior IUGR infant
    c. Prior stillborn after 20 weeks' gestation
    d. Three or more consecutive spontaneous abortions

78. Any three of the following:
    a. Prepregnant weight
    b. Cigarette smoking
    c. Alcohol consumption
    d. Illicit drug use

79. a. Placenta previa
    b. Preeclampsia
    c. Multiple gestation
    d. Elevated maternal serum α-fetoprotein

80. a. Low maternal weight gain
    b. Leopold maneuvers
    c. Fundal height

81. Fundal height

82. Measure from the uppermost border of the symphysis pubis to the uppermost border of the fundus in the center of the abdomen.

83. a. Lagging by more than 3 cm
    b. Increasing in disparity

84. Ultrasound

85. Any five of the following:
    a. To determine gestational age
    b. To identify fetal anomalies
    c. To calculate amniotic fluid volume
    d. To grade the placenta
    e. To estimate fetal weight
    f. To determine adequate fetal growth
    g. To assess fetal well-being

86. 8 to 13 weeks

87. 18 to 20 weeks

88. A

89. Fetal growth is a dynamic process and requires more than one ultrasound. This enables comparison of growth and decreases error.

90. 2 to 4 weeks

91. 1. b
    2. c
    3. a
    4. d
    5. f
    6. d
    7. a
    8. a
    9. d
    10. d
    11. e

92. Estimated fetal weight (EFW)

93. Oligohydramnios

94. a. The two perpendicular plane method—Measure the largest pocket of fluid in two perpendicular planes. If at least one pocket measuring at least 2 cm is identified, the volume is normal. If a 1- to 2-cm pocket is seen, it is considered marginal. If less than a 1-cm pocket is noted, it is considered decreased.
    b. The four-quadrant method—Measure the largest pool of fluid in each of four quadrants in the uterus. Add theses numbers to get the amniotic fluid index. If the total is less than 10, it is considered decreased. If the total is less than 5, it is identified as significantly decreased.

95. B

96. a. Eliminate contributing factors.
    b. Increase uterine blood flow and improve fetal oxygenation
    c. Perform fetal surveillance testing
    d. Include treatment therapies
    e. Deliver at appropriate time and place

97. a. Underweight: 28 to 40 pounds
    b. Normal weight: 25 to 35 pounds
    c. Overweight: 15 to 25 pounds
    d. Carrying twins: 35 to 45 pounds

98. B

99. a. To improve uteroplacental perfusion
    b. To increase amniotic fluid volume

100. To prevent fetal death

101. Fetal karyotype

102. a. Cordocentesis
     b. Amniocentesis

103. A decrease in maternal perception of fetal movement often, but not invariably, precedes fetal death.

104. Nonstress test

105. In a 20-minute period, there must be at least two fetal heart rate accelerations of at least 15 beats per minute above the normal baseline lasting at least 15 seconds (from beginning to end).

106. 32

107. a. Contraction stress test
     b. Biophysical profile

108. a. Nipple stimulation
     b. IV oxytocin

109. *Negative:* No late or significant variable decelerations are noted.
     Positive: Late decelerations follow 50% or more of the contractions (even if the contraction frequency is less than three in 10 minutes).

110. a. Preterm labor (or those at risk for preterm labor)
     b. Premature rupture of membranes
     c. History of extensive uterine surgery or classical cesarean section
     d. Known placenta previa

111. a. Nonstress test
     b. Fetal breathing
     c. Fetal movement
     d. Fetal tone
     e. Qualitative amniotic fluid volume

112. To score a 2, there needs to be at least one or more episodes of rhythmic fetal breathing movements lasting 30 seconds or longer and occurring within 30 minutes.

113. Three

114. To score a 2, there needs to be one or more episode of extension of a fetal extremity with return to flexion, or opening or closing of a hand, within 30 minutes.

115. To score a 2, a single vertical pocket of amniotic fluid exceeding 2 cm must be measured.

116. 8

117. Oligohydramnios

118. Fetal heart rate reactivity; fetal breathing movements

119. B

120. RBCs; downstream resistance; placental circulation

121. Decreased; absent; reversed

122. Corticosteroids

123. B

124. The risks of prematurity versus a deteriorating intrauterine environment

125. a. 38 weeks' gestation
     b. Documented fetal lung maturity
     c. Positive CST
     d. Low BPP score
     e. "Severe" oligohydramnios
     f. Complete cessation of fetal growth
     g. Absent or reversed umbilical Doppler flow studies

126. Continuous electronic fetal monitoring, left lateral position, IV hydration, oxygen therapy, epidural for pain, availability of adequate personnel and functioning equipment at the delivery

127. a. Thick meconium
     b. Presence of variable decelerations

128. B

129. A

130. A

131. A

REFERENCES

1. Spellacy, W. N. (1999). Fetal growth retardation. In J. R. Scott, P. J. DiSaia, C. B. Hammond, & W. N. Spellacy (Eds.), *Danforth's obstetrics & gynecology* (pp. 279–285). Philadelphia: Lippincott Williams & Wilkins.

2. Lin, C., & Santolaya-Forgas, J. (1998). Current concepts of fetal growth restriction: Part I. Causes, classification, and pathophysiology. *Obstetrics & Gynecology, 92*(6), 1044–1052.

3. ACOG Practice Bulletin. (2000, January). *Intrauterine growth restriction* (Issue Number 12). Washington, DC: Author.

4. Vandenbosche, R. C., & Kirchner, J. T. (1998). Intrauterine growth retardation. *American Family Physician, 58*(6), 1384–1390.

5. Peleg, D., Kennedy, C. M., & Hunter, S. K. (1998) Intrauterine growth restriction: Identification and management. *American Family Physician, 58*(2), 453–460.

6. Perry, S. (2000). Nursing care of the high risk newborn. In D. L. Lowdermilk, S. E. Perry, & I. M. Bobak (Eds.), *Maternity and women's health care* (7th ed., pp. 1097–1133). St. Louis: Mosby.

7. Goldberg, R. L., & Dolan-Mullen, P. (2000, November). Convincing pregnant patients to stop smoking. *Contemporary OB/GYN, 45*(11), 35-44.

8. Blatt, S. D., Meguid, V., & Church, C. C. (2000, September). Prenatal cocaine: What's known about outcomes? *Contemporary OB/GYN, 45*(9), 67–81.

9. Henriksen, T. (1999). Foetal nutrition, foetal growth restriction and health later in life. *Acta Pediatrica Supplement, 429,* 4–8.

10. Platt, L. D. (1998, March). Assessment of gestational age. *Contemporary OB/GYN, 43*(3), 15–26.

11. Lin, C., & Santolaya-Forgas, J. (1999). Current concepts of fetal growth restriction: Part II. Diagnosis and management. *Obstetrics & Gynecology, 93*(1), 140–145.

12. ACOG Practice Bulletin. (1999, October). *Antepartum fetal surveillance* (Issue Number 9). Washington, DC: Author.

13. Fattal-Valevski, A., Leitner, Y., Kutai, M., Tal-Posener, D., Tomer, A., Lieberman, D., Jaffa, A., Many, A., & Harel, S. (1999). Neurodevelopmental outcome in children with intrauterine growth retardation: A 3-year follow-up. *Journal of Child Neurology, 14*(11), 724–727.

14. Zubrick, S. R., Kurinczuk, J. J., McDermott, B. M., McKelvey, R. S., Silburn, S. R., & Davies, L. C. (2000). Fetal growth and subsequent mental health problems in children aged 4 to 13 years. *Developmental Medicine and Child Neurology, 42,* 14–20.

SUGGESTED READINGS

ACOG Practice Bulletin. (2000, January). *Intrauterine growth restriction* (Issue Number 12). Washington, DC: Author.

Cunningham, F. G., MacDonald, P. C., Gant, N. F., Leveno, K. J., Gilstrap, L. C., Hankins, G. D., & Clark, S. L. (1997). Fetal growth restriction. In *Williams obstetrics* (20th ed., pp. 839–852). Norwalk, CT: Appleton & Lange.

Phillitieri, A. (1999). Nursing care of the high risk newborn and family. In *Maternal and child care nursing: Care of the childbearing and childrearing family* (3rd ed., pp. 696–741). Philadelphia: Lippincott Williams & Wilkins.

Woods, J. R., Jr. (1998). Substance abuse in pregnancy. *Obstetrics and Gynecology Clinics of North America, 25*(1), 1–268.

MODULE 11

Caring for the Laboring Woman With HIV Infection or AIDS

MARY COPELAND MYERS

As you complete this module, you will learn:

1. The current status of the HIV/AIDS epidemic
2. Recommendations by the U.S. Public Health Service for HIV screening of pregnant women
3. The pathogenic process of HIV
4. How to correctly diagnosis HIV infection
5. Risk factors for HIV infection
6. The current definition of *AIDS* and common opportunistic infections
7. How HIV infection is transmitted horizontally
8. The timing and mechanisms of vertical transmission
9. Methods to prevent vertical transmission
10. The impact of HIV infection on pregnancy
11. The impact of pregnancy on HIV infection
12. Recommendations for delivery of a newborn of an HIV-infected pregnant woman
13. Pharmacotherapeutic treatment recommendations for the HIV-infected pregnant woman
14. Diagnosis of HIV infection in the infant of an HIV-infected mother
15. How to use universal precautions recommended by the Centers for Disease Control and Prevention
16. Intrapartum and immediate postpartum management of the HIV-infected mother and newborn
17. Psychosocial issues related to the care of the HIV-infected mother
18. Ethical issues related to the care of the HIV-infected mother
19. Educative issues to discuss with the HIV-infected mother

When you have completed this module, you should be able to recall the meaning of the following terms. You should also be able to use the terms when consulting with other health professionals. The terms are defined in this module or in the glossary at the end of this book.

AIDS
antiretroviral therapy
AZT (or ZVD or Retrovir)
CD4+ T cell
confirmatory test
EIA (formerly called the ELISA)
HAART
HIV DNA PCR test
HIV-1
HIV-2

HIV RNA test (or viral load or RNA)
horizontal transmission
perinatal transmission
sensitivity
specificity
SUDS (Single Use Diagnostic System) HIV-1 test
vertical transmission
Western blot test

Epidemiology and Pathophysiology of HIV

■ What is known about the epidemiology of HIV?

The human immunodeficiency virus was first identified in the early 1980s; ever since, it has been the focus of worldwide medical, political, and research efforts. Unfortunately, today it is believed that all cases of AIDS will eventually result in the death of the infected person. Worldwide, based on estimates from the Joint United Nations Programme on HIV/AIDS (UNAIDS), as of December 2000, a total of 36.1 million people are living with HIV or AIDS. Of these, 16.4 million are women and 1.4 million are children (younger than 15 years of age). In the year 2000, 600,000 children were newly diagnosed with HIV infection.[1]

In the United States, through June 2000, the Centers for Disease Control and Prevention (CDC) reported a cumulative number of 753,907 AIDS cases, with 124,911 cases in females and 8,804 cases in children younger than 13.[2] African American and Hispanic women have been disproportionately affected by the epidemic. At the end of 1999, an estimated 8,000 perinatally acquired AIDS cases were reported, with an 84% incidence among Black and Hispanic children.[2]

From 1985 to 1995, approximately 6,000 to 7,000 HIV-infected women gave birth in the United States. The CDC estimates that each year (as of 1999), 300 to 400 babies will be born with HIV infection.[3] The dramatic decreases in the number of HIV infections in infants born to HIV-infected women is attributable mainly to the rapid implementation of zidovudine (ZDV) treatment according to the U.S. Public Health Service Guidelines for the Prevention of Perinatal HIV Transmission. This decline could be even more dramatic; however, all pregnant women are not offered HIV testing. Many pregnant women who are HIV positive are not diagnosed during their pregnancy. Therefore, they do not receive the appropriate treatment to reduce the risk of transmitting HIV to their babies.

Risk Factors for HIV Infection

As health care providers evaluate pregnant women, they must be aware of certain factors and behaviors that place women at risk for becoming HIV infected. Assessment is essential throughout pregnancy and on admission for delivery. *A complete history and assessment of risk factors must be accomplished.* It is essential to formulate a plan of care that will provide for the special needs of the woman, her infant, and the hospital staff.

Some of the factors that place women at risk for HIV infection include a history of the following:

- **Intravenous (IV) drug use**—One way HIV is transmitted is through blood. Because drug users often share syringes and needles without adequate cleaning, the virus can be transferred from one person to another in this manner.
- **Multiple sexual partners**—Having multiple sexual partners increases the risk of exposure to HIV.
- **Sex with partners who are infected or at risk for infection**—Partners at risk include people with hemophilia, bisexual men, IV drug users, and partners who have or have had multiple sexual partners.
- **Receiving a blood transfusion before blood was being screened *but after* HIV infection occurred in the United States (1978–1985)**—Before 1986, no tests were available to detect HIV in blood. Consequently, people who received blood during this period are at increased risk for HIV infection.
- **Multiple sexually transmitted diseases (STDs)**—Infection with multiple STDs is often associated with other risk factors such as multiple sexual partners, IV drug use, and high-risk partners.
- **Currently living in or born in communities or countries where there is a known or suspected high prevalence of HIV infection**—There is more opportunity for exposure to HIV.

■ What are the recommendations for HIV screening of pregnant women?

In 1995, after studies showed that treatment with ZDV decreased perinatal HIV transmission by 67.5%, the U.S. Public Health Service published guidelines recommending the following:

- Universal HIV counseling of all pregnant women
- Voluntary HIV testing of all pregnant women
- Voluntary treatment of pregnant women infected with HIV

Health care providers rapidly implemented these guidelines. Compared with the incidence in 1992, pediatric AIDS cases declined by 75% in 1998.[3] However, infants are still becoming infected. Review of the trends during the past years shows that many women are not tested for HIV during pregnancy. Reasons for not being tested include the following[3]:

- Lack of prenatal care (especially among women who use illicit drugs)
- Lack of strong recommendation by the health care provider
- Perception of low risk by the patient and the provider
- Provider perception of the difficulties and complexity of required counseling
- Misunderstanding of counseling requirements by providers
- Complex logistics of testing

Therefore, in October 2000, the U.S. Public Health Service published the following *revised* recommended guidelines for HIV screening of pregnant women in the United States[3]:

1. All pregnant women should be tested for HIV. This should be a routine part of prenatal care.
2. Written informed consent *should* be included to ensure that women have been informed about the procedure and of their right to refuse the test. If written informed consent is a barrier to testing, verbal consent with documentation is sufficient.
3. Although testing is recommended, it should be a *voluntary decision* by the pregnant woman. No testing should be done without the patient's knowledge. Women should be allowed to refuse testing.
4. Before HIV testing, the basic information should be provided in the form of a brochure, pamphlet, or video.
5. HIV testing for consenting women should be performed as early as possible, and retesting in the third trimester is recommended in women who are at high risk for acquiring HIV.
6. After consent is obtained, HIV status should be assessed immediately in women admitted for labor and delivery with an unknown status of HIV.
7. In accordance with the policies of the organization legally responsible for the infant, HIV testing is recommended for infants with unknown HIV status who are in foster care.
8. The mother should be informed that knowing her newborn's HIV infection status has benefits for the infant. She should be informed that a positive HIV antibody test for her newborn indicates that she has HIV.

Health care providers should be familiar with their state and local laws, regulations, and policies concerning HIV screening of pregnant women and infants. The revised guidelines also provide recommendations on HIV prevention, counseling and education, interpretation of HIV test results, recommendations for HIV-infected pregnant women, and recommendations for postpartum follow-up of HIV-infected women and perinatally exposed infants.[3]

■ Is the United States blood supply safe?

The U.S. blood supply is one of the safest in the world. As of March 1985, all donations were screened for HIV-1 antibodies. In addition, as of June 1992, all donations were screened for HIV-2 antibodies. An estimated 1 in 450,000 to 1 in 660,000 donations per year are infected with HIV but are not detected by the current antibody screening test. Therefore, in August of 1995, the U.S. Food and Drug Administration (FDA) recommended that all donated blood and plasma also be screened for HIV-1 p24 antigen. The HIV-1 p24 antigen test detects the HIV-1 antigen instead of antibodies. Because the antigen is present before the antibodies are formed in the course of infection (before seroconversion), the addition of this test allows for earlier detection of the virus by 6 to 12 days.[4]

Pathophysiology of HIV Infection

■ What is the human immunodeficiency virus?

The human immunodeficiency virus (HIV-1) is one of five known retroviruses. These viruses store genetic information in the form of RNA. The five known retroviruses are as follows[5]:

1. Human T-cell lymphotrophic virus (HTLV)-I   Causes adult T-cell leukemia/lymphoma

2. HTLV-II   Causes hairy cell leukemia
3. HTLV-III   Causes HIV-1 (previously called human
                  T-cell lymphotrophic virus type III)
4. HTLV-IV   Causes HIV-2
5. HTLV-V   Causes cutaneous T-cell
                  lymphoma/leukemia

> In the United States, and in most of the world, HIV infection is usually caused by HIV-1. HIV-2 infection is predominantly found in West Africa.

> HIV-1 was discovered in 1984.
> HIV-2 was discovered in 1986.

Because of the extremely high replication rate of the HIV, there is substantial genetic variation of HIV. Within HIV-1, the two major groups are group M and group O. HIV-1 group M consists of nine subtypes, which are subtypes A though I.[6]

Findings reported at the Sixth Conference on Retroviruses and Opportunistic Infections in 1999 indicate that HIV-1 originated in nonhuman primates, that is, chimpanzees. The establishment of HIV-1 in humans is likely to have resulted from the cross-species transmission. The origin of HIV-2 has been identified with the sooty mangabey, another monkey species.[7]

> Both HIV-1 and HIV-2 have the same modes of transmission, cause similar opportunistic infections, and cause AIDS.

HIV-2 seems to develop more slowly. It is milder and is less infectious early in the course of infection. As disease advances, the duration of increased infectiousness is shorter. HIV-2 infection in children is rare. When compared with HIV-1, it seems to be less transmissible from mother to child. ZVD treatment is recommended for HIV-2–infected pregnant women. Because epidemiologic data indicate that the prevalence of HIV-2 is very low in the United States, *the CDC does not recommend routine HIV-2 testing at HIV counseling and test sites or in settings other than blood centers.*[8]

The Pathogenic Processes in HIV Infection

HIV has a great affinity for a protein complex called CD4, which is an antigen on the surface of certain cells.

The following cells have extremely high levels of CD4 surface antigen[9]:

Lymphocytes (especially CD4+ T cells)
Monocytes
Neural cells

> Cells with a high surface density of CD4 are most at risk for invasion.

The following cells also have high levels of CD4 surface antigen[9]:

- Macrophages
- Langerhans' cells
- Endothelial cells
- Cells of the placenta

The large number of cell types affected by the virus explains the wide range of organs/systems affected by HIV infection.

Infection occurs when the human immunodeficiency virus envelope glycoprotein attaches itself to the CD4 receptors on the cellular membrane of its target cell. The virus then enters the cell. Because the virus carries only RNA, it must invade the nucleus, accessing DNA of a host cell, to replicate. The following outlines the process of HIV replication.

1. After entering the host cell, the virus uses an enzyme called reverse transcriptase to convert its RNA to DNA. This process is called *reverse transcription.*

2. The new viral DNA is incorporated into the host cell's chromosomal DNA, where it forms a provirus.
3. Transcription of the viral DNA begins and results in multiple copies of viral RNA. This RNA codes for the production of viral proteins and enzymes.
4. Viral RNA and proteins are packaged as budding viruses. They are released from the host lymphocyte surface. They can now invade other host cells.

New viral particles that leave the infected cell destroy part of the host cell's outer membrane. As a consequence of this viral replication, the host cell dies. **Declining numbers of CD4+ T cells result in the progressive decline of the individual's immune response.** Replication of HIV in macrophages can occur *without cellular destruction.*[10] Because macrophages are widely distributed throughout the body, they may play a critical role in the persistence of HIV infection because they provide reservoirs for chronically infected cells. *Viral replication is active throughout the course of the infection, and replication proceeds at a faster rate than what was predicted before the more sensitive tests were developed to detect viral loads.* Ongoing HIV replication in an active but incompletely effective immune system is probably responsible for secondary manifestations of HIV disease such as wasting and dementia.[11]

The impact of HIV infection is related to its effect on the normal function of the CD4+ T cells. These cells play an essential role in orchestrating the body's immune responses. When CD4+ T cells decline from cellular death or injury, the person becomes more susceptible to opportunistic infections. Progression of HIV infection varies among individuals.

- The average time of progression from the initial infection to AIDS, without antiretroviral therapy or with monotherapy, is approximately 10 to 11 years.
- Approximately 20% of individuals will develop AIDS within 5 years.
- Less than 5% have sustained long-term asymptomatic HIV infection without a decline in CD4+ T-cell counts to less than 500 cell/mm^3.[12,13]

This great variation in disease development depends on several factors, including the following:

- Health of the immune system
- Virulence of the HIV strain
- Viral concentration
- Mode of transmission

With disease advancement, there is increased susceptibility to infection and increased incidence of neoplasms, particularly Kaposi's sarcoma, B-cell lymphoma, non-Hodgkin's lymphoma, and some carcinomas.

Diagnosis of HIV Infection and AIDS

■ How is the diagnosis of HIV infection made?

The standard algorithm (step-by-step procedure) for HIV testing consists of the following:

1. An initial screening with a sensitive FDA-licensed enzyme immunosorbent assay (EIA), *followed by*
2. Confirmation with the specific FDA-licensed Western blot test

The initial test to screen for HIV antibody status in the adult is the EIA. The EIA detects antibodies produced in response to HIV. The HIV infection causes a reaction in the EIA; therefore, a positive result is called *reactive.* The EIA is sensitive in that it identifies almost all blood containing antibodies to HIV (true-positive test), but the EIA is not specific. It sometimes produces false-positive results.

False-positive results with the EIA can be caused by the following conditions[14]:

- Contamination in the laboratory
- Multiple pregnancies
- Hemophilia
- Alcoholism with hepatitis

• Cross-reactivity with other retroviruses
• History of injected drug use

• Hemodialysis

> A **false-positive test** is a positive reading on a blood specimen that *does not* contain antibodies to HIV (the patient does *not* have HIV).

> A **false-negative test** is a negative reading on a blood specimen that *does* contain HIV (the patient does have HIV).

False-negative results are rare with the EIA. False-negative results can occur in the early stage of HIV infection or in the late stage of HIV infection. In early infection, there is an interval in which the test can be negative because the patient has not yet produced antibodies against HIV.

> The average time to develop detectable antibodies is 25 days.[15] At the point in time when antibodies are detectable by testing, it is said that **seroconversion** has occurred.

Although an initial EIA may be reactive, it should not be considered a positive test until another EIA is repeated on the same blood sample. If the two tests are reactive, the test is reported as repeatedly reactive and the results are confirmed using a second, more specific antibody test called the *Western blot*. The Western blot is not used as the initial screening test because it is expensive and time-consuming. The Western blot is an immunoelectrophoresis procedure that identifies antibodies to nine specific viral proteins. Western blot test results are reported as unequivocal positive or indeterminate.

- An *unequivocal positive result* means that HIV antibody–positive serum reacts with all nine viral antigens. This means the patient is infected with HIV.
- An *indeterminate result* means that there are not enough detectable antibodies to the viral antigens. Retesting in 1 month is recommended.[16]
- If the test results are indeterminate, the test can mean that either it is too early to detect HIV antibodies or the blood has produced something to cause a test reaction.
- When the test remains indeterminate for 6 months or longer, it is called a *stable indeterminate*. If the results remain stable indeterminate for 6 months or longer, the patient is considered uninfected *unless* clinical conditions of HIV infection are present.

> When used together, the EIA and Western blot are greater than 99% accurate.[17]

■ What other tests are available to diagnose HIV?

In addition to blood test for the diagnosis of HIV, the FDA has also approved tests that detect HIV antibodies using oral fluids and urine. These tests were developed because many patients are more willing to have these tests, which are less invasive compared with the blood test.

The *immunofluorescent antibody (IFA) test* can be used to confirm the results if an EIA is repeatedly reactive and an indeterminate Western blot is obtained. The IFA is highly sensitive and specific. Although the IFA is less likely than the Western blot to yield indeterminate results, it is rarely used because it is difficult to perform.

Additional tests that are less commonly used to identify HIV infection include the following:

- HIV-1 p24 antigen assays
- Viral load assays
- Viral culture
- Polymerase chain reaction (PCR)

These tests are used most often to clarify an indeterminate Western blot, to monitor therapeutic intervention, to monitor disease progression, and to identify the infected neonate or infant.[3,16]

The *SUDS (Single Use Diagnostic System) HIV-1 test* is the only rapid HIV test that is licensed by the FDA for use in the United States. This rapid HIV test is easier to perform when compared with the EIA. The sensitivity and specificity are equal to those of the EIA. Although the SUDS test costs more than the EIA, research indicates that rapid HIV testing is more cost-effective than the current EIA/Western blot testing. The rapid test can usually be performed in 5 to 30 minutes, as opposed to several days with the EIA. Patients learn their results at the initial visit. Because it does not require a second visit to obtain the results, patient compliance is better.[14,16] As with the EIA, a negative test does not require a confirmation, yet a positive or reactive test does require a confirmation with the Western blot or IFA.

■ Can HIV be accurately diagnosed during pregnancy?

HIV infection during pregnancy can usually be diagnosed using the standard algorithm consisting of the EIA and Western blot. Before the development of more sensitive HIV antibody test, the estimated time between exposure and HIV antibody seroconversion was 2.4 months. Now, with more sensitive tests, detection of HIV antibody is approximately 20 days earlier.[16]

Individuals at risk for HIV infection should have repeated testing at appropriate intervals. Rarely, HIV detection can take up to 6 months. The period between actual infection with HIV until the time when enough antibodies are produced by the body to cause a positive HIV test result is called the *latency period*. Because of this period, the CDC recommends testing for HIV at 6 months after the possible exposure.[4]

Because some common complaints and problems associated with pregnancy are similar to those seen in the initial phase of HIV infection, accurate differential diagnosis can be difficult and thus delayed. Problems common to both early HIV infection and pregnancy are fatigue, malaise, anemia, and dyspnea. If an individual has a recent history of known or possible exposure to HIV and has a negative HIV-1 test, a false-negative result should be considered. Additional testing should be performed, including testing for HIV-2 and HIV-1 group O infections.

■ What is AIDS?

AIDS is the result of advanced HIV infection. Recent studies have suggested that all HIV-positive individuals will *eventually* develop AIDS. At present, AIDS is considered a lethal disease. In January 1993, the CDC expanded the AIDS surveillance case definition to include (a) laboratory evidence of infection, (b) laboratory evidence of severe immunosuppression, and/or (c) one or more of the 26 identified clinical conditions for AIDS.[19] Display 11.1 presents an outline of the most current CDC diagnostic criteria (definition) for AIDS in adults and adolescents.

DISPLAY 11.1 Current Diagnostic Criteria for AIDS in Adults and Adolescents

Laboratory evidence of HIV infection

1. Repeatedly reactive EIA
2. Subsequent confirmatory Western blot or immunofluorescence assay

plus

Laboratory evidence of severe immunosuppression

1. Less than 200 CD4+ T lymphocytes
2. CD4+ T lymphocytes less than 14% of total lymphocytes

and/or

One or more of the following:

1. Candidiasis of the bronchi, trachea, or lungs
2. Candidiasis, esophageal
3. Recurrent pneumonia (bacterial, more than one episode)

4. Invasive cervical cancer (diagnosed by biopsy)
5. Coccidioidomycosis, disseminated or extrapulmonary
6. Cryptococcosis, extrapulmonary
7. Cryptosporidiosis, chronic intestinal (of at least 1 month's duration)
8. Cytomegalovirus disease (other than liver, spleen, or nodes)
9. Cytomegalovirus, retinitis (with loss of vision)
10. HIV encephalopathy
11. Herpes simplex: chronic ulcer(s) (of at least 1 month's duration); or bronchitis, pneumonitis, or esophagitis
12. Histoplasmosis, disseminated or extrapulmonary
13. Isosporiasis, chronic intestinal (of at least 1 month's duration)
14. Kaposi's sarcoma
15. Lymphoma, Burkitt's (or equivalent term)
16. Lymphoma, immunoblastic (or equivalent term)
17. Lymphoma, primary, of brain
18. *Mycobacterium avium-intracellulare* complex or *Mycobacterium kansasii,* disseminated or extrapulmonary
19. *Mycobacterium tuberculosis,* disseminated or extrapulmonary
20. *Mycobacterium,* other species or unidentified species, disseminated or extrapulmonary
21. *Pneumocystis carinii* pneumonia (PCP)
22. Progressive multifocal leukoencephalopathy
23. *Salmonella* septicemia, recurrent
24. Toxoplasmosis of the brain
25. Wasting syndrome due to HIV
26. Pulmonary tuberculosis

■ What are opportunistic infections?

Opportunistic infections are caused by organisms that a healthy immune system, under normal situations, could easily destroy on its own or manage to overcome with the assistance of medication. However, with HIV infection, the immune system is compromised. *An opportunistic infection can be deadly.* Some of the most common opportunistic infections that often occur early in HIV infection are the following:

- Thrush
- Shingles
- Herpes simplex
- Pneumococcal pneumonia
- Oral hairy leukoplakia
- Thrombocytopenic purpura

Opportunistic infections that occur late in the course of HIV infection are the following[20]:

- *Pneumocystis carinii* pneumonia (PCP)
- Kaposi's sarcoma
- Tuberculosis
- Toxoplasmosis
- Cryptococcosis
- Cryptosporidiosis

Methods of HIV Transmission

HIV can be transmitted through the following three routes:

1. Sexual contact
2. Exposure to infected blood or blood products
3. Perinatally from an infected mother to her baby

HIV has been isolated from the following:

- Blood
- Semen
- Vaginal secretions
- Saliva
- Tears
- Breast milk
- Cerebrospinal fluid
- Amniotic fluid
- Urine

However, evidence reveals that it is transmitted only by the following[21]:

- Blood
- Semen

- Vaginal secretions
- Breast milk
- Body fluids such as amniotic fluid and urine that contain visible blood

---

The two methods of transmission for HIV are:

1. Horizontal transmission
2. Vertical transmission

Horizontal Transmission of HIV

Horizontal transmission **means that the virus is transmitted from one person to another by direct contact.** Examples of such contact include the following:

- **Intimate sexual contact (oral, anal, or vaginal) with someone infected with the human immunodeficiency virus**—Studies demonstrate that the receptive partner in intercourse has a greater chance of acquiring HIV infection than does the insertive partner. Receptive rectal intercourse has an approximate risk of 0.1% to 3% per episode, whereas receptive vaginal intercourse has an approximate risk of 0.1% to 0.2% per episode. Insertive rectal intercourse has an approximate risk of 0.06% per episode, and insertive vaginal intercourse has an approximate risk of 0.1% per episode.[22,23] Other factors associated with an increased risk of HIV infection are exposure to blood, such as with genital ulcer disease, trauma during sex, and menstruation of the HIV-infected woman, and exposure to inflammation of the genital or rectal mucosa, which can occur with STDs.[24] Open-mouth kissing is considered very low risk; however, prolonged open-mouth kissing could damage the mouth or lips and allow HIV transmission through bloody saliva. Therefore, the CDC recommends against open-mouth kissing with an infected partner.[4]
- **Sharing of drug needles and syringes with an infected individual**—Sharing IV drug paraphernalia has an approximate risk of 0.67% per exposure.[25]
- **Receipt of a blood transfusion that contains HIV**—Risk from blood transfusions has been virtually eliminated through careful screening procedures now done on all donated blood and plasma.
- **Inadvertent contamination of mucous membranes or breaks in the skin (e.g., of a nurse or other health care provider) by the blood or body fluid of the infected person.** The overall risk for HIV infection after percutaneous exposure to HIV-infected blood is approximately 0.3% and is 0.09% after mucous membrane exposure.[26] The Public Health Service provides specific management guidelines for postexposure antiretroviral intervention. Every institution should use these guidelines.

Vertical Transmission of HIV

Vertical transmission of HIV occurs when the virus is passed from the mother to her infant during the perinatal period. Transmission can occur during the antepartum, intrapartum, or postpartum period. HIV has been isolated from many sources (early gestational embryo, blood, breast milk, amniotic fluid, cord blood, and the placenta), which indicates multiple potential routes of fetal or neonatal transmission. The virus has been isolated in 13- to-20-week-old fetuses, but **transmission is generally believed to occur most often in late pregnancy.**[27–29] In nonbreastfeeding populations, antepartum transmission accounts for 25% to 40% of infections, and intrapartum transmission accounts for 60% to 75% of HIV infections.[30] In breastfeeding populations, antepartum transmission accounts for 20% to 25% of infections, intrapartum transmission accounts for 60% to 70% of infections, and postpartum transmission accounts for 10% to 15% of infections.[31]

The HIV-1 vertical transmission rate *in the absence of antiretroviral use* is approximately 16% to 20% in large cohort studies in Europe and North America, 25% to 40% in Africa, and 19% to 24% in Thailand.[30] In the United States, the introduction of ZDV treatment of HIV (which decreases the risk of mother-to-infant transmission) has resulted in a dramatic decline in the risk of transmission. **Recent studies have reported transmission rates of 5% to 6% and as low as less than 2% among women with undetectable viral plasma loads.**[30]

Mechanisms of Vertical Transmission

Antepartum transmission most likely occurs through transplacental transmission of HIV. An example is when HIV is transmitted after placental disruption, as in placental abruption or during amniocentesis. *Intrapartum transmission* can occur through maternal–fetal transfusion of blood during labor and through contact of the infant with infected blood or other maternal secretions during delivery. *Postpartum transmission* can occur though breastfeeding because of prolonged exposure of the infant's oral and gastrointestinal tracts to infected breast milk. Most studies indicate that transmission by breastfeeding occurs during the early weeks of breastfeeding.[30]

Risk Factors for Vertical Transmission

The following are risk factors for vertical transmission:

- **Demographic and behavioral**—Maternal age, ethnicity, parity, and race are *not* associated with an increased risk for vertical transmission of HIV. However, some behavioral risk factors that increase the risk for vertical transmission are smoking, using illicit drugs, having multiple sexual partners and not using barrier protection, and breastfeeding.[3,30]
- **Clinical**—Clinical factors that have been related to the increased risk for transmission are maternal anemia, low maternal vitamin A levels among women in developing countries, severity of maternal HIV disease (high viral load and a low CD4+ count), presence of other STDs, and not receiving the ZDV chemoprophylaxis.[3,30]
- **Immunogenetics**—Researchers have examined the importance of immunogenetics in perinatal transmission. Two areas of research that are currently under study are human leukocyte antigens (HLAs) and the role of chemokine receptor 5 gene (CCR5). These factors have an effect on the transmission of HIV infection. Further investigation hopes to reveal how immunogenetics can play a role in medication and vaccine development.
- **Obstetric**—Obstetric factors that have been associated with an increased risk of HIV transmission include preterm delivery, delivery 4 hours after rupture of membranes, cervicovaginal infection, chorioamnionitis, presence of meconium, and use of invasive procedures (e.g., amniocentesis, fetal scalp electrodes, use of forceps, performance of episiotomy).[3,30]

Prevention of Perinatal HIV Transmission

Perinatal HIV transmission can be reduced by the following methods:

- Reducing the viral load
- Reducing the exposure of the fetus to HIV during delivery
- Reducing the risk to the fetus if exposed to HIV
- Reducing exposure to HIV infection during the postpartum period

Reducing the Viral Load

The *viral load* (also called the HIV-RNA test) is a measurement of the magnitude of active HIV replication. The viral load assesses the relative risk for disease progression and assesses the efficacy of antiretroviral therapies. The *CD4+ T-cell count* is an indicator of the extent of immune system damage. The CD4+ T-cell count assesses the risk of developing specific opportunistic infections and other sequelae of HIV infection. *When the viral load and the CD4+ T-cell count are used together, the risk for disease progression and death can be predicted.*

As in the nonpregnant patient, the viral load should be monitored every 3 months in pregnant women.

The viral load correlates with the risk of perinatal transmission.

At a viral load of less than 1,000 copies per milliliter, the incidence of vertical transmission was about 2%.[34-36] However, *perinatal transmission has occurred in women with viral loads below the level of detection.* This indicates that other factors must play a role in the transmission.[37-39]

Current therapeutic intervention goals are as follows[40]:

1. Early initiation of an aggressive combination of antiretroviral regimens to maximally suppress viral replication
2. Preservation of immune function
3. Reduction in the development of resistance to drug therapy

Potent antiretroviral drugs (which can inhibit the protease enzyme of HIV-1) used in combination with nucleoside analog reverse transcriptase inhibitors can reduce viral loads to undetectable levels for prolonged periods. **The current recommended standard treatment for HIV-1–infected women who are *not* pregnant is a combination of two nucleoside analog reverse transcriptase inhibitors and one protease inhibitor.** *Although pregnancy should not preclude the use of this standard, considerations must be made for potential dosing changes due to the physiologic changes of pregnancy and for potential short- and long-term effects of drugs on the fetus and newborn.*[39]

Reducing Exposure of the Fetus to HIV During Delivery

Because not all babies born to HIV-positive mothers are infected with HIV, care must be taken to protect and prevent further exposure of these babies to the virus. Avoiding procedures that represent an increased risk for infection is an important element in reducing the risk. Procedures that increase the risk of HIV infection to the infant include invasive procedures and extended exposure to potentially infected body fluids. Invasive procedures include the following:

- **Internal fetal heart monitoring**—The electrode pierces the scalp of the fetus and permits exposure to bloody maternal amniotic fluid. As a result, the risk of contracting HIV is greatly increased.
- **Fetal pH scalp sampling**—Fetal scalp sampling involves breaks in the skin surface of the fetus. It can increase the potential for inoculation with HIV. Unless an urgent medical reason exists for performing this procedure, it is not recommended in the HIV-infected patient.
- **Eye prophylaxis, the giving of injections, or drawing of blood from the newborn before removal of maternal body fluids and blood**—Before these procedures are done, the newborn must be bathed with soap and water. Alcohol should be used afterward to prepare the injection site. The alcohol should be allowed to dry completely before the puncture is made to prevent possible skin contamination and body fluids from being transmitted into the tissues.
- **Cutting the cord with contaminated instruments**—Use sterile instruments to cut and clamp the cord after delivery. This reduces the risk of cross-contamination from instruments that have been in contact with maternal tissues and body fluids. After cutting the cord, apply an antimicrobial agent to the cord.

Newborns can also be infected during the birth process by exposure to the mother's infected body fluids. The following guidelines should be used to reduce the length of neonatal exposure to these fluids.

- Avoid cutting an episiotomy.
- Avoid using forceps or vacuum extraction.
- Dry the infant immediately after the delivery to remove all maternal blood and amniotic fluid.
- Gently remove excess fluid and blood from the nares and oropharynx with a bulb syringe, mucus extractor, or meconium aspirator with wall suction set on the low setting. Because of the operator's risk of exposure to body fluids, do not use a suction device that requires the operator to provide suction by placing one end of the device in his or her mouth.
- Bathe the newborn under a radiant warmer as soon as the newborn is stable. Thorough cleansing with a mild nonmedicated soap removes amniotic fluid and blood from the body surface, which is essential in reducing the chance of infection.

- Thoroughly clean the eye area before applying antibiotic prophylaxis. Failure to remove the maternal fluids from the ocular area before prophylaxis placement can result in exposure of the mucous membranes to the virus.
- Instruct the mother to avoid breastfeeding.
- Perform cesarean delivery for women with a high viral load. Pregnant women with HIV should be counseled with the following information:
  - Without ZDV therapy, the risk of vertical transmission is approximately 25%.
  - With ZDV therapy, the risk is reduced to 5% to 8%.
  - With both ZDV therapy and a scheduled cesarean delivery (delivery before the onset of labor and before rupture of membranes), the risk is approximately 2%.
  - With a viral load of less than 1,000 copies per milliliter, a vaginal delivery has a risk of 2% or less.
  - If a cesarean delivery is planned, delivery is recommended at 38 completed weeks of gestation. For women receiving ZDV therapy, adequate levels of the drug in the blood should be obtained *by starting the IV infusion 3 hours preoperatively.* Because morbidity is increased, prophylactic antibiotics should be considered. The risk of maternal morbidity associated with cesarean delivery should also be discussed with the woman. Her decision regarding the method of delivery should be respected.[41]

Reducing Risk of Infection If Exposed to HIV

In some cases, antiretroviral therapy given during or after an infant's exposure to HIV during labor and delivery blocks infection. For example, if HIV-infected women are treated only with ZDV within 24 hours of birth, only 9% of infants are infected, as opposed to 25% of infants who are infected if no treatment is given.[42] In Africa, the effectiveness of neonatal antiretroviral prophylaxis in infants who received either ZDV-3TC or nevirapine during labor and delivery and during the first week of life was demonstrated.[30,43]

Reducing Exposure to HIV During the Postpartum Period

Infants are at risk for HIV infection if they are breastfed by HIV-infected mothers. Most infection from breastfeeding occurs during the first few weeks to the first few months of life.[44,45] **In the United States, where safe alternative sources of nutrition are available, breastfeeding is contraindicated in mothers with HIV infection.**[46,47]

A worldwide policy statement was issued in May 1997 by UNAIDS and cosponsored by the World Health Organization (WHO) and the United Nations Children's Fund (UNICEF). The guidelines state the following[48]:

- HIV infection can be transmitted though breastfeeding.
- Appropriate and affordable alternatives to breastfeeding should be available to HIV-infected women.
- HIV-positive women should be assisted in making fully informed decisions about the best way to feed their infants. This includes weighing the risk of (a) illness/death from infectious diseases and (b) the availability of safe alternatives to breastfeeding to reduce the risk of HIV transmission through breastfeeding.
- Women need to know and accept their HIV status.
- More voluntary and confidential counseling and testing needs to be available to women and their partners.
- Primary prevention of HIV infection is an essential priority for all adults of reproductive age and young people.

To counter the negative effects of the introduction of breast milk substitutes in developing countries, the International Code of Marketing of Breastmilk Substitutes was developed by WHO in 1981.[48,49]

Management of the HIV-Infected Pregnant Woman

■ What is the effect of pregnancy on HIV infection?

Even though pregnancy is accompanied by a mildly immunosuppressive state, **no conclusive evidence exists that pregnancy aggravates the health of the expectant woman who has**

early HIV infection.[50] During pregnancy, a decline in absolute CD4 cell counts is seen in both HIV-positive and HIV-negative women. It is thought to be secondary to hemodilution of pregnancy. Therefore, the use of a percentage of CD4 cells, rather than an absolute number of CD4 cells, is the most accurate method to measure immune function.[51] Pregnancy does not accelerate a decline in CD4 cells, and HIV RNA levels remain relatively stable during pregnancy.[52,53]

■ What is the effect of HIV infection on pregnancy?

HIV-infected women often have multiple coexisting problems that negatively affect pregnancy, including STDs, malnutrition, poverty, substance abuse, domestic violence, and inadequate or no prenatal care. These problems are often difficult to separate from problems stemming from the HIV infection.

Older studies that investigated the effects of early HIV infection on pregnancy suggested an increased risk for poor pregnancy outcomes, such as low birth weight and premature rupture of membranes. These studies were flawed because they did not take into account the impact of other coexisting problems on pregnancy outcome. Even today, it is difficult to evaluate the effect of many potential confounding factors such as IV drug use, STDs, lack of prenatal care, smoking, and maternal malnutrition. Also, adverse pregnancy outcomes may occur not only because of secondary disease processes but also because of antiretroviral therapy side effects and complications.

In regard to fertility, with HIV, the incidence of pregnancy is decreased by 12 per 100 persons.[54] The United States and underdeveloped countries have reported fetal loss associated with HIV infection. In West Africa, higher rates of both spontaneous abortion and stillbirths are found in women infected with HIV-1 or HIV-2.[55]

Many studies have revealed no increased risk of adverse outcome of asymptomatic or mildly symptomatic HIV-infected women. Reports regarding infant outcomes in underdeveloped countries indicate reduced birth weight for infants exposed to or infected with HIV-1. In the United States, mean birth weight was reported as 0.28 kg lighter and length was 1.64 cm shorter in HIV-infected infants. However, two confounding factors were maternal drug use and limited maternal antiretroviral therapy.[56]

Contradicting data exist on the impact of HIV infection on preterm delivery. Industrialized nations report an incidence of preterm labor as 5%; however, underdeveloped nations report an incidence of preterm labor as high as 26%. Moreover, underdeveloped nations also have been shown to have an increase in infant mortality among HIV-infected women. However, many coexisting medical problems contribute to the mortality.[57] HIV infection may predispose pregnant women to a variety of poor outcomes, such as preterm labor, prematurity, low-birth-weight infants, and postpartum endometritis. However, these poor obstetric outcomes occur mostly in women who are severely immunocompromised.[58]

In addition, some common infections often seen in HIV-negative women are more prevalent and often more severe in HIV-positive pregnant women. These infections include the following:

- Genital herpes simplex
- Human papillomavirus
- Syphilis
- Cytomegalovirus
- Hepatitis B
- Hepatitis A
- Vulvovaginal candidiasis

In conclusion, the effect of HIV infection on pregnancy is difficult to measure because of many confounding factors. The risk varies depending on the following factors:

- Population location (developed or underdeveloped countries)
- Clinical stage of HIV
- Availability of antiretroviral treatment
- Availability of obstetric care

Assessment and Monitoring of HIV-Infected Pregnant Women and Their Infants

Along with an initial social, emotional, and nutritional assessment, the initial medical assessment of the HIV-infected woman should include the following:

- CD4+ T-cell count to evaluate the degree of existing immunodeficiency
- Viral load to evaluate the risk for disease progression
- History of prior and current antiretroviral medications

The decision to initiate therapy or alternative therapy should be the same for women who are not receiving antiretroviral therapy and who are not pregnant. The discussion should include the following:

- Potential impact of therapy on the baby
- Ability to adhere to the prescribed regimen
- Long-term treatment plans for the mother

The final decision regarding treatment is the responsibility of the woman. The decisions regarding the use and choice of drugs are becoming increasingly complicated.

> The standard of care is the simultaneous use of multiple antiretroviral drugs to suppress the viral load below detectable limits.

Although the standard of care is the simultaneous use of multiple antiretroviral drugs to suppress the viral load below detectable limits, a decision by the woman (a) to refuse treatment of ZDV, (b) to only use ZDV, or (c) to refuse other antiretroviral drugs should not result in denial of care or punitive action.

The initial medical assessment should also include a review of the current status of vaccinations. *Immunizations should be given as early as possible in the course of HIV infection because the ability to form specific antibodies after immunizations becomes progressively impaired as the disease advances. (Remember that immune system function declines as the disease advances.)* Live pathogen vaccines, such as the MMR (measles-mumps-rubella), are contraindicated, but killed or inactivated vaccines are considered safe.

Recommended vaccines include the following[59]:

- Pneumococcal vaccine
- Hepatitis B immunization series (in the presence of a negative screen)

Vaccines to consider are as follows[59]:

- Influenza vaccine
- *Haemophilus influenzae* type B (Hib) vaccine
- Tetanus-diphtheria vaccine
- Hepatitis A vaccine
- Polio vaccine

In addition to the aforementioned assessments and a physical examination, the following laboratory data should be evaluated:

- All routine prenatal laboratory tests, including blood type and Rh, antibody screen, rubella, urine culture, gonorrhea/chlamydia screening, Pap smear, syphilis serology, and hemoglobin electrophoresis (as indicated)
- Complete blood count (CBC) every 3 months
- Hepatitis serology to screen for vaccine candidates
- Serum chemistry panel to screen for adverse effects of some drug therapies
- Purified protein derivative (PPD) skin test for tuberculosis
- Cytomegalovirus IgG
- Toxoplasmosis IgG if with a low CD4 count
- Maternal serum α-fetoprotein if patient desires
- Glucose challenge test at 24 to 28 weeks (Remember that protease inhibitors are diabetogenic, so repeat if indicated.)
- Group B streptococcal culture

During pregnancy, **continued monitoring should include measurement of CD4+ T-cell counts and an HIV-RNA test approximately every 3 months** to determine whether:

- Antiretroviral therapy is needed
- Current therapy needs to be altered
- Prophylaxis against *Pneumocystis carinii* pneumonia should be started

Although ZDV is not associated with an increased risk for fetal complications, less is known about the effect of combination antiretroviral therapy on the fetus. **More intensive fetal surveillance is recommended with the use of combination antiretroviral therapy,** including the following[39]:

- Assessment of fetal anatomy with a level II ultrasound
- Assessment of fetal growth
- Assessment of fetal well-being during the third trimester, with fetal kick counts, nonstress tests, or biophysical profiles

For the postpartum woman, comprehensive care and support services are required to optimize the woman's own medical care and to provide proper family planning assistance. Services must be coordinated between the obstetrician and the HIV specialist. It must be determined whether continuing antiretroviral treatment is required for the woman's health. If continuing antiretroviral treatment is best for the woman, compliance with drug therapy is essential.

The following guidelines should be used for initial assessment and for follow-up monitoring of newborns of HIV-infected women[39]:

- A baseline CBC and differential should be determined before the initial administration of ZDV.
- Hemoglobin measurements are required (at a minimum) after the completion of the 6-week ZDV regimen and again at 12 weeks of age. *ZDV can cause anemia complications in the newborn.*
- Newborns who are anemic at birth or who are born premature need more intensive hemoglobin monitoring.
- If the infant's mother used combination antiretroviral therapy, more intensive monitoring of hematologic and serum chemistry values are advised.
- To prevent *P. carinii* pneumonia, all infants should begin prophylaxis at 6 weeks of age after the completion of ZDV therapy.
- Infants with negative virologic tests during the first 6 weeks of life should have the evaluation repeated after the completion of neonatal antiretroviral prophylaxis therapy. The effect of combination therapy on the sensitivity of infant virologic diagnostic testing is not known.[39]

Pharmacotherapeutic Treatment for HIV Infection

> **In 1994, during the PACTG 076 study, the use of zidovudine (ZDV, Retrovir, AZT) therapy in pregnant women who were HIV positive resulted in a 67.5% reduction in the risk of HIV perinatal transmission. The estimated risk of perinatal transmission without ZDV therapy was 25.5% compared with an 8.3% risk of transmission with ZDV therapy.[60]**

ZDV is an antiretroviral drug that attacks the HIV virus. It is a nucleoside analog whose action inhibits viral replication in the cells by incorporating itself into the replicating RNA of the virus and causing an interruption of viral replication. Since 1994, major advances in the understanding of the pathogenesis of HIV-1 infection, the treatment, and monitoring of the disease have been made. Given that the mean half-life of plasma virions (a complete virus particle) is estimated at only 6 hours, the focus of intervention is to initiate aggressive combination antiretroviral regimens quickly to maximally suppress viral replication, preserve immune function, and reduce the development of drug resistance.[40] *Maximal suppression of viral replication is now recommended.*

> Potent protease inhibitors (which inhibit the protease enzyme of HIV-1) along with nucleoside analog reverse transcriptase inhibitors can reduce plasma HIV-1–RNA to undetectable levels for prolonged periods.

In making decisions regarding treatment in a pregnant patient, the following must be considered:

- The treatment of HIV infection
- Reduction of the risk of perinatal transmission
- The known and unknown benefits and risks of therapy

> Although unique considerations associated with pregnancy should be discussed, pregnancy is not a reason to defer antiretroviral treatment.

Antiretroviral monotherapy is now considered suboptimal treatment for pregnant women with HIV infection. Along with ZDV chemoprophylaxis, standard antiretroviral therapy should be offered to HIV-infected pregnant women.

Combination antiretroviral therapy is often called *highly active antiretroviral therapy* **(HAART).**

> The current HAART standard of care for HIV-1–infected adults who are not pregnant consists of two nucleoside analog reverse transcriptase inhibitors and one protease inhibitor.

Guidelines for initiation and optimal antiretroviral therapy for pregnant women should be the same as guidelines for nonpregnant adults. The primary issues to consider in guiding treatment decisions are the woman's clinical, virologic, and immunologic status. However, the potential effect on the fetus must also be considered.

In the first trimester of pregnancy, women who have not begun antiretroviral therapy may wish to delay initiation of therapy until after 10 to 12 weeks' gestation. This is the period of organogenesis, when major organs are developing. Some women who are already receiving antiretroviral therapy may consider temporarily stopping therapy until after the first trimester; however, most experts recommend continuation of maximally suppressive therapy.

> If antiretroviral therapy is discontinued for any reason, all agents should be stopped and restarted simultaneously to prevent the development of drug resistance.

Currently, minimal data exist on the pharmacokinetics and safety of antiretroviral agents used during pregnancy. Drug choice needs to be individualized based on the patient's status. **The combination of medications that seems to work best in many people and is strongly recommended consists of a choice of one protease inhibitor** *plus* **a choice of two nucleoside analog reverse transcriptase inhibitors**[61] (Table 11.1). Alternative recommendations are available (refer to ATIS, 2000, *Guidelines for the Use of Antiretroviral Agent in HIV-Infected Adults and Adolescents* for further details).

TABLE 11.1 Recommended HAART Regimens	
PROTEASE INHIBITORS	**NUCLEOSIDE ANALOG REVERSE TRANSCRIPTASE INHIBITORS**
Efavirenz	Stavudine + lamivudine
Indinavir	Stavudine + didanosine
Nelfinavir	Zidovudine + lamivudine
Ritonavir + saquinavir	Zidovudine + didanosine

There are currently six approved nucleoside analog reverse transcriptase inhibitors (Table 11.2). ZDV and d4T *should not* be used together.[61]

TABLE 11.2 Nucleoside Analog Reverse Transcriptase Inhibitors	
NAME OF DRUG	**FDA PREGNANCY CATEGORY**
Zidovudine (Retrovir)	C
Didanosine (Videx, ddi)	B
Lamivudine (Epivir, 3TC)	C
Stavudine (Zerit, d4T)	C
Zalcitabine (HIVID, ddc)	C
Abacavir (Ziagen, ABC)	C

There are three non-nucleoside analog reverse transcriptase inhibitors (Table 11.3).[61] Nevirapine has been evaluated, and to date, no adverse effects have been seen in women or infants. Because of teratogenic effects seen in primate studies with efavirenz, pregnancy should be avoided in women receiving this drug. No studies are currently planned with efavirenz in pregnant women.

TABLE 11.3 Non-nucleoside Analog Reverse Transcriptase Inhibitors	
NAME OF DRUG	**FDA PREGNANCY CATEGORY**
Delavirdine (Rescriptor)	C
Efavirenz (Sustiva)	C
Nevirapine (Viramune)	C

There are five approved protease inhibitors (Table 11.4). In the United States, the use of four protease inhibitors is currently being studied in pregnant women and their infants. No data are available at this time. Amprenavir has not been studied in pregnant women.[61]

TABLE 11.4 Protease Inhibitors	
NAME OF DRUG	**FDA PREGNANCY CATEGORY**
Indinavir (Crixivan)	C
Nelfinavir (Viracept)	B
Ritonavir (Norvir)	B
Saquinavir (Fortovase)	B
Amprenavir (Agenerase)	C

At present, if combination antiretroviral drugs are going to be used during the antepartum period, *whenever possible*, ZDV should be included as a component of the antenatal therapeutic regimen. During the intrapartum and neonatal period, ZDV should be used to reduce the risk of perinatal transmission.

The current standard ZDV dosing regimen for the antenatal period is 200 mg three times daily or 300 mg twice daily. This is a change from the regimen used in the PACTG 076 study, which used 100 mg five times a day. The current regimen has shown comparable clinical responses and is expected to enhance maternal adherence.[39]

Recommendations for the Use of Antiretroviral Drugs to Reduce Perinatal HIV Transmission

The Public Health Service Task Force has made the following recommendations regarding the use of antiretroviral drugs to reduce perinatal transmission[39]:

1. *If an HIV-infected pregnant woman has not received prior antiretroviral therapy, the three-part ZDV chemoprophylaxis regimen should be recommended.* The three-part ZDV regimen consists of the following:
   - **An antepartum regimen**—The dosage is zidovudine 200 mg three times daily or 300 mg twice daily.
   - **An intrapartum regimen**—The dosage is an initial loading dose of zidovudine 2 mg/kg intravenously followed by a continuous infusion of 1 mg/kg per hour until delivery.
   - **A neonatal regimen**—The dosage is zidovudine syrup 2 mg/kg orally four times a day for 6 weeks. Treatment of the newborn must begin as soon as possible after delivery. Optimally, treatment should begin within 12 to 24 hours after birth.

   The combination of additional antiretroviral drugs should be discussed and recommended based on the woman's clinical, immunologic, and virologic status. A woman in the first trimester may consider delaying initiation of treatment until after 10 to 12 weeks' gestation.

2. *If an HIV-infected pregnant woman has already been receiving antiretroviral therapy during the current pregnancy, the following recommendations are:*
   - If past the first trimester, the woman should continue with her therapy.
   - If in the first trimester, the woman should be counseled on the risks versus the benefits of antiretroviral therapy during this period. Continuation of therapy should be considered. If therapy is discontinued, all drugs should be stopped simultaneously and restarted simultaneously to prevent the development of drug resistance.
   - If the current regimen does not contain ZDV, the addition of ZDV (or substitution of another nucleoside analog reverse transcriptase inhibitor) is recommended after 14 weeks' gestation. Also, ZDV administration is recommended during the intrapartum period and for the newborn.

3. *If an HIV-infected pregnant woman presents in labor with no prior therapy, the following recommendations are:*
   - A single dose of nevirapine at the onset of labor, followed by a single dose of nevirapine for the newborn at 48 hours of age **OR**
   - Oral ZDV and 3TC during labor, followed by 1 week of oral ZDV-3TC for the newborn **OR**
   - Intrapartum IV ZDV, followed by 6 weeks of ZDV for the newborn **OR**
   - The two-dose nevirapine regimen combined with intrapartum IV ZDV and 6 weeks of ZDV for the newborn
   - *The woman should be assessed in the immediate postpartum period to determine whether antiretroviral therapy is necessary for her health.*

4. *If an infant is born to a mother who has received no antiretroviral therapy during her pregnancy or intrapartum period, the following recommendations are:*
   - A 6-week course of ZDV therapy for the infant should be offered and discussed with the mother.
   - ZDV should be initiated as soon as possible (within 12 to 24 hours of birth).
   - The appropriate dosing for premature infants is currently being studied in infants less than 34 weeks' gestation. The regimen being studied is 1.5 mg/kg body weight orally or intravenously every 12 hours for the first 2 weeks of life, then increased to 2 mg/kg body weight every 8 hours for infants 2 to 6 weeks of age.

5. *The woman should be assessed in the immediate postpartum period to determine whether antiretroviral therapy is recommended for her health.*[39]

Serious Side Effects of Antiretroviral Therapy

ZDV has been associated with hematologic toxicity, including granulocytopenia and severe anemia (especially in patients with advanced HIV disease). Prolonged use has also been associated with symptomatic myopathy. Rare occurrences of potentially fatal lactic acidosis and severe hepatomegaly with steatosis have been reported. Nucleoside analog drugs are also known to cause mitochondrial dysfunction. Toxicity related to mitochondrial dysfunction has been reported in patients who have received long-term treatment. It has resolved with discontinuation of the drugs.

Protease inhibitors have been reported to cause hyperglycemia, new-onset diabetes mellitus, exacerbation of existing diabetes mellitus, and diabetic ketoacidosis. Because pregnancy can also cause hyperglycemia (as seen with gestational diabetes), pregnant women receiving protease inhibitor drugs should be monitored closely for hyperglycemia.[62]

■ Does zidovudine present any threat to the fetus?

Studies of ZDV use at recommended dosages during pregnancy indicate that it is well tolerated by adults and term infants. Long-term data are not available, but short-term data are reassuring. Infants who were exposed to ZDV in utero have been followed for up to 6 years. They show no significant findings in immunologic, neurologic, or growth parameters. In the PACTG 076 study, the only significant side effect observed with ZDV use in infants was the presence of anemia. The anemia was mild and resolved spontaneously without transfusions.[60]

> Providers who are treating HIV-infected pregnant women and their infants are advised to report cases of prenatal exposure to antiretroviral drugs to the Antiretroviral Pregnancy Registry.

The Antiretroviral Pregnancy Registry

The Antiretroviral Pregnancy Registry is an epidemiologic project to collect observational, nonexperimental data on the use of antiretroviral drugs during pregnancy and their potential teratogenicity. The registry is a collaborative project between pharmaceutical companies, the CDC, the National Institutes of Health, and obstetric and pediatric practitioners.

The registry data will be used to supplement animal studies and assist providers in evaluating the risks and benefits of treatment for their patients. *The registry does not use patient names.* Information is obtained from reporting providers who call the project office at 800-258-4263, fax the enrollment form to 800-800-1052, or mail the form to Antiretroviral Pregnancy Registry, Pharma Research Corporation, 115 North Third Street, Wilmington, NC 28401.

Current Recommendations Regarding the Delivery the Woman With HIV Infection

Transmission of HIV to the infant can occur by transplacental–maternal–fetal microtransfusion of HIV-contaminated blood during a uterine contraction or by prolonged mucocutaneous exposure to maternal blood and vaginal secretions during labor. Because of these findings, studies that examine the delivery method and transmission have been conducted. **A significant relationship has been noted between the mode of delivery and vertical transmission.** Research indicates that scheduled cesarean delivery reduces risk of vertical transmission compared with vaginal delivery or unscheduled cesarean delivery; however, maternal morbidity is increased with cesarean delivery compared with vaginal delivery. The postpartum morbidity is greatest among HIV-infected women with low CD4+ T-cell counts.[41]

The American College of Obstetricians and Gynecologists released the following recommendations regarding mode of delivery[41]:

- Without ZDV treatment, vertical transmission is approximated 25%.
- With ZDV treatment, vertical transmission is reduced to 5% to 8%.
- With ZDV treatment and a scheduled cesarean delivery, the risk of vertical transmission is approximately 2%.
- If a woman's viral load is less than 1,000 copies per milliliter, the risk of vertical transmission with a vaginal delivery is approximately 2%.
- Women with viral loads greater than 1,000 copies per milliliter should be counseled on the potential benefit of a scheduled cesarean delivery.
- *No therapies guarantee a 0% risk of vertical transmission.*

- *The highest risk for vertical transmission is among women with relatively high plasma viral loads.*
- The patient must be respected in her decision regarding the route of delivery she prefers.
- The patient should receive antiretroviral chemotherapy during pregnancy according to the current guidelines. Adequate ZDV levels should be achieved if the IV infusion is begun 3 hours preoperatively.
- Prophylactic antibiotics should be considered during all cesarean deliveries.
- Cesarean delivery is recommended at 38 completed weeks of gestation to reduce the likelihood of onset of labor or rupture of membranes.
- There is no reduction in the transmission rate if cesarean delivery is performed after the onset of labor or after rupture of membranes.
- Amniocentesis to determine fetal lung maturity *should be avoided*. The expected date of confinement should be made on clinical estimates.
- Plasma viral load should be evaluated every 3 months or following changes in therapy. The most recent viral load should be used when counseling regarding mode of delivery.

Risks associated with a cesarean delivery should be discussed with all women. The choice of delivery must be individualized.

■ How is HIV infection diagnosed in the newborn?

The presence of maternal HIV antibodies is a normal finding in babies born to HIV-infected mothers, regardless of whether the newborn is infected. These passively acquired maternal antibodies may persist for up to 15 to 18 months of age. Because these antibodies form the basis for standard HIV testing with the EIA and Western blot, these tests are invalid in the determination of whether the newborn has contracted HIV. **Using viral diagnostic assays, HIV infection can be diagnosed in most infants by 1 month of age and in virtually all infants by 6 months of age.** Diagnostic testing should be performed at the following times:

- 48 hours of age
- 1 to 2 months of age
- 3 to 6 months of age

The following tests are available for the diagnosis of HIV infection in infants[65]:

- **HIV-DNA PCR is the *preferred* virologic method for diagnosing HIV infection in infants.** It is both sensitive and specific.
- HIV-RNA plasma assays may also be useful in the diagnosis of HIV infection in infants; however, data are limited regarding its sensitivity and specificity.
- HIV culture has a similar sensitivity compared with DNA PCR, but the culture is more complex and expensive to perform. Furthermore, the HIV culture takes 2 to 4 weeks for a final result.
- The p24 antigen test is another highly specific test for HIV infection, but the sensitivity is less than for the other HIV virologic test. The use of p24 antigen alone is not recommended for the diagnosis because of the high frequency of false-positive results in infants younger than 1 month of age.

Initial testing is recommended by 48 hours of age. Infants with positive virologic test at or before 48 hours are considered to have *intrauterine* or *antepartum infection*. Infants with positive virologic test during the first week of life or later are considered to have *intrapartum infection*.[63] Because the sensitivity of virologic assays increases at age 2 weeks, repeat diagnostic testing should be repeated at 14 days of age if the infant had a prior negative test. Infants with initially negative test should be retested at 1 to 2 months of age. HIV-exposed infants who have had repeatedly negative virologic assays at birth and 1 to 2 months of age should be retested at 3 to 6 months of age.

HIV infection in the infant is diagnosed with two positive HIV virologic tests performed on separate blood samples.

HIV infection in the infant can be reasonably excluded in the following situations:

- An infant has two or more negative virologic tests performed at 1 month of age or greater, with one performed at 4 months of age or greater.
- An infant has two or more negative HIV IgG antibody test performed at greater than 6 months of age with an interval of at least 1 month between tests, *and* the infant has no clinical evidence of HIV infection.

HIV infection in the infant can be *definitely* excluded in the following situations[65]:

- HIV IgG antibody is negative in the absence of hypogammaglobulinemia at 18 months of age, AND
- The infant has no clinical symptoms of HIV infection, AND
- HIV virologic assays are negative.

Special Issues to Consider in the Intrapartum and the Immediate Postpartum Management of HIV-Infected Women

The following factors must be addressed so that an effective, individualized plan of care can be developed and implemented:

- Infection control
- Pharmacotherapeutic options (as previously outlined)
- Psychosocial needs
- Ethical issues
- Patient education

Infection Control

Infection control measures must be a primary concern when providing care for the pregnant HIV-positive patient. The potential for infection of hospital personnel is certainly important; however, it is not the only consideration in the labor management of these patients. Obvious concerns are for fetal infection with HIV and for maternal infection because of potential immunocompromise and anemia. The following procedures are meant to help protect the HIV-positive woman from infection:

- **Reduce exposure to opportunistic organisms**—Limit vaginal examinations, avoid invasive procedures, avoid episiotomies and lacerations, attend to aseptic and sterile technique when performing procedures, and use the proper suturing techniques when episiotomy or laceration repair is necessary.
- **Monitor the patient closely for signs of infection**—Check vital signs and be especially alert for increasing temperature and pulse. Perform respiratory auscultation at regular intervals. Inspect laboratory results closely.
- **Review the patient's chart for a history of infection** (especially a history of recent infections and evidence of cure).
- **Be alert for signs of chorioamnionitis**—The higher incidence of STDs combined with the potential for immunocompromise in HIV-positive women place the woman at risk for ascending infection. These infections have been implicated as possible causes of premature rupture of the membranes. These women require close monitoring of maternal vital signs (especially elevations of temperature and pulse), antibiotic usage when chorioamnionitis occurs, and continuous external intensive fetal surveillance to detect a signs of infection (e.g., increasing baseline rate, tachycardia, or decreasing variability).
- **Screen for colonization of group B streptococcus at 35 to 36 weeks' gestation**—If cultures are positive, provide chemoprophylaxis during labor.

Additional guidelines for the delivery of a mother at high risk or infected with HIV include the following:

- Follow universal precautions carefully to protect *yourself* from accidental needlesticks, splatter, or contact with body fluids.
- Carefully maintain patient hygiene. Keep the skin and perineum as clean and dry as possible. Change disposable underpads frequently. Closely follow institutional guidelines for care of urinary catheters and intravenous lines.
- Review the woman's chart for evidence of normal or abnormal fetal growth (ultrasound reports, maternal weight gain, and fundal height measurements). Palpate the mother's

abdomen to obtain an estimation of the fetal weight. Many factors associated with HIV infection, such as drug use, poverty, and inadequate prenatal care, have an impact on the weight and condition of the baby at birth.

- Carefully monitor for blood loss, contraction pattern, and fetal heart rate pattern during labor.
- Observe the patient and laboratory values for signs of thrombocytopenia and anemia (common side effects of ZDV therapy).
- Handle blood and body fluid–stained linen according to institutional infection control guidelines. Dispose of soiled linens promptly after use to reduce the chance of accidental contact with personnel.
- Precisely follow the recommended guidelines of the institution for sterilization, disinfection, and housekeeping.
- Inform the nursery staff of the mother's HIV status.
- Use universal precautions when caring for the newborn.

Psychosocial Needs

For most people, the birth of a baby is a time of happiness, joy, and celebration. **However, the HIV-positive mother *might* have ambivalent feelings about the whole process.** She might feel happy about motherhood *but* at the same time be worried about her health and her baby's health. This can interfere with bonding and can contribute to the development of postpartum blues or depression. The following actions can help promote maternal–infant bonding.

- Encourage the new mother to hold her baby as soon as possible after delivery.
- Personalize the baby. Reinforce positive qualities of the newborn (e.g., pretty eyes, hair; has all her fingers and toes) and call the newborn by name.
- Encourage maternal–infant interaction. Encourage the mother to touch, talk to, and examine the baby.
- Promote family involvement in the birth process by allowing family attendance. Encourage participation in the labor, delivery, and postpartum period.

Many emotional and psychological adjustments are also occurring during this critical time. The following actions can help promote psychological adjustment.

- If a psychiatric professional or a social worker has followed the mother, with her permission, notify that person of her status.
- Allow the mother to verbalize her feelings. Listening to her concerns will often help reduce her anxiety and assist her in coming to terms with issues she must face.
- Do not avoid the mother because of her HIV status. Your time with her is therapeutic because women like her often feel isolated and are commonly ostracized by others.
- Avoid judgmental behavior and attitudes when providing care.
- Keep the new mother informed of both her status and that of her baby (before and after delivery). Counsel the mother regarding necessary health screenings for her newborn and herself.

> Remember that HIV is a family disease. It affects every family member, regardless of whether they are infected.

Ethical Issues

The care of the HIV-positive patient includes many emotionally charged issues for both patients and staff. These issues demand recognition and consideration to ensure that optimal care is provided to patients. The following are some of the key issues that affect both the patient and staff in the care of IV-positive patients.

- **Confidentiality**—It is a central issue in the treatment of HIV/AIDS patients. Unauthorized disclosure of a patient's HIV status by health care workers is not only unethical but can cause irreparable damage to the patient by affecting social, occupational, and personal relationships. **If a breach of confidentiality occurs, it can serve as grounds for legal action.** Fear of disclosure can also keep patients from seeking early prenatal care, from receiving any prenatal care, and from consenting to testing for HIV.

- **Advance directives**—They provide the patient with an opportunity to direct her own care in advance. All health care facilities that receive federal money must follow guidelines set by the Federal Patient Self-Determination Act of 1991. This act requires institutions to make information available to all patients regarding options available to them for care if they become unable to make their own decisions. Staff members should be aware of these options and should respect the patient's plans, values, and beliefs.
- **Right to medical care**—This means that each individual has a right to expect the best possible health care regardless of his or her disease state.
- **Consent and coercion issues**—These include the fact that each patient has the right to full information regarding treatment options available. Decisions made by HIV-positive patients about their care should be with the full knowledge of the potential benefits, risks, indications, and side effects for both her and her unborn or newborn baby. Threat, coercion, and incomplete information have no place in patient care. Health care professionals have the opportunity and responsibility to help the woman understand options and implications of treatment.

Patient Education

Because the laboring woman might have a limited ability to concentrate on complex or lengthy explanations, effective patient education during labor and delivery can be difficult. In addition to standard labor and delivery information, the following material should be presented in a thorough, but concise, manner.

- Risks and benefits of drug therapy
- Contraindications to breastfeeding
- Immediate care of the newborn
- Immediate care of the mother after delivery

As long as the mother and baby are stable, the primary focus in the immediate postpartum period should be on the promotion of bonding. Extensive information concerning self-care, baby care, contraception, lifestyle, nutrition, and transmission of HIV should be covered later.

Universal Precautions Recommended by the CDC

Medical and nursing histories, as well as physical examinations, do not identify all individuals who might be infected with HIV, hepatitis B virus, or other bloodborne pathogens.

> All health care workers (medical, nursing, housekeeping, and allied health personnel) should always use precautions when dealing with blood and other body fluids containing visible blood.

The CDC first recommended this approach in 1987. It is referred to as universal blood and body fluid precautions or universal precautions. **Universal precautions recommend that you consider all patients as potentially infected with HIV, hepatitis B virus, or other bloodborne pathogens.** These precautions are standards of practice for all health care personnel and must be used with every patient. In addition, *hepatitis B vaccine is recommended as an important adjunct to universal precautions for all health care workers who are exposed to blood.*[66]

Nursing, medical, and housekeeping personnel on an obstetrics unit are exposed on a daily basis to a variety of body fluids. The following precautions should be followed rigorously to minimize the risk of exposure to blood and body fluids of all patients.

- Universal precautions apply to blood and other body fluids containing visible blood.
- Universal precautions apply to semen, vaginal secretions, tissue, cerebrospinal fluid, synovial fluid, pleural fluid, peritoneal fluid, and amniotic fluid.
- Universal precautions do *not* apply to feces, nasal secretions, sputum, sweat, tears, urine, and vomitus, unless they contain visible blood. The risk of transmission of HIV and hepatitis B virus from these fluids and materials is extremely low.

- Although universal precautions do not apply to human breast milk, gloves may be worn in situations in which exposures to breast milk might be frequent, such as with breast milk banking.
- Use protective barriers such as gloves, gowns, masks, and protective eyewear to reduce the risk of exposure of skin or mucous membranes to these fluids. The type of barrier should be appropriate for the procedure and type of exposure anticipated.
- Be careful when using needles, scalpels, and other sharp instruments. Use caution when handling or cleaning sharp instruments. Do not recap, bend, or break needles after use. In addition, do not recap Vacutainer devices. Dispose of used syringes immediately after use in a designated waste container designed for sharp hazardous waste materials. These special containers should be readily accessible to the staff to prevent accidental punctures during transport. They should be available in every patient room, examination room, treatment room, and delivery area. They should be emptied often to prevent accidental sticks when trying to push needles into an overflowing container.
- Immediately and thoroughly wash hands and other skin surfaces that are contaminated.
- Wear gloves during phlebotomy. Gloves should be made of latex or vinyl. Never wash or disinfect surgical or examination gloves for reuse.

Additional considerations include the following measures:

- Wear vinyl or latex gloves when contact with blood, amniotic fluid, mucous membranes, broken skin, or other body fluids is anticipated. To reduce the chance of exposure caused by tears or imperfections in the gloves, some institutions recommend double gloving when exposure to these substances will be prolonged or intense. Examples of intense exposure include surgery, delivery, episiotomy repair, and placement of internal monitoring devices. Gloves should also be worn when changing dressings, underpads, perineal pads, and diapers and when giving perineal care.
- Remove gloves and wash hands immediately after giving care to one patient and before giving care to another patient. A single pair of gloves should not be repeatedly used because potential defects could render the gloves useless as a protective barrier.
- Always wear protective coverings such as gloves, impervious gowns/aprons, masks, and eye/face shields when doing invasive procedures that can contaminate you. This includes births (both vaginal and cesarean) and cleaning procedures that can cause splashing of blood and body fluids.
- Use protective eyeglasses or a face shield during any procedure that could result in contamination of the eyes. Providing goggles for employees is a responsibility of the employing institution.
- Refrain from all direct patient contact and from handling potentially contaminated equipment if you have exudative lesions, weeping dermatitis, or breaks in the skin that cannot be adequately covered.
- Wear gloves when inserting and discontinuing an IV catheter.
- Remove a glove torn by a needlestick or other injury and cleanse the area immediately. Report all accidents and follow institutional protocol.
- Place all specimens of blood and body fluids in containers with secure lids or sealed plastic bags to prevent leaking during transport. Care should be taken when collecting each specimen to prevent contamination of the outside of the container and the laboratory form.
- Blood and body fluid, soiled linen, and other potentially contaminated articles from all patients should be handled according to the infection control measures recommended by your institution.
- If you are pregnant, there are no special guidelines to follow. You should use the same universal precautions for patient care as other staff members.

Conclusion

HIV infection and AIDS remain major worldwide health concerns. The number of women and children infected with HIV continues to grow. **Much has been learned about this virus, but far more must be learned before a cure is found for this devastating killer.** Until then, health care providers need to keep abreast of the latest advances, findings, and treatment modalities available to these patients and their families.

Resources for Current HIV Information

AIDS Education Global Information System (AGEiS)
A comprehensive website of HIV information and resources.
www.aegis.com

AIDS Treatment Information Service (ATIS)
Provides all the Public Health Service treatment guidelines and up-to-date information.
Contains the Living Document—New data is reviewed by the Perinatal HIV Guidelines
Working Group and regular updates to the guidelines are made.
www.hivatis.org
Phone: 800-HIV-0440

Association of Nurses in AIDS Care (ANAC)
Professional association that provides information and advises members about clinical and
policy issues related to nursing and HIV care.
www.anacnet.org
Phone: 800-260-6780

The Body
A comprehensive website of HIV information and resources.
www.thebody.com

Centers for Disease Control and Prevention National Prevention Information Network
Offers up-to-date epidemiologic information, daily updates on HIV/AIDS, and patient-
oriented information.
www.cdcnpin.org

HIV Medication Guide
A website providing drug information.
www.jag.on.ca/asp_bin/Main.asp

International Association of Physicians in AIDS Care (IAPAC)
This organization provides a website with policy information about ongoing efforts to expand access to health care services and lifesaving drugs and technologies.
www.iapac.org
Phone: 312-795-4930

Important Phone Numbers
AIDS Clinical Trials Information Services (ACTIS): 800-874-2572
CDC National Prevention Information Network: 800-458-5231
HIV/AIDS Treatment Information Service (ATIS): 800-448-0440
National AIDS Hotline: 800-342-2437
STD Hotline: 800-227-8922

PRACTICE/REVIEW QUESTIONS
After reviewing this module, answer the following questions.

1. What is the causative agent of AIDS? _____

2. What three parameters does the CDC use in its definition of AIDS?

    a. _____

    b. _____

    c. _____

3. What is the difference between AIDS and HIV infection? _____

_____

_____

_____

4. Why are most of the effects of HIV infection on the immune system?

    _____

    _____

    _____

    _____

    _____

5. State five ways in which HIV can be transmitted.

    a. _____

    b. _____

    c. _____

    d. _____

    e. _____

6. The standard algorithm for HIV testing consists of which two tests?

    a. _____

    b. _____

7. Having a sexually transmitted disease increases a person's chance of getting HIV infection.

    A. True

    B. False

8. Give two reasons why HIV in pregnant women can go undetected.

    a. _____

    b. _____

9. The primary cause of HIV infection in children is _____.

10. According to the PACTG 076 study, the rate of HIV transmission from an infected mother to her infant without ZDV treatment is estimated to be _____%. The rate of HIV transmission from an infected mother to her infant with ZDV treatment is estimated to be _____%.

11. What is meant by the *latency period*?

    _____

    _____

12. A negative HIV antibody testing may need to be repeated in 3 to 6 months after a high-risk exposure.

    A. True

    B. False

13. State three ways in which newborns can acquire HIV from their mother.

    a. _____

    b. _____

    c. _____

14. Breastfeeding is permitted for an HIV-infected mother in the United States.

    A. True

    B. False

15. Breastfeeding should be encouraged for all women in the United States.

    A. True

    B. False

16. What is the primary means of postpartum vertical transmission of HIV?

    _____

17. What is the World Health Organization position on breastfeeding and HIV infection?

    _____

    _____

18. What does practicing "universal precautions" as recommended by the CDC mean?

    _____

    _____

19. What are five characteristics or factors in a woman's history that increase her risk for contracting HIV?

    a. _____

    b. _____

    c. _____

    d. _____

    e. _____

20. Which body fluid has the highest concentration of the human immunodeficiency virus?

    _____

21. The concept of universal precautions presumes that _____

    _____.

22. List those body fluids to which universal precautions apply. _____

    _____

    _____

    _____

23. List body fluids to which universal precautions do not apply. (Presume none of these contain blood.)

    _____

    _____

24. Regarding universal precautions:

    a. When will you wear gloves? _____

    _____

    b. How often should gloves be changed? _____

    _____

    c. What rule will guide you in handwashing? _____

    _____

    d. When should protective coverings such as gloves, impervious gowns/aprons, masks, and eye/face shields be used?   _____

    _____

    e. How should one dispose of used needles? _____

    _____

    f. How should specimens of blood and body fluids be handled?_____

    _____

    g. What specimens require special infection warning labels?   _____

    _____

25. Pregnant health care workers are at greater risk of contracting HIV infection than non-pregnant health care workers.

    A. True

    B. False

26. The CDC recommends routine HIV antibody testing of all health care workers.

    A. True

    B. False

27. Explain why invasive procedures on the fetus during labor should be avoided if possible.

    _____

    _____

28. List six steps you need to take in caring for the delivering woman who has HIV.

    a. _____

    b. _____

    c. _____

    d. _____

    e. _____

    f. _____

29. List six steps you should take while caring for the newly delivered baby that can reduce the risk of HIV transmission to the newborn.

    a. _____

    b. _____

    c. _____

    d. _____

    e. _____

    f. _____

30. What should guide you in deciding whether the mother with HIV infection or AIDS should have close contact with her baby? _____

_____

31. Isolation is not necessary for the HIV-infected mother or mother with AIDS.

    A. True

    B. False

32. Mother and infant should avoid direct contact if the mother has skin lesions.

    A. True

    B. False

PRACTICE/REVIEW ANSWER KEY

 1. The human immunodeficiency virus (HIV)

 2. a. Laboratory evidence of infection, plus
    b. Laboratory evidence of severe immunosuppression, and/or
    c. One or more of the 26 identified clinical conditions for AIDS

 3. HIV infection occurs when an individual is infected with the human immunodeficiency virus. This individual has no clinical signs or symptoms of the disease. *AIDS* is the term used to denote the disease stage when individuals develop a severely weakened immune system and opportunistic infections occur.

 4. HIV has a great affinity for the CD4 antigen. This antigen is largely found on the surface of lymphocytes. The virus attaches itself to these cells, enters the cell, completes viral replication, and causes cell destruction when it exits the cell. Lymphocytes are precursors to other cells that are important in the body's defense against infection. When lymphocyte numbers are significantly reduced, the body is no longer able to adequately protect itself from infection.

 5. a. Intimate sexual contact (oral, anal, or vaginal) with someone infected with HIV
    b. Sharing of drug needles and syringes with an infected person
    c. Receipt of a blood transfusion that contains HIV
    d. Inadvertent contamination of either mucous membranes or breaks in the skin with the blood or body fluid of an infected person
    e. Vertical transmission from a mother who transfers the virus to the fetus during the perinatal period

 6. a. Enzyme immunosorbent assay (EIA)
    b. Western blot

 7. A

 8. a. Testing too soon before the antibodies develop will result in a false-negative test.
    b. Some signs and symptoms of pregnancy (e.g., anemia, fatigue, dyspnea) are similar to symptoms of progressing HIV infection and AIDS and can mask or delay the diagnosis.

 9. Perinatal transmission from mother to child

10. a. 25.5
    b. 8.3

11. The latency period is the period between actual infection with the virus through the time when enough antibodies are produced by the body to cause a positive HIV test result.

12. A

13. a. Vertical transmission during pregnancy
    b. Through contact with infected blood and body fluids during delivery
    c. Breastfeeding

14. B

15. B

16. Breastfeeding

17. Women at risk for HIV infection should feed their babies infant formula if it is easily accessible. In areas where accessibility of formula is a problem, it is recommended that women, even those at risk for HIV infection, breastfeed their infants.

18. All health care workers should use precautions when dealing with blood and body fluids on all patients. All patients should be considered as potentially infected with HIV, hepatitis B virus, or other bloodborne pathogens.

19. a. Is an IV drug user
    b. Has had multiple sexual partners
    c. Has had sexual partners who are infected or at risk for infection because they are hemophiliacs, bisexual, or IV users or they have had multiple sexual partners
    d. Had a blood transfusion received before blood was being screened but after HIV infection occurred in the United States
    e. Had or has multiple STDs
    f. Currently living in or born in communities or countries where there is a known or suspected high prevalence of HIV infection

20. Blood

21. All patients are considered potentially infected with a bloodborne pathogen such as HIV or hepatitis B virus. No distinction is made among patients as needing precautionary care by the health care worker.

22. Blood and other body fluids containing visible blood; semen; vaginal secretions; tissues; cerebrospinal fluid; synovial fluid; pleural fluid; peritoneal fluid; pericardial fluid; amniotic fluid

23. Feces, nasal secretions, sputum, sweat, tears, urine, vomitus

24. a. Wear gloves when contact with blood, amniotic fluids, mucous membranes, broken skin, or other body fluids is anticipated or when giving baths if your hands are cut, are chapped, or have abrasions.
    b. Gloves should be changed after giving care to one patient and before providing care to another. A single pair of gloves should *not* be used repeatedly in giving care to a single patient because defects can occur.
    c. Handwashing occurs after gloves are removed and after care is rendered to each patient.
    d. Protective coverings should be used when carrying out or assisting with invasive procedures that might contaminate an individual with droplets or splashing of body fluids or tissue.
    e. Never recap, bend, or break needles. Dispose of needles immediately in a designated container. Keep needle disposal containers in each patient's room. Avoid overfilled containers. Also, do not recap Vacutainer devices. Either remove the needles with a hemostat or dispose of the unit according to your institution's protocol.
    f. Place specimens in containers with secure lids or sealed plastic bags to prevent leaking during transport. Avoid contaminating the outside of the container.
    g. None. Blood and body fluids from all patients should be considered infective.

25. B

26. B

27. Some infants can be infected with HIV by inoculation during an invasive procedure.

28. a. Follow universal precautions to protect yourself from splatter or contact with body fluids.
    b. Maintain patient hygiene carefully.
    c. Promote maternal–infant bonding by all possible means as you would in any birthing situation.
    d. Handle blood and body fluid–stained linen as you would for any infection control measure.
    e. Follow institutional recommended sterilization, disinfection, or housekeeping guidelines.
    f. Alert nursery staff to expect the newborn and of the HIV infection status of the mother.

29. a. Assign one nurse to attend to the newborn after delivery.
    b. Dry the infant immediately after the delivery to remove all maternal blood and amniotic fluid.
    c. Gently remove excess fluid and blood from the nares and oropharynx.
    d. Aspirate stomach contents using a bulb syringe, mucus extractor, or meconium aspirator with wall suction on a low setting.
    e. Delay administration of vitamin K until after the infant is bathed.
    f. Bathe the newborn early and thoroughly with a mild, nonmedicated soap under radiant heat as soon as the infant is stable.

30. If the mother does not have an opportunistic infection or skin lesions and she and the baby are physically able, she should be encouraged to hold and cuddle the baby.

31. A

32. A

REFERENCES

1. UNAIDS. (2000, December). *Report on the global HIV/AIDS epidemic: December 2000* [On-line]. Available at: www.unaids.org/wac/2000/wad00/files/WAD_epidemic_report.htm.
2. Centers for Disease Control and Prevention. (2000). *HIV/AIDS Surveillance Report, 12*(1), 1–44. Available at: www.cdc.gov/hiv/stats/hasr1201/notice.htm. Accessed January 17, 2001.
3. Centers for Disease Control and Prevention. (2000). *Revised US Public Health Service recommendations for human immunodeficiency virus screening of pregnant women* [On-line]. Available at: ftp.cdcnpin.org/Guidelines/perinatal.pdf.
4. Centers for Disease Control and Prevention. (1998). *Frequently asked questions on HIV/AIDS.* Available at: www.cdc.gov/hiv/pubs/faqs.htm.
5. Minkoff, H. (1994). Human immunodeficiency virus. In R. K. Creasy & R. Resnick (Eds.), *Maternal-fetal medicine principles and practice* (3rd ed., Rev., pp. 1310–1312). Philadelphia: WB Sanders.
6. Hardy, W. (1996). Management of the HIV-infected patient, part 1. *Medical Clinics of North America, 80*(6), 1239–1261.
7. Centers for Disease Control and Prevention. (1999, January). *CDC statement in response to presentation on origin of HIV-1 at 6th conference on retroviruses and opportunistic infections* [On-line]. Available at: www.cdcnpin.org/hiv/faq/virus.htm.
8. Centers for Disease Control and Prevention. (1998). *Human immunodeficiency virus type 2* [On-line]. Available at: www.cdc.gov/hiv/pubs/facts/hiv2.htm.
9. Maury, W., Potts, B., & Rabson, A. (1989). HIV-1 infection of the first trimester and term human placental tissue: A possible mode of maternal-fetal transmission. *Journal of Infectious Diseases, 164*(4), 583–588.
10. Green, W. (1991). The molecular biology of the human immunodeficiency virus type-1 infection. *New England Journal of Medicine, 324*(5), 308–317.

11. Centers for Disease Control and Prevention. (1998). Report of the NIH panel to define principles of therapy of HIV infection. *Morbidity and Mortality Weekly Report, 47*(RR-5), 1–41. Available at: http://aepo-xdv-www.epo.cdc.gov/wonder/prevguid/m0052295/m0052295.asp. Accessed November 27, 2000.

12. Enger, C., Graham, N., Peng, Y., Chmiel, J. S., Kingsley, L. A., Detels, R., & Munoz, A. (1996). Survival from early, intermediate, and late stages of HIV infection. *Journal of the American Medical Association, 275,* 1329–1334.

13. Haynes, B., Panteleo, G., & Fauci, A. (1996). Toward an understanding of the correlates of protective immunity to HIV infection. *Science, 271,* 324–328.

14. Centers for Disease Control and Prevention. (1997). *Gateway to AIDS knowledge: accuracy of tests.* Available at: http://hivinsite.ucsf.edu/topics/testing/2098.3075.html. Accessed January 26, 2001.

15. Centers for Disease Control and Prevention. (1998). *Frequently asked questions about HIV and AIDS—HIV testing.* Available at: www.cdcnpin.org/hiv/faq.

16. Centers for Disease Control and Prevention. (2000). *Revised guidelines for HIV counseling, testing, and referral* [On-line]. Available at: www.cdc.gov/hiv/frn/hivctr.pdf.

17. CDCNAC. (1997). *Guide to information and resources on HIV testing.* Atlanta: CDC National AIDS Clearinghouse.

18. Centers for Disease Control and Prevention. (1998). Update: HIV counseling and testing using rapid tests—United States, 1995. *Morbidity and Mortality Weekly Report, 47*(11), 211–215. Available at: http://aepo-xdv-www.epo.cdc.gov/wonder/prevguid/m0051715/m0051718.asp. Accessed November 17, 2000.

19. Centers for Disease Control and Prevention. (1992). 1993 revised classification system for HIV infection and expanded surveillance case definition for AIDS among adolescents and adults. *Morbidity and Mortality Weekly Report, 41*(RR-17), 1–11.

20. COHIS. (2000, May). *AIDS/HIV opportunistic infections.* Available at: www.medvalet.com/index.html. Accessed January 21, 2001.

21. Centers for Disease Control and Prevention. (1987). Recommendations for prevention of HIV transmission in health-care settings. *Morbidity and Mortality Weekly Report, 36*(SU02), 1–19.

22. Mastro, T., & de Vinceni, I. (1996). Probabilities of sexual HIV-1 transmission. *AIDS, 10*(Suppl. A), S75–S82.

23. Vittinghoff, E., Douglas, J., Judson, F., McKirnan, D., MacQueen, K., & Buchbinder, S. P. (1999). Per-contact risk of human immunodeficiency virus transmission between male sexual partners. *American Journal of Epidemiology, 150*(3), 306–311.

24. Anderson, J. (Ed.) (2000). *A guide to the clinical care of women with HIV: 2000 preliminary edition* [On-line]. Available at: http://hab.hrsa.gov/womencare.htm.

25. Kaplan, E., & Heimer, R. (1992). A model-based estimate of HIV infectivity via needle sharing. *Journal of Acquired Immune Deficiency Syndromes, 5,* 1116–1118.

26. Centers for Disease Control and Prevention. (1998). Public Health Service guidelines for the management of health-care worker exposures to HIV and recommendations for postexposure prophylaxis. *Morbidity and Morality Weekly Report, 47*(RR-7), 1–28.

27. Chin, J. (1994). The growing impact of HIV/AIDS pandemic on children born to HIV-infected women. *Clinics in Perinatology, 21*(1), 111–114.

28. Goedert, J., Mendez, H., & Drummond, J. (1989). Mother-to-infant transmission of human immunodeficiency type-1: Association with prematurity or low anti-gp 120. *Lancet, 336,* 1351–1354.

29. Barkowsky, W., Krasinski, K., Pollack, H., Hoover, W., Kaul, A., & Ilmet-Moore, T. (1992). Early diagnosis of human immunodeficiency virus infection in children less than 6 months of age: Comparison of polymerase chain reaction, culture, and plasma antigen captive techniques. *Journal of Infectious Diseases, 166*(3), 616–619.

30. Fowler, M., Simonds, R., & Roongpisuthipong, A. (2000). HIV/AIDS in infants, children, and adolescents: Update on perinatal transmission. *Pediatric Clinics of North America, 47*(1), 21–38.

31. Bertolli, G., St. Louis, M. E., Simonds, R. J., Nieburg, P., Kamenga, M., Brown, C., Tarande, M., Quinn, T., & Ou, C. Y. (1996). Estimating the timing of mother-to-child transmission of human immunodeficiency virus in a breastfeeding population in Kinshasa, Zaire. *Journal of Infectious Diseases, 174*(4), 722–726.

32. Kostrikis, L. G., Neumann, A. U., Thomson, B., Lew, J. F., McIntosh, K., Pollack, H., Palumbo, P., Ho, D. D., & Moore, J. P. (1999). *Polymorphism in the regulatory regions of the CCR5 influence of perinatal transmission of HIV (abstract 263) Presented at the 6th Conference on Retroviruses and Opportunistic Infections.* Chicago.

33. MacDonald, K. S., Embree, J., Njenga, S., Nagelkerke, N. J., Ngatia, I., Mohammed, Z., Barber, B. H., Ndinya-Achola, J., Bwayo, J., & Plummer, F. A. (1998). Mother-child class I HLA concordance increases perinatal human immunodeficiency virus type 1 transmission. *Journal of Infectious Disease, 177*(3), 551–556.

34. Mofenson, L., Lambert, J. S., Stiehm, E. R., Bethel, J., Meyer, W. A., 3rd, Whitehouse, J., Moye, J. Jr., Reichelderfer, P., Harris, D. R., Fowler, M. G., Mathieson, B. J., & Nemo, G. J. (1999). Risk factors for perinatal transmission of human immunodeficiency virus type 1 in women treated with zidovudine. Pediatric AIDS clinical trials study 185 team. *New England Journal of Medicine, 341*(6), 385–393.

35. Garcia, P., Kalish, L. A., Pitt, J., Minkoff, H., Quinn, T. C., Burchett, S. K., Kornegay, J., Jackson, B., Moye, J., Hanson, C., Zorrilla, C., & Lew, J. F. (1999). Maternal levels of plasma human immunodeficiency virus type 1 RNA and the risk of perinatal transmission. Women and Infants Transmission Study Group. *New England Journal of Medicine, 341*(6), 394–402.

36. Maternal viral load and vertical transmission of HIV-1: an important factor but not the only one: The European collaborative study. (1999). *AIDS, 13,* 1377–1385.

37. Mock, P., Shaffer, N., Bhadrakom, C., Siriwasin, W., Chotpitayasunondh, T., Chearskul, S., Young, N. L., Roongpisuthipong, A., Chinayon, P., Kalish, M. L., Parekh, B., & Mastro, T. D. (1999). Maternal viral load and timing of mother-to-child transmission. *AIDS, 13,* 407–414.

38. Shaffer, N., Roongpisuthipong, A., Siriwasin, W., Chotpitayasunondh, T., Chearskul, S., Young, N. L., Parekh, B., Mock, P. A., Bhadrakom, C., Chinayon, P., Kalish, M. L., Phillips, S. K., Granade, T. C., Subbarao, S., Weniger, B. G., & Mastro, T. D. (1999). Maternal virus load and perinatal human immunodeficiency virus subtype E transmission, Thailand. *Journal of Infectious Disease, 179,* 590–599.

39. Public Health Service Task Force. (2000, November). *Public Health Service Task Force recommendations for the use of antiretroviral drugs in pregnant HIV-1 infected women for maternal health and interventions to reduce perinatal HIV-1 transmission in the United States* [On-line]. Available at: http://hivatis.org/guidelines/perinatal/Nov_00/text/index.html.

40. Centers for Disease Control and Prevention. (1998). Public Health Service Task Force recommendations for the use of antiretroviral drugs in pregnant women infected with HIV-1 for maternal health and for reducing perinatal HIV-1 transmission in the United States. *Morbidity and Mortality Weekly Report, 47*(RR-2), 1–31.

41. American College of Obstetricians and Gynecologist. (2000, May). *ACOG committee opinion: Scheduled cesarean delivery and the prevention of vertical transmission of HIV infection* [On-line]. Available at: www.acog.com/publications/committee_opinions/bco234.htm.

42. Wade, N. A., Birkhead, G. S., Warren, B. L., Charbonneau, T. T., French, P. T., Wang, L., Baum, J. B., Tesoriero, J. M., & Savicki, R. (1998). Abbreviated regimens of zidovudine prophylaxis and perinatal transmission of human immunodeficiency virus. *New England Journal of Medicine, 339,* 1409.

43. Saba, J. (1999, February). *Interim analysis of early efficacy of three short ZVD/3TC combination regimens to prevent mother-to-child transmissions of HIV-1: The PETRA trial* [6th Conference on Retroviruses and Opportunistic Infections]. Chicago.

44. Miotti, P. G., Taha, T. E., Kumwenda, N. I., Broadhead, R., Mtimavalye, L. A., Van der Hoeven, L., Chiphangwi, J. D., Liomba, G., & Biggar, R. J. (1999). HIV transmission through breastfeeding: a study in Malawi. *Journal of the American Medical Association, 282,* 744–749.

45. Nduati, R., John, G., Mbori-Ngacha, D., Richardson, B., Overbaugh, J., Mwatha, A., Ndinya-Achola, J., Bwayo, J., Onyango, F. E., Hughes, J., & Kreiss, J. (2000). Effect of breastfeeding and formula feeding on transmission of HIV-1: A randomized clinical trial. *Journal of the American Medical Association, 283,* 1167–1174.

46. American Academy of Pediatrics. (1997). AAP policy statement: Breastfeeding and the use of human milk. *Pediatrics, 100*(6), 1035–1039. Available at: www.aap.org/policy/re9729.htm.

47. American College of Obstetricians and Gynecologist. (2000, July). *ACOG news release: ACOG issues guidelines on breastfeeding* [On-line]. Available at: www.acog.org/from_home/publications/press_releases/nr07-01-00.htm.

48. WHO, UNAIDS, & UNICEF. (1998). *Technical consultation on HIV and infant feedings, Geneva* [On-line]. Available at: www.unaids.org/publications/documents/mtct/meetrev.html.

49. The Linkages Project. (1998). *Frequently asked questions on breastfeeding and HIV/AIDS* [On-line]. Available at: http://linkagesproject.org/FAQ_Html/FAQ_HIV.htm.

50. Minkoff, H. (1998). HIV and women and pregnancy: the relationship of pregnancy to HIV disease. *Immunology and Allergy Clinics of North America, 18*(2), 329–344.

51. Brettle, R. P., Raab, G. M., Ross, A., Fielding, K. L., Gore, S. M., & Bird, A. G. (1995). HIV infection in women: Immunological markers and the influence of pregnancy. *AIDS, 9,* 1177–1184.

52. O'Sullivan, M., Lai, S., Yasin, S., & Hefgott, A. (1995). The effect of pregnancy on lymphocyte counts in HIV infected women. HIV Infectious Women Conference S20. February 22–24, 1995.

53. Burns, D., Landesman, S., Minkoff, H., Wright, D. J., Waters, D., Mitchell, R. M., Rubinstein, A., Willoughby, A., & Goedert, J. J. (1998). The influence of pregnancy on human immunodeficiency virus type-1 infection: Antepartum and postpartum changes in human immunodeficiency virus type-1 viral load. *American Journal of Obstetrics and Gynecology, 178,* 355–359.

54. De Vicenzi, I., Jadand, C., Couturier, E., Brunet, J. B., Gallais, H., Gastaut, J. A., Goujard, C., Deveau, C., & Meyer, L. (1997). Pregnancy and contraception in a French cohort of HIV-infected women: SEROCO Study Group. *AIDS, 11*(3), 333–338.

55. De Cock, K. M., Zadi, F., Adjorlolo, G., Diallo, M. O., Sassan-Morokro, M., Ekpini, E., Sibailly, T., Doorly, R., Batter, V., Brattegaard, K., & Gayle, H. (1994). Retrospective study of maternal HIV-1 and HIV-2 infection and child survival in Abidjan, Cote d'Ivoire. *British Medical Journal, 308,* 441–443.

56. Moye, J., Jr., Rich, K. C., Kalish, L. A., Sheon, A. R., Diaz, C., Cooper, E. R., Pitt, J., & Handelsman, E. (1996). Natural history of somatic growth in infants born to women infected by human immunodeficiency virus: Women and infants transmission study group. *Journal of Pediatrics, 128*(58), 58–69.

57. Hanson, C. (1998). HIV and women and pregnancy: Effect of HIV infection on pregnancy outcome. *Immunology and Allergy Clinics of North America, 18*(2), 345–353.

58. Landers, D., Martinez de Tejada, B., & Coye, B. (1997). HIV disease in pregnancy. Immunology of HIV in pregnancy: The effect of each on the other. *Obstetrics and Gynecology Clinics, 24*(4), 821–831.

59. Libman, H. (1999, January). *Beth Israel Deaconess Medical Center: Healthcare associates HIV guidelines—Immunizations in HIV-infected adults.* Available at: http://clinical.caregroup.org/guidelines/hiv/hivvactable1.htm. Accessed January 20, 2001.

60. Connor, E., Sperling, R. S., Gelber, R., & the Pediatric AIDS Clinical Trials Group Protocol 076 Study Group (1994). Reduction of maternal-infant transmission of human immunodeficiency virus type 1 with zidovudine treatment: Pediatric AIDS Clinical Trials Group Protocol 076 Study Group. *New England Journal of Medicine, 331,* 1173–1180.

61. ATIS. (2000). *Guidelines for the use of antiretroviral agents in HIV-infected adults and adolescents* [On-line]. Available at: www.thebody.com/hivatis/agents1/agents01.html.

62. Glaxo Wellcome Inc. (2000). *Antiretroviral pregnancy registry.* Available at: www.glaxowellcome.com/preg_reg/antiretroviral.html. Accessed January 20, 2001.

63. Semprini, A. E., Castagna, C., Ravizza, M., Fiore, S., Savasi, V., Muggiasca, M. L., Grossi, E., Guerra, B., Tibaldi, C., Scaravelli, G., et al. (1995). The incidence of complications after cesarean section in 156 HIV-positive women. *AIDS, 9,* 913–917.

64. Bryson, Y., Luzuriaga, K., Sullivan, J., & Wara, D. (1993). Proposed definitions for in utero versus intrapartum transmission of HIV-1. *New England Journal of Medicine, 327,* 1246–1247.

65. The Working Group. (2000). *Guidelines for the use of antiretroviral agents in pediatric HIV infection* [On-line]. Available at: www.thebody.com/hivatis/pediatric/ped1.html.

66. Centers for Disease Control and Prevention. (1988). Perspectives in disease prevention and health promotion update: Universal precautions for prevention of transmission of human immunodeficiency virus, hepatitis B virus, and other bloodborne pathogens in health-care settings. *Morbidity and Mortality Weekly Report, 37*(24), 377–388.

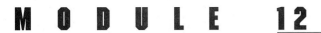

MODULE 12

*Hepatitis B
Infection:
Maternal–Newborn
Management*

*(Hepatitis A and C
addressed)*

E. JEAN MARTIN

A word to the reader:
This topic is extremely complex. Understanding the concepts presented might take several thought-
ful readings. DO NOT become discouraged if on the first read-through you feel a bit overwhelmed.
This will probably be the experience of many. Regarding the diagnostic markers, keep relating the
antigens to the schematic drawing of the virus. Try to see them in the context of being pieces of
the virus. Appreciate that each antigen is capable of inducing a physiologic immune response in
an individual, which gives rise to a unique antibody. The antigens and/or antibodies are referred
to as serologic markers because most of them can be identified by laboratory analysis of exposed
individuals' blood. Some readers might not feel the need to master the diagnostic interpretation of
the serologic markers. Knowing the risk factors, clinical features, and implications for care in vari-
ous settings may suffice. However, if your level of practice requires an interpretation of laboratory
reports, you do need to understand the significance of serologic markers in the report or in the pa-
tient's history.

The sad truth is that this disease will be with us for a while, so it behooves health care professionals
to stay informed.

OBJECTIVES

As you complete this module, you will learn:

1. The distinctions between major forms of viral hepatitis (hepatitis A, B, C, D, and E), that is, how to distinguish each form according to infecting organism, mode of transmission, diagnostic workup, and risks during pregnancy
2. To identify forms of viral hepatitis that can confer a carrier state
3. Immunization recommendations for hepatitis A viral infection, including implications for pregnant women
4. Important information about hepatitis C: epidemiology, pathophysiology, causes of the disease, risk factors, diagnosis, treatments, and implications for pregnant women
5. How hepatitis B antigens and antibodies are used in laboratory tests to identify individuals who are acutely infected, immune, or carriers
6. Facts about the course of hepatitis B disease, including the timing and sequence of serologic titers beginning with exposure
7. The epidemiology of the hepatitis B carrier state
8. Diagnostic markers for the carrier state
9. Transmission risks for the fetus and newborn when the pregnant woman has acute hepatitis B or is a carrier
10. To identify those woman who are at high risk of being hepatitis B carriers
11. Clinical implications for mother and fetus during the antepartum period
12. About products for active and/or passive immunization: hepatitis B vaccines and hepatitis B immune globulin
13. Facts about hepatitis B vaccine and recommendations by the Centers for Disease Control and Prevention (CDC) for preexposure immunization
14. CDC recommendations for appropriate hepatitis B status screening in pregnant women
15. Recommendations for hepatitis B screening in women being admitted to the labor unit
16. Risk of hepatitis B transmission to health care personnel and precautions that medical and nursing personnel need to take while caring for the hepatitis B carrier woman in the perinatal setting

17. Nursing care of the mother and newborn during labor, during delivery, and postpartum
18. Treatments and precautions to use in reducing hepatitis B transmission to the newborn
19. Current breastfeeding recommendations for the hepatitis B–infected mother
20. CDC recommendations for immunization treatment of individuals needing preexposure or postexposure immunization for hepatitis A and hepatitis B:
    a. Preexposure immunization
       - Newborns
       - Adolescents
       - Adults
       - Pregnant or lactating women
    b. CDC recommendations for employees in exposure-prone occupations
    c. CDC recommendations for hepatitis B and hepatitis C exposure
    d. Nonresponder management guidelines
    e. Booster recommendations

KEY TERMS

When you have completed this module, you should be able to recall the meaning of the following terms. You should also be able to use the terms when consulting with other health professionals. An understanding of the terms will be important in interpreting prenatal and neonatal laboratory results. The terms are defined in this module or in the glossary at the end of this book.

alanine aminotransferase (ALT)	inoculate
antibody	lochia
antigen	nosocomial infections
aspartate aminotransferase (AST)	plasma-derived vaccine
carrier	prevalence
Engerix-B (Engerix-B, Pediatric/ Adolescent)	Recombivax HB (Recombivax HB, Pediatric)
Havrix	seronegative
hepatitis B immune globulin (HBIG)	seroprotective
hepatocellular carcinoma	serous exudates
horizontal transmission	serum
immune serum globulin (ISG)	Vaqta
immunization	vertical transmission

The topic of hepatitis infection, its various forms, and how it can affect a pregnancy outcome is a complex one. Several terms needed for a clear understanding of this module's content are defined here. You may want to refer to these definitions throughout this module until you become familiar with them.

Terms to Know
- **Antigen**—a substance that, when introduced in a host, is capable of inducing the production of antibodies. An antigen can be introduced into the host, or it can be formed within the body. Bacteria and viruses are examples of antigens.

- **Antibody**—protein substances developed by the body in response to the presence of an antigen. Antibodies are produced to inhibit or destroy the antigen and are a defense against foreign substances such as bacteria and viruses.
- **Carrier**—an individual who harbors a pathogen and is capable of transmitting a disease caused by this pathogen to another person. Often, carriers do not experience any significant illness and have no idea that they are capable of spreading the disease.
- **Plasma**—the fluid part of blood.
- **Serum**—that fluid part of blood that remains after clotting has occurred.
- **Inoculate**—to introduce a substance (the inoculum) into the body, which can produce a disease or an immunity to the disease, depending on the circumstances and the substance. The inoculate is sometimes a cultured substance.

Facts About the Major Hepatitis Infections

■ What is viral hepatitis?

Viral hepatitis has the following characteristics:

- It is an infection that occurs in the liver.
- The clinical features in each type of viral hepatitis are similar and are uniquely derived from the consequences of liver cell injury.
- Jaundice, low-grade fever, abdominal pain, or "flulike" symptoms may or may not accompany hepatitis infection. Most people do not develop clinically apparent disease.
- It can exist as an acute or a chronic disease.
- Viral hepatitis is a major cause of death and morbidity in third world countries.
- Infection can occur any time during pregnancy.
- Hepatitis A, B, and D viral infections can be prevented by immunization in most cases.
- Vaccines do not exist for hepatitis C or E.
- Hepatitis is a major public health problem.
- Chronic liver disease is the tenth leading cause of death among adults in the United States.

Viral hepatitis diseases differ in mode of transmission, diagnostic criteria, pathophysiology, and infectivity states and how they can affect people in disease outcome. Five major forms of hepatitis exist, all of which are caused by a virus or "viruslike" particles:

- Hepatitis A virus (HAV), formerly known as "infectious hepatitis"
- Hepatitis B virus (HBV), formerly known as "serum hepatitis"
- Hepatitis C virus (HCV), formerly known as "non-A, non-B"
- Hepatitis D virus (HDV), known as "delta hepatitis"
- Hepatitis E virus (HEV)

> **NOTE:** *Other viral agents such as the herpes simplex virus (HSV), cytomegalovirus (CMV), and Epstein-Barr virus (EBV) can cause acute liver disease but are not included in this module.*

HAV and HEV initially enter the body by way of the gut, where they begin to multiply. HBV, HCV, and HDV enter the body via the bloodstream, eventually passing to the liver, where they begin to reproduce. The body's immune response to any of these viruses residing in the liver is to produce inflammation, thereby setting up the potential of mild or severe liver damage.

With HBV infection, the liver is usually able to repair itself readily. However, with HCV infection, resolution of liver damage may not occur. Over many years, unresolved damage may lead to severe liver pathology. Therefore, the quality of life resulting from these two viral infections is usually very different.

Although this module is especially concerned with the impact of HBV on pregnant women and newborns, considerable content has been added on HAV and HCV.

Hepatitis A, C, D, and E

Hepatitis A (HAV) Infection[1-4]

- In the United States, about one third of acute hepatitis cases are caused by HAV.
- In the United States, the incidence of acute HAV infection in pregnancy is approximately 1 per 1,000. Pregnant women at greatest risk are those who have recently traveled to or emigrated from developing nations such as Southeast Asia, Africa, Central America, Mexico, and the Middle East, where HAV infection is endemic.[5]
- This disease is spread through the fecal–oral route, usually by person-to-person contact (i.e., horizontal transmission) or ingestion of contaminated food or water.
- Outbreaks are common in winter and spring.
- The incubation period averages 28 days (15 to 50 days).
- Transmission by blood transfusion or injection is rare.
- Risk factors for HAV infection include personal contact with infected individuals (26%), employment in a day care center (14%), intravenous drug use (11%), travel to an area where HAV infection is prevalent (4%), and consumption of food or water contaminated with feces (3%).[2]
- Acute infection is diagnosed by the identification of antibody IgM anti-HAV in the individual's blood (serum). This is always present at the first sign of the disease and remains present for several months to a year.
- IgG anti-HAV develops during convalescence. This antibody persists and is responsible for the individual's subsequent immunity to HAV infection.
- There is no chronic carrier state that can transmit HAV to others after recovery from acute infection.
- HAV infection in pregnant women is generally no more severe than in nonpregnant women.
- There is no evidence that this viral infection is teratogenic in pregnancy.
- Pregnancy can be complicated by poor outcomes from this disease in vulnerable populations in third world countries. Perinatal and maternal morbidity can be increased.
- Pregnant women exposed to HAV should be given human serum immunoglobulin containing antibodies to the virus (confers passive immunization).
- Hepatitis A vaccines contain formalin-inactivated virus and *are safe for use in pregnant women* (active immunization). Two vaccines, called Havrix and Vaqta, were released in 1995. They both require two doses. A single dose provides immunity for 1 year. A booster dose administered 6 to 12 months after the initial injection provides protection for approximately 15 years.

Immunization Recommendations[1]

Current recommendations include routine hepatitis A vaccination of children in states, countries, and communities with infection rates that are twice the 1987 to 1997 national average or greater (greater than or equal to 20 cases per 100,000 population) and consideration of routine vaccination of children in states, countries, and communities with rates exceeding the 1987 to 1997 national average (greater than or equal to 10 but no less than 20 cases per 100,000 population). This is expected to reduce the overall incidence of HAV infection.

NOTE: Hepatitis A immunization in selected populations may begin with 24-month-old infants through to young adulthood at 18 years of age. Local public health authorities should be consulted for policy and practice.

Recommendations for vaccinating individuals in groups known to be at high risk for HAV infection remain a focus. This includes travelers to countries with high or intermediate infections incidence, men who have sex with men, persons with occupational risk exposure (e.g., certain research laboratories, sewage disposal personnel), injecting drug users, persons with clotting disorders, persons with chronic liver disease, and children living in communities with high rates of the disease.

Hepatitis C (HCV) Infection[4,6-8]

HCV infection is a major cause of acute and chronic hepatitis, both of which are asymptomatic in most individuals.

Epidemiology

Worldwide, it is estimated that 170 million people are infected (3% of the world's population)—many of whom have no idea they are infected. In some endemic regions of the world (e.g., Egypt), prevalence rates range from 10% to 30%. The CDC reports a seroprevalence rate in the United States of 4 million chronically infected Americans.[7] The incidence rate in the United States is 200,000 new infections each year, and about 30% of these are symptomatic. Approximately 8,000 to 10,000 deaths from chronic HCV infection occur yearly.[7]

Pregnancy

Seroprevalence rates among the pregnant population have been found to range from 1.9% to 5.2% in reported studies. Lower rates are found among the private patient population.[4] Vertical transmission rates (pregnant mother to newborn) are reported to be around 6% in HIV-negative women. Investigators find significantly higher rates of transmission (14% to 17%) in women coinfected with HIV. This is thought to be due to higher maternal hepatitis C viremia.[7]
NOTE: Maternal antibodies to HCV (anti-HCV) are not protective!

Perinatal outcomes appear to be no different than among mothers who do not have the infection. Universal screening is not recommended.

Breastfeeding

The average rate of HCV infection in both bottle-fed and breastfed infants is 4%. It appears that breastfeeding does not appreciably increase transmission risk to the newborn.[7,8]

Transmission

Transmission modes appear to be the same as for HBV infections, that is, parenteral; contact with infected blood (as in intravenous drug blood use); and use of contaminated needles, razors, tattoo equipment, acupuncture needles, and shared straw use among cocaine users. It is not nearly as easily spread through sexual contact as is HBV infection. Health care workers are at risk through needlesticks and other exposures.

Blood transfusion was a significant source of HCV transmission before 1992, at which time routine screening of blood donors was initiated. Blood transfusion from an anti-HCV–positive donor results in very high infectivity for recipients (more than 80%). Since the advent of rigorous screening procedures, transfusion transmission in the United States is very low. However, the risk is not 0%; one source states a 4% transmission risk.[6]

Infection

There are 10 or more types and numerous subtypes of this virus, some of which appear uniquely in different geographic regions of the world. Most infected individuals are not symptomatic, and most do not know they are infected. Symptoms are the same as with HBV infection. Sequelae are very serious in that 75% to 85% of infected persons develop chronic infection and a very high percentage (about 70%) develop chronic liver disease, eventually leading to the need for transplantation or to death. The likelihood of developing chronic HCV infection is a function of the following:

- Viral genotype (certain types are correlated with high chronicity rates)
- Mode of acquisition (e.g., a transfusion with HCV-contaminated blood is associated with a greater risk of chronic infection versus a lower risk with a small amount of inoculate involved in illicit drug use)
- Host immune response (the more vigorous the antibody and T-cell responses to severe acute infections, the more likely there will be a spontaneous resolution of the infection)[6]

Serologic Markers

Infection with HCV results in the presence of unique serologic markers to indicate the virus' presence. Two major markers are actual viral material called HCV RNA and the antibody anti-HCV, produced by the host immunologic response. *Research indicates that a large percentage of anti-HCV–positive individuals do not clear HCV RNA; in other words, they are HCV RNA positive and can transmit the infection to others.*

Diagnosis

Diagnosis is made by detecting the antibody to hepatitis C through enzyme immunoassay (EIA). All positive EIA results are verified with a supplemental assay called the recombinant immunoblot assay (RIBA). Sensitivity is 97% or greater.[7] *This test does not distinguish between acute, chronic, or resolved infection.*

Another diagnostic test can be done to quantify or qualify the amount of HCV RNA by using gene amplification techniques (e.g., polymerase chain reaction [PCR]). The PCR process takes a very small amount of viral or bacterial content not detectable in usual laboratory analysis and multiplies the content to detectable levels. HCV RNA analysis measures a part of the hepatitis C virus.

The gold standard in diagnostic workup for individuals with HCV infection is a liver biopsy, especially when treatment is being considered for a person with suspected chronic hepatitis C.

Recommendations for routine testing for HCV are shown in Display 12.1. Postexposure follow-up recommendations are given in Display 12.2.

DISPLAY 12.1   Testing for Hepatitis C Virus

PERSONS WHO SHOULD BE TESTED ROUTINELY FOR HEPATITIS C VIRUS (HCV) INFECTION BASED ON THEIR RISK FOR INFECTION

- Persons who ever injected illegal drugs, including those who injected once or a few times many years ago and do not consider themselves as drug users
- Persons with selected medical conditions, including the following:
  –Persons who received clotting factor concentrates produced before 1987
  –Persons who were ever on chronic (long-term) hemodialysis
  –Persons with persistently abnormal alanine aminotransferase levels
- Prior recipients of transfusions or organ transplants, including the following:
  –Persons who were notified that they received blood from a donor who later tested positive for HCV infection
  –Persons who received a transfusion of blood or blood components before July 1992
  –Persons who received an organ transplant before July 1992

PERSONS WHO SHOULD BE TESTED ROUTINELY FOR HCV INFECTION BASED ON A RECOGNIZED EXPOSURE

- Health care, emergency medical, and public safety workers after needlesticks, sharps, or mucosal exposures to HCV-positive blood
- Children born to HCV-positive women

PERSONS FOR WHOM ROUTINE HCV TESTING IS NOT RECOMMENDED

- Health care, emergency medical, and public safety workers
- Pregnant women
- Household (nonsexual) contacts of HCV-positive persons
- The general population

Reprinted with permission from Centers for Disease Control and Prevention. (1998). Recommendations for prevention and control of hepatitis C virus (HCV) infection and HCV-related chronic disease. *MMWR Morbidity and Mortality Weekly Report, 47*(RR-19), 21, 24.

DISPLAY 12.2   Postexposure Follow-up

POSTEXPOSURE FOLLOW-UP OF HEALTH CARE, EMERGENCY MEDICAL, AND PUBLIC SAFETY WORKERS FOR HEPATITIS C VIRUS (HCV) INFECTION

- For the source, baseline testing for anti-HCV
- For the person exposed to an HCV-positive source, baseline and follow-up testing, including the following:
  –Baseline testing for anti-HCV and ALT activity
  –Follow-up testing for anti-HCV (e.g., at 4–6 months) and ALT activity (If earlier diagnosis of HCV infection is desired, testing for HCV RNA may be performed at 4–6 weeks.)
- Confirmation by supplemental anti-HCV testing of all anti-HCV results reported as positive by enzyme immunoassay

Reprinted with permission from Centers for Disease Control and Prevention. (1998). Recommendations for prevention and control of hepatitis C virus (HCV) infection and HCV-related chronic disease. *MMWR Morbidity and Mortality Weekly Report, 47*(RR-19), 24.

Treatment

Current treatments with interferon–ribavirin combinations are having encouraging success. However therapies are fairly toxic and accompanied by severe side effects. "Cure" is currently defined as a loss of detectable HCV RNA in serum using a sensitive PCR assay at least 6 months after cessation of therapy.

Currently, there are insufficient data to recommend treatment of acute HCV infection. HCV-positive persons should be referred for ongoing evaluation to detect the presence or development of chronic disease and treatment according to current practice guidelines. Counseling is needed to prevent further liver damage. Counseling for reducing the risks of HCV transmission to others is critical.[7]

Immunization

No vaccine exists for hepatitis C. Development of a vaccine is complicated by the fact that antibodies to HCV are not protective against the infection. In addition, the virus has a rapid mutation rate, especially when under efforts to eradicate it (i.e., during treatment).

Hepatitis D (HDV) Infection (Delta Hepatitis)[2,4]

The virus was named "delta" virus, hence hepatitis D. It is caused by a defective virus that can replicate and cause infection only in the presence of an active HBV infection; therefore, it never outlasts HBV infection. HDV infection occurs worldwide but is most common in nations bordering the Mediterranean Sea and is less common in the United States. It exists as an acute coinfection acquired simultaneously with hepatitis B, or it can be a superinfection in a chronic hepatitis B carrier and can produce more severe disease.

HDV is diagnosed in the following ways:

- By detecting the antibody to the delta virus antigen (anti-HDV) in blood
- By liver biopsy, which identifies the delta antigen
- By identifying the IgM antibody to the hepatitis D virus in blood

HDV is transmitted by exposure to blood and blood products and by sexual contact (similar to HBV transmission). It is most prevalent in intravenous drug users, patients with hemophilia, and patients who have received multiple blood transfusions. It is highly infectious and associated with serious illness.

Hepatitis B vaccination usually protects against hepatitis D. There is no cure for or prevention of HDV infection in hepatitis B carriers.

Hepatitis E (HEV) Infection[2,4,5]

Hepatitis E is an enteric disease associated with large epidemics from sewage-contaminated food and water. It is widespread in developing countries, such as India, Southeast Asia, Africa, and South America. The disease is characterized by acute infection similar to that of hepatitis A and affects primarily persons of childbearing age (ages 15 to 40). Hepatitis E does not exist as a chronic infection. The development of antibodies to the hepatitis E antigen (IgG anti-HEV) confers immunity.

Although the disease is usually characterized by a mild illness, there is a high mortality rate for fulminant hepatic failure in pregnant women. The reason for this is unknown. Infection in the third trimester of pregnancy is associated with an increased incidence of fetal complications. Neonates die from HEV infection much more than from any other type of viral hepatitis. Vertical transmission of HEV has been reported.[5]

Acute infection can be diagnosed by a positive serum test for IgM anti-HEV antibody, but this test is not available in most laboratories, especially in developing countries. Diagnosis is made by the signs and symptoms of liver disease, excluding other causes such as HAV, HBV, cytomegalovirus, and Epstein-Barr virus.

Hepatitis B (HBV) Infection

Hepatitis B infection is caused by the hepatitis B virus. It is found in liver cells (hepatocytes), where it replicates (reproduces itself). The virus also travels to the bloodstream. Infection often goes unrecognized.

Epidemiology[9,10]

More than 1.25 million people are chronically infected with HBV *in the United States alone.* The annual number of new infections is 335,000. Estimates are that chronic hepatitis B results in 4,000 deaths annually from cirrhosis and 800 deaths from hepatocellular carcinoma.[10]

The prevalence (number of existing infections in a given population over 1 year) differs greatly among countries, ethnic groups, and ages. For example, drawing from a national health survey under vital statistics in 1992, the infection rate (present or past) in the United States is 3% for Whites, 12% for Blacks, 3% for Mexican Americans, and 17% for Asian Pacific Islanders, Native Americans, and Native Alaskans.[10]

Clinical Features[9,10]

Clinical features of HBV infection include the following:

- The virus has been found in body fluids such as saliva, menstrual and vaginal discharge, semen, colostrum, breast milk, and serous exudates. These have been implicated as vehicles of infection transmission.[9] There is no evidence that the infection is spread by an airborne route.[9]
- The incubation period ranges from 14 to 180 days.
- Most patients have no symptoms.
- One third of patients with symptoms have jaundice (evident in the skin and eyes).
- Some individuals will experience fatigue, lassitude, loss of appetite, nausea, vomiting, and/or abdominal pain.
- Occasionally, joint pain (arthralgia) and a rash can be present.
- The symptoms are often misdiagnosed as "the flu," especially if no jaundice is present.
- Liver enzymes, **alanine aminotransferase** (ALT) and **aspartate aminotransferase** (AST), are elevated (e.g., above 1,000 U/mL in the acute phase of viral hepatitis).
- Acute infection generally runs its course over a 3- to-4 week period, but symptoms can remain for as long as 6 months.
- For pregnant women, the disease generally does not assume any greater virulence, but there are serious implications for transmission to the newborn.
- In vulnerable populations, such as third world counties, fulminant hepatitis B results in increased perinatal and maternal mortality.
- When individuals develop the disease (symptomatic or not), they experience complete resolution or they might retain the virus in their bodies in a chronic state. Individuals who retain the virus in a chronic state are at risk for two potential situations:
  1. They are chronic active hepatitis carriers who can transmit the disease to others under certain conditions.
  2. They are at risk for developing cirrhosis and/or hepatocellular carcinoma (cancer of the liver).

Mothers who develop the disease (symptomatic or not) might recover completely, or they might retain the virus in their bodies in a chronic state. These hepatitis B carriers can transmit the disease to others, including the newborn.

Diagnosis

■ **What laboratory tests are used to diagnose hepatitis B active disease or carrier status?**

Identifying the antigens and antibodies for HBV that are found in the blood of infected individuals confirms that the individual is:

- In the active disease state
  or
- A carrier
  or
- Immune

HBV contains three antigens. These antigens are protein particles that derive from the virus, as shown in Figure 12.1. When found in blood, they are called *serologic markers*. As you study the following antigen names and characteristics, refer to Figure 12.1 to identify from where they derive.

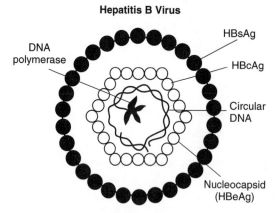

Hepatitis B Virus

DNA polymerase

HBsAg

HBcAg

Circular DNA

Nucleocapsid (HBeAg)

HBV Antigen Serologic Markers

Hepatitis B surface antigen **(HBsAg)**—protein coat

Hepatitis B core antigen **(HBcAg)**—core of the virus

Hepatitis B e antigen **(HBeAg)**—part of the core

> Study these abbreviations so that you know exactly what each stands for as you read on.

FIGURE 12.1 Hepatitis B virus and serologic markers.

Hepatitis B Antigens

Hepatitis B Surface Antigen (HBsAg)
- Is the protein coat of the virus
- Is detectable in large quantities in serum because more HBsAg is produced than is needed to cover the core
- Can be present in the absence of any symptoms of the disease
- Has several subtypes detectable only in research laboratories
- Is associated with chronic hepatitis B and denotes a carrier state when its presence persists in blood

> *Laboratory studies of blood serum can identify the presence of HBsAg in infected persons. This is one of the earliest indications of HBV infection.*

> *The persistent presence of HBsAg in serum is associated with chronic hepatitis B.*

Hepatitis B Core Antigen (HBcAg)
- Comes from the center, or core, of the virus
- Is not found in the blood, and therefore, no commercial test is available to detect this antigen in infected persons; is located in the nuclei of liver cells (hepatocytes)
- Can be detected by a liver biopsy

> HBcAg cannot be found in the blood serum of infected persons.

Hepatitis B e Antigen (HBeAg)
- Is found only in association with the surface antigen HBsAg in the blood
- Evidence suggests that it derives from the core antigen or a breakdown product of the core antigen
- Its presence correlates with high titers of hepatitis B viral DNA and an increased infectivity state

> *HBeAg is found in serum during the early part of the acute phase of the infection and then disappears. This antigen is never found alone. It always occurs after HBsAg is present and the infection state has begun.*

> *Laboratory studies of blood serum can identify the presence of HBeAg in infected persons.*

> *If a pregnant women has HBsAg in her blood at the time of birthing, she has HBV infection. She may not have symptoms. If the mother is positive for only HBsAg, the rate of transmission to the baby who is not immunized is about 10% to 20%.[5]*

> *If a pregnant woman has both HBsAg and HBeAg at the time of birthing, the risk of perinatal transmission of HBV to her infant, if not immunized, is approximately 90%.[5,9]*

> MORE THAN 90% OF WOMEN FOUND TO BE HBsAg POSITIVE ON ROUTINE SCREENING WILL BE HEPATITIS B CARRIERS.[11]

Antigen levels tend to be high in early and midstages of a disease and then fall to levels so low that they cannot be detected by laboratory examination. During the recovery phase of HBV infection, HBsAg is cleared and not detectable.

Hepatitis B Antibodies

Most individuals infected with HBV are capable of producing antibodies against the viral antigens. Because three **antigens** have been identified, it is not surprising to learn that there are three **antibodies** that the human body can produce against the antigens. These antibodies also can be detected in blood and are referred to as *serologic markers*.

Combinations of antigen and antibodies tell us whether an individual is:

- Infectious
    or
- A carrier
    or
- Immune

HBV Antibody Serologic Markers:
Antibody to HBsAg (**anti-HBs**)

Antibody to HBcAg (**anti-HBc**)

Antibody to HBeAg (**anti-HBe**)

> Study these abbreviations so that you know exactly what each stands for as you read on.

Antibody to the Surface Antigen (Anti-HBs)

Anti-HBs can be present 2 to 6 weeks after the disappearance of HBsAg. The surface antigen (HBsAg) and surface antibody (anti-HBs) do NOT exist together. Study Figure 12.2 to see the timing and rise and fall of titers for these two markers. Note: an exceptioin to this diagram (and laboratory findings) occur in the presence of both a subtype HBsAg and an anti-HBs produced from a different subtype. In such occasional situations both markers could exist together.

> When anti-HBs is found alone without HBsAg, the individual:
>
> - Has developed immunity to the disease
> - Is not infectious
> - Is not a carrier

Antibody to the Core Antigen (Anti-HBc) [12]

- Can be easily detected in blood
- Appears in blood around the time of onset of symptoms
- Refers to one or both immunoglobulins (i.e., IgM and IgG)
- Can indicate a convalescent stage after acute infection
  - This period lasts for several weeks but can persist for several months or more before anti-HBs develops.
- Can, in rare instances, be passively transferred to adults during a blood transfusion
  - With current blood screens, this no longer occurs. Persons with passively acquired anti-HBs are not infectious and should receive vaccine if indicated.
- Can persist alone in a chronic pattern and can indicate a low-level carrier state
  - Such persons are presumably minimally contagious.
- **According to the CDC:**
  "In settings where small amounts of blood or body secretions are transferred, such as in needlesticks or sexual and household exposures, persons with anti-HBc alone can be considered noninfectious, and their contacts do not need postexposure prophylaxis or vaccine." [12]

Sometimes neither the hepatitis B surface antigen (HBsAg), the hepatitis B e antigen (HBeAg), nor the antibodies for these are found in blood serum. However, if the hepatitis B core antibody is found, it is evidence that the individual has encountered the hepatitis B virus. The antibody to hepatitis B core antigen is the only factor that is detectable by laboratory studies during all phases of the infection.

The presence of the antibody to hepatitis B core antigen (anti-HBc):
- Can remain for an individual's lifetime
- Can indicate a carrier state postinfection if the hepatitis B surface antigen (HBsAg) is also present
- Can indicate the possibility of passing the infection on to the baby at birth if the surface antigen (HBsAg) is present

---

Antibody to the Hepatitis B e Antigen (Anti-HBe)

- Appearance of this antibody occurs as levels of HBsAg are diminishing and the disease is resolving.
- This antibody develops in most hepatitis B infections.
- It can persist along with HBsAg in the carrier state.
- The presence of anti-HBe correlates with low levels of hepatitis viral DNA.

Timing and Titers in Hepatitis B Virus Infection

Figure 12.2 demonstrates the timing and sequence of titers in the majority of patients with acute HBV infection who go on to resolution with resulting immunity. Immunity is indicated by the sustained rise in the antibody to the surface antigen (anti-HBs) and/or core antibody (anti-HBc). Study the graph carefully and, as you do, try to relate the following facts correlating with the graph.

- The incubation period is long, varying from 14 to 180 days and averaging about 120 days.
- Symptoms do not appear for at least 1 to 3 months after exposure.
- Symptoms, if present, can last for several weeks.
- HBsAg can be identified in blood anywhere from 1 to 2 months after exposure.
- HBeAg appears after HBsAg *and never exists without the presence of HBsAg.*
- The presence of HBeAg is associated with high levels of circulating HBsAg. This indicates a highly infectious state.
- By the time symptoms appear, it is usually possible to detect HBsAg and HBeAg in blood.
- Detectable levels of HBsAg generally disappear by 6 months after exposure.

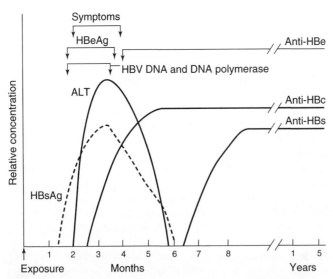

FIGURE 12.2 Course of hepatitis B disease. (Adapted with permission from Cohen, M., & Cohen, H. [1990]. Current recommendations for viral hepatitis. *Contemporary OB/GYN, 35*[11], 65.)

- The antibody to the core antigen, anti-HBc, begins to appear during the acute viremic phase (high virus levels), can be detected easily, and can persist for an individual's lifetime.
- The antibody to the e antigen, anti-HBe, appears before the production of the surface antibody, anti-HBs, but after production of anti-HBc; it can persist indefinitely.
- The appearance of anti-HBs does not occur until many weeks or months after the appearance and eventual disappearance of HBsAg. Titers for the surface antigen and antibody do not exist together. This antibody (anti-HBs) indicates that the individual has developed an immunity to hepatitis B infection. The antibody can persist for a lifetime.
- Diminishing of anti-HBs after a resolved infection to below-detectable levels can occur over many years, but immunity is believed to be retained ("immune memory").
- HBV is associated with several serologic subtypes and is now known to have mutations associated with its replication. This may be related to recurrent disease, failure to clear the virus, or altered response to therapy in chronic infection.[3]

Carrier State[9,10,13,14]

> ■ **How serious is the carrier state, and what impact does it have on pregnancy?**

An estimated 400 million people worldwide are carriers of HBV.[10] Carriers have the potential of transmitting the disease to others under certain circumstances. In the United States, more than 1.25 million people are chronically infected.[10] Carriers have a 12 to 30 times higher risk of developing primary liver cancer than noncarriers. Approximately 800 people die from hepatocellular carcinoma each year. An even larger number, 4,000 persons, die yearly from HBV infection–related cirrhosis, and 350 die of fulminant hepatic failure (i.e., rapid, overwhelming system involvement within a few days to weeks).[10]

The patterns of transmission and prevalence of hepatitis B carrier states vary markedly in geographic locations. In areas where the disease is highly prevalent, perinatal transmission is the primary transmission route. In low endemic areas, sexual contact in the high-risk adult population is the predominant route. The disease is highly endemic in China, Southeast Asia, most of Africa, most Pacific Islands, the Middle East, and the Amazon Basin. The infection is acquired at birth or during childhood in these areas. An estimated 8% to 15% of the population becomes chronic carriers. However, in the United States, Western Europe, and Australia, the infection is contracted primarily during adulthood. The prevalence of the *carrier state* is much lower, at only 0.2% to 0.9%.[13]

Unfortunately, the risk of becoming chronically infected varies inversely with the age at which the infection occurs. Newborns who contract the disease have a 90% carrier rate, whereas the carrier rate of those infected before they are 5 years of age is between 25% and 50%. Only 6% to 10% of acutely infected adults become carriers.[13]

Hepatitis B Carriers[13,14]

- Hepatitis B carriers are unable to clear HBsAg from their blood, and they harbor the virus in a chronic state.
- They can have an intermittent but chronic symptomatic infection. These individuals have serologic evidence of HBsAg, constant or intermittent elevations of liver enzymes, and evidence of liver inflammation. Symptoms come and go, but liver biopsies reveal a chronic form of hepatitis.
- Carriers can be asymptomatic. This state is characterized by a "healthy" carrier who has no symptoms and usually has normal liver studies but continues to be HBsAg positive serologically. Liver biopsies show evidence of viral infection.
- These patients are frequently also immunocompromised (e.g., HIV-infected individuals).
- Carriers can include infants infected at birth, who have a high likelihood of becoming carriers.
- Typically, carriers have high titers of anti-HBc and *do not have anti-HBs.*
- Carriers who demonstrate the presence of HBeAg are considered to have a high degree of infectivity.

■ How is the carrier state diagnosed?

When detectable levels of HBsAg are found in an individual on at least two occasions, at least 6 months apart, that individual probably is a carrier. This means the individual will indefinitely be capable of transmitting the disease to others through blood and other body fluids and through sexual contact.

Certain immunoglobulins serve as serologic markers, which also denote infectiousness and the carrier state. Immunoglobulins are unique types of antibodies. Different antigens are capable of stimulating the body's production of immunoglobulins in response to foreign antigenic substances. These immunoglobulins or antibodies inactivate the foreign antigen as part of the body's defense system. Currently, five classes of antibodies (immunoglobulins) have been identified.

The two classes of immunoglobulins relevant to hepatitis B are called IgG and IgM.

NOTE: When a laboratory report identifies the presence of the antibody to the core antigen, anti-HBc, it refers to the "total" amount of anti-HBc. Depending on the individual's disease state, the "total" anti-HBc may contain either IgG or IgM antibodies or both. This is an important concept to understand as you read on about these two unique and different immunoglobulins, which serve as important diagnostic markers for the hepatitis B carrier state.

IgG Immunoglobulins

- These are the major immunoglobulins in the blood, comprising approximately 75% to 80% of the total antibodies in a normal individual. Because of relatively small molecular size, these are the only immunoglobulins capable of crossing the placenta.
- IgG immunoglobulins are protein complements specific to the antigen responsible for their production. Numerous IgG immunoglobulins exist for different diseases, including one for hepatitis B. It is referred to as **IgG anti-HBc. IgG blood levels of individuals exposed to a given antigen may remain present for years or a lifetime.** The presence of IgG to a specific antigen simply means that the individual has been exposed to that antigen (e.g., bacteria, virus).
- Because IgG is usually produced as a response to a disease, it is associated with resolving or postinfectious states and in many diseases signals postinfection immunity.

IgM Immunoglobulins

- These are the *first immunoglobulins produced during the body's immune response.*
- There are specific IgM complements for individual antigens, including one for hepatitis B, called **IgM anti-HBc.**
- IgM levels rise, peak, and fall within a few weeks or months of contracting a disease.
- IgM immunoglobulins serve as important markers for the acute phase of a disease.

Figure 12.3 represents a chronic carrier state with persisting HBsAg, HBeAg, and anti-HBc titers.

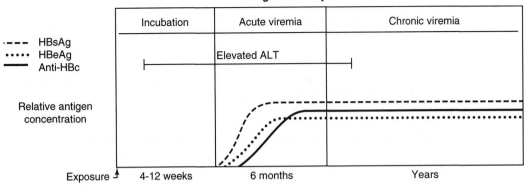

High Infectivity Potential

FACTS

*All three serologic markers persist: HBsAg, HBeAg, and Anti-HBc.

*It is the continued presence of HBeAg along with HBsAg that indicates high blood levels of HBsAg and therefore an elevated degree of infectivity.

*Liver enzymes (e.g., ALT) will be elevated in the chronic, active, and highly infectious carrier.

FIGURE 12.3 Hepatitis B titers of a chronic carrier.

The following additional serologic markers play a role in diagnosing the hepatitis B carrier state:

- IgM class of anti-HBc
- IgG class of anti-HBc

When patients have an *acute* or *recent* HBV infection, *the IgM class of anti-HBc is present* in the blood. However, if patients have the *chronic* form of the disease or have recovered from the acute disease, the IgM anti-HBc is absent and the *IgG class of anti-HBc is present.*
REMEMBER: *When a report identifies "anti-HBc," it refers to "total" anti-HBc. Depending on the patient's disease state (active or chronic), this "total" may include both IgM anti-HBc and IgG anti-HBc. The distinction is made by a laboratory order to identify the IgM anti-HBc marker.*

IgM Anti-HBc
- Is an immunoglobulin produced by the body's defense system early in the disease
- Is an immunoglobulin or antibody to the core antigen HBcAg
- Indicates recent infection with HBV
- Is detectable for several weeks to months after infection

NOTE: Absence of the IgM class antibody means there is no acute infectious process present.
To summarize:

A carrier is a person who is either HBsAg positive on at least two occasions at least 6 months apart or **who is anti-HBc positive and IgM anti-HBc negative when only a single blood serum specimen is tested.**[13]
CAUTION: Chronic active carriers who are having an exacerbation of the disease will test positive for IgM anti-HBc.

Care must be exercised when labeling an individual a carrier. Occasionally, 6 to 8 months may be required to clear the system of HBsAg. HBsAg-positive individuals should be tested after 6 months to establish chronicity.

■ **If the pregnant woman has had hepatitis B, will she necessarily be a carrier?**

Fortunately no. Sometimes individuals completely recover from the disease, and when tested, HBsAg and HBeAg are not present. These individuals are not carriers and will not transmit the disease.

■ How common is the infection in pregnant women?

Annually, approximately 22,000 women with chronic hepatitis B deliver infants in the United States. Approximately 0.1% to 0.5% of the population in the United States are carriers. However, in some populations, such as in Southeast Asia, the population carrier rate is 10% to 20%.[10]

Recent migrations to the United States of high-carrier populations, such as Vietnamese, Haitians, and Africans, might lead to an increased frequency of maternal hepatitis B encountered in perinatal units in the United States.

Hepatitis B is also a sexually transmitted disease. Recent epidemiologic studies indicate that male homosexuality, drug abuse, and heterosexual exposure with a hepatitis B carrier or with multiple partners account for the major modes of transmission in individuals.

> *One of the major risk factors for hepatitis B currently is intravenous drug abuse.*

> The proportion of individuals whose risk factor for hepatitis B is heterosexual exposure has increased.

■ Can pregnant women who have acute hepatitis B or who are carriers give the disease to the newborn?

Yes, these mothers can transmit this disease to the newborn. This mother-to-infant transmission process is known as **vertical transmission.** Transmission of HBV by carrier mothers to their babies occurs during the perinatal period, and this appears to be the single most important factor in the prevalence of the infection in some regions, such as in China and Southeast Asia.

Vertical transmission most likely occurs in the following ways:

- Through small breaks in the placental membrane—As pregnancy progresses, the placenta becomes more porous and is then more susceptible to microscopic breaks with maternal–fetal bleeds. The mother's infected blood can mix with fetal blood before or during labor.
- Contact of the baby with infected amniotic fluid or blood during the process of birth.

Transmission risk is highest in the following cases[2,5,9]:

- When infection occurs during the third trimester
- When the mother is in an especially acute infectious state, with her blood testing positive for both HBsAg and HBeAg serologic markers

The acute infectious state occurs when the mother's blood has two serologic markers:

HBsAg positive and HBeAg positive   = 90% to 95% risk of perinatal transmission
HBsAg positive and HBeAg negative   = 10% risk of perinatal transmission

■ Which women are at high risk of being hepatitis B carriers?

Woman in any of the following categories are at high risk for being hepatitis B carriers[4,10]:

- Drug abusers who inject drugs under the skin or into veins (needles can be contaminated)
- Women who are partners of intravenous drug abusers or bisexual men or who have multiple partners
- Health care workers such as nurses, physicians, medical technologists, dentists, and dental hygienists (because of exposure to blood or to blood-tinged saliva)
- Southeast Asians, Native Alaskans, Pacific Islanders, Haitians, and sub-Saharan Africans (owing to epidemic/endemic exposure in their mother country or refugee camps)
- Women with active disease or a history of hepatitis (can be a chronic carrier)
- Women with a history of venereal disease
- Women rejected as blood donors (these individuals might have had HBsAg detected)
- Women who work in a renal dialysis unit (includes partners of men who are receiving dialysis treatment as a result of frequent exposure to blood and semen)
- Workers in institutions for the retarded (as a result of inadequate hygiene habits and biting and breaking of skin)

- Women living with hepatitis patients or carriers
- Women who have received many blood transfusions (as a result of receiving donated blood)
- Women with acute and chronic liver disease

NOTE: *The CDC Immunization Practices Advisory Committee recommends routine screening of all pregnant women as the only strategy that will provide control of perinatal transmission of HBV infection in the United States.*[13,15]

Antepartum Care

■ **What are the maternal complications and clinical implications during the antepartum period?**

Maternal complications are not common. The following facts are known about the course of HBV infection during pregnancy[2,10,11]:

- Pregnancy is *not* thought to aggravate the course of the disease.
- Most infections go unrecognized.
- Fifty percent or fewer of HBV infections are accompanied by clinical signs and symptoms.
- Usual *clinical signs* are jaundice, hepatitic tenderness, and weight loss.
- Most symptoms appear 45 to 180 days after exposure. These symptoms include anorexia, nausea, malaise, weakness, and abdominal pain.
- Acute infection lasts 3 to 4 weeks.
- Mothers rarely need hospitalization unless dehydration or marked liver damage has occurred.
- No special dietary prescriptions are needed.
- In the event of severe symptoms of anorexia, nausea, vomiting, and diarrhea, hospitalization is recommended to do the following:
  –Correct fluid and electrolyte imbalance
  –Assess for liver damage
  –Conserve energy
  –Minimize infection transmission

> Fulminant hepatitis with encephalopathy can be a complication of hepatitis B.

Screening

During pregnancy, every woman should be screened for hepatitis B. This is done by testing for the surface antigen, HBsAg. The presence of HBsAg in serum identifies any infected person in either an acute or carrier state. *The test does not differentiate members of the two groups.*

If HBsAg is present, additional tests need to be carried out to identify the following:

- The degree of infectivity
- Whether the mother is in the acute or chronic carrier state

The hepatitis B laboratory panel for disease identification includes the following serologic markers:

- HBsAg
- anti-HBs
- anti-HBc

NOTE: *HBeAg and anti-HBe are looked for only when HBsAg is found. They are prognostic indicators of degree of infectivity.*

Although the presence of the marker IgM anti-HBc would identify acute or recent (within the last 4 to 6 months) infection, this is not routinely included in initial laboratory panels.

If a mother tests positive for HBsAg, her liver biochemistry should be analyzed to determine whether any liver damage has occurred. If the results are abnormal or if her liver is enlarged, she should be further evaluated to assess whether the disease is acute or chronic.

Hepatitis B is a sexually transmitted disease. The presence of one sexually transmitted disease in an individual indicates the possibility of others. HBsAg-positive mothers should be screened for gonorrhea, syphilis, chlamydial infection, HIV, herpes, and human papillomavirus. An additional disease, group B streptococcus, has seen a striking increase in incidence among young sexually active persons over the last decade. It can be sexually transmitted. Because this organism is currently the most common cause of sepsis and meningitis in the neonate and young infant, GBS screening in pregancy is recommended.[16] (See Appendix A.)

Women who are HBsAg negative but at high risk of contracting HBV infection need to be counseled that vaccination is recommended during pregnancy. Health care providers need to be aware that recent findings indicate that maternal obesity, advancing age, and smoking tend to reduce the efficacy of HBV vaccination in pregnant women.[17]

Screening mothers also means that families of infected or carrier patients can then be tested and immunized. Thus, this becomes an important case-finding tool as well.

Counseling and testing are recommended in all prenatal settings, whether private or clinic services, where women who are at risk for hepatitis B are encountered. In addition, women should be educated about the following:

- A description of the infection
- Risk behaviors associated with contracting or transmitting the infection
- Potential social and family implications (carrier transmission risks in home and employment settings)
- Testing and immunization benefits for family members and sexual contacts

Immunization

Products for Active and/or Passive Immunization

Two types of immunizing products are available for prophylaxis against hepatitis B. These are *vaccines, which confer active immunization, and hepatitis B immune globulin, which confers passive immunization.*

Hepatitis B Vaccines

Recombinant vaccines are produced by inserting the HBsAg gene into *Saccharomyces cerevisiae,* common baker's yeast cells, which are capable of synthesizing large quantities of HBsAg in the host cell. Purified HBsAg is obtained by lysing the yeast cell and extracting the surface antigen particles. Hepatitis B vaccines are packaged to contain 10 to 40 mg of HBsAg protein per milliliter. The HBsAg is absorbed to aluminum hydroxide and preserved through the addition of thimerosal. Currently licensed recombinant vaccines are Recombivax HB (Merck & Co., West Point, PA) and Engerix-B (SmithKline Beecham, Philadelphia, PA).[18]

Plasma-derived vaccines are produced from pooled serum of hepatitis B–infected individuals. There are 15 or more different types of plasma-derived vaccines produced and licensed throughout the world.[19]

Both plasma-derived vaccine and recombinant vaccine are used throughout the world; 80% of hepatitis B vaccine production is plasma derived. Both vaccines confer equal and long-term protection.[3]

Clinical trials have established that the achievement of a level of 10 mIU/mL of anti-HBs in a vaccinated individual is associated with protection against clinical infection.[3,20]

A series of three IM doses of hepatitis B vaccine induces a protective antibody response (anti-HBs ≥95% of infants, children, and adolescents).[3]

NOTE: *Viruses that use RNA and reverse transcriptase for replication are capable of multiple mutations. There is concern about HBV mutants that may develop vaccine and treatment resistance. Preliminary data on enhancing hepatitis B vaccine immune-producing capabilities against one or more of these mutants has been established, but no such vaccines are as yet licensed in the United States.[3]*

Some childhood vaccines used since the 1930s have contained a weak nonbacterial agent and preservative called *thimerosal*. It has come under criticism in recent years because it contains ethyl mercury, a neurotoxin. Although effective in preventing bacterial contamination, it metabolizes to organic mercury, which is readily absorbed through the skin (as well as by ingestion and inhalation). The central nervous system, kidney, and immune system are the most commonly affected systems at toxicity levels.[21] The CDC reports that there is no current evidence of any harm to children in these recent years of vaccine exposure to thimerosal.[22] Although the use of thimerosal-containing vaccines should be reduced or eliminated, the use of vaccines containing thimerosal is considered preferable to withholding vaccinations against disease that could pose immediate and serious risk (e.g., newborns of hepatitis B carrier mothers).[21]

Early in 2001, thimerosal-free vaccines became available. For example, Recombivax HB, Pediatric (Merck), and Engerix-B, Pediatric/Adolescent (SmithKline Beecham), are now produced as thimerosal-free vaccines. Combination thimerosal-free vaccines are also being produced (e.g., thimerosal-free hepatitis B and *Haemophilus influenzae* type b [Hib] vaccine called COMVAX [Merck]).[21]

Hepatitis B Immune Globulin

Hepatitis B immune globulin (HBIG) is prepared from the plasma of donors known to contain a high titer of antibody against HBsAg. This human plasma is carefully screened for antibodies to HIV and HCV. In addition, the process used to prepare HBIG actually inactivates and eliminates HIV from the final globulin product. The final product is also free of HCV RNA. Since 1999, all products available in the United States have been manufactured by methods that inactivate HCV and other viruses.[23] No evidence exists that HIV can be transmitted by HBIG. Because administration of HBIG confers antibodies to the recipient directly, immediate passive protection is received that is temporary (3 to 6 months) and is usually recommended prophylactically in the case of newborn exposure risk or health care personnel parental exposure (e.g., needlestick) or within hours after exposure in certain postexposure situations. This serves as an intermediate and transient step while the individual begins to develop his or her own antibodies after immunization with hepatitis B vaccine.

CDC Recommendations for Hepatitis B Preexposure Immunization

Facts About HBV Vaccine[18]

- The usual schedule for both children and adults is three intramuscular (IM) injections, the second and third administered 1 month and 6 months, respectively, after the first. Engerix-B has a four-dose schedule that is supposed to allow a more rapid induction of immunity. However, when used for preexposure prophylaxis, no clear evidence exists that this dosage schedule provides greater protection than the three-dose schedule.
- The third dose confers optimal protection, acting as a booster dose. Long intervals between the second and third doses (4 to 12 months) result in higher final titers of anti-HBs.
- When Engerix-B is administered in four doses at 0, 1, 2, and 12 months, the last dose is necessary to ensure an optimal final antibody titer.
- Administration of HBV vaccine at the same time as other vaccines does not interfere with the antibody response of any of the vaccines.
- Hemodialysis patients often require larger vaccine doses or an increased number of doses to induce a protective antibody response. This might be true of other immunocompromised individuals.
- When one or two doses of a vaccine produced by one drug manufacturer are followed by subsequent doses from a different drug manufacturer, the immune response has been shown to be comparable to that resulting from a full course of vaccination with a single vaccine.
- Should the vaccination series be interrupted after the first dose, the second dose should be administered as soon as possible. The second and third doses should be separated by an interval of at least 2 months. If only the third dose is delayed, it should be administered as soon as convenient.
- Current recombinant hepatitis B vaccines should not be administered through an intradermal route. The CDC Advisory Committee on Immunization Practices (ACIP) has recommended the IM route only. The U.S. Food and Drug Administration (FDA) has not licensed the vaccine for intradermal use because this can fail to induce immunity in a substantial portion of those vaccinated.[24] Intradermal vaccines are under study.

Recent Research Findings [17,25]

- Adults younger than 40 years of age tend to have a better immune response than older persons.
- Studies regarding vaccination during pregnancy indicate that some pregnant women who received a three-dose series at 0, 1, and 6 months not only achieved **seroprotective** titers (i.e., conferring immunity) at the time of delivery but also had cord blood titers indicating seroprotective levels, which means immune protection for the newborn.
- Thimerosal, a mercury-based compound, *is no longer being used as a preservative in any pediatric vaccines* licensed in the United States. The preservative-free pediatric vaccines are referred to as Engerix-B, Pediatric/Adolescent, and Recombivax HB, Pediatric.[26] *Pediatric HBV vaccines should not be used for adult immunization; failure to induce adequate immunizing titers can result.*
- Currently recommended three-dose schedules achieve seroprotective levels, that is, 10 mIU/mL or higher, in 95% of younger, healthy immunocompetent individuals. Severely immunosuppressed persons may not respond.
- The need for booster doses in healthy individuals is uncertain. Studies show that in approximately 40% of vaccinated individuals, anti-HBs may disappear from the serum within 10 years of a vaccination. **However, immunity against the disease persists for years after the loss of detectable circulating anti-HBs and may be lifelong in healthy individuals.** This is because immune cells "remember" that they were vaccinated—this is called "immune memory." When exposed to HBV, they begin rapidly making antibodies. The long incubation period for HBV infection allows time for the immune system to mount a protective response.[27]

NOTE: To date there are no data to support the need for booster doses in immunocompetent individuals who have responded to a primary course of hepatitis B vaccination.[28]

- Boosters are definitely recommended for immunosuppressed individuals in whom the anti-HBs levels have fallen below 10 mIU/mL.
- Hepatitis B vaccination is safe and capable of producing immunity in individuals with chronic hepatitis C.[29]

Intrapartum Care

■ How is the disease transmitted to others, including health care personnel?

HBV is viable in blood and in secretions containing serum or those derived from serum. Transmission of the virus can be by one of five routes[30]:

1. Direct inoculation through the skin (percutaneous) of infected serum or plasma or by transfusion of infected blood or blood products
2. Indirect inoculation through the skin of infected serum or plasma through abrasions or small skin cuts
3. Absorption of infected serum or plasma through mucosal surfaces (e.g., eye, mouth)
4. Absorption of infective secretions (e.g., saliva, semen) through mucosal surfaces (could occur during vaginal, anal, or oral sexual contact)
5. Transfer of infected serum or plasma by way of inanimate surfaces or possibly vectors

Besides blood, body fluids include the following:

Serous fluid (e.g., cerebrospinal fluid, synovial fluid, pleural fluid, peritoneal fluid)	Breast milk
	Vaginal secretions
	Semen
Amniotic fluid	Urine
Saliva	Sweat
Tears	Feces

Universal precautions involve a mindset that incorporates practices performed every hour of the professional day to be used consistently to reduce transmission of bloodborne pathogens, whether that be from patients to health care workers, from health care workers to patients, or from patient to patient. Precautions include appropriate use of barrier equipment such as gloves, gowns, face shields, and goggles, as well as proper instrument/equipment cleaning, disinfection, or sterilization.

Precautions Recommended for Hospital Personnel[30,31]

Nursing, medical, and housekeeping personnel are exposed to a variety of body fluids on an obstetrics unit during an average workday.

HBV has been isolated from blood, semen, urine, breast milk, saliva, tears, and brain tissue of infected individuals. However, research to date indicates that the virus is not transmitted to individuals through saliva, sweat, tears, urine, or stool.

> The concentration of HBV in bodily fluids is proportional to the number of white blood cells in the fluid. Blood has the highest concentration of HBV, whereas saliva and tears have much lower concentrations.

Precautions do not apply to feces, nasal secretions, sputum, sweat, tears, urine, and vomitus *unless they contain gross, visible blood.*

> The risk of HBV transmission from these fluids and material is low or nonexistent.

Pregnant health care workers have additional motivation for adhering to universal precautions because of the risk of perinatal transmission to the fetus.

> The CDC strongly recommends hepatitis B vaccination for all at-risk health care workers.

> Pregnant women who are considered at high risk of becoming infected with HBV should be considered for HBV immunization. Pregnancy is not a contraindication to the use of hepatitis B vaccine.[13,15]

A major aim of appropriate intrapartum care is the prevention of nosocomial infection in patients and health care workers. **Nosocomial infections** are acquired while in and as a result of being in a hospital, as opposed to community-acquired infections. The infection is neither present nor in the incubation stage at the time the patient is admitted to the hospital. Symptoms of a nosocomial infection are not necessarily present during hospitalization but can become evident after discharge.

Basic guidelines are as follows:

- Universal precautions should be followed by all medical and nursing staff, as well as allied health workers and housekeeping personnel.
- Focusing only on patients known to be infected puts the health care provider at risk from patients infected but not yet identified and who, therefore, are not being properly treated.
- Hospital personnel who are at high risk of exposure to blood and other body fluids should have hepatitis B screening and immunization made available to them.

Hospital Admission Screening

■ Which women require hepatitis B screening on admission?

- All pregnant women should have prenatal screening for hepatitis B infection.
- Women who present with no prenatal care or without documentation of prenatal care and laboratory testing results should have a hepatitis B screen done immediately.
- Women who have incomplete documentation of their hepatitis B status should have the remaining serologic markers evaluated to determine their infectious and/or carrier state. (For example, an HBsAg-positive marker documented from a screening examination always needs further evaluation. Is HBeAg present? Has the HBsAg marker cleared and is anti-HBs present, denoting immune status? Has the HBsAg marker persisted for more than 6 months, indicating a carrier state?)

REMEMBER: *Many persons clear their system of HBsAg over a 6-month period and go on to develop an immune state.*

Therefore, when admitting a pregnant woman who is at increased risk for being a hepatitis B carrier, the following should be done:

- Review her prenatal record to determine the results of her hepatitis screen.
- If no record is available, contact the primary care provider immediately.
- If no documentation can be obtained for her hepatitis B status, HBsAg testing on the mother should be done immediately.
- After an initial positive test for HBsAg on a laboring woman, treatment of the infant should begin within 24 hours of birth.
- **If a hospital does not possess the capacity to do the hepatitis B screen and the mother has no documentation of her status, the infant should be presumed to be at risk. Treatment with both HBIG and hepatitis B vaccine should begin within 24 hours of birth.**[18]

Prevention of Perinatal Transmission

■ **How can the risk of transmission of hepatitis B to the newborn be reduced?**

In 1991 and 1995, the CDC Immunization Practices Advisory Committee[18,32] recommend strategies to eliminate HBV transmission in infancy and childhood, as well as in adolescence and adulthood. Immunization of all susceptible persons will prevent new infections. **Therefore, routine vaccination of children born to HBsAg-negative mothers is now recommended.** Infants and children should receive the vaccine during routine visits to clinical or private practices.

THE PRIMARY GOAL IN TREATING THE NEWBORN IS PREVENTION OF THE INFANT BECOMING A CARRIER OF HEPATITIS B. NINETY PERCENT OF INFECTED INFANTS BECOME CHRONIC CARRIERS OF HBsAg. APPROXIMATELY 25% OF THESE INFANTS WILL DIE FROM CIRRHOSIS OF THE LIVER OR LIVER CANCER.

> **The best newborn treatment to prevent acute or chronic hepatitis B infection is timely immunization using a combination of HBIG and hepatitis B vaccine.**

CAUTION: Currently the American Academy of Pediatrics and the CDC recommend delaying the initiation of hepatitis B immunization beyond the first week of life for premature infants at low risk for hepatitis B infection, especially those weighing less than 1,700 g at birth. Studies indicate an inadequate immune response in these infants. Vaccination can be considered once the infants reach 2,200 g of weight or until 2 months of age.[33]

Because newborns are most often infected by exposure to the mother's infected secretions during the birthing process, *the following guidelines are intended to reduce that risk in infants of carrier mothers.* Remember that blood and amniotic fluid are the predominant contaminants in this situation.

Precautions aimed at preventing the spread of infection from the mother to the newborn during the intrapartum period include the following:

- Consider the intact fetal skin as a protective barrier. *Maintain the integrity of the skin when possible.*
- Avoid invasive procedures. These should be performed only after careful assessment of risks versus benefits. Examples include the following:
  – Internal scalp electrode monitoring
  – Fetal scalp blood sampling
  – Internal uterine pressure monitoring
  – Vaginal examination after rupture of membranes
  – Vacuum extraction
  – Forceps delivery
- Studies do not demonstrate that cesarean section lowers the risk of neonatal hepatitis B infection. Therefore, this route of delivery should be reserved for obstetric indications only.

- Women admitted for delivery who have no record of prenatal HBsAg testing should have blood drawn for testing. While awaiting the test results and within the first 12 hours of birth, the infant should receive hepatitis B vaccine.
  - –If the mother is found to be HBsAg positive, the infant should also receive HBIG as soon as possible and within 7 days of birth. If for some reason HBIG is not given, it is important that the infant be given the second vaccination treatment at 1 month and no later than 2 months of age because the risk of infection is somewhat greater when HBIG has not been given.
  - –Even if the mother tests negative for HBsAg, the infant should continue with the vaccination schedule.
- In populations where pregnant women are not routinely screened for HBsAg, all newborns should receive the first dose of hepatitis B vaccine and HBIG within 12 hours of birth, the second dose at 1 to 2 months of age, and the third dose at 6 months of age.

Guidelines for Delivery of At-Risk Newborns

- Obtain informed consent for treatment of the infant before delivery.
- Assign one nurse to attend to the newborn after delivery when possible.
- Dry the infant immediately after the delivery to remove all maternal blood and amniotic fluid.
- Mucous membrane exposure should be reduced by careful suctioning of the nares and oropharynx. Gently remove excess fluid and blood from the nares and oropharynx.

> Take care to avoid traumatizing the mucous membranes.

- Aspirate stomach contents using a mucus extractor or meconium aspirator with wall suction on a low setting.

> Always use wall suction or newly devised mucus extractors, which prevent potentially contaminating fluids from coming in contact with the mouth.

- **Delay administration of vitamin K until after the infant is bathed.**
- Bathe the newborn early and thoroughly with a mild, nonmedicated soap under radiant heat as soon as possible.

> Prompt removal of infectious fluids reduces the chance of exposing both the infant and caregivers to infection. Attention should also be given to cleansing around the eyes.

- Remove potentially infectious maternal blood and secretions before any application of eye medications.
- Begin immunization treatment immediately on infants of hepatitis B–infected or carrier mothers.
- If the infant is born with additional problems, any life-threatening situation takes priority.

> In performing invasive procedures, avoid introducing the mother's blood or amniotic fluid into the baby.

- If the baby must be transported:
  - –Inform the receiving physician/flight nurse/hospital that the baby's mother is infected with hepatitis B or is a carrier.

–Label the maternal blood as HBsAg positive before transport.

–Inform the transport team of what has been done for the baby regarding the prevention of transmission of the infection.

–Document all steps taken in the newborn's chart.

Guidelines for At-Risk Newborn Vaccine Administration[18]

STUDIES DEMONSTRATE THE HIGHEST EFFICACY (85% TO 95%) OF COMBINED HBIG AND HEPATITIS B VACCINE PROPHYLAXIS WHEN HBIG IS ADMINISTRATED WITHIN 1 TO 12 HOURS AFTER BIRTH.[18]

Newborns at risk should receive a three-dose series of Recombivax HB, Pediatric, or Engerix-B, Pediatric/Adolescent. The first dose, which is given at birth, should be combined with a single dose of HBIG given intramuscularly at another site. The second dose of Recombivax HB, Pediatric, or Engerix-B, Pediatric/Adolescent is administered at 1 to 2 months of age and the third dose at 6 months of age.[18] There is a four-dose series with Engerix-B, Pediatric/Adolescent .[32]

Treatment

One dose at birth: HBIG 0.5 mL intramuscularly. Use the anterolateral thigh muscle in the newborn.

Passive immunity is developed with the dose of HBIG. This gives babies the antibodies needed immediately to protect them from infection with HBV through maternal blood and body fluids.

Treatment

Dose: Recombivax HB, Pediatric,
5 μg/dose, 0.5 mL intramuscularly
OR
Engerix-B, Pediatric/Adolescent,
10 μg/dose, 0.5 mL intramuscularly
Use the *other* anterolateral thigh muscle.

Active immunity is developed by the administration of hepatitis B vaccine. This simulates the baby's immune system to begin producing its own hepatitis B antibody protection.

NOTE: *Infants born to HBsAg-negative mothers should receive 2.5 μg of Recombivax-HB, Pediatric, or 10 μg of Engerix-B, Pediatric/Adolescent, ideally at birth or before discharge. The second dose should be administered at least 1 month after the first dose. The third dose should be at least 2 months after the first dose but not before 6 months of age.*

Failures of immunization for some newborns are believed to occur because a small percentage of these babies probably acquired the infection transplacentally before birth. Testing for efficacy of immunization in the infant is usually done at 9 months of age.

REMEMBER:

* *These medications should be administered within 12 hours after delivery. Recent studies indicate that administration of the first does of hepatitis B vaccine at birth is associated with increased likelihood of completion of the hepatitis B vaccination series.[34]*
* *Different sites for each injection should be used. In the newborn, only the anterolateral thigh muscles should be used.*
* *Be sure the baby has been bathed thoroughly before the injections are given.*
* *The baby will require two additional immunizations: one at 1 month of age and one at 6 months of age.*

Communication with private physicians and community health departments is important. Arrangements can be made for babies to receive their second and third doses of the vaccine at the public health immunizations clinic.

■ Can hepatitis B be diagnosed in the newborn?

Currently, there are no available methods for prenatal diagnosis of fetal HBV infection. It is generally believed that vertical transmission occurs primarily at birth (85% to 95%).[5] Although transplacental passage of viral particles can occur, it is rare. Hepatitis B viral particles, including the surface antigen, are too large to pass through the placenta easily. Exceptions to this can occur in situations of maternal–fetal bleeds such as in microplacental abruptions.[10]

Obtaining a definite diagnosis of HBV infection in the newborn is also a problem. Infected infants cannot be distinguished from noninfected infants through testing. Laboratory testing of newborns in the first few months of life is not conclusive because transplacentally acquired maternal HBsAg or anti-HBs in the infant's blood complicates the diagnosis. Basically, all infants born to mothers who are positive for hepatitis B antigens or antibodies will be seropositive for those markers at birth. The exception to this will be IgM markers, whose large molecular size does not permit transplacental passage. IgG immunoglobulins are of smaller size and are passed from mother to newborn.

CDC Recommendations for Vaccination

The following doses and schedules (Tables 12.1, 12.2, and 12.3) are CDC recommendations for vaccination of newborn infants and children younger than 11 years:

- Individual vaccines have been evaluated to determine the age and dosage at which the best antibody response is achieved.
- The highest titers of anti-HBs are achieved when the last two doses of vaccine are spaced at least 4 months apart. However, schedules with 2-month intervals between doses, which would be congruent with schedules for other childhood vaccines, have been proven to produce a good antibody response. This latter schedule may need to be used in populations in which it is uncertain that infants will be brought back for all of their vaccinations.[18]
- A protective antibody response is achieved when anti-HBs serum levels are at or above 10 IU/mL. The various schedules and doses given have all been shown to produce effective antibody levels for immunity.
- When hepatitis B vaccine is administered at the same time as other vaccines, there is no interference with antibody response in any of the vaccines.
- Studies demonstrate that the current hepatitis vaccines produce seroconversion in more than 95% of individuals vaccinated.

The vaccines in the following schedules should be noted as available in thimerosal-free formulations. It is imperative to consult the current CDC periodic publication of immunization schedules under the leadership of the ACIP to remain informed of new vaccines and combination vaccines with the appropriate administration schedule.[21,22,35]

TABLE 12.1	Hepatitis B Immunoprophylaxis: Infants of HBsAg-Positive Mothers[a]	
TREATMENT	**AGE OF INFANT**	**VACCINES**
First vaccine dose (IM)	Birth (within 12 hours)	Recombivax HB, Pediatric dose (5 μg or 0.5 mL) OR Engerix-B, Pediatric/Adolescent dose (10 μg or 0.5 mL)
HBIG (IM)	Birth (within 12 hours)	0.5 mL
Second vaccine dose (IM)	1–2 months	As above
Third vaccine dose (IM)	6 months	As above

NOTE: Use the anterolateral thigh muscle in the newborn. Use the other anterolateral thigh muscle for the HBIG injection.

[a]An alternative schedule: repeat at 1, 2, and 12 to 18 months of age.

Adapted with permission from Centers for Disease Control and Prevention. (1991). Hepatitis B infection: A comprehensive strategy for eliminating transmission in the United States through universal childhood vaccinations–Recommendations of the Immunization Practices Advisory Committee (ACIP). *MMWR Morbidity and Mortality Weekly Report, 40*(RR-13), 1–25; and current ACIP Recommendations for Childhood Immunization Schedule, January–Decemeber 2001.

TABLE 12.2	Hepatitis B Immunoprophylaxis: Infants Born to Mothers Whose Status Is Unknown[a]	
TREATMENT	**AGE OF INFANT**	**VACCINES**
First vaccine dose (IM)	Birth (within 12 hours)	Recombivax HB, Pediatric dose (5 µg or 0.5 mL) OR Engerix-B, Pediatric/Adolescent dose (10 µg or 0.5 mL)
HBIG (IM)	Maternal blood should be drawn upon admission, and if the mother tests positive for HBsAg, administer dose to infant as soon as possible, and no later than 1 week of age	0.5 mL
Second vaccine dose (IM)	1–2 months if mother is HBsAg positive	Recombivax HB, Pediatric dose (5 µg or 0.5 mL) OR Engerix-B, Pediatric/Adolescent dose (10 µg or 0.5 mL)
	1–2 months OR 1–4 months if mother is HBsAg negative	Recombivax HB, Pediatric dose (2.5 µg or 0.25 mL) OR Engerix-B, Pediatric/Adolescent dose (10 µg or 0.5 mL)
Third vaccine dose (IM)	6 months if the mother is HBsAg positive; if the mother is HBsAg negative, this should be at least 2 months after second dose but not before 6 months of age for infants	As in the second vaccine dose outlined for the infant born of an HBsAg-positive mother

[a]An alternative schedule: repeat at 1, 2, and 12 months of age.

Adapted with permission from Centers for Disease Control and Prevention. (1991). Hepatitis B infection: A comprehensive strategy for eliminating transmission in the United States through universal childhood vaccinations–Recommendations of the Immunization Practices Advisory Committee (ACIP). *MMWR Morbidity and Mortality Weekly Report, 40*(RR-13), 1–25; and current ACIP Recommendations for Childhood Immunization Schedule, January–Decemeber 2001.

TABLE 12.3	Hepatitis B Prophylaxis: Other Infants and Children Younger Than 11 Years of Age	
TREATMENT	**AGE OF INFANT**	**VACCINES**
Option 1		
First vaccine dose (IM)	Birth, before hospital discharge OR with unvaccination, children begin series at any visit	Recombivax HB, Pediatric dose (2.5 µg or 0.25 mL) OR
Second vaccine dose (IM)	1–4 months (at least 1 month after the first dose)[a]	Engerix-B, Pediatric/Adolescent dose (10 µg or 0.5 mL)
Third vaccine dose (IM)	6–18 months after second dose	

Resources:

1. Centers for Disease Control and Prevention. (1991). Hepatitis B infection: A comprehensive strategy for eliminating transmission in the United States through universal childhood vaccinations–Recommendations of the Immunization Practices Advisory Committee (ACIP). *MMWR Morbidity and Mortality Weekly Report, 40*(RR-13), 1–25.
2. Centers for Disease Control and Prevention. (1995). Recommended childhood immunization schedule–United States. *MMWR Morbidity and Mortality Weekly Report, 44*(RR-5), 1–9.
3. Current ACIP Recommendations for Childhood Immunization Schedule, January–December 2001.
   - In an alternative four-dose schedule using Engerix-B, the second and third doses should be administered at 1 and 2 months of age, respectively, and the fourth dose at 12 to 18 months of age.
   - In preterm infants, hepatitis B vaccination should be delayed until they are of term gestational age and a minimum weight of 2,500 g.
   - All children and adolescents (through 18 years of age) who have not been immunized against hepatitis B may begin the series during any visit. Special efforts should be made to immunize children who were born in or whose parents were born in areas of the world with moderate to high endemicity of hepatitis B virus infection.

[a]See ACIP Immunization Schedule for Combination Vaccines.

Postpartum Care

■ What are the important aspects of postpartum care?

There is no reason to separate the mother and infant after the infant has been bathed. **NOTE:** *Mothers should be permitted to hold their infants immediately after birth, even though the baby has not been bathed.*

Only infants who are stable and able to tolerate the heat loss that occurs with bathing should be given a bath.

Until a complete bath is given, strict isolation procedures for the infant should be instituted. Before the baby is bathed, health care personnel should do the following:

REMEMBER: *The reason for isolation procedures is to prevent transmission of the infection to staff or other patients through contact with the mother's infected blood or amniotic fluid.*

- Wear gown and gloves when handling the baby.
- Wear masks and goggles or large-size glasses if there is a possibility of blood being spattered during a particular procedure.
- Consider all linens and other articles that come in contact with the baby to be sources of contaminated blood and/or amniotic fluid.

Handle these linens and other discarded articles according to infection control guidelines.

Once the infant has been thoroughly bathed with a detergent soap and water, there is no need to isolate the baby.

The production of viruses in an infant who is infected with HBV does not occur for several weeks.[35]

Although there is no urgent need to place the mother in a private room, it might be reasonable and prudent to do so when possible because a shared bathroom is probably the most likely source of contamination. Heavy lochia can contaminate the toilet, her hands, and anything that she might touch before washing her hands. If she is sharing a bathroom, she should be taught to report any contamination with blood immediately.

After the infant has been bathed, teach the mother the following:

- To wash her hands before handling the baby
- Precautions for blood spills, lochia, and perineal pads
- To avoid letting the baby come in contact with soiled linen
- Why it is important to delay breastfeeding for 48 hours after administration of HBIG to the baby
- To inspect her breasts and nipples for infection or breaks in the skin if she is breastfeeding (The nurse should make this inspection with the mother once a day.)

Education is a critical part of the mother's care after delivery. Be sure that the mother and her family members understand the following:

- Her hepatitis carrier status
- How the infant is infected and the importance of proper handwashing after handling blood-soiled materials (e.g., in changing her perineal pads before handling the baby)
- The potential for transmission via saliva
- The risks her hepatitis carrier status poses for the infant
- The risks and benefits of immunization for the infant
- The need for complete immunization plans for the baby over the next 6 months

Breastfeeding

> ### ■ What are the breastfeeding recommendations for the infant of a carrier mother?

The CDC states that the infant of a hepatitis B–infected or carrier mother is not likely to be at risk for contracting the disease through breastfeeding. The infant has already received intense exposure to the virus during the birth process.[11]

> **However, it is recommended that breastfeeding be delayed for 48 hours after HBIG treatment of the infant. This precaution ensures the conferring of passive immunity to the infant.**

Breastfeeding is not contraindicated unless the mother develops any of the following:

- Cracked nipples
- Mastitis
- Other breast lesions

Feeding from the breast with any of these problems must be stopped because highly infectious discharge from the lesions can mix with breast milk.

Teach the breastfeeding mother the following:

- Nipple care
- Good breastfeeding techniques to prevent nipple trauma
- To stop breastfeeding the baby on the breast that develops a cracked nipple, mastitis, or other lesions and to express milk from that breast to prevent engorgement; to feed the infant from the unaffected breast (*The mother does not have to stop breastfeeding.*)

> Engorgement slows the healing in breasts affected with these problems. Good circulation is important to maintain.

Discharge Planning

> ### ■ What unique components need to be incorporated in discharge planning?

Essential discharge preparation for the postpartum hepatitis B–positive mother and her infant include the following:

- Education about self-care
- Guidance to reduce transmission risks for household members
- Screening needs of household members, including sexual partner
- Scheduling the newborn for HBV immunization
- Counseling about safer sexual practices and contraceptive methods

Education About Self-Care

In addition to instructions concerning nutrition and perineal and breast care, stress must be placed on sources of contamination, such as body fluids, especially blood. Proper handling and use of sanitary pads, razor blades, toothbrushes, and bathroom facilities need to be reviewed. Handwashing practices related to handling objects that could be sources of contamination (e.g., a sanitary pad) should be explained. At the same time, it should be made clear that urine, tears, and stool are not sources of contamination. Giving the mother and family balanced perspective for a reasonable and responsible lifestyle is important.

The mother should be encouraged to seek regular, ongoing medical follow-up for herself. If she is in the acute infectious stage, periodic screening will eventually reveal seroconversion to an immune or carrier state. She needs to know her postinfection status when the acute stage passes so that appropriate medical interventions can be instituted. If she is a carrier, periodic medical follow-up is imperative. She is at risk for long-term sequelae resulting in cirrhosis of the liver and/or hepatocellular carcinoma.

Guidance to Reduce Transmission Risks for Household Members

Teach the hepatitis B–positive mother that her hands and other skin surfaces should be washed immediately and thoroughly if contaminated with her blood. Warm water and soap suffice. Waterless antiseptic hand cleaners are appropriate if handwashing facilities are not available. Household surfaces should be cleaned with an Environmental Protection Agency (EPA)-approved germicide solution or a 1:100 solution of a household bleach when any blood is spilled. Blood-soiled linen can be contaminated with HBV, but the risk of actual disease transmission is negligible. The linen should be handled as little as possible and washed quickly. Normal laundry cycles and detergent can be used.

EVERY HOSPITAL CARING FOR OBSTETRIC PATIENTS SHOULD HAVE WRITTEN UNIVERSAL PRECAUTIONS GUIDELINES FOR NURSES, PHYSICIANS, ALLIED HEALTH WORKERS, AND HOUSEKEEPING PERSONNEL TO FOLLOW WHEN CARING FOR MOTHERS AND THEIR INFANTS ON INTRAPARTUM AND POSTPARTUM UNITS.

Preexposure and Postexposure Immunization Recommendations

Immunization of Adolescents

Universal immunization of adolescents is encouraged. Risk factors among this population can be difficult to identify, and yet it is known that adolescents and young adults can exhibit high-risk behaviors. Clearly at risk are injecting drug users or those with multiple sex partners (the CDC defines this as more than one partner in 6 months). In communities where teenage pregnancy, drug use, and sexually transmitted diseases are frequent, HBV immunization is strongly recommended. The schedule of 0, 1, and 6 months is preferred for adolescents.[18] For normal adolescents (as well as adults), vaccination dosages are 10 μg of Recombivax HB or 20 μg of Engerix-B given intramuscularly into the deltoid at 0, 1, and 6 months.[10]

Immunization of Pregnant or Lactating Women

When a pregnant woman is at risk for exposure to bloodborne pathogens because of her occupation, lifestyle behaviors, or intravenous drug–abusing sexual partners, she should be considered a candidate for HBV immunization. Neither pregnancy nor lactation is considered a contraindication to receiving HBV vaccination. Evidence to date indicates no adverse effects on the developing fetus. The vaccine contains noninfectious HBsAg particles sufficient to induce an appropriate antibody response in most adults. On the other hand, HBV infection in the pregnant woman places both the mother and the fetus at risk from disease and chronic infection.[18]

Management of Employees in Exposure-Prone Occupations

In June 2001, the CDC released updated guidelines for the management of occupational exposures to HBV, HCV, and HIV, as well as recommendations for postexposure prophylaxis.[23] The following comments reflect these recommendations and report.

The CDC defines *health care personnel* as those persons whose activities involve contact with patients or with blood or other body fluids from patients in a health care setting or a laboratory or public safety setting. This includes employees, students, contractors, attending clinicians, public safety workers, or volunteers in any of these settings.

Occupational exposure is defined as exposure that could reasonably be anticipated from skin, eye, mucous membrane, or parenteral contact with blood or other potentially infectious materials resulting from the performance of an employee's duties. Exposures placing a worker at risk for HBV, HCV, or HIV infection could be a percutaneous injury such as a needlestick or contact of mucous membranes or nonintact skin (chapped, abraded, or affected with dermatitis) with potentially infectious blood, tissue, or other body fluids.

Facts About Occupational Exposure[23]

*   Blood contains the highest HBV titers of all body fluids.
*   Semen and vaginal secretions are considered potentially infectious.
*   Other potentially infectious fluids are cerebrospinal fluid, synovial fluid, pleural fluid, peritoneal fluid, pericardial fluid, and amniotic fluid. *The risk for transmission of HBV, HCV, or HIV infection from these fluids is unknown.*
*   Feces, nasal secretions, saliva, sputum, sweat, tears, urine, and vomitus *are not considered potentially infectious unless they contain visible blood.* Transmission risk from these fluids and materials is extremely low. It appears that the risk of acquiring HBV infection is higher than that for acquiring HIV or HCV. Also, the risk of acquiring HCV is greater than that the risk of contracting HIV.[36]
*   Occupational exposure should be considered an urgent medical concern with the appreciation for the need of timely postexposure management.

HBV infection is the major infectious risk for health care personnel. There has been a 90% decrease in the number of health care workers infected between 1985 and 1993. During 1993, an estimated 1,450 workers became infected through exposure to blood and serum-derived body fluids.

There is no doubt that regulations issued under the Occupational Safety and Health Act,[37,38] making HBV vaccine available to all occupationally-exposed health care personnel, have been instrumental in this marked improvement. It is unsettling, however, to see recent surveys indicating continuing gaps in adequate coverage among health care personnel.[39,40]

Studies indicate that 5% to 10% of HBV-infected workers become chronically infected. These individuals are at risk for chronic liver disease (e.g., cirrhosis, primary hepatocellular carcinoma) and are potentially infectious for their lifetime. Current estimates indicate that 100 to 200 health care personnel have died each year during the past decade owing to consequences of HBV infection, yet vaccines exist that could prevent most of those deaths.[38]

Important Data Cited by the CDC[23]

*   The risk of HBV infection is primarily related to the degree of contact with blood in the workplace.
*   In needlestick injuries, the risk of developing *clinical* HBV infection (with signs and symptoms) from a contaminated needle was 22% to 31% if the blood contained both HBsAg and HBeAg.
*   The risk of developing serologic evidence of HBV infection (i.e., the laboratory markers such as HBsAg, etc., can be identified) was 37% to 62%.
*   When the surface antigen was present (HBsAg positive) without the e antigen (HBeAg negative), the risk was considerably lower: *Clinical* evidence of infection is 1% to 6%, and *serologic* evidence of infection is 23% to 37%. Considering that 5% to 10% of those infected will become chronically infected, these numbers are sobering and should motivate all "at-risk" personnel to seek vaccination.
*   Having hepatitis B–vaccinated personnel reduces the risk of infection transmission to patients.
*   HBV has been demonstrated to survive in dried blood at room temperature on surfaces for as long as 1 week and is seen as a potential for infection transmission.
*   HCV is not efficiently transmitted through *occupational exposure* to blood, including blood on environmental surfaces. One study indicates that percutaneous transmission occurred only with hollow-bore needles as compared with other sharps.

Postexposure Recommendations

Since 1992, with the Occupation Safety and Health Administration's (OSHA) bloodborne pathogen standard, employers are required to establish a control plan for cases of exposure that includes postexposure follow-up for employees. This includes the following:

*   Availability of postexposure care during all working hours, including night and weekends
*   Provision of HBIG, HBV vaccine, and antiretroviral agents for HIV postexposure treatment *for timely administration*

NOTE:

*   *Prescreening is not required as a condition for receiving the vaccine.*
*   *Employees must sign a form stating that they decline the vaccine if they choose not to be vaccinated.*
*   *If booster doses are later recommended by the U.S. Public Health Service, employees must be offered them.*

The control plan, among many stipulations, requires the following:

- That employers identify tasks, procedures, and job classification where occupational exposure to blood occurs
- That evaluation plans be developed for postexposure circumstances
- The use of universal precautions in all exposure-prone work settings
- That engineering and work-practice controls be implemented (e.g., procedures to minimize needlesticks and splashing and spraying of blood)
- Appropriate packaging and labeling of specimens and waste

■ Who should have postvaccination testing?[18,23]

- **Health care personnel who are in contact with patients and/or blood and are at ongoing risk for percutaneous injuries should be tested for anti-HBs 1 to 2 months after they have completed the three-dose vaccination series; includes surgeons and dentists**
- Infants born to HBsAg-positive mothers (Knowledge of their immune status will dictate subsequent clinical management.)
- Dialysis patients and staff
- HIV-infected individuals

TABLE 12.4	Recommended Postexposure Prophylaxis for Exposure to Hepatitis B Virus		
	TREATMENT		
VACCINATION AND ANTIBODY RESPONSE STATUS OF EXPOSED WORKERS[a]	**SOURCE HBsAG POSITIVE**	**SOURCE HBsAG NEGATIVE**	**SOURCE UNKNOWN OR NOT AVAILABLE FOR TESTING**
Unvaccinated	HBIG[b] × 1 and initiate HB vaccine series[c]	Initiate HB vaccine series	Initiate HB vaccine series
Previously vaccinated			
Known responder[d]	No treatment	No treatment	No treatment
Known nonresponder[e]	HBIG × 1 and initiate revaccination or HBIG × 2[f]	No treatment	If known high-risk source, treat as if source were HBsAg positive
Antibody response unknown	Test exposed person for anti-HBs 1. If adequate,[d] no treatment is necessary 2. If inadequate,[e] administer HBIG × 1 and vaccine booster	No treatment	Test exposed person for anti-HBs 1. If adequate,[d] no treatment is necessary 2. If inadequate,[e] administer vaccine booster and recheck titer in 1–2 months

[a]Persons who have previously been infected with HBV are immune to reinfection and do not require postexposure prophylaxis.
[b]Dose is 0.06 mL/kg intramuscularly.
[c]Hepatitis B vaccine.
[d]A responder is a person with adequate levels of serum antibody to HBsAg (i.e., anti-HBs ≥10 mIU/mL).
[e]A nonresponder is a person with inadequate response to vaccination (i.e., serum anti-HBs <10 mIU/mL).
[f]The option of giving one dose of HBIG and reinitiating the vaccine series is preferred for nonresponders who have not completed a second three-dose vaccine series. For persons who previously completed a second vaccine series but failed to respond, two doses of HBIG are preferred.
Reprinted with permission from Centers for Disease Control and Prevention. (2001). Updated U.S. Public Health Service guidelines for the management of occupational exposures to HBV, HCV, and HIV and recommendations for postexposure prophylaxis. *MMWR Morbidity and Mortality Weekly Report, 50*(RR-11), 22.

Management of Nonresponders[23]

Important information:

Nonresponders to the primary hepatitis B vaccination series are those who do not develop an antibody titer (anti-HBs) at a level equal to or above 10 mIU/mL. A second three-dose vaccine series should be given, or the nonresponder should be evaluated to determine whether he or she is HBsAg positive. See Table 12.4 for options with known nonresponders.

A second vaccine series for nonresponders has a 30% to 50% chance of producing appropriate antibody levels.

Nonresponders who are determined to be HBsAg positive need to be counseled regarding further medical evaluation and how to prevent transmission to others.

Nonresponders who are determined to be HBsAg negative are at risk for contracting HBV and need to be counseled regarding precautions and the need to obtain HBIG prophylaxis in the event of any parenteral exposure to HBsAg-positive blood.

For any occupational exposure, the infectious status of the source should be determined for the presence of the following:

- HBsAg
- HCV antibody
- HIV antibody

Hepatitis B Virus Exposure Treatment

- Prophylactic treatment to prevent infection after exposure should be considered in situations involving the following:
  - Percutaneous (e.g., needlestick, lacerations, bites) or perimucosal (ocular or mucosal) exposure to HBsAg-positive blood
  - Perinatal exposure of an infant born to an HBsAg-positive mother
  - Sexual exposure to an HBsAg-positive person
  - Household exposure of an infant younger than 12 months to a primary caretaker who has acute HBV infection
- In situations of perinatal exposure to an HBsAg-positive, HBeAg-positive mother, treating the newborn with HBIG and initiation of hepatitis B vaccine at birth is 85% to 95% effective in preventing infection.
- Regimens of either multiple doses of HBIG alone or the hepatitis B vaccine series alone are 70% to 75% effective in preventing infection.
- In occupational settings, the combination HBIG plus hepatitis B vaccine is recommended, as cited in Table 12.4, with the following guidelines:
  - Administer HBIG as soon as possible after exposure (preferably within 24 hours). Effectiveness is unknown when HBIG is administered later than 7 days.
  - Administer hepatitis B vaccine as soon as possible after exposure (preferably within 24 hours); it can be administered simultaneously with HBIG at a separate site.
  - Administer the vaccine only in the deltoid muscle using a 1- to 1.5-inch-long needle.
  - Persons exposed to HBsAg-positive blood or body fluids who are nonresponders to a primary vaccine series should receive a single dose of HBIG and the three-dose vaccine series initiated.

Booster Recommendations

A booster dose constitutes the amount of vaccine used in the vaccine dose for the three-dose series.[18]

In current guidelines, the CDC states that booster doses of hepatitis B vaccine are not necessary and that periodic serologic testing to monitor antibody concentrations after completion of the vaccine series is not recommended.[23] *To date, there appears to be no data to support the need for booster doses in immunocompetent individuals who have responded to a primary vaccine series. Immunity is long term and may be lifelong.*[27,28]

For *immunocompromised individuals* (e.g., hemodialysis patients whose anti-HBs levels fall below 10 mIU/mL), booster doses and periodic serologic testing are recommended.[3,28]

Occupational exposure–prone individuals need to know their hepatitis B serologic status. Postvaccination serologic testing for anti-HBs is strongly recommended by some authors. Nonresponse rates have been demonstrated in several studies. One study cites a 29% nonresponse rate among health care workers who were vaccinated against hepatitis B. Booster vaccination response in 6 of 6 subjects in this study suggests immunity. These authors recommend the following[39]:

- Post vaccination testing within 1 to 2 months to document immunity
- Periodic anti-HBs monitoring
- Booster vaccination to maintain protective titer levels

Hepatitis C Virus Exposure Treatment[23]

- After accidental percutaneous exposure from a hepatitis C–positive source, an average of 1.8% persons demonstrate anti-HCV seroconversion. Transmission rarely occurs from mucous membrane exposure to blood; no transmission has been documented from intact or nonintact skin exposures to blood.
- Immune globulin and antiviral agents such as interferon with or without ribavirin *are not recommended for postexposure treatment.*
- The HCV infection status of the source and the person exposed should be evaluated. If the source tests anti-HCV, follow-up testing of the exposed person should be performed to determine whether infection develops. This is intended to identify chronic hepatitis C infection early so that referral for treatment can be made. Currently, data are insufficient to recommend treatment of acute HCV infection; that is, HCV RNA is first detected, but no evidence of liver disease is seen (normal ALT levels).
- Review Display 12.2 (p. 479) for CDC recommendations on postexposure follow-up.

PRACTICE/REVIEW QUESTIONS

After reviewing this module, answer the following questions. ONE OR MORE THAN ONE of the choices may be correct.

1. List the five major forms of hepatitis:

   a. _____

   b. _____

   c. _____

   d. _____

   e. _____

2. All forms of hepatitis are caused by a(n) _____ or _____.

3. The five major forms of hepatitis differ in:

   A. Mode of transmission

   B. How they affect people

   C. How they are diagnosed

   D. All of these

   E. None of these

4. Which of the following statements about hepatitis A reflect current knowledge?

   A. The disease is spread by the fecal–oral route or ingestion of contaminated food or water.

   B. The disease is commonly contracted through contaminated blood.

   C. About one third of acute hepatitis cases in the United States are caused by HAV.

   D. The infection is much more severe when contracted by pregnant women.

   E. No vaccine exists for this disease.

   F. Viral infection in pregnancy is not associated with teratogenicity.

   G. Persistent antibody after infection (IgG anti-HAV) means the individual is immune.

   H. Absence of the IgG anti-HAV antibody after infection indicates a carrier state.

5. HCV is estimated to have infected about _____ people worldwide or _____ % of the world's population.

6. In the United States, the CDC reports that about _____ people are chronically infected with HCV.

7. Annually, approximately _____ deaths occur from chronic HCV infection.

8. Most hepatitis C–infected individuals are:

   A. Symptomatic

   B. Not symptomatic

9. Of hepatitis C–infected persons, _____ % to _____ % develop chronic liver disease, leading to the need for a liver transplant or resulting in death.

10. Hepatitis C postinfected persons who test positive for anti-HCV are:

    A. Infectious

    B. Immune

11. Hepatitis _____ exists as an acute coinfection acquired simultaneously with hepatitis B or as a superinfection in a chronic hepatitis B carrier.

12. Hepatitis _____ has a high mortality rate for fulminant hepatic failure in pregnant women, is associated with serious neonatal mortality, and does not exist as a chronic infection.

13. An *antigen* is defined as: _____

    _____ .

14. An *antibody* is defined as: _____

    _____ .

15. Match the symbols in Column B with the appropriate hepatitis B antigen or antibody term listed in Column A.

Column A

_____ 1. Surface antigen

_____ 2. Core antigen

_____ 3. e antigen

_____ 4. Antibodies to the surface antigen

_____ 5. Antibodies to the core antigen

_____ 6. Antibodies to the e antigen

Column B

a. HBcAg

b. anti-HBe

c. HBeAg

d. HBsAg

e. anti-HBs

f. anti-HBc

16. Match the terms in Column B with the appropriate characteristic or definition in Column A.

Column A

_____ 1. The protein coat of the virus can be found in infected persons.

_____ 2. This antigen cannot be found in the blood of infected persons.

_____ 3. The presence of this antigen in serum indicates that hepatitis B infection is one of the earliest indicators of the infection.

_____ 4. This antigen is never found alone. It always occurs after HBsAg is present and the infection state has begun.

_____ 5. When this antibody is found alone with HBsAg, the individual has developed an immunity to the disease and is neither infectious nor a carrier.

_____ 6. The detection of this antibody indicates that the core antigen is or was present in the body at one time (i.e., the individual has had hepatitis B).

_____ 7. This antibody is the only one that is detectable by the laboratory studies during all phases of a hepatitis B infection.

_____ 8. Whenever this antibody is found together with the HBsAg surface antigen, the individual is a carrier of hepatitis B infection but is of decreased infectiousness.

_____ 9. The presence of this antibody can remain for an individual's lifetime, can indicate a carrier state after infection, and in a pregnant woman, can indicate the possibility of passing the infection to the baby if the HBsAg surface antigen is also present.

_____ 10. The persistent presence of this antigen occurs in chronic hepatitis B.

Column B

a. HBcAg

b. anti-HBe

c. HBeAg

d. HBsAg

e. anti-HBs

f. anti-HBc

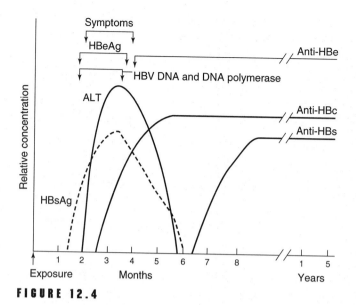

FIGURE 12.4

17. Mark an "X" beside those statements that accurately reflect what Figure 12.4 depicts about the course of hepatitis B infection.

_____ a. Symptoms appear approximately 1 to 3 weeks after exposure.

_____ b. The appearance of symptoms (if any) usually correlates with the ability to detect HBsAg and HBeAg in blood.

_____ c. HBcAg is not detectable in blood.

_____ d. Detectable levels of HBsAg generally disappear after 6 months.

_____ e. The antibody to the core antigen begins to appear during the symptom phase and can be detected easily. It can persist for a lifetime.

_____ f. HBsAg and anti-HBs do not exist together.

18. Carrier states:

A. Are a key factor in the spread of hepatitis B worldwide

B. Pose minimal problems for individual carriers themselves

C. Are associated with high prevalence rates in most populations worldwide

D. Are easily identified through symptoms of the disease

19. A child's best chances of avoiding the hepatitis B carrier state would be if he or she were born in:

A. The Philippines

B. East Africa

C. Hong Kong

D. Canada

20. Children in endemic areas of hepatitis B carriers, such as in the Pacific Islands or Southeast Asia:

A. Develop an immunity to the disease in the majority of cases

B. Have the greatest risk of contracting the infection at birth

C. Have the greatest risk of contracting the infection as adults

D. Can contract the infection but rarely become carriers

21. The major influences on the increase of hepatitis B in the United States are

    _____ and _____.

22. List eight groups of women who are at high risk for hepatitis B carrier status during pregnancy.

    a. _____

    b. _____

    c. _____

    d. _____

    e. _____

    f. _____

    g. _____

    h. _____

Select from the following list the serologic marker to complete the statement(s) in questions 23 through 25:

    HBsAg   anti-HBs
    HBeAg   anti-HBe
    HBcAg   anti-HBc

23. A highly infectious carrier has HBsAg and _____ in his or her blood.

24. A carrier of diminished infectivity has HBsAg and _____ in his or her blood.

25. An immune state exists when _____ is found in the blood.

26. Mothers who have had hepatitis B:

    A. Will always be carriers

    B. Can recover completely from the disease and not be carriers

27. There is no evidence that hepatitis B is transmitted to the fetus through the placenta during pregnancy.

    A. True

    B. False

28. Transmission from an infected or carrier mother to the baby is most likely to occur as the baby comes into contact with infected amniotic fluid or blood during the birth process.

    A. True

    B. False

29. In the United States, hepatitis B is contracted most often during adulthood.

    A. True

    B. False

30. Infants who contract hepatitis B are less likely to become chronic carriers than are adults who contract the disease.

    A. True

    B. False

31. Carriers are the predominant vehicle by which the hepatitis B virus is passed on from person to person.

    A. True

    B. False

32. Many carriers are asymptomatic and do not know that they have been exposed to the virus.

    A. True

    B. False

33. A patient's hepatitis B screen shows the presence of HBsAg. Which of the following serologic markers should be ordered to identify whether the patient might be a carrier?

    A. anti-HBc

    B. IgM anti-HBc

    C. HBeAg

    D. anti-HBe

34. IgM anti-HBc and IgG anti-HBc serologic markers are requested on the patient referred to in question 33. The report reads as follows: *IgG anti-HBc = positive; IgM anti-HBc = negative.* Which of the following are the correct diagnostic interpretations?

    A. Carrier state

    B. Immune

    C. Infectious

    D. Recently infected

35. A patient's laboratory report reads as follows: *Anti-HBs = present; IgG anti-HBc = present.* Which of the following is the appropriate interpretation?

    A. Carrier state

    B. Immune state

    C. Minimally infectious

    D. Recent infection

36. Betty Lou's hepatitis B screen reads as follows: *HBsAg = positive.* A correct conclusion includes that she is:

    A. Infected

    B. A carrier

    C. Immune

    D. Susceptible

37. In a follow-up test on Betty Lou (the patient referred to in question 36) the following report is sent: *HBsAg = positive; HBeAg = positive; IgM anti-HBc = positive.* You can correctly conclude that she is:

    A. Acutely infected

    B. Chronically infected

    C. Of a lower infectivity level

    D. Not infectious at all

38. Despite the 1988 universal screening guidelines for pregnant women, transmission during the perinatal period still occurs in the United States because:

    A. A relatively high percentage of women do not receive prenatal care

    B. Hepatitis B immunization is not 100% effective

    C. There is a high rate of viral transmission across the placenta

    D. There is a high viral transmission rate to newborns from infected health care personnel

39. Which of the following pregnant women should be screened for hepatitis B?

    A. 35-year-old mother of four children, married to the same man for 16 years

    B. 29-year-old lawyer in a monogamous relationship

    C. 20-year-old college graduate who tested negative for HBsAg 1 year ago

    D. 25-year-old nurse who tested anti-HBs positive 1 month ago

40. Which of the following women need liver function tests?

    A. 16-year-old at 16 weeks' gestation with a palpable liver and who is positive for HBsAg, IgG anti-HBc, and anti-HBe

    B. 18-year-old at 39 weeks' gestation who is positive for anti-HBs

    C. 30-year-old at 18 weeks' gestation who is negative for HBsAg and positive for anti-HBc

    D. 21-year-old at 6 weeks' gestation who tests positive for HBsAg on her hepatitis screen

41. Jane Rupp is a 20-year-old woman, gravida 1, at 7 weeks' gestation. Her hepatitis B screen reads as follows: *HBsAg = negative.* You interpret this to mean that she is:

    A. Highly infectious

    B. Immune

    C. Needs no further workup

    D. Infectious but not acutely so

42. Mandy Soffit is a 26-year-old woman, gravida 1, who is at 9 weeks' gestation. Her hepatitis B screen is reported as HBsAg = positive. You interpret this to mean that:

    A. She is infectious

    B. Further workup is needed

    C. She is immune

    D. A risk of perinatal transmission exists

43. Hettie Swan is a 30-year-old woman, gravida 3, who is 32 weeks pregnant. Late entry to prenatal care leads to her hepatitis workup being received today. The report reads as follows: *HBsAg = positive; HBeAg = negative; anti-HBe = positive.* You interpret this to mean that:

    A. There is a 10% risk of perinatal transmission

    B. She has a history of hepatitis B but is now immune

    C. There is a 90% risk of perinatal transmission

    D. There is no risk of perinatal transmission

44. Ida Plano is the mother of a 3-year-old and is approximately 34 weeks pregnant. Her hepatitis B screen at 12 weeks' gestation was negative. Owing to a recent exposure through a new sexual partner, she is tested again. Today, the results read as follows: *HBsAg = positive; HBeAg = positive.* Perinatal transmission risk is:

    A. *Low* because maternal infectiousness is occurring during the third trimester

    B. *Low* because of the presence of HBeAg

    C. *High* because maternal infectiousness is occurring during the third trimester

    D. *High* because of the presence of HBeAg

45. Appropriate follow-up to Ida Plano's test result is to:

    A. Test her 3-year-old immediately if never immunized with hepatitis B vaccine

    B. Immunize Ida immediately

    C. Arrange for hepatitis B testing for Ida's recent sexual partner and other intimate household contacts

    D. Order liver tests for Ida

46. When caring for infants of hepatitis B carrier mothers, what is your primary goal?

    _____

47. State seven steps, other than the immunization treatment, that are aimed at reducing the risk of transmission of the disease to the infant of a carrier mother or a mother of unknown HBV status.

    a. _____

    b. _____

    c. _____

    d. _____

    e. _____

    f. _____

    g. _____

48. The immunization treatment for the newborn of a carrier mother includes administering both _____ and _____ within _____ after delivery.

49. _____ is given at birth only and ideally within 12 hours of delivery.

50. In recommendations for vaccination of infants and children younger than 11 years, _____ is administered in two additional doses at _____ months of age and at _____ months of age.

51. The correct dose of HBIG for the newborn given at birth is _____.

52. The correct dose of Recombivax HB, Pediatric, given in three doses (birth, 1 month later, 5 months later) is _____.

53. HBIG and Recombivax HB, Pediatric (or Engerix-B, Pediatric/Adolescent), should always be administered to the newborn in the same site.

    A. True

    B. False

54. Should the baby be bathed before or after the injections of HBIG and Recombivax HB, Pediatric, or Engerix-B, Pediatric/Adolescent? _____

55. The appropriate injection sites to use for administration of HBIG and Recombivax HB, Pediatric, or Engerix-B, Pediatric/Adolescent, are in the _____ muscles.

56. HBIG confers _____ immunity in the newborn, whereas Recombivax HB, Pediatric, or Engerix-B, Pediatric/Adolescent, confers _____ immunity in the newborn.

57. There are never any justifiable reasons for waiving risk reduction measures for hepatitis B transmission in the newborn.

    A. True

    B. False

58. If the baby must be transported, besides preparing the infant for transport, what additional steps would you take with the infant of a carrier mother?

    a. _____

    b. _____

    c. _____

59. If an infant is born to a mother who has not been screened for hepatitis B but belongs to one of the risk groups, the recommendation(s) is(are):

    A. Obtain a blood specimen from the mother for a hepatitis B screen

    B. Obtain a blood specimen from the baby for a hepatitis B screen

    C. Give the baby HBIG 0.5 mL intramuscularly within 12 hours of birth

    D. Give Recombivax HB, Pediatric, or Engerix-B, Pediatric/Adolescent, to the newborn within 12 hours of birth

60. Select the statements that reflect what is known about newborn testing for HBV.

    A. Accurate methods exist for testing the newborn within the first month of life.

    B. Transplancentally acquired maternal HBsAg or anti-HBs in the newborn's blood complicates the diagnosis.

    C. All infants born to mothers who are positive for hepatitis B antigens or antibodies will be seropositive for these markers at birth.

    D. The maternal IgM marker can be identified in the newborn's blood.

61. Active immunization can be conferred in most newborns through the administration of:

    A. Hepatitis B immune globulin (HBIG)

    B. Recombivax HB, Pediatric

    C. Engerix-B, Pediatric/Adolescent

    D. Vitamin K

62. The treatment regimen used to confer active immunity on the newborn is:

    A. An initial 0.5-mL dose of Recombivax HB, Pediatric, intramuscularly within 12 hours of birth, followed by two additional immunizations at 1 month of age and 6 months of age

    B. An initial 0.5-mL dose of HBIG intramuscularly within 12 hours of birth, followed by immunizations with Recombivax HB, Pediatric, at 1 month and 5 months of age

    C. A single immunization with Recombivax HB, Pediatric, within 12 hours of birth

    D. An initial 0.5-mL dose of HBIG intramuscularly within 12 hours of birth, followed by immunization with HBIG at 1 and 6 months of age

63. A Vietnamese patient who has no record of having a hepatitis B screening delivers a healthy 7-pound infant. While awaiting the results from the mother's hepatitis B test, the recommendation(s) for care of this infant is(are):

   A. That no special care is required

   B. Isolation should be maintained after bathing the infant

   C. 0.5 mL of Recombivax HB, Pediatric, should be administered intramuscularly within 12 hours of birth

   D. 0.5 mL of HBIG should be administered intramuscularly within 12 hours of birth

64. An analysis of a newborn's cord blood for hepatitis B markers reveals the following results: *HBsAg = negative; anti-HBc = positive; anti-HBs = positive.* Which of the following conclusions can be drawn?

   A. The mother is an HBV carrier.

   B. The baby is immune.

   C. The mother is immune.

   D. The baby is infected with HBV.

65. Select those practices that correctly reflect universal precautions.

   A. Gloves are worn when bathing newly delivered babies.

   B. Gown, face shields, and goggles are worn while performing an amniotomy.

   C. Full-size eye glasses are used for eye protection during a vaginal birth.

   D. Double gloving is done when discontinuing a woman's IV line.

   E. Gloves are worn while giving an HBsAg-positive laboring woman a bedpan.

66. A registered nurse works in a labor and delivery unit in a busy metropolitan area. Select the following activities that are likely to put her at risk of contracting HBV infection.

   A. Screening high-risk patient charts to identify patients most at risk for being infected with HBV

   B. Recapping all needles carefully after use

   C. Choosing to wear gloves only while bathing babies who have been born of intravenous drug users or of women who are partners of intravenous drug users

   D. Hugging a hepatitis B carrier mother after the birth of her child

67. You are going to give a bath to a newly delivered hepatitis B carrier mother. After the bath, you need to begin an IV line. Which sequence of steps is recommended in the universal precautions guidelines?

   A. Wash hands, put on gloves, remove gloves after the bath, immediately put on another pair of gloves prior to starting the IV line.

   B. Continue to use the same pair of gloves without interrupting for handwashing.

   C. Wash hands, put on gloves for the bath, remove gloves, wash hands, and put on the same pair of gloves if you see no tears.

   D. Remove gloves after the bath, wash hands immediately, and put on another pair of gloves before starting the IV line.

68. A pregnant nurse working on a labor and delivery, nursery, or postpartum unit should:

   A. Request a change to another hospital unit

   B. Be assigned to low-risk patients on those units

   C. Know her hepatitis B status

   D. Use universal precautions

69. List five areas of education that should be addressed with the newly delivered hepatitis B carrier mother and her family.

    a. _____

    b. _____

    c. _____

    d. _____

    e. _____

70. Indicate whether the following statements are true (T) or false (F):

    _____ a. Infants who are not bathed need to be kept isolated from their hepatitis B carrier mothers in the delivery or birthing room.

    _____ b. An unstable newborn who has not been able to be bathed should be kept in isolation after being brought from the delivery or birthing room.

    _____ c. Nursing and medical staff to the nursery should use gowns and gloves when handling a baby who has not been bathed.

    _____ d. The reason for any isolation procedure used with the baby is to prevent transmission of hepatitis B to the baby.

    _____ e. Even if a baby has been infected with HBV, the baby will not be infectious to nurses and medical personnel after a thorough bathing.

    _____ f. Hepatitis B carrier mothers need not be placed in a private room.

71. Explain why a baby of a hepatitis B carrier mother, after being thoroughly bathed, need not be kept isolated from other mothers or babies in the nursery or on the postpartum unit.

    _____

72. List four areas of self-care and precautions about which you need to instruct the newly delivered hepatitis B carrier mother.

    a. _____

    b. _____

    c. _____

    d. _____

73. Which of the following mothers have contraindications to any breastfeeding throughout the postpartum course?

    A. Angie is a known hepatitis B carrier mother who has just delivered her third child this morning. The baby received HBIG after birth.

    B. Mary Beth is an intravenous drug abuser who tested positive for both HBV and HIV. Her newborn is doing well at 2 hours of age and has received HBIG.

    C. Claire has recently tested positive for HBsAg and HBeAg but has no clinical signs or symptoms of infection. She delivered a healthy newborn yesterday. The baby received HBIG after birth.

    D. Isun is a nurse who works on a labor and delivery unit. Because she was found to be susceptible (no history of immunization and no anti-HBs), she received the full course of hepatitis B immunization during the last 6 months of her pregnancy. She delivered a healthy baby today.

    E. Teryl, a carrier mother, delivered by cesarean birth 4 days ago. The baby was given HBIG after birth. Today both of Teryl's nipples are cracked, with a slight serosanguinous discharge.

74. Which of the following statements best applies to recombinant vaccines?

    A. Production involves HBsAg gene manipulation in a yeast host cell.

    B. They confer short-term, passive immunity.

    C. They are no longer being produced in the United States.

    D. Production involves using the plasma of chronically infected persons.

75. Recombivax HB was administered *to a population of infants and young children* in a series of three IM injections according to recommended dose and interval. Current research predicts that:

    A. 90% of the population will be successfully immunized

    B. 95% of the population will be immunized

    C. 100% of the population will be immunized

    D. It is not possible to project the efficacy of the immunization process on the population

76. Choose the statements that best describe Engerix-B.

    A. Engerix-B is a plasma-derived vaccine.

    B. Engerix-B is given in a three-dose series.

    C. When given in a four-dose series, the last dose ensures an optimal final antibody titer.

    D. Engerix-B is not as effective in producing an immune response as Recombivax HB.

77. Isabella brings her 6-month-old child into the Health Department to receive his third dose of Recombivax HB, Pediatric. The child is also due for his DPT booster. You know that:

    A. The antibody response of one vaccine can interfere with the other vaccine

    B. These vaccines should not be given together because of potential side effects

    C. Administration of both vaccines is appropriate

    D. The DPT vaccine should be delayed at least 1 month after administration of the hepatitis B vaccine

78. The following individuals receive a complete series of hepatitis B vaccine.

    1. Baby Donald, whose mother was HBsAg positive at the time of birth

    2. A medical technologist

    3. Damion, who is 28 years old and HIV positive

    4. Theresa, a 16-year-old adolescent

    Which of these individuals should have postvaccination testing?

    A. 1, 2, and 4

    B. 1, 2, and 3

    C. 2 and 4

    D. All of them

79. Studies indicate that approximately 5% to 10% of infected health care workers become carriers.

    A. True

    B. False

80. An unvaccinated health care worker could potentially infect susceptible patients with the hepatitis B virus.

    A. True

    B. False

81. The gluteal muscle is not recommended for HBV vaccination in children or adults.

    A. True

    B. False

82. Which of the following statements accurately profile the recommended use of HBIG in postexposure treatment?

    A. When HBIG is given in conjunction with hepatitis B vaccine, efficacy of the immune response is improved.

    B. An exposed health care worker's immune response is improved if given HBIG 2 weeks after a documented percutaneous exposure to HBsAg-positive blood.

    C. HBIG is administered in postexposure situations in calculated amounts based on the body weight of the individual at risk.

    D. HBIG may be given in two doses, 1 month apart, to a vaccinated individual who shows inadequate anti-HBs levels (a nonresponder) and who suffers an inadvertent exposure to HBsAg-positive blood.

83. When a health care worker accidentally receives a needlestick from a needle used on an individual with unknown serologic status, appropriate actions include:

    A. Obtaining an immediate hepatitis B blood (and HIV) workup of the health care worker to assess immune status

    B. Beginning hepatitis B immune globulin injections only after the health care worker's and the patient's status are known

    C. Evaluating the patient's hepatitis B status immediately

    D. Giving the health care worker HBIG immediately and beginning immunization within 7 days if the patient is a carrier and the worker is nonimmune

PRACTICE/REVIEW ANSWER KEY

1. a. Hepatitis A virus (HAV)
   b. Hepatitis B virus (HBV)
   c. Hepatitis C virus (HCV)
   d. Hepatitis D virus (HDV)
   e. Hepatitis E virus (HEV)

2. virus; viruslike particles

3. D

4. A, C, F, and G

5. 170 million; 3

6. 4 million

7. 8,000 to 10,000

8. B

9. 75; 85

10. A

11. D

12. C

13. A substance that, when introduced into a host, is capable of producing antibodies; bacteria and viruses are examples of antigens.

14. A protein substance developed in response to the presence of an antigen; they are part of the body's defense against foreign substances such as bacteria and viruses.

15. 1. d
    2. a
    3. c
    4. e
    5. f
    6. b

16. 1. d
    2. a
    3. d
    4. c
    5. e
    6. f
    7. f
    8. b
    9. f
    10. d

17. X at b, c, d, e, and f

18. A and C

19. D

20. B

21. Drug abuse; migration of high-carrier populations, such as Vietnamese, Haitians, and Africans, to the United States

22. a. Drug abusers who inject drugs under the skin or into veins
    b. Women who are partners of intravenous drug abusers or bisexual men or those who have multiple partners
    c. Health care workers such as nurses, physicians, medical technologists, dentists, dental hygienists
    d. Southeast Asians, Native Alaskans, Pacific Islanders, and Haitians
    e. Those with active disease or a history of hepatitis
    f. Those with a history of venereal disease
    g. Those rejected as blood donors—these individuals might have had the hepatitis surface antigen (HBsAg) detected
    h. Those who work in a renal dialysis unit (this also includes wives of men who are receiving dialysis)

23. HBeAg

24. Anti-HBe

25. Anti-HBs

26. B

27. B

28. A

29. A

30. B

31. A

32. A

33. B

34. A and C

35. B

36. A

37. A

38. A and B

39. A, B, and C

40. A, D

41. C

42. A, B, and D

43. A

44. C and D

45. A, C, and D

46. Prevention of the infants from becoming carriers of hepatitis B

47. Any seven of the following:
    a. Obtaining informed consent for treatment of the infant before delivery
    b. Avoiding invasive procedures on the fetus during the labor and birth period if possible
    c. Assigning one nurse to attend to the newborn after delivery
    d. Drying the infant immediately after the delivery to remove all maternal blood and amniotic fluid
    e. Gently removing excess fluid and blood from the nares and oropharynx
    f. Aspirating stomach contents using a mucus extractor or meconium aspirator with wall suction on a low setting
    g. Delaying the administration of vitamin K until after the infant is bathed
    h. Bathing the newborn early and thoroughly with a mild, nonmedicated soap under radiant heat as soon as the infant is stable
    i. Treating the infant of a hepatitis B infectious or carrier mother immediately

48. HBIG; Recombivax HB, Pediatric, or Engerix-B, Pediatric/Adolescent; 12 hours

49. HBIG

50. Recombivax HB, Pediatric, or Engerix-B, Pediatric/Adolescent; 1 to 4; 6 to 18

51. 0.5 mL

52. 5 µg (0.5 mL) of Recombivax HB, Pediatric, or 10 µg (0.5 mL) of Engerix-B, Pediatric/Adolescent

53. B

54. Before

55. Anterolateral thigh

56. Passive; active

57. B (life-threatening situations take priority)

58. a. Inform the receiving physician/flight nurse/hospital that the baby's mother is infected with hepatitis B or a carrier.
    b. Label the maternal blood as HBsAg positive before making the transport.
    c. Inform the transport team of what has been done for the baby regarding the prevention of transmission of the infection.

59. A, C, and D

60. B, C

61. B and C

62. A

63. C and D

64. C

65. A, B, and C (Also see Module 11 p. 460)

66. A and C (These activities represent selective identification of some women and not others for the practice of universal precautions. Treat all patients as if they were potentially infected with a bloodborne pathogen.)

67. D (See module 11)

68. C and D

69. a. How hepatitis B could be transmitted to the infant and the importance of proper hand-washing after handling blood-soiled materials (e.g., in changing the mother's perineal pads before handling the baby)
    b. The potential for saliva causing transmission of the infection
    c. The risks the mother's hepatitis carrier status poses for the infant
    d. The risks and benefits of immunization for the infant
    e. The need for complete immunization plans for the baby over the next 6 months

70. a. F
    b. T
    c. T
    d. F
    e. T
    f. T

71. Because the production of viruses in an infant who is infected with hepatitis B does not occur for several weeks

72. Any four of the following:
    a. To wash her hands before handling the baby
    b. Precautions for blood spills, lochia, and perineal pads
    c. To avoid letting the baby come in contact with soiled linen
    d. Why it is important to delay breastfeeding for 48 hours after administration of HBIG to the baby
    e. To inspect her breasts and nipples for infection or breaks in the skin if she is breast-feeding (maternal HIV infection is a contraindication to breastfeeding)

73. B and E

74. A

75. B (90% applies to a population of adults.)

76. B and C

77. C

78. D

79. A

80. A

81. A

82. A and C

83. A, C, and D

REFERENCES

1. Centers for Disease Control and Prevention. (1999). Prevention of hepatitis A through active or passive immunization: Recommendations of the Advisory Committee on Immunization Practices (ACIP). *MMWR Morbidity and Mortality Weekly Report, 48*(RR-12), 1–37.
2. Reinus, J. F., & Leiken, E. L. (1999). Viral hepatitis in pregnancy. *Clinics in Liver Disease, 3*(1), 115–130.
3. Regev, A., & Schiff, E. R. (2000). Viral hepatitis A, B, and C. *Clinics in Liver Disease, 4*(1), 47–71.
4. Cunningham, F. G., Gant, N. F., Leveno, K. J., Gilstrap, L. C., Hauth, J. C., & Wenstrom, K. D. (2001). *Williams obstetrics* (21st ed., pp. 1289–1293). New York: McGraw-Hill.
5. American College of Obstetricians and Gynecologists. (1998). ACOG educational bulletin: Viral hepatitis in pregnancy. No. 248. *International Journal of Gynaecology and Obstetrics, 63*(2), 195–202.
6. Bonkovsky, H. L., & Mehta, S. (2001). Hepatitis C: A review and update. *Journal of the American Academy of Dermatology, 44*(2),159–179.
7. Centers for Disease Control and Prevention. (1998). Recommendations for prevention and control of hepatitis C virus (HCV) infection and HCV-related chronic disease. *MMWR Morbidity and Mortality Weekly Report, 47*(RR-19), 1–39.
8. American College of Obstetricians and Gynecologists. (1998). ACOG committee opinion: Breastfeeding and the risk of hepatitis C virus transmission. No. 220. *International Journal of Gynaecology and Obstetrics, 66*(3), 307–308.
9. Zuckerman, J. N., & Zuckerman, A. J. (1999). The epidemiology of hepatitis B. *Clinics in Liver Disease, 3*(2), 179–187.
10. Befeler, A. S., & Di Bisceglie, A. M. (September, 2000). Hepatitis B. *Infectious Disease Clinics of North America, 14*(3), 617–619.
11. Centers for Disease Control and Prevention. (1988). Recommendations of the Immunization Practices Advisory Committee: Prevention of perinatal transmission of hepatitis B virus—Prenatal screening of all pregnant women for hepatitis B surface antigen. *MMWR Morbidity and Mortality Weekly Report, 37*(22), 341–346, 351.
12. Centers for Disease Control and Prevention. (1989). *Hepatitis surveillance report.* No. 52. Atlanta: Author.
13. Centers for Disease Control and Prevention. (1990). Protection against viral hepatitis: Recommendations of Immunization Practices Advisory Committee (ACIP). *MMWR Morbidity and Mortality Weekly Report, 39*(RR-2), 1–26.

14. Arevalo, J. A. (1989). Hepatitis B in pregnancy. *Western Journal of Medicine, 150*(6), 668–674.

15. Committee on Obstetrics: Maternal and Fetal Medicine. (March, 1992). Guidelines for hepatitis B virus screening and vaccination during pregnancy. ACOG Committee Opinion. No. 103. Washington, DC: American College of Obstetricians and Gynecologists.

16. Centers for Disease Control and Prevention. (1996). Prevention of perinatal group B streptococcal disease: A public health perspective. *MMWR Morbidity and Mortality Weekly Report, 45*(RR-7), 1–24.

17. Ingardia, C. J. (1999). Hepatitis B vaccination in pregnancy: Factors influencing efficacy. *Obstetrics and Gynecology, 93*(6), 983–986.

18. Centers for Disease Control and Prevention. (1991) Hepatitis B virus: A comprehensive strategy for eliminating transmission in the United States through universal childhood vaccination—Recommendations of the Immunization Practices Advisory Committee (ACIP). *MMWR Morbidity and Mortality Weekly Report, 40*(RR-13), 1–25.

19. Jefferson, T., Demicheli, V., Deeks, J., MacMillan, A., Sassi, F., & Pratt, M. (2000). Vaccines for preventing hepatitis B in health-care workers. *Cochrane Database System Review,* (2), CD000100.

20. Ellis, R. W. (1990). New and improved vaccines against hepatitis. In G. C. Woodrow & M. M. Levine (Eds.), *New generation of vaccines* (pp. 439–445). New York: Marcel Dekker.

21. Kimmel, S. R. (2000). Immunizations. *Clinics in Family Practice, 2*(2), 369–389.

22. Centers for Disease Control and Prevention. (1999). Thimerosal in vaccines: A joint statement the American Academy of Pediatrics and the Public Health Service. *MMWR Morbidity and Mortality Weekly Report, 48*(26), 563.

23. Centers for Disease Control and Prevention. (June 29, 2001). Updated U.S. Public Health Service guidelines for the management of occupational exposures to HBV, HCV, and HIV and recommendations for postexposure prophylaxis. *MMWR Morbidity and Mortality Weekly Report, 50*(RR-11), 1–52.

24. Centers for Disease Control and Prevention. (1991). Inadequate immune response among public safety workers. Reviewing intradermal vaccination against hepatitis B—United States, 1990-1991. *MMWR Morbidity and Mortality Weekly Report, 40*(33), 569–572.

25. Ingardia, C. J., Kelley, L., Lerer, T., Wax, J. R., & Steinfeld, J. D. (1999). Correlation of maternal and fetal hepatitis B antibody titers following maternal vaccination in pregnancy. *American Journal of Perinatology, 16*(3), 129–132.

26. Centers for Disease Control and Prevention. (2000) Update: Expanded availability of thimerosal preservative-free hepatitis B vaccine. *MMWR Morbidity and Mortality Weekly Report, 49*(28), 642, 651.

27. Margolis, H. J. (May 18, 1999). Testimony of Harold S. Margolis, M.D., Chief Hepatitis Branch, National Center for Infectious Diseases, Centers for Disease Control and Prevention (CDC) before the U.S. House of Representatives Committee on Government Reform, Subcommittee on Criminal Justice, Drug Policy, and Human Resources (pp. 1–10). Available at: www.cdc.gov/ncidod/diseases/hepatitis/margolis.htm

28. European Consensus Development Conference. (2000). Are booster immunizations needed for lifelong hepatitis B immunity? *Lancet, 355*(9203), 561–565.

29. Lee, S. D., Chan, C. Y., Yu, M. I., Lu, R. H., Chan, F. Y., & Lo, K. J. (1999). Hepatitis B vaccination in patients with chronic hepatitis C. *Journal of Medical Virotology, 59*(4), 463–468.

30. Centers for Disease Control and Prevention. (1989). Guidelines for the prevention of transmission of human immunodeficiency virus and hepatitis B virus to healthcare and public safety workers. *MMWR Morbidity and Mortality Weekly Report, 38*(S-6), 177.

31. Department of Labor, Occupational Safety and Health Administration. (1991). OSHA blood-borne pathogens final rule. *Federal Register, 56*(235, Pt II, excerpts), 64175–64182.

32. Centers for Disease Control and Prevention. (1995). Recommended childhood immunization schedule—United States. *MMWR Morbidity and Mortality Weekly Report, 44*(RR-5), 1–9.

33. Losonsky, G. A., Wasserman, S. S., Stephens, I., Mahoney, F., Armstrong, P., Gumpper, K., Dulkerian, S., West, D. J., & Gewolb, I. H. (1999). Hepatitis B vaccination of premature infants: A reassessment of current recommendations for delayed immunizations. *Pediatrics Electronic Pages, 103*(2), E14.

34. Yusuf, H. R., Daniels, D., Smith, P., Coronado, V., & Rodewald, L. (2000). Association between administration of hepatitis B vaccine at birth and completion of the hepatitis B and 4: 3: 1: 3 vaccine series. *Journal of the American Medical Association, 284*(8), 978–983.

35. Centers for Disease Control and Prevention. (1981). Hepatitis in Indo-Chinese refugees. *Hepatitis Surveillance, 46*, 26, 351–356.

36. American College of Obstetricians and Gynecologists. (1998). Hepatitis virus infections in obstetricians-gynecologists. ACOG committee opinion. *International Journal of Obstetrics and Gynecology, 63*, 203–204.

37. Department of Labor, Occupational Safety and Health Administration. (1991). (29 CFR Part 1910. 1030.) Occupational exposure to bloodborne pathogens: Final rule. *Federal Register, 56*, 64004–64182.

38. Centers for Disease Control and Prevention. (1997). Immunization of health-care workers: Recommendations of the Advisory Committee on Immunization Practices (ACIP) and the Hospital Infection Control Practices Advisory Committee (HICPAC). *MMWR Morbidity and Mortality Weekly Report, 46*(RR-18), 1–42.
39. Barash, C., Conn, M. I., DiMarino, A. J., Jr., Marzano, J., & Allen, M. L. (1999). Serologic hepatitis B immunity in vaccinated health care workers. *Archives of Internal Medicine, 159*(13), 1481–1483.
40. Rosen, E., Rudensky, B., Paz, E., Isacohn, M., Jerassi, Z., Gottehrer, N. P., & Yinnon, A. M. (1999). Ten-year follow-up study of hepatitis B virus infection and vaccination status in hospital employees. *Journal of Hospital Infection, 41*(3), 245–250.

MODULE 13

Caring for the Pregnant Woman With Diabetes

MARY COPELAND MYERS

As you complete this module, you will learn:

1. The epidemiology of diabetes mellitus and gestational diabetes
2. Perinatal consequences for women with preexisting diabetes and gestational diabetes
3. Preconception health care issues for diabetic women
4. Current classification and diagnostic criteria for diabetes mellitus
5. Characteristics of type 1 diabetes
6. Characteristics of type 2 diabetes
7. Characteristics of secondary diabetes
8. Characteristics of gestational diabetes
9. Physiology of normal glucose metabolism
10. Physiology of glucose metabolism during pregnancy
11. Pathophysiology of type 1, type 2, and gestational diabetes
12. Effect of pregnancy on preexisting diabetes
13. Effect of preexisting diabetes on pregnancy
14. Antepartum management goals for women with preexisting diabetes
15. Intrapartum management for women with preexisting diabetes
16. Postpartum management for women with preexisting diabetes
17. The pathophysiology of gestational diabetes
18. Diagnostic criteria for gestational diabetes
19. Antepartum management of pregnancy complicated by gestational diabetes
20. Intrapartum management of pregnancy complicated by gestational diabetes
21. Postpartum management of pregnancy complicated by gestational diabetes
22. Blood glucose goals during pregnancy
23. Signs and symptoms of hypoglycemia and proper treatment
24. Medical nutritional therapy requirements for diabetes during pregnancy
25. Exercise guidelines for women with diabetes during pregnancy
26. Insulin types and treatment regimens

When you have completed this module, you should be able to recall the meaning of the following terms. You should also be able to use the terms when consulting with other health professionals. The terms are defined in this module or in the glossary at the end of this book.

diabetic ketoacidosis (DKA)
diabetogenic
endogenous insulin
euglycemia
exogenous insulin
hemoglobin A_{1c} (HbA$_{1c}$)
hyperglycemic hyperosmolar nonketotic syndrome (HHNS)
hyperpnea
maturity-onset diabetes of youth (MODY)

nephropathy
neuropathy
organogenesis
polydipsia
polyphagia
polyuria
postprandial
preexisting diabetes or pregestational diabetes
proliferative retinopathy
retinopathy

Epidemiology of Diabetes

Diabetes is a significant public health challenge for the United States. In the United States, 15.7 million people (5.9% of the population) have diabetes. Of these people, 10.3 million are diagnosed and 5.4 million are undiagnosed. Approximately 8.2% of all women have diabetes. Each day, approximately 2,200 people are diagnosed with diabetes.[1,2] Diabetes is becoming more common, with an increase in both prevalence and incidence. Currently, it is a chronic disease that has no cure and is the seventh leading cause of death in the United States.

Age, sex, and race affect the prevalence of diabetes. Prevalence increases with age (Table 13.1). In women age 20 and older, the prevalence increases to 8.1 million, compared with 7.5 million men. Diabetes is increased in African Americans, Mexican Americans, Hispanic/Latino Americans, American Indians, Alaska Natives, Asian Americans, and Pacific Islanders (Table 13.2).[2]

TABLE 13.1 Age and Prevalence of Diabetes		
AGE	**PERCENTAGE OF PEOPLE WITH DIABETES**	**NUMBER OF PEOPLE WITH DIABETES**
<20	0.16	123,000
20–64 years	8.2	15.6 million
>65	18.4	6.3 million

TABLE 13.2 Race/Ethnicity and Prevalence of Diabetes		
RACE/ETHNICITY	**PERCENTAGE WITH DIABETES**	**INCREASED RISK OVER WHITES**
Whites	7.8	—
African Americans	10.8	1.7
Mexican Americans	10.6	1.9
Hispanic/Latino Americans	Insufficient data	2.0
American Indians and Alaska Natives	9	2.8

During pregnancy, approximately 2% to 5% (depending on race and ethnicity of the population) of women are diagnosed with gestational diabetes. Approximately 0.2% to 0.3% of all pregnancies are in women with type 1 diabetes. *In addition, approximately 2% of all women of childbearing age in the United States have undiagnosed type 2 diabetes mellitus.* Risks to the fetus depend on maternal glucose control during the time of conception and throughout the pregnancy.

Perinatal Consequences of Diabetes

Perinatal consequences depend on blood glucose control. In addition, the consequences differ depending on the gestational age when glycemic control is poor. If glycemic control is poor during conception and in the first trimester during organogenesis (first 8 weeks of gestation, when major organs are developing), congenital anomalies or miscarriage can occur. If glycemic control is poor during the second and third trimester, metabolic consequences occur. The metabolic problems are attributable to increased insulin production by the fetus in response to the elevated blood glucose of the mother. However, in gestational diabetes, which usually develops and is diagnosed after 24 weeks' gestation, congenital anomalies are not a consequence. However, metabolic problems can be encountered.

> If blood glucose is controlled during conception and throughout the pregnancy, perinatal consequences can be minimal.

The U.S. Public Health Service endorses preconception health as an integral component of care for all women contemplating pregnancy.[3] The March of Dimes Birth Defects Foundation recommends that preconception (prepregnancy planning) visits become a standard component of care.[4] *Unfortunately, preconception health care has not become a standard of care, and unplanned pregnancies occur in about two thirds of women with diabetes.[5]*

> Preconception care is recommended as a standard of care for all women of childbearing age.

> All women of childbearing age should be placed on a daily multivitamin with 0.4 mg of folic acid. Folic acid helps reduce the risk of neural tube defects.

Preconception health care management for diabetic women should include the following:

- Patient education about the interaction of diabetes and pregnancy
- Education about diabetes self-management skills
- Medical care and laboratory testing
- Counseling by a mental health professional, as necessary, to reduce stress and improve adherence to the treatment plan.

The specific goal is to lower the HbA$_{1c}$ before conception to a level that is associated with optimal development during organogenesis. Organogenesis is the time of organ development and occurs 17 to 56 days after conception. HbA$_{1c}$ levels that are less than 1% above the normal range are desirable.[5] Normal values are 4% to 6%.

The following assessment should be completed:

- **Complete history and physical examination.**
- **Laboratory testing**—This should include Pap smear, complete blood count (CBC), HbA$_{1c}$, serum creatinine, thyroid studies, and 24-hour urine evaluation for total protein, creatine clearance, and microalbumin.
- **Medication usage**—Example: Angiotensin-converting enzyme (ACE) inhibitors should not be used during pregnancy. Patients taking these medications should be assessed to determine whether the drug should be stopped or switched to another hypertensive medication.
- **Current insulin regimen**—The blood glucose log should be reviewed and insulin adjustments made for optimal control. If oral diabetic agents are being used, the patient should be switched to insulin therapy because *oral agents are contraindicated during pregnancy.*
- **Dilated retinal examination**—This should be performed by an ophthalmologist. Assess for retinopathy.
- **Screening test for coronary artery disease if cardiac or vascular diseases are present**—Testing includes a lipid panel (cholesterol, high-density lipoprotein, low-density lipoprotein, very-low-density lipoprotein, and triglycerides), electrocardiogram (ECG), and blood pressure. This will evaluate whether the patient can tolerate the increased cardiac demands of pregnancy.
- **Neurologic examination**—Assess for signs of autonomic neuropathy.
- **Referral to a diabetes educator and a registered dietitian**—They will assist the patient with her diet, exercise, and self-management skills.
- **Counseling regarding risks associated with the effects of diabetes on the pregnancy and the effects of pregnancy on diabetes.**
- **Counseling regarding lifestyle changes to enhance health**—Examples include daily exercise, smoking cessation, cessation of alcoholic beverage intake, and adequate rest.
- **Contraception**—Stress the importance of using effective contraception while obtaining optimal glycemic control. There are no specific contraceptive methods that are contraindicated in women with diabetes. The woman's support system must be explored. She should be seen every 1 to 2 months after the initial visit to determine whether goals are being achieved and to assess for the presence of other coexisting medical complications. *Once goals are achieved, contraception may be discontinued.* Once conception

has been achieved, the woman should be evaluated as early as possible to confirm her pregnancy and reinforce goals and management plans. She and her partner need to understand that even with **euglycemia** (normal blood glucose levels), it is not possible to reduce the incidence of congenital anomalies to zero. There remains the 2% to 3% incidence of congenital malformations found in the general population.[6]

Classification and Physiology of Diabetes

■ How is diabetes diagnosed?

In 1997, the Expert Committee on the Diagnosis and Classification of Diabetes Mellitus updated the classification and diagnostic criteria for diabetes and impaired glucose homeostasis (Display 13.1). The committee also recommended eliminating the old categories of insulin-dependent diabetes mellitus (IDDM) and non–insulin-dependent diabetes mellitus (NIDDM). The new recommendations use the Arabic 1 and 2 (type 1 and type 2) instead of the Roman numerals I and II.

DISPLAY 13.1 Diagnostic Criteria for Diabetes Mellitus

Diabetes can be diagnosed using any of the following three methods and **must** be confirmed on a subsequent day.

1. Acute symptoms of diabetes (polyuria, polydipsia, and polyphagia) plus a random plasma glucose greater than or equal to 200 mg/dL

2. Fasting (no calorie intake for 8 hours) plasma glucose greater than or equal to 126 mg/dL

3. 2-Hour plasma glucose greater than or equal to 200 mg/dL during an oral glucose tolerance test (the glucose load is 75 g anhydrous glucose dissolved in water)

The committee also recognized two categories that indicate prediabetic conditions in which glucose metabolism is impaired: impaired fasting glucose and impaired glucose tolerance (Display 13.2). Clinicians who care for pregnant women with these laboratory findings need to be aware of their relationship to a prediabetic condition.[7]

DISPLAY 13.2 Diagnostic Criteria for Impaired Glucose

---

1. Impaired fasting glucose is diagnosed when the fasting glucose levels are greater than 110 mg/dL but less than 126 mg/dL.

2. Impaired glucose tolerance is diagnosed when the 2-hour oral glucose tolerance values are greater than or equal to 140 mg/dL but less than 200 mg/dL.

NOTE: Impaired fasting glucose and impaired glucose tolerance are not categories of diabetes mellitus.[7]

■ What are the classifications of diabetes?

Type 1 diabetes is defined by the following characteristics:

- It develops at any age, but most cases are diagnosed before the age of 30.
- Symptoms include significant weight loss, polyuria, and polydipsia with significant hyperglycemia.
- **Diabetic ketoacidosis** (DKA) can occur.
- The patient is dependent on **exogenous insulin** to prevent ketoacidosis and sustain life.
- Coma and death can result if diagnosis and/or treatment are delayed.

Type 2 diabetes is defined by the following characteristics:

- It accounts for 90% of all cases of diabetes among people in the United States.
- It is usually diagnosed after the age of 30 but can occur at any age.

- Often, patients are asymptomatic at the time of diagnosis, but 20% of patients have end-organ complications such as retinopathy, neuropathy, or nephropathy at the time of diagnosis.
- Endogenous insulin levels may be increased, normal, or decreased. The need for exogenous insulin is variable.
- Insulin resistance with impaired glucose tolerance is usually seen in the first stages.
- The patient is not prone to ketosis.
- Hyperglycemic hyperosmolar nonketotic syndrome (HHNS) may develop.
- At the time of diagnosis, approximately 80% of patients are obese.

Secondary diabetes is diagnosed when diabetes occurs as the result of other disorders or treatment of disorders. Diabetes resulting from the following is classified as secondary diabetes.

- Genetic defects associated with **maturity-onset diabetes of youth** (MODY), glycogen synthase deficiency, and mitochondrial DNA markers
- Pancreatic disorders such as hemochromatosis, chronic pancreatitis, and pancreatectomy
- Concomitant diabetogenic drug therapy
- Disorders such as cystic fibrosis, congenital rubella syndrome, and Down's syndrome
- Hormonal disorders such as Cushing's syndrome, thyrotoxicosis, and acromegaly

Gestational diabetes has the following characteristics:

- Glucose intolerance develops or is first discovered during pregnancy.
- After pregnancy, the diagnostic classification may be changed to type 1, type 2, impaired glucose tolerance, impaired fasting glucose, or normoglycemic.
- The occurrence of gestational diabetes increases the future risk for progression to type 2 diabetes.

NOTE: Impaired fasting glucose and impaired glucose tolerance are not to be confused with a medical diagnosis of glucose intolerance (diabetes mellitus).

Many classification systems have been developed to assist the health care provider in identifying risk factors. Priscilla White first published one commonly used classification system in 1932. It classifies patients on the basis of age at onset of diabetes, duration of disease, and secondary vascular and other end-organ complications (Table 13.3).

TABLE 13.3	White's Classifications of Diabetes		
CLASS	**DIABETES ONSET AGE (yr)**		**DURATION (yr)**
Gestational Diabetes			
A1	Any		Any
A2	Any		Any
Pregestational Diabetes			
B	>20	*or*	<10
C	10–19	*or*	10–19
D	<10	*or*	>20
F	Any		Any
R	Any		Any
T	Any		Any
H	Any		Any

From White, P. (1949). Pregnancy complicating diabetes. *American Journal of Medicine 7,* 609–616.

Normal Glucose Metabolism

Normal glucose metabolism involves the following pathways[8]:

1. After eating, carbohydrates are broken down into glucose.
2. The glucose is absorbed into the blood.

3. The glucose in the blood stimulates the pancreas to release insulin.
4. The insulin is released from the beta cells in the islets of Langerhans. Insulin is released in two phases:

   - A bolus release is the immediate rapid spike insulin response due to hyperglycemia caused by the meal.
   - A basal release is the gradual release of insulin and is under the feedback control of the blood glucose. As glucose increases, the insulin release is increased. As glucose decreases, the insulin release is decreased.

5. Insulin causes the following actions:

   - Stimulates entry of glucose into cells for utilization as energy
   - Promotes the storage of glucose as glycogen in muscles and liver cells
   - Inhibits release of glucose from the liver or muscle glycogen
   - Stimulates entry of amino acids into cells
   - Enhances fat storage and prevents the mobilization of fat for energy
   - Inhibits the formation of glucose from noncarbohydrates (e.g., amino acids)

Normal Glucose Metabolism During Pregnancy

Many metabolic changes occur during pregnancy to optimize the growth of the fetus. Because the fetus depends entirely on the mother for its supply of energy, maternal adaptations must occur to increase glucose supply to the fetus.

Early in pregnancy, glucose homeostasis is altered by the increases in estrogen and progesterone that cause pancreatic beta-cell hyperplasia (the cells multiply), with subsequent increased insulin secretion.

At the end of the first trimester, preexisting diabetic patients will often experience hypoglycemia as a result of the following factors:

   - Increased glucose utilization (results in approximately a 10% reduction of maternal glucose)
   - Increased insulin secretion (results in increased glycogen stores and decreased hepatic glucose production)

In the second and third trimesters, levels of estrogen, progesterone, human placental lactogen (HPL), cortisol, and prolactin increase progressively and cause increasing tissue resistance to insulin action. (Insulin resistance is caused by a defect in the insulin receptor sites on cells. The defect does not allow the insulin to transport glucose into the cell. This causes a decrease in insulin function or sensitivity.) If a patient has preexisting borderline beta-cell reserve, hyperglycemia will result.[9] The following changes are seen:

   - Increased basal insulin level requirements due to insulin resistance
   - Increased bolus insulin level requirements due to insulin resistance
   - Increased infant glucose utilization

> As pregnancy progresses, insulin production is increased to more than twice the nonpregnant levels.[10]

Throughout pregnancy, there is an increased risk for DKA and fasting ketosis due to the following factors:

   - Decreased levels of alanine (a gluconeogenetic amino acid that is able to form glucose from substances other than carbohydrates such as fats and protein)
   - Increased levels of fatty acids
   - Increased triglycerides
   - Increased ketones

These metabolic factors cause increased fat catabolism (breakdown), and decreased maternal glucose production in the fasting state. This allows for increased utilization of fat stores for energy, therefore protecting muscle mass breakdown.

Pathophysiology of Type 1, Type 2, and Gestational Diabetes

Type 1 diabetes is a result of an autoimmune attack on the beta cells in the pancreas. The stages of development involve a genetic predisposition, an environmental trigger, active autoimmunity directed against the beta cells, progressive beta-cell dysfunction, and then the clinical onset of diabetes.

Type 2 diabetes is a result of abnormal insulin secretion and resistance to insulin action in target tissue. The following three phases occur before overt diabetes presents.[11]

1. In phase one, insulin resistance begins but plasma glucose remains normal because of an elevated insulin level.
2. In phase two, insulin resistance increases and **postprandial** (following a meal) hyperglycemia develops.
3. In phase three, insulin resistance remains the same but declining insulin secretion causes fasting hyperglycemia and overt diabetes.

Gestational diabetes is a result of the combination of insulin resistance and a diminished insulin secretion. *Pregnancy hormones such as estrogen, progesterone, prolactin, cortisol, and HPL are responsible for the increase in insulin resistance that is found later in pregnancy as the fetal placental unit grows.*[12] HPL is a hormone produced by the placenta. It is found in increasing levels as the pregnancy progresses and the placenta grows.

> Human placental lactogen (HPL) has the greatest influence on insulin resistance and is found in increasing levels as pregnancy progresses.[13]

NOTE: Preexisting (type 1 and type 2) diabetes and pregnancy cause multiple effects on each other. Pregnancy affects insulin requirements, retinopathy, nephropathy, coronary artery disease, neuropathy, and DKA. In addition, diabetes can cause both maternal and fetal complications.

■ What is the effect of pregnancy on preexisting diabetes?

Insulin requirements undergo many changes throughout pregnancy (Table 13.4). During the first trimester, the effect of morning sickness on nutritional intake may cause necessary changes in insulin requirements. By the end of the first trimester (10 to 16 weeks), because of metabolic changes, insulin needs may slightly decrease; however, from that point onward, insulin requirements steadily increase. During the third trimester, a twofold to threefold increase in insulin requirements may be seen.[14] After delivery, insulin requirements dramatically decrease because the insulin resistance caused by HPL, estrogen, progesterone, prolactin, and cortisol is decreased.

TABLE 13.4	Insulin Requirements During Pregnancy
GESTATIONAL PERIOD	**INSULIN REQUIREMENTS**
First trimester	Same or may be decreased (because of decreased nutritional intake from nausea and vomiting)
End of first trimester	Decreased
Second trimester	Increased
Third trimester	Increased
Postpartum	Decreased

Retinopathy (damage to the retina of the eye caused by microvascular deterioration from elevated blood glucose levels) **tends to progress during pregnancy.** *HPL causes vascular changes that accelerate retinopathy.* A woman with background retinopathy at the beginning of her pregnancy has a 16% to 50% risk of progression during pregnancy. In most situations, background retinopathy regresses after delivery.[14] In addition, *a rapid change in glycemic control of the blood glucose can cause progression of retinopathy.* This is often the situation encountered when the patient begins pregnancy in poor control, and because of the risks of congenital anomalies, she is encouraged to obtain quick glycemic control. Women with untreated **proliferative** retinopathy should receive laser photocoagulation to stabilize their eyes before pregnancy. Risk of progression can be as high as 63% with proliferative retinopathy.[14] During pregnancy, close surveillance must be maintained by an ophthalmologist.

> Because of the increased pressure in the eyes caused by pushing during the second stage of labor, vaginal delivery is **contraindicated** in a woman with untreated proliferative retinopathy.

The most serious consequence of **diabetic nephropathy** during pregnancy is *preeclampsia.* Nephropathy is disease of the kidneys caused by microvascular changes. Research has found the following[14]:

- If initial proteinuria is less than 190 mg/day, 7% of women had preeclampsia.
- If proteinuria is between 190 and 499 mg/day, 31% of women had preeclampsia.
- If proteinuria is greater than 500 mg/day, 38% of women had preeclampsia.

Renal function should be assessed every trimester. With overt nephropathy, studies indicate that the rate of renal function *does not deteriorate* with pregnancy. Nephropathy without hypertension does not affect fetal outcome unless the kidney function is more than 50% impaired. A creatinine clearance below 50 mL per minute implicates an increased risk of fetal loss.[15] Nephropathy with hypertension can have serious **cardiovascular complications,** including the following:

- Chronic hypertension
- Pregnancy-related hypertension
- Heart disease

In regard to chronic hypertension, ACE inhibitors are contraindicated in pregnancy. They cause fetal hypotension and oligohydramnios. Methyldopa and hydralazine have been proven safe for use in pregnancy. **Perinatal complications encountered with hypertension include intrauterine growth restriction (IUGR), preeclampsia, and abruptio placenta.**

> Coronary heart disease during a pregnancy complicated with diabetes is a serious situation. The maternal mortality rate is 75%, and the perinatal loss rate is 29%.[10]

Diabetic neuropathy is a disease of the nervous system that involves peripheral nerve dysfunction. Potential complications from diabetic neuropathy in the pregnant woman may involve the following:

- Gastroparesis
- Urinary retention
- Hypoglycemia unawareness
- Orthostatic hypotension
- Carpal tunnel syndrome

Metoclopramide (Reglan) can be used for women with gastroparesis. This may aid in improving nutritional status and glucose control. Both family and patient education regarding safety must be provided for those with hypoglycemia unawareness, orthostatic hypotension, and carpal tunnel syndrome. Hand braces may provide some relief for patients with carpal tunnel syndrome.

DKA is seen is 1% to 3% of pregnancies complicated by diabetes. Maternal loss resulting from DKA is 4% to 15%. Historically, fetal loss was reported at 30% to 90%; however, in the past decade it was approximately 9%.[16] Most cases of DKA are in patients with undiagnosed new-onset diabetes. **The most common cause of DKA is infection.** *The hallmarks of DKA treatment consist of fluid replacement and insulin therapy.*

■ What is the effect of preexisting diabetes on pregnancy?

The effect of diabetes on pregnancy impacts both the mother and the fetus. The following risks are increased:

Maternal Consequences
- Preeclampsia
- Bacterial infections
- Polyhydramnios
- Birth trauma from macrosomic infants
- Cesarean delivery
- Postpartum hemorrhage

Fetal Consequences
- Congenital anomalies
- Spontaneous abortion
- Macrosomia
- Intrauterine fetal death (IUFD)
- Delayed pulmonary maturity
- Hypoglycemia at birth
- Hyperbilirubinemia and polycythemia
- Hypocalcemia
- Decreased magnesium serum levels
- IUGR

> Congenital anomalies and spontaneous abortion are the two major fetal complications seen in women who have poor glycemic control during the period of fetal organogenesis.

Hyperglycemia in the first trimester can result in numerous complications. **Organogenesis** is the development of the major organs of the fetus and occurs during the first 8 weeks of gestation. The rate of risk of structural anomaly with hyperglycemia is increased fourfold to eightfold. Structural anomalies *mainly* involve the following:

- Central nervous system
- Cardiovascular system
- Skeletal system

During the first trimester, the rate of anomalies is only 3.4% with an HbA_{1c} of 8.5 or less, but the rate of anomalies increases to 22.4% with an HbA_{1c} greater than 8.5.[17]

In regard to spontaneous abortion, rates also correlate with blood glucose control at the time of conception. Ensuring normal blood glucose values at the time of conception and during the first trimester, when organ development occurs, can reduce the risk of both spontaneous abortion and congenital anomalies.

Hyperglycemia in the second and third trimesters results in metabolic complications. If maternal physiologic glucose control is lacking, maternal hyperglycemia occurs. Pathologic elevated glucose levels leads to higher amounts of glucose transfer across the placenta to the fetus. Because the fetal pancreas begins to function at approximately 13 weeks' gestation, the fetal pancreas responds to the elevated fetal glucose levels. Fetal hyperglycemia results in increased fetal insulin output (i.e., fetal hyperinsulinism). The outcome of the fetal response is accelerated fetal growth, resulting in large-for-gestational-age (LGA) infants and macrosomia. *Macrosomia* is generally defined as an infant weight above the 90th percentile or greater than 4,000 g. Macrosomic infants and LGA infants have an increased requirement for oxygen. If the increased demand for oxygen exceeds the supply available, fetal distress or IUFD may occur. Hyperglycemia also causes an increase in fetal erythropoietin production, which leads to polycythemia and hyperbilirubinemia.

When delivery plans are being made, **pulmonary maturity of the infant** must be ensured. Infant pulmonary maturity in the nondiabetic patient is achieved at a mean gestational age of

34 to 35 weeks. By 37 weeks' gestation, more than 99% of infants have mature pulmonary profiles. However, **with diabetic mothers, the risk of pulmonary immaturity is not passed until after 38.5 weeks' gestation.**[18]

> In all deliveries of diabetic women before 38.5 weeks, lung maturity must be assessed through amniocentesis.

In addition, at the time of delivery, the infant must be assessed carefully for signs of hypoglycemia. *Hypoglycemia* is a plasma glucose level of less than 35 mg/dL in the term infant and less than 25 mg/dL in the premature infant. Hypoglycemia is caused by the elimination of excess maternal blood glucose when the cord is cut and the continued excess production of insulin by the infant. *The peak incidence of neonatal hypoglycemia is 6 to 12 hours after birth.*[14]

In regard to future implications for infants of diabetic mothers, both an increased risk for glucose intolerance and obesity have been noted.[19] Infants of diabetic mothers have a 1.2% risk of impaired glucose tolerance before 5 years of age, a 5.4% risk at 5 to 9 years of age, and a 19.3% risk at 10 to 16 years of age.[20] The risk that a mother with IDDM would have a diabetic child is approximately 1%; if both parents are diabetic, this risk increases to approximately 6%.[21]

Management of Diabetes in the Pregnant Woman

Preexisting Diabetes

Antepartum Management for Mothers With Preexisting Diabetes
The three hallmarks in the treatment of diabetes during pregnancy include the following:

1. Medical nutritional therapy (MNT)
2. Exercise
3. Insulin therapy

Careful attention to each component is essential for optimal glucose control.

Antepartum management includes the evaluation, education, and/or treatment for the following factors:

- MNT
- Exercise
- Self-management of blood glucose (SMBG)
- Insulin regimen
- Medications
  - All women should continue a prenatal vitamin, which contains 0.4 mg of folic acid.
  - All medications should be assessed for their safety during pregnancy.
  - ACE inhibitors are contraindicated during pregnancy.
- Prenatal laboratory tests
  - In addition to routine prenatal laboratory tests, an HbA_{1c}, thyroid panel, serum creatinine, 24-hour urine for total protein, microalbumin, and creatinine should be obtained.
- ECG
  - A baseline ECG should be obtained to rule out a preexisting cardiac problem.
- Ophthalmology examination
  - A thorough baseline examination is needed to determine the existence or extent of retinopathy.
- Maternal serum α-fetoprotein (MSAFP)
  - MSAFP should be offered to all patients between $15^{0}/_{7}$ and $20^{6}/_{7}$ weeks' gestation because of the increased risk of neural tube defects.
- HbA_{1c}
  - Repeat every 4 to 6 weeks to monitor glucose control.
- Ultrasound
  - An ultrasound should be done initially to confirm viability. It should be repeated at approximately 18 to 20 weeks for anatomic survey. A screening fetal echocardiogram is indicated. Cardiac views are best imaged near 20 to 22 weeks of pregnancy.

–Growth should be assessed every 4 weeks as clinically indicated.
- Fetal kick counts
  –Fetal kick counts should be taught to the patient and should begin daily at 28 weeks' gestation.
- Nonstress test (NST)
  –NSTs should begin weekly at 32 weeks and twice a week at 36 weeks. With poor glycemic control, NSTs may begin as early as 28 weeks' gestation. If the test is nonreactive, a biophysical profile should be obtained.
- Delivery plan
  –The timing of delivery should be based on maternal glucose control and fetal status.
  –As a general rule, diabetic patients should be delivered between 39 and 40 weeks. If delivery is planned electively before 38.5 weeks, an amniocentesis must be performed to confirm lung maturity.

Intrapartum Management for Mothers With Preexisting Diabetes

Timing of delivery and the route of delivery should be based on clinical judgment. Indications for delivery include the following:

- Nonreassuring fetal status
- Arrest or decline in fetal growth rate
- Macrosomia with fetal lung maturity
- Severe preeclampsia
- Decreased maternal renal function
- Preterm labor with failure of tocolysis
- Fetal maturity greater than 38.5 weeks

> Intrapartum management goals include providing adequate carbohydrate intake for energy requirements and maintaining maternal glucose control.

In patients with excellent glucose control, delivery may be delayed; **however, after 40 weeks' gestation, the benefits of delivery outweigh the benefits of conservative management because of the danger of fetal compromise.**

A protocol for insulin infusion to maintain glycemic control includes the following algorithm[22]:

- Withhold the morning subcutaneous insulin.
- Begin and maintain a glucose infusion of D_5W at 100 mL per hour throughout labor.
- Begin an infusion of regular insulin. Adjust the insulin infusion to maintain maternal glucose at 80 to 120 mg/dL (Table 13.5).
- Monitor maternal blood glucose every hour.

TABLE 13.5	Insulin Drip Rates to Maintain Maternal Blood Glucose at 80 to 120 mg/dL	
MATERNAL BLOOD GLUCOSE	**INSULIN DRIP**
80 mg/dL	**Stop drip**
80–100 mg/dL	0.5 U/hr
101–140 mg/dL	1.0 U/hr
141–180 mg/dL	1.5 U/hr
181–220 mg/dL	2.0 U/hr
>220 mg/dL	2.5 U/hr

In addition to using an intravenous insulin drip, the insulin pump may also be used to maintain euglycemia during labor and delivery. For type 2 diabetic patients in excellent control, blood glucose control may be achieved by avoiding dextrose intravenous fluids. Blood glucose must be monitored hourly. At delivery, the newborn must be assessed for hypoglycemia. The degree of hypoglycemia in the newborn correlates approximately with the degree of glycemic control by the mother over the prior 6 to 12 weeks.[10]

Continuous fetal monitoring should be used during labor to monitor the infant closely for signs of distress. **The provider must watch carefully for indications of shoulder dystocia because many infants are macrosomic.** Indications of shoulder dystocia include an estimated fetal weight of more than 4,000 g, a dysfunctional labor curve, a prolonged second stage, and the turtle sign occurring with the delivery of the head (the head is extremely tight against the perineum).

Postpartum Management for Mothers With Preexisting Diabetes

The management issues during the postpartum period include insulin adjustment, care of the newborn, breastfeeding, and balancing of self-care needs of the mother with the needs of her newborn.

> **After the delivery, insulin requirements decrease dramatically. Often, very little or no insulin is required for the first 24 to 72 hours.**

If required, insulin requirements should be recalculated as follows[14]:

- 0.6 units per kg of current weight for nonlactating women
- 0.4 units per kg of current weight for lactating women

Oral agents cannot be used while lactating. Breastfeeding patients should also be informed that lactating women have reported 50- to 100-mg/dL drops in blood glucose over a 30-minute nursing session.[14] Caloric requirements are approximately 25 kcal/kg per day for nonlactating women and 27 kcal/kg per day for lactating women.[15]

At the postpartum visit, a complete physical examination should be performed, and education on contraceptive methods, diet, exercise, insulin regimen, glucose control, and HbA_{1c} should be assessed. Counseling regarding future pregnancies is important. Last, assurance must be made that the woman has a health care provider to monitor and assist her with diabetes care between pregnancies.

Gestational Diabetes

Gestational diabetes consists of both insulin resistance and diminished insulin secretion during pregnancy. It has implications for both the mother and the baby. The mother has an increased risk for the following:

- Preeclampsia
- Polyhydramnios
- Operative delivery because of fetal macrosomia
- Urinary tract infections

Of great significance is the risk for the mother to develop type 2 diabetes or glucose intolerance later in life (Table 13.6).

TABLE 13.6 Risk of Developing Type 2 Diabetes After Gestational Diabetes	
YEARS AFTER DIAGNOSIS OF GESTATIONAL DIABETES MELLITUS	**RISK OF DEVELOPING TYPE 2 DIABETES (%)**
0–2	6
3–4	13
5–6	15
7–10	30

Data from Coustan, D., Carpenter, M., O'Sullivan, P., & Carr, S. (1993). Gestational diabetes mellitus: Predictors of subsequent disordered glucose metabolism. *American Journal of Obstetrics and Gynecology, 168,* 1139–1145.

Approximately 6% of women will progress within 0 to 2 years, 13% of women within 3 to 4 years, 15% of women within 5 to 6 years, and 30% of women within 7 to 10 years.[23]

The fetus has an increased risk for the following:

- Macrosomia
- Shoulder dystocia
- Hypoglycemia
- Hypocalcemia
- Hyperbilirubinemia

Long-term implications for the offspring are an increased risk for obesity and impaired glucose tolerance or diabetes later in life.[24]

■ How is gestational diabetes diagnosed?

The diagnosis of gestational diabetes is a two-step process[14]:

1. An initial screening test—1-hour glucose challenge test (GCT) (Table 13.7)
2. A diagnostic test—3-hour glucose tolerance test (GTT) (for those who fail the screening test) (Table 13.8)

TABLE 13.7	Implications of 1-Hour Glucose Challenge Test (GCT)
GCT RESULTS	**IMPLICATION**
140–185 mg/dL	Requires 3-hour GTT
>185–200 mg/dL	Treat for gestational diabetes; do not perform a 3-hour GTT

TABLE 13.8	Cut-off Values for the 3-Hour Glucose Tolerance Test (GTT)	
TIME	**NATIONAL DIABETES DATA GROUP**	**CARPENTER AND COUSTAN**
Fasting	105 mg/dL	95 mg/dL
1 hour	190 mg/dL	180 mg/dL
2 hour	165 mg/dL	155 mg/dL
3 hour	145 mg/dL:	140 mg/dL

All women should be screened by either their history, clinical risk factors, or laboratory screening. The optimal method of screening is controversial; therefore, many providers elect to screen all their patients by laboratory testing. Women are considered low risk if they meet the following criteria:

1. Younger than 25 years of age
2. Body mass index of 25 or less
3. No first-degree relatives with diabetes mellitus
4. Not of an ethnic group that is at increased risk of type 2 diabetes mellitus (This includes Latinos, Native Americans, Asians, Africans, African Americans, Pacific Islanders, indigenous Australians, and women from the Indian subcontinent.[7])
5. No previous history of abnormal glucose tolerance.
6. No previous history of adverst obstetric outcomes usually associated with gestational diabetes.[31]

Screening with a **1-hour GCT** is recommended between 24 and 28 weeks' gestation. At this time, the production of HPL is increased to a level high enough to cause impaired insulin sensitivity. The screening 1-hour Glucola test consists of having the woman drink a 50-g glucose solution and drawing a venous plasma glucose measurement in 1 hour. The screening test can be done at any time of the day. The woman does not need to be fasting before the test. According to the Second, Third, and Fourth International Workshop Conferences on gestational diabetes, a value below 140 mg/dL is considered normal. A value of 140 to 185 mg/dL requires further evaluation with a 3-hour oral GTT. If the test is greater than 185 mg/dL, the 3-hour GTT is contraindicated and the patient is diagnosed and treated for gestational diabetes.[14]

The **3-hour GTT** consists of obtaining a fasting (at least 8 hours but no more than 14 hours) blood glucose level followed by having the patient drink 100 g of glucose. The venous blood glucose is drawn at 1 hour, 2 hours, and 3 hours. The diagnosis of gestational diabetes can be made with the diagnostic criteria of the National Diabetes Data Group (NDDG) *or* the diagnostic criteria of Carpenter and Coustan. **If two or more values are met or exceeded, the patient is diagnosed with gestational diabetes.** Another method for diagnosing gestational diabetes is based on the results of a 75-g

GTT based on the World Health Organization (WHO) criteria. It is most commonly used outside of the United States.

Antepartum Management for Mothers With Gestational Diabetes

Treatment of gestational diabetes includes the following:

- MNT
- SMBG
- Exercise
- Insulin therapy if indicated
- Fetal surveillance

MNT, exercise, and SMBG are usually the first line of therapy. Exercise, if not medically contraindicated, does improve insulin sensitivity. MNT based on maternal weight and height is recommended. **Among obese women, a reduction of carbohydrates to 35% to 40% of calories has been shown to decrease maternal glucose levels and improve maternal and fetal outcomes.**[25]

> The recommended blood glucose goals for gestational diabetes are as follows[9]:
> - Fasting levels less than 105 mg/dL
> - 2-Hour postprandial values less than 120 mg/dL

If blood glucose values are repeatedly above the desired goal even with diet and exercise, insulin therapy should be initiated. The choice of insulin type and regimen should be based on the patient's glucose profile and lifestyle. *The same calculations used in calculating insulin requirements for type 1 and type 2 diabetes are used to calculate insulin requirements for gestational diabetes.* Although research has been done to compare the use of glyburide (an oral diabetogenic medication) with insulin use among women with gestational diabetes, its use during pregnancy has *not* been approved by the U.S. Food and Drug Administration.

Much controversy remains regarding the criteria for initiation and timing of fetal testing.[26] Patients with well-controlled diabetes are at low risk for fetal death. Fetal surveillance for patients without insulin therapy usually consists of weekly NSTs from 36 weeks' gestation until delivery; however, some providers begin NSTs at 40 weeks' gestation if the patient has uncomplicated gestational diabetes. *Fetal surveillance for patients receiving insulin therapy is managed in a manner similar to the management in preexisting diabetes.* An NST is performed each week from 32 weeks until 36 weeks and then twice a week until delivery.

Fetal movement counts are taught to all patients and should begin on a daily basis at 28 weeks' gestation until delivery. The most common technique is the "count to 10" technique, which involves the mother monitoring the time it takes to feel 10 fetal movements. If 10 movements are not felt within a 2-hour limit, the patient is to call her provider. In addition to the NSTs and fetal movement counts, an ultrasound examination is often completed to evaluate fetal growth. Frequency of performing ultrasound is based on clinical judgment.

Delivery plans are based on glucose control and cervical evaluation. Elective delivery at term should be considered if the following conditions are true:

- Glycemic control is suboptimal.
- The patient requires insulin.
- Fetal monitoring is not reassuring.
- The patient has a history of stillbirth.
- Other complications exist (e.g., hypertension, preeclampsia).

> If delivery is planned before the thirty-ninth week of gestation, lung maturity should first be assessed.[27]

Expectant management can be used if blood glucose is well controlled, but fetal growth must be monitored carefully because of the risk of macrosomia with advancing gestational age.[9] Induction should not be based only on suspected fetal macrosomia. Current evidence from multiple studies does not support a policy of early induction of labor for suspected fetal macrosomia.[28]

Intrapartum Management for Mothers With Gestational Diabetes

The goals of glucose management during labor are the same as those for preexisting diabetes. The blood glucose should be monitored and, if necessary, an insulin drip initiated. With diet-controlled gestational diabetes, rarely is glucose control a problem during labor. **A major risk factor during delivery for all diabetic patients is shoulder dystocia.** Risk factors for shoulder dystocia are multifactorial and include the following:

- Fetal macrosomia
- Maternal diabetes
- Maternal obesity
- Excessive maternal weight gain
- Multiparity
- Advanced gestational age

- Prolonged second stage of labor
- Midpelvic delivery
- Postdate pregnancy
- Previous macrosomia
- Previous shoulder dystocia

In addition, infants of mothers with either gestational or preexisting diabetes usually weigh more than infants of nondiabetic mothers. These infants often display asymmetric growth in which there is a disproportionate increase in chest and shoulder size related to the head circumference.[29] Although the occurrence of shoulder dystocia is often difficult to predict, health providers should always be aware of its potential effect on the delivery and know the proper techniques to manage it.

Postpartum Management for Mothers With Gestational Diabetes

With the delivery of the fetal–placental unit, the diabetogenic (diabetic-causing) effect of HPL and the counterregulatory hormones are diminished. Therefore, women with gestational diabetes usually regain glycemic control. To ensure that this occurs, blood glucose values should be assessed in the immediate postpartum period by checking postprandial glucose values. Assessment of maternal glycemic status should be reevaluated at approximately 6 weeks.

> **All women with gestational diabetes should receive a 2-hour oral glucose tolerance test with 75 g of glucose during the postpartum period.**

Because breastfeeding can cause a lower blood glucose reading, the 2-hour GTT should be performed after the patient has stopped breastfeeding. Upon testing, the woman should be reclassified as either diabetic, impaired fasting glucose, impaired glucose tolerance, or normoglycemic (normal blood glucose). All patients should also be educated regarding lifestyle modifications such as exercise and diet. Exercise, proper diet, and breastfeeding will help the mother maintain normal body weight, which will help decrease insulin resistance. Symptoms of hyperglycemia should be reviewed with her. If these symptoms occur later in life, medical attention should be obtained. Annual assessment of glucose control should be recommended. Future pregnancy plans and contraceptive methods should also be discussed. Future pregnancy plans should be reviewed, with emphasis on ensuring optimal glycemic control before the next conception.[30]

■ What are blood glucose goals during pregnancy?

SMBG is an *essential* element in the treatment plan of patients with diabetes. It provides the patient with immediate feedback. It assists her in achieving and maintaining her blood glucose goals; in preventing and detecting hypoglycemia; and in determining necessary adjustments in pharmacologic therapy, diet, and exercise. Remember, however, that the accuracy of the values obtained depends on the accuracy of the blood glucose meter. All patients should be taught how to properly do the following:

- Use the meter
- Check the meter calibration
- Use control solutions
- Store reagent strips

- Perform proper fingerstick technique
- Clean the meter
- Dispose of lancets
- Interpret data

The American Diabetes Association recommendations for maternal glucose goals during pregnancy are shown in Table 13.9.

TABLE 13.9	ADA Maternal Glucose Goals During Pregnancy
TIME	**BLOOD GLUCOSE VALUES**
Fasting blood glucose	60–90 mg/dL
Premeal blood glucose	60–105 mg/dL
1-Hour postprandial blood glucose	100–120 mg/dL
2-Hour postprandial blood glucose	60–120 mg/dL

Data from Jornsay, D. (1998). Pregnancy: Preconception to postpartum. In M. Funnell, C. Hunt, K. Kulkarni, R. Rubin, & P. Yarborough (Eds.), *A core curriculum for diabetes education* (3rd ed., pp. 570–629). Chicago: American Association of Diabetic Educators.

The frequency and timing of SMBG must be individualized. The best method of SMBG requires obtaining both premeal and postprandial glucose levels; however, few patients are willing to collect all of these samples. Most patients taking insulin prefer to obtain premeal blood glucose values because it is the most convenient. They administer their insulin before meals. A premeal blood glucose reading allows them to adjust their insulin according to their current blood glucose. However, patients following diet restrictions or taking oral medications should obtain postprandial blood glucose values. This value will allow them to observe how their blood glucose responded to the carbohydrate content of the meal.

An additional method used to monitor glucose control over an extended period is the **glycosylated hemoglobin (HbA$_{1c}$).** The HbA$_{1c}$ measures the percentage of glycosylation that occurs in red blood cells (RBCs). Glycosylation is the linkage of hemoglobin to glucose.

Most of the hemoglobin in adults is hemoglobin A. Glycosylated hemoglobin can be separated from hemoglobin A by a laboratory technique called electrophoresis. The three separated factions of hemoglobin A are HbA$_{1a}$, HbA$_{1b}$, and HbA$_{1c}$. Normally, only HbA$_{1c}$ is measured.

Glycosylation of hemoglobin is a slow, continuous process throughout the replenishing of RBCs during their 120-day life span. The more RBCs are exposed to glucose, the higher the percentage of glycosylated hemoglobin. Because the RBC has a life span of approximately 120 days, the test is able to reflect the blood glucose control during this time (Table 13.10).

TABLE 13.10	Blood Glucose and HbA$_{1c}$ Correlation
HBA$_{1c}$	**BLOOD GLUCOSE WEIGHTED MEAN**
10.0%	240 mg/dL
9.0%	210 mg/dL
8.0%	180 mg/dL
7.0%	150 mg/dL
6.0%	120 mg/dL
5.0%	90 mg/dL

Although this test is useful to providers and patients as a method to measure overall blood glucose control, it is not useful in adjusting insulin levels on a daily basis. SMBG must be performed daily.

The HbA$_{1c}$ reflects the weighted mean of blood glucose over the previous 4 to 6 weeks. A normal HbA$_{1c}$ is 4% to 6%.

Signs and Symptoms of Hyperglycemia and Hypoglycemia

Hyperglycemia, or **high blood glucose,** can be caused by either too much food, too little insulin, illness, or stress. Symptoms of hyperglycemia include the following:

- Polydipsia (extreme thirst)
- Polyuria (frequent urination)
- Polyphagia (hunger)
- Blurred vision

- Headache
- Drowsiness
- Hyperpnea (deep respirations)
- Nausea

> If not treated, prolonged hyperglycemia can lead to diabetic ketoacidosis or hyperglycemic hyperosmolar nonketotic syndrome.

DKA is most common with type 1 diabetes and is characterized by hyperglycemia, ketosis, acidosis, and dehydration. DKA is caused by insulin deficiency and often occurs as a result of illness or infection. Because of the insulin deficiency, the body uses stored fat for energy. The use of stored fat causes ketone buildup. Polyuria, nausea, and vomiting cause dehydration and electrolyte imbalance. DKA is a medical emergency. If not properly treated, ketoacidosis can lead to coma and eventually death.

During pregnancy, DKA affects only 1% to 3% of diabetic women[16]; however, it is an acute medical emergency that can threaten the life of both the mother and baby. Treatment of DKA includes correction of fluid and electrolyte imbalances, initiation of insulin to restore normal glucose metabolism and to correct acidosis, and prevention of further complications.

Hyperglycemic/hyperosmolar nonketotic syndrome (HHNS) occurs in type 2 diabetes and is characterized by extreme hyperglycemia, absence of ketosis, severe dehydration, and decreased consciousness. The hyperglycemia causes polyuria, nausea, and vomiting, which lead to extreme dehydration. HHNS is usually caused by infection, illness, or medications that cause impaired glucose tolerance or increased fluid loss. It is also seen in noncompliant patients or undiagnosed diabetic patients. Prompt medical attention is needed to prevent these adverse outcomes.

Hypoglycemia, or **low blood glucose,** is a blood glucose level of 70 mg/dL or lower. It can be caused by too little food, too much insulin or diabetic medication, or extra exercise. The initial symptoms are as follows:

- Shakiness
- Sweating
- Tachycardia

- Hunger
- Irritability
- Light-headedness

As the blood glucose continues to drop, confusion, inability to concentrate, slurred speech, irrational behavior, blurred vision, or extreme fatigue may be exhibited. If left untreated, a continued drop in blood glucose can lead to seizures or loss of consciousness.

Hypoglycemia treatment must be initiated quickly. If the patient is alert, hypoglycemia should be treated by having the patient eat a simple, fast-acting source of carbohydrate. The lower the drop in blood glucose, the greater the amount of carbohydrate needed to raise the blood glucose. Foods with a high fat content should be avoided because fat slows the absorption of glucose, which slows the rise in blood glucose. General guidelines for hypoglycemia treatment are as follows:

1. Check the blood glucose.
2. If the blood glucose is 70 mg/dL or less, treat with a simple, fast-acting carbohydrate. The amount of carbohydrate depends on the blood glucose value. Approximately 15 g of carbohydrate will raise the blood glucose by 20 mg/dL. Examples of 15 g of glucose include 4 ounces of apple juice, four Dex-4 tablets, or five LifeSavers.
3. Wait 10 to 15 minutes, then check the blood glucose. If the blood glucose is not above 70 mg/dL, re-treat with carbohydrates.
4. Repeat the previous step. Continue the treatment until the blood glucose is above 70 mg/dL.

During severe hypoglycemia, the patient may become uncooperative, combative, unresponsive, or unconscious or may have seizures. If it is not possible to give the patient a carbohydrate source by mouth, the patient should be given an intramuscular injection of glucagon and emergency services called.

Glucagon is a hormone that stimulates hepatic glucose production. To administer, mix the solution and inject 1.0 mg (all the solution) in the arm, thigh, or buttock. If there is no response, the injection may be repeated in 15 minutes. When the patient is awake and alert, treat with 15 g of carbohydrates. Continue to check the blood glucose and treat appropriately until the blood glucose is above 70 mg/dL.

See Appendix B for details on treatment of diabetes during pregnancy.

PRACTICE/REVIEW QUESTIONS

After reviewing this module, answer the following questions.

1. How is diabetes diagnosed?

   a. _____

   b. _____

   c. _____

2. What are the characteristics of type 1 diabetes?

   a. _____

   b. _____

   c. _____

   d. _____

   e. _____

3. What are the characteristics of type 2 diabetes?

   a. _____

   b. _____

   c. _____

   d. _____

   e. _____

   f. _____

   g. _____

   h. _____

4. What is *gestational diabetes?*_____

   _____

5. What are fasting blood glucose goals during pregnancy? _____

6. What are premeal blood glucose goals during pregnancy? _____

7. What are 2-hour postprandial blood glucose goals during pregnancy? _____

8. What does the HbA$_{1c}$ measure? _____

9. What is *hypoglycemia?* _____

10. What are the calorie requirements for a type 2 diabetic pregnant woman who is 5 feet, 2 inches tall and weighs 258 pounds? _____

11. What are the general guidelines that should be followed during exercise in pregnancy?

    a. _____

    b. _____

    c. _____

    d. _____

    e. _____

12. What is the major complication of insulin therapy? _____

13. Can oral diabetic medications be used during pregnancy? _____

14. What changes in insulin requirements occur during the first, second, and third trimesters?

    _____

    _____

15. What conditions of diabetes are affected by pregnancy?

    a. _____

    b. _____

    c. _____

    d. _____

    e. _____

    f. _____

16. When does the fetal pancreas begin to function? _____

17. When and how often should NSTs begin in pregestational diabetes?

    _____

18. Can oral diabetic medications be used while breastfeeding? _____

19. How is gestational diabetes diagnosed? _____

    _____

    _____

    _____

20. Who should be offered preconception health care?

    _____

21. Who should be placed on 0.4 mg of folic acid?

    _____

PRACTICE/REVIEW ANSWER KEY

1. Diabetes can be diagnosed using any of the following three methods and must be confirmed on a subsequent day:

    a. Acute symptoms of diabetes plus a casual plasma glucose concentration that is greater than or equal to 200 mg/dL

    b. Fasting plasma glucose that is greater than or equal to 126 mg/dL

    c. 2-Hour plasma glucose that is greater than or equal to 200 mg/dL during an oral GTT

2. a. It develops at any age, but most cases are diagnosed before the age of 30.
   b. Symptoms include significant weight loss, polyuria, and polydipsia with hyperglycemia.
   c. DKA is possible.
   d. The patient is dependent on exogenous insulin.
   e. Coma and death can result if diagnosis and/or treatment are delayed.

3. a. It accounts for 90% of all diabetes in the United States.
   b. It is usually diagnosed after the age of 30 but can occur at any age.
   c. Often, patients are asymptomatic at the time of diagnosis, but 20% have end-organ complications at the time of diagnosis.
   d. Endogenous insulin levels may be increased, normal, or decreased. The need for exogenous insulin is variable.
   e. Insulin resistance with impaired glucose tolerance is usually seen in the first stages.
   f. The patient is not prone to ketosis.
   g. HHNS may develop.
   h. Approximately 80% of patients are obese at the time of diagnosis.

4. Glucose intolerance develops or is first discovered during pregnancy; insulin resistance and diminished insulin secretion is usually seen.

5. 60 to 90 mg/dL

6. 60 to 105 mg/dL

7. 60 to 120 mg/dL

8. The HbA_{1c} reflects the weighted mean of blood glucose over the past 4 to 6 weeks.

9. Blood glucose level of 70 mg/dL or lower

10. 258 pounds = 117 kg
    117×12 kcal/kg per day = 1,404
    117×18 kcal/kg per day = 2,106
    Her requirements range from 1,404 to 2,106 calories each day.

11. a. Obtain metabolic control before exercising.
    b. Avoid exercising if fasting blood glucose is greater than 250 mg/dL and ketones are present. Use caution if blood glucose is greater than 300 mg/dL and no ketones are present. Treat with carbohydrates if blood glucose is less than 100 mg/dL.
    c. Monitor blood glucose before and after exercise.
    d. Monitor necessary food intake. Always have carbohydrates available during and after exercise.
    e. Include a warm-up and cool-down period with each exercise session.

12. Hypoglycemia

13. No. Oral diabetic agents cross the placenta and may have teratogenic effects on the fetus. Currently, researchers are investigating the use of glyburide.

14. Usually in the first trimester, insulin requirements are slightly decreased, but they increase in the second and third trimesters. They again decrease during the immediate postpartum period.

15. a. Insulin requirements
    b. Retinopathy
    c. Nephropathy
    d. Coronary artery disease
    e. Neuropathy
    f. DKA

16. Approximately 13 weeks

17. Usually begin NSTs at 32 weeks' gestation on a weekly basis and increase to twice a week at 36 weeks' gestation

18. No. The oral medications are secreted through the breast milk and may affect the infant.

19. Gestational diabetes is diagnosed by an elevated 1-hour screening glucose challenge test of 140 mg/dL or greater, which is followed by a diagnostic 3-hour glucose challenge test. The patient is diagnosed with gestational diabetes if two or more values exceed the following: NDDG criteria: fasting, 105 mg/dL; 1 hour, 190 mg/dL; 2 hour, 165 mg/dL; and 3 hour, 145 mg/dL; Carpenter and Coustan criteria: fasting, 95 mg/dL; 1 hour, 180 mg/dL; 2 hour, 155 mg/dL; and 3 hour, 140 mg/dL.

20. All women of childbearing age who are planning a pregnancy

21. All women of childbearing age

REFERENCES

1. American Diabetes Association. (2000). *Diabetes facts and figures* [On-line]. Available at: www.diabetes.org/ada/facts.asp.
2. Centers for Disease Control and Prevention. (1998). *Diabetes public health resource: National diabetes fact sheet* [On-line]. Available at: www.cdc.gov/diabetes/pubs/facts98.htm.
3. United States Public Health Service. (1989). *Expert panel on the content of prenatal care: Caring for the future—The content of prenatal care.* Washington, DC: US Public Health Service.
4. March of Dimes Birth Defects Foundation. (1993). *Towards improving the outcome of pregnancy—The 90s and beyond.* White Plains, NY: March of Dimes Birth Defects Foundation.
5. American Diabetes Association. (2001). Preconception care of women with diabetes. *Diabetes Care, 24* (Suppl. 1). Available at: http://journal.dibetes.org/FullText/Supplements/DiabetesCare/Supplement101/S66.htm. Accessed February 16, 2001.
6. Cefalo, R., & Moos, M. (1995). *Preconceptional health care: A practical guide* (2nd ed.). St. Louis: Mosby.
7. Expert Committee on the Diagnosis and Classification of Diabetes Mellitus. (1997). Report of the expert committee on the diagnosis and classification of diabetes mellitus. *Diabetes Care, 20,* 1183–1197.
8. White, J., Campbell, R., & Yarborough, P. (1998). Therapies: Pharmacologic therapies. In M. Funnell, C. Hunt, K. Kulkarni, R. Rubin, & P. Yarborough (Eds.), *A core curriculum for diabetes education* (3rd ed., pp. 295–360). Chicago: American Association of Diabetes Educators.
9. Landon, M. (1996). Diabetes mellitus and other endocrine diseases. In S. Gabbe, J. Niebyl, & J. Simpson (Eds.), *Obstetrics: Normal and problem pregnancies* (3rd ed., pp. 1037–1081). New York: Churchill Livingstone.
10. Moore, T. (1999). Diabetes in pregnancy. In R. Creasy & R. Resnik (Eds.), *Maternal-fetal medicine* (4th ed., pp. 964–995). Philadelphia: WB Saunders.
11. Foster, D. (1999). Diabetes mellitus. *Harrison's Online, Chapter 334.* Available at: www.harrisononline.com/marketing/sample/entrypages/public/ch334/334_pathi-main.htm. Accessed September 21, 1999.
12. Kuhl, C. (1998). Etiology and pathogenesis of gestational diabetes. *Diabetes Care, 21*(Suppl. 2), B19–B26.
13. Ryan, E. (1998). Prevention and treatment of diabetes and its complications: Pregnancy and diabetes. *Medical Clinics of North America, 82*(4), 823–845.
14. Jornsay, D. (1998). Pregnancy: Preconception to postpartum. In M. Funnell, C. Hunt, K. Kulkarni, R. Rubin, & P. Yarborough (Eds.), *A core curriculum for diabetes education* (3rd ed., pp. 570–629). Chicago: American Association of Diabetic Educators.
15. Jovanovic, L. (2000). Acute complications of diabetes: medical emergencies in the patient with diabetes during pregnancy. *Endocrinology and Metabolism Clinics, 29*(4), 771–787.
16. Ramin, K. (1999). Diabetic ketoacidosis in pregnancy. *Obstetrics and Gynecology Clinics, 26*(3), 481–488.
17. Miller, E., Hare, J. W., Cloherty, J. P., Dunn, P. J., Gleason, R. E., Soeldner, J. S., & Kitzmiller, J. L. (1981). Elevated maternal hemoglobin A1c in early pregnancy and major congenital anomalies in infants of diabetic mothers. *New England Journal of Medicine, 304,* 1331–1334.
18. Kulovich, M., & Gluck, L. (1979). The lung profile: II. Complicated pregnancy. *American Journal of Obstetrics and Gynecology, 135,* 64–70.

19. Whitaker, R., & Dietz, W. (1998). Role of the prenatal environment in the development of obesity. *Journal of Pediatrics, 132*(5), 768–776.
20. Silverman, B., Metzger, B., Cho, N., & Loeb, C. (1995). Impaired glucose tolerance in adolescent offspring of diabetic mothers. Relationship to fetal hyperinsulinism. *Diabetes Care, 18*(5), 611–617.
21. Warram, J., et al. (1984). Difference in risk of insulin-dependent diabetes in offspring of diabetic mothers and diabetic fathers. *New England Journal of Medicine, 311,* 149–156.
22. Jovanovic, L., & Peterson, C. (1983). Insulin and glucose requirements during the first stage of labor in insulin-dependent diabetic women. *American Journal of Medicine, 75*(4), 607–612.
23. Coustan, D., Carpenter, M., O'Sullivan, P., & Carr, S. (1993). Gestational diabetes mellitus: Predictors of subsequent disordered glucose metabolism. *American Journal of Obstetrics and Gynecology, 168,* 1139–1145.
24. Petitt, D., et al. (1985). Gestational diabetes mellitus and impaired glucose tolerance during pregnancy: Long-term effects on obesity and glucose tolerance in the offspring. *Diabetes, 34,* (Suppl. 2), 119–122.
25. Major, C., Henry, M., De Veciana, M., & Morgan, M. (1998). The effects of carbohydrate restriction in patients with diet-controlled gestational diabetes. *Obstetrics and Gynecology, 91*(4), 600–604.
26. ACOG. (1994). *ACOG technical bulletin: diabetes and pregnancy* (No. 200). Danvers, MA: ACOG Committee on Technical Bulletins.
27. Landon, M., & Gabbe, S. (1996). Fetal surveillance and timing of delivery in pregnancy complicated by diabetes mellitus. *Obstetrics and Gynecology Clinics, 23*(1), 109–123.
28. ACOG. (2000). *ACOG practice bulletin: Fetal macrosomia* (No. 22). Danvers, MA: ACOG Committee on Practice Bulletins.
29. Bennett, B. (1999). Shoulder dystocia: an obstetric emergency. *Obstetrics and Gynecology Clinics, 26*(3), 445–458.
30. American Diabetes Association. (2001). Position statement: Gestational diabetes. *Diabetes Care, 24* (Suppl. 1). Available at: http://journal.diabetes.org/FullText/Supplements/DiabetesCare/Supplement 101/S77.htm. Accessed February 5, 2001.
31. ACOG. (2001). *ACOG practice bulletin: Gestational diabetes* (No. 30). Danvers, MA: ACOG Committee on Technical Bulletins.

MODULE 14

Delivery in the Absence of a Primary Care Provider

MARCELLA T. HICKEY

As you complete this module, you will learn:

1. Those situations that can result in an emergency delivery
2. Signs of an impending birth
3. What equipment should always be ready and available for an emergency delivery (emergency delivery pack)
4. How to deliver the baby
5. Precautions taken for the safety of the mother and baby
6. What to do when there is meconium-stained amniotic fluid, difficulty delivering the baby's shoulders, excessive maternal bleeding, hidden maternal bleeding (hematoma), or a newborn with difficulty breathing
7. What should alert the nurse to the possibility of excessive maternal bleeding
8. What to do if the emergency delivery is a breech
9. Dangers of an improperly conducted delivery
10. Immediate care of the newborn
11. Immediate care of the mother
12. Information that must be charted on the hospital record

KEY TERMS

When you have completed this module, you should be able to recall the meaning of the following terms. You should also be able to use the terms when consulting with other health professionals. The terms are defined in this module or in the glossary at the end of this book.

hematoma	restitute
lochia	shoulder dystocia
nasopharynx	thermoregulation
nuchal cord	uterine atony
oropharynx	

■ Why is it important for you to be able to deliver a baby in the absence of a primary care provider?

The maternity nurse has a responsibility to provide safe care for the mother and baby. If the nurse makes the assessment that a woman will give birth before her primary care provider arrives, the nurse must be prepared to instruct and assist the woman as well as care for the newborn.

> Comprehensive protocols addressing emergency delivery in the absence of the primary care provider should be developed by each institution.

DO NOT WAIT TO PREPARE for the delivery in the hope that the primary care provider will arrive momentarily. Prepare the woman, the place of delivery, yourself, and an assistant.

■ Which women are at risk for delivery before the arrival of their primary care provider?

Women who are at risk include those who:

- Have a history of rapid labors
- Have made rapid progress during the current labor
- Are in active labor and must travel a great distance to the hospital
- Have an unexpectedly small baby

The Delivery Process

Signs of an Impending Delivery

- Nausea and retching as the cervix reaches full dilatation
- Increased bloody show
- Strong urge to "push" or to bear down with contractions
- Feelings expressed by the mother that "the baby is coming!"
- Separation or parting of the labia (Fig. 14.1)

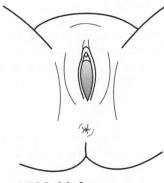

FIGURE 14.1

• Increased fullness and pressure against the perineum (bulging perineum) (Fig. 14.2)

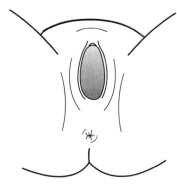

FIGURE 14.2

• Relaxation and bulging of the anus, with or without loss of stool (Fig. 14.3)

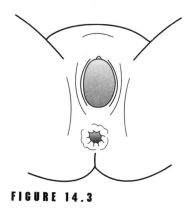

FIGURE 14.3

The Nurse's Role

■ What must you do to assist with the delivery?

If the primary care provider is not yet present, you should do the following:

• Call for assistance. Have another staff member in the room to help with the care of mother and newborn.
• Inform the woman and her support person that the birth is about to take place.
• Reassure the woman that she will be assisted and will not be left unattended.
• Instruct the woman to "feather blow" with each contraction, *unless* told to push.
• Cleanse the perineal area thoroughly.
• Open the emergency delivery pack at the bedside. It should contain the following:
  −A package of 4" × 4" gauze sponges
  −Two absorbent towels
  −A soft bulb syringe
  −A small drape or sterile field barrier
  −Two clamps, such as Kelly or Rochester
  −A cord clamp or umbilical tape
  −Scissors
  −Baby blanket
  −Gloves
  −Mucus extractor (DeLee mucus trap)—in cases when there is meconium-stained amniotic fluid
• Put on sterile gloves, place the sterile barrier under the woman's hips, and prepare to control the delivery of the baby.

Remember to observe universal precautions.

■ Why should you instruct the laboring woman to feather blow rather than push with some contractions?

When a woman pushes, she uses abdominal muscles and increases intraabdominal pressure. This enhances the expulsive action of the contracting uterus. Feather blowing helps the woman control the urge to push. Because you want to protect maternal tissue and the baby from trauma, a controlled delivery with gradual stretching of perineal tissue is desired.

■ What is the recommended method of aseptic skin preparation before delivery?

- Tell the woman that skin cleansing is being done and that the solution will feel extremely cold (unless, of course, a system has been devised to use a warm solution, which is preferable).
- **Wash your hands and forearms thoroughly before putting on sterile gloves.**
- Soak sterile swabs with antiseptic solution.
- Scrub the woman's pubis, thighs, and perineal and rectal areas thoroughly. Use the pattern noted in Figure 14.4. Each number indicates the use of a new sterile swab. Of course, this complete scrub is done only when time permits and the baby is not delivering.

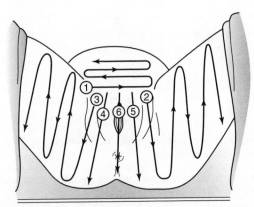

FIGURE 14.4 Systematic aseptic perineal skin preparation before delivery.

■ Why is control of the head so important?

If the head is delivered too rapidly or with too much force, it can tear the mother's tissues and traumatize the baby's brain. The fetal skull is not fully calcified and is unable to absorb the pressures of sudden decompression (during delivery) and expansion (immediately after the birth of the head).

■ Why is it important not to hold back the delivery of the baby's head by pushing against it or crossing the mother's thighs?

Once it is clear that birth is about to occur, preparation must be made toward a safe and satisfying delivery experience. Pushing back on the head to prevent its delivery can seriously traumatize the baby and maternal tissues.

The nurse should use the pads of the thumb, index, and middle fingers (Fig. 14.5) OR the cupped palm of the hand (Fig. 14.6) to maintain flexion of the head and to provide control as the head delivers.

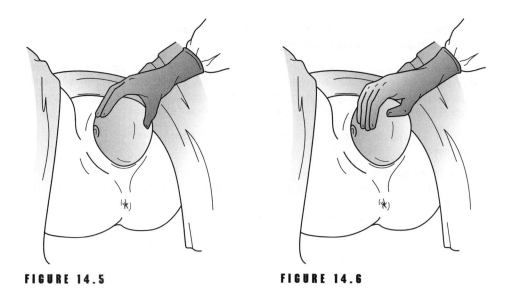

FIGURE 14.5   **FIGURE 14.6**

Never try to hold the head back from delivering!

■ **What other safety measures must you take to protect the mother during an emergency delivery?**

Position the mother comfortably so that the perineum, to which you must have access, can easily be viewed. Most often this will be:

- **In the labor bed,** on her back, with her head elevated to a semisitting position (45-degree angle) (Fig. 14.7).

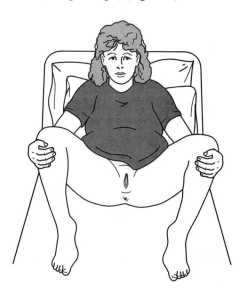

FIGURE 14.7 Position in the labor bed.

OR

- **In the delivery room.** If the mother has been moved to the delivery room table, the nurse should not "break the table" completely unless skilled in conducting a delivery in this position. Rather, the leg extension should remain partly out to provide safety for the baby with the mother's legs supported by the table stirrups (Fig. 14.8).

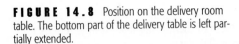

FIGURE 14.8 Position on the delivery room table. The bottom part of the delivery table is left partially extended.

Some women may select alternate positions such as side-lying or squatting. The side-lying position is usually comfortable for the mother and helps reduce stress on the stretching perineum.

Maintain asepsis (clean technique). Careful handwashing, perineal skin cleansing, and the use of a sterile emergency pack and sterile gloves will help reduce the possibility of maternal infection.

Allow delivery of the placenta without manipulation. Do not tug on the cord or massage the uterus.

REMEMBER: If the nurse is observing the progress of the mother's labor and watching closely for signs of an impending birth, the emergency delivery can:
- Be well planned and conducted in such a way to eliminate last-minute rushing about
- Provide a safe, satisfying experience for the woman

■ What safety measures should be taken to protect the newborn?

In addition to careful control of the delivery of the head, you should do the following:

- Inspect the baby for any cord around the neck as the head emerges.
- Wipe off the baby's face and head as soon as possible after delivery. Remove any mucus coming from the nose and mouth.
- Suction the oropharynx and nasopharynx with a bulb syringe to ensure the airway is clear.
- Prevent body heat loss by drying the baby thoroughly, placing the dry baby in the heated crib or directly on the skin of the mother's chest or abdomen, and covering them both well **(thermoregulation).**

Managing Problems

Meconium-Stained Amniotic Fluid[1]

- Occurs more often in high-risk pregnancies
- May be found in the presence of uterine hyperstimulation
- May be associated with maternal hypertension
- Is seen more often when the woman has a biophysical profile (BPP) of less than 6
- Occurs more often in postdate pregnancies
- May be associated with fetal hypoxic episodes
- May also be found with decreased variability in fetal heart rate baseline; late declinations do not have to be present

- May be a physiologic indicator of a mature gastrointestinal tract
- Is not absolutely associated with fetal acidosis

Critical Interventions When Meconium Stained Amniotic Fluid Is Noted

As soon as the baby's head is delivered and before the shoulders deliver, the baby's oropharynx and then the nasopharynx must be well suctioned, using a DeLee mucus trap. To prevent aspiration of the meconium, this should be done before the baby starts to breathe. Have the woman feather blow to avoid pushing.

Shoulder Dystocia[2]

- This condition cannot reliably be predicted.
- Risk does increase with high birth weight (macrosomia) and diabetes mellitus.
- A substantial number of cases occur among women who do not have diabetes and with infants of birth weights less than 4,000 g.
- Ultrasonography is not an accurate predictor of macrosomia.
- There are no studies documenting the usefulness of identifying macrosomic fetuses for planned cesarean delivery among women with diabetes.

A review of the woman's prenatal history will identify antepartum risk factors associated with shoulder dystocia. These factors are as follows[3]:

- Glucose intolerance
- Excessive maternal weight or weight gain
- Previous birth of a macrosomic infant
- Abnormal pelvic shape/size
- Short stature
- Male fetus
- Gestational age of more than 42 weeks (postterm)
- Previous delivery with shoulder dystocia

> ■ **What should you do if the baby's shoulders become "stuck" (shoulder dystocia)?**

Important steps to take include the following:

- **Be prepared.**
- Identify which maternal side the fetal back is facing.
- Position a stool on the side of the mother where the fetal back is lying.
- Ensure that the bladder is empty by catheterization.
- Lower the maternal head (i.e., avoid a full Fowler's position).
- Have two nurses assist the mother to sharply flex her knees and hips (McRoberts maneuver) by pulling back on her legs. This action flattens the lumbosacral spine and rotates the symphysis pubis anteriorly. This may dislodge the fetal anterior shoulder (Fig. 14.9).
- Suprapubic pressure is applied by the nurse who is on the side of the mother where the fetal back lies. This is done while standing on a stool. Using the palmar surface of the hands placed above the pubic bone, apply reasonable pressure straight down (Fig. 14.10). This pressure causes flexion of the shoulder toward the fetal chest, decreasing the diameter of the shoulders. This may aid in the delivery of the shoulder.
- Consider not suctioning the baby's mouth after the head delivers, but instead take advantage of the baby's rotating shoulders moving to the anteroposterior (AP) position. Do not let the shoulders become directly AP. Shoulders should be delivered in the oblique position.

Bleeding

> ■ **If the postpartum mother bleeds excessively, what should you do while waiting for the primary care provider to arrive?**

Attempt to discover the source of the bleeding and perform the corresponding nursing interventions (Table 14.1).

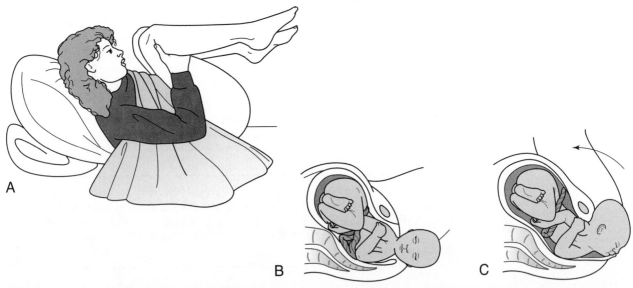

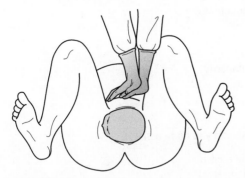

FIGURE 14.9 McRoberts maneuver. **A.** McRoberts maneuver position. **B.** Normal position of the symphysis pubis and the sacrum. **C.** The symphysis pubis rotates and the sacrum flattens. (Adapted with permission from Naef, R. W., & Martin, J. N. (1995). Emergent management of shoulder dystocia. *Obstetrics and Gynecology Clinics of North America, 22*[2], 252.)

FIGURE 14.10 Pressure is applied by pushing down just above the pubic bone onto the fetal shoulder.

> Suprapubic pressure is most effective when the person applying it is positioned higher than the maternal body. Never use fundal pressure.

TABLE 14.1	Signs and Symptoms of and Interventions for Active Maternal Bleeding	
SOURCE	**SIGNS AND SYMPTOMS**	**NURSING INTERVENTION**
Uterine atony OR Retained pieces of placenta	1. Soft and poorly contracting uterus 2. Dark red vaginal bleeding 3. Clots	1. Massage the top of the uterus to stimulate a contraction and express clots 2. Give oxygen if needed 3. Increase rate of intravenous fluids 4. Take and record blood pressure and pulse
Laceration of cervix or vagina	1. Firm uterus 2. Bright red vaginal bleeding	1. Place woman flat or in Trendelenburg position 2. Give oxygen if needed 3. Increase rate of administration of intravenous fluids
Laceration of perineum or labia	1. Firm uterus 2. Obvious tear of tissue 3. Bright red bleeding from tear	1. Apply pressure using a sterile pad 2. Place woman flat or in Trendelenburg position 3. Increase rate of administration of intravenous fluid

Hematoma (Hidden Bleeding)

It is possible for some bleeding to occur under the surface of the tissues (hematoma of the perineum or vagina). The woman might complain of increasing pelvic pain or rectal pressure. A reddish blue mass might be seen in the vagina or at the perineum. This must be noted and observed over several hours.

Additional actions to take include the following:

- Send another person to find a physician.
- Increase administration of intravenous fluids to more than 125 mL per hour.
- Take and record the woman's blood pressure and pulse.
- Note on the chart the amount, color, and type of blood loss.

> To treat a decreasing blood volume caused by excessive bleeding, lactated Ringer's solution should be administered for immediate fluid replacement and prevention of shock. Extreme caution should be used if a large volume of physiologic normal saline is used because it can increase the risk for electrolyte imbalance, coagulation problems, and renal failure.

■ **Which women are at greatest risk to bleed excessively after the birth?**

Women at greatest risk for excessive bleeding include those women who have had the following:

- A large baby, multiple pregnancy, or hydramnios
- A long labor
- A rapid labor
- Oxytocin induction/augmentation
- A history of many pregnancies (grandmultiparity)
- A history of excessive postpartum bleeding

Breech Delivery

■ **If the emergency delivery is a breech, what should you do to assist it?**

- Avoid excessive handling of the delivering breech.
- Prevent stress on the cord (gently pull a loop free).
- After the breech is delivered, keep the exposed baby warm by carefully applying a warm towel.

> The towel is used to support the infant's lower body *without* grasping the infant's abdomen.

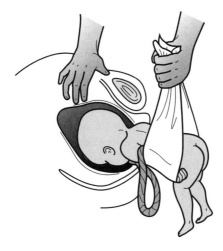

FIGURE 14.11 Use a warm towel and lift the body.

- Lift the body, using the towel, to deliver the shoulders. To avoid abdominal trauma, do not grasp the baby's abdomen.
- Lower the body after delivery of the shoulders.
- Keep the head flexed using suprapubic pressure. Another nurse may apply this pressure.
- Using the towel, **raise the body once the hairline is visible;** deliver the chin, mouth, nose, forehead, and top of the head.
- A second nurse may clear the airway as soon as the mouth and nose are visible.

Review

Immediate Care of the Newborn

Immediate care of the newborn involves safety measures discussed previously:

- Maintain a clear airway.
- Maintain body heat (thermoregulation).
- Assess general health status (i.e., inspect for any birth injuries or abnormalities).
- Observe vital signs.
- Assess 1- and 5-minute Apgar scores.

In addition, the following must be done:

- Clamp and cut the umbilical cord with sterile scissors.
- Note the number of vessels in the cord (two arteries and one vein).
- Identify the mother/baby unit (mother's fingerprints and baby's footprints, as well as matching namebands for each).

Postpartum Care of the Mother

- Assess firmness and position of the uterus.
- Note the color and quantity of the lochia.
- Note any lacerations.
- Observe and record vital signs every 15 minutes.
- Assess the status of the bladder.
- Provide warmth and rest.

The birth of a baby is a powerful emotional as well as physical experience. Studies indicate a most sensitive period exists immediately after the infant's birth. It is during this time that the parents are most likely to develop strong emotional ties ("bond") with their child. Touching, skin-to-skin contact, holding, nursing, and eye contact all help to develop this tie.

An emergency birth can often be so rushed and hectic that parents miss the opportunity to bond with their baby. The nurse's attitude toward every family's birth should be one of concern for health and safety and a commitment to promote family bonding.

Documentation

Information you should note in the legal record of the birth includes the following:

- Presentation and position of the baby
- Date and time of the birth
- Sex of the baby
- Apgar scores at 1 minute and 5 minutes
- Presence of cord around the baby's body and the number of times the cord encircles the part (e.g., neck, shoulder, leg)
- Any lacerations to the maternal tissue
- The presence of birth injuries or abnormalities in the baby
- Time of delivery of the placenta

- Appearance of the placenta and membranes (intact, color, abnormalities)
- Appearance of the cord (number of vessels, abnormalities)
- Estimated blood loss
- Any drugs administered to the mother or baby
- Anything unusual about the birth
- First stooling or voiding by the baby
- Vital signs of the mother and the baby
- Name of the person conducting the birth

PRACTICE/REVIEW QUESTIONS

After reviewing this module, answer the following questions. ONE OR MORE THAN ONE of the choices may be correct.

1. Which of the following situations could result in delivery of the baby before the arrival of the primary care provider?

   A. An unexpectedly small baby

   B. Rapid progress during labor

   C. Multigravida

   D. History of rapid labors

2. List six signs of impending delivery.

   a. _____

   b. _____

   c. _____

   d. _____

   e. _____

   f. _____

3. List the supplies and equipment that should be available in the sterile emergency delivery pack.

   _____

   _____

   _____

   _____

4. Feather blowing may help the laboring woman control the urge to push.

   A. True

   B. False

5. The woman's thighs and perineal and rectal areas should be cleansed in all situations.

   A. True

   B. False

6. If the baby's head is delivering too fast, you should hold it back.

   A. True

   B. False

7. List at least six things you should do once the baby is delivered to ensure its safety.

   a. _____

   b. _____

   c. _____

   d. _____

   e. _____

   f. _____

8. Meconium-stained amniotic fluid may be associated with:

   A. Exercise

   B. Abnormal glucose tolerance test results

   C. Postdated pregnancies

   D. Decreased variability in fetal heart rate baseline

9. What should you do to the baby if the amniotic fluid is stained with meconium?

   _____

   _____

   _____

10. Shoulder dystocia should be a concern when caring for a woman with:

    A. History of shoulder dystocia

    B. Height less than 5 feet

    C. Glucose intolerance this pregnancy

    D. Meconium-stained fluid

11. What should you do if the baby's shoulders become stuck?

    _____

    _____

    _____

12. Match the signs and symptoms in Column B with the source in Column A.

    Column A

    _____ 1. Retained placenta

    _____ 2. Lacerations of cervix or vagina

    _____ 3. Laceration of perineum or labia

    Column B

    a. Uterus feels firm but bleeding easily seen from torn tissue

    b. Bright red vaginal bleeding

    c. Soft uterus and dark red bleeding and/or clots

    d. Watery discharge

13. If the source of excessive postpartum bleeding is retained pieces of placenta, what should you do?

    a. _____

    b. _____

    c. _____

    d. _____

14. Which of the following situations place the woman at risk for excessive bleeding after the birth?

    A. Grandmultiparity

    B. Short rapid labor

    C. Small baby

    D. Oxytocin induction/augmentation

15. What should you do to assist a breech delivery?

    a. _____

    b. _____

    c. _____

    d. _____

PRACTICE/REVIEW ANSWER KEY

1. A, B, and D

2. Any six of the following:
   a. Nausea and retching
   b. Increased bloody show
   c. Strong urge to push
   d. Separation of the labia
   e. Increased pressure against the perineum
   f. Bulging of the anus
   g. Mother's feelings

3. 4" × 4" gauze sponges, two absorbent towels, soft bulb syringe, small drape, two clamps, scissors, baby blanket, gloves, mucus trap (e.g., DeLee mucus trap)

4. A

5. B

6. B

7. Any six of the following:
   a. Wipe the baby's face and head.
   b. Inspect the baby's neck for the cord.
   c. Suction the baby's oropharynx and nasopharynx.
   d. Check the airway.
   e. Dry the baby.
   f. Cut the umbilical cord.
   g. Prevent heat loss.

8. C and D

9. Use the mucus trap to suction the baby's oropharynx and nasopharynx before the shoulders deliver.

10. A, B, and C

11. Have the mother sharply flex her knees and hips, bringing the thighs alongside her abdomen. Occasionally, it may also be necessary to ask another staff member to apply suprapubic pressure.

12. 1. c
    2. b
    3. a

13. a. Massage the top of the uterus.
    b. Administer oxygen, if needed.
    c. Increase the rate of administration of intravenous fluid.
    d. Take and record blood pressure and pulse

14. A and D

15. a. Avoid excessive handling of the baby.
    b. Prevent stress on the cord.
    c. Lift the baby's body using a towel to help deliver the shoulders and head.
    d. Perform other safety measures, as with a normal delivery.

Managing an Unexpected Delivery
SKILL UNIT 1

The birth of a baby should be planned and conducted to ensure safety for the mother and child and to promote bonding for the family. A birth conducted by the primary care provider who has cared for the woman throughout her pregnancy is ideal. Sometimes, however, circumstances prevent this, and it is then the nurse in the labor and delivery unit who often assists the mother. The labor and delivery nurse must be prepared and have the necessary skills to provide the woman and her baby with the safest and most satisfying experience possible.

The section details how to use the necessary equipment and control the delivery itself. The preceptor will demonstrate the use of hand maneuvers and equipment. You will then be expected to demonstrate *your* skill using a doll.

ACTIONS	REMARKS
Assemble Equipment	
Sterile skin prep kit	It is important to maintain asepsis and prevent infection for both mother and child.
Sterile emergency delivery pack	USE UNIVERSAL PRECAUTIONS.
Prepare for the Delivery	
1. Call for assistance.	A second person can help care for the newborn, assist the nurse conducting the delivery, and help with any unexpected events.
2. Position the woman.	Position the woman on her back with her head elevated, with or without her legs in stirrups—whichever provides the greatest safety and comfort for the woman.
3. Cleanse the perineum.	Use the recommended aseptic skin preparation technique to ensure adequate cleansing.

Controlling the delivery of the baby's head is most important. Do not take time to do a thorough "skin prep" if the baby is delivering.

4. Open the sterile emergency delivery pack wherever the birth will take place.	You need to have the pack within easy reach. It is important to maintain sterile technique. This will help decrease the chances of infection.
5. Put on the sterile gloves. Place the sterile barrier under the buttocks and use the available sterile drapes.	

> Be sure you know the presentation of the baby. If you are uncertain about the presentation, a vaginal examination should be done to see whether the baby is vertex or breech.

Conduct the Emergency Delivery

6. As the head crowns, break the bag of waters if it does not break by itself.

   The bag of waters will usually break by itself, but if not, it must be cut or torn to prevent aspiration of fluid at birth.

7. Using the nondominant hand, support the perineum with a sterile towel or 4″ × 4″ gauze squares.

   This protects the sterile glove while supporting the stretching perineum.

8. In the groin area adjacent to the perineum, place the thumb on one side and fingers on the opposite (Fig. 14.12). Exert pressure by drawing the thumb and fingers together. This action is aimed at trying to create a pouch of the perineum.

   This relieves pressure on the stretching perineal body.

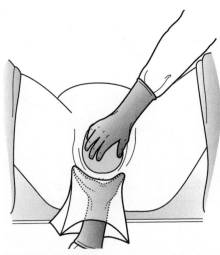

FIGURE 14.12

9. Instruct the woman when to feather blow and when to push.

10. Gently maintain pressure on the fetal head, using a cupped hand or the pads of the fingers until most of the head is delivered. Then gently assist the head to extend and deliver the forehead, face, and chin.

    This helps prevent uncontrolled, rapid delivery of the head.

    Keep the head flexed by slowly allowing it to rise under your palm or fingers. Assist extension by raising the head as the forehead comes over the perineum. It is sometimes helpful to have the woman push or bear down after the contraction is over.

> Be clear when telling the woman what to do. Make your instructions short and easy to understand.

11. Slide your fingers down around the baby's neck to inspect for a cord as soon as the head has delivered (Fig. 14.13).

    Need to determine whether cord is present.

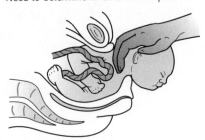

FIGURE 14.13

If loose cord is felt around the baby's neck, gently pull a loop down over the head (Fig. 14.14).

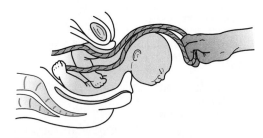

FIGURE 14.14

If a tight cord is felt, put two clamps on the cord (approximately 1 inch apart) and then cut between the clamps (Fig. 14.15). Quickly loosen the cord from around the neck.

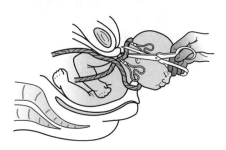

FIGURE 14.15

12. Wipe the head and face dry, paying special attention to mucus coming from the nose and mouth.

Mucus is forced out of the nose and mouth as the baby squeezes through the birth canal. If the mucus is not wiped away, the baby can aspirate it when the baby begins to breathe. At this point, use a bulb syringe to suction out the mouth and nose.

13. Allow the head to **restitute.** Place the hand palm-side up and with the fingers toward the face, under the head for support (Fig. 14.16).

Head and shoulders are resuming normal alignment. The baby's head will turn slightly.

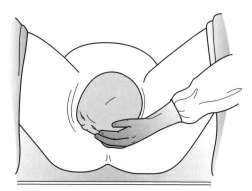

FIGURE 14.16

Allow the shoulders to rotate *externally* (Fig. 14.17).

As the shoulders move into position for birth, you will observe another slight turn of the baby's head. The shoulders are now in the AP diameter of the maternal pelvis.

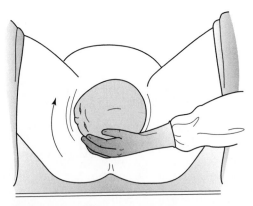

FIGURE 14.17

14. Place the second hand on the other side of the baby's head and, with downward, outward traction on the head, deliver the anterior shoulder (Fig. 14.18).

Keep your fingers flat on the sides of the head. *Do not* grab the baby around the neck.

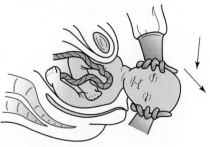

FIGURE 14.18

15. As soon as the anterior shoulder delivers, provide upward, outward traction to the head to deliver the posterior shoulder (Fig. 14.19).

Keep fingers away from eyes and neck.

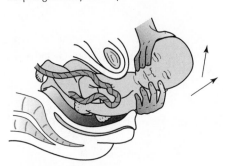

FIGURE 14.19

16. As the shoulder clears the perineum, support the head with the heel of your hand and thumb. Using the fingers of this hand, grasp the baby's arm to the chest wall (Fig, 14.20). Support the baby in your lower hand.

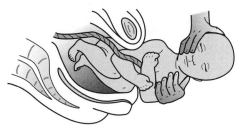

FIGURE 14.20

17. As the body delivers, slide the upper hand down the baby's back to grasp the feet (Fig. 14.21).

Holding the arm to the chest helps prevent laceration of the perineum by the elbow.

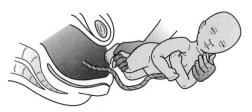

FIGURE 14.21

18. As the feet deliver, turn the baby in an arm hold, with the head turned slightly and the head slightly lower than the feet (Fig. 14.22).

This helps drain the airway. The nose and mouth can be suctioned with a bulb syringe. Keep the baby close to the perineum to prevent excess pulling on the cord. Avoid grasping the baby's neck and compressing carotid arteries.

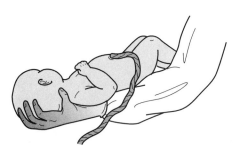

FIGURE 14.22

19. Double clamp the umbilical cord. Cut the cord between the two clamps (Fig. 14.23).

Take care to avoid wide spraying of the blood.

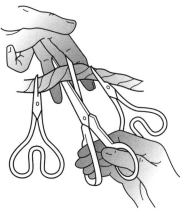

FIGURE 14.23

Care of the Newborn

20. Place the baby directly on the mother's warm chest or abdomen.

   This assists in maintaining the baby's body heat with skin-to-skin contact (or a heated crib).

21. With skin-to-skin contact, cover the newborn and mother with warm towels or a blanket.

   This helps prevent heat loss in the newborn.

22. Dry the baby thoroughly.

   Wet babies lose a great deal of heat. It is important to replace wet towels immediately.

23. Collect blood from the cord attached to the placenta.

   Because the amount of cord blood drawn will depend on the tests needed, check the mother's chart and your hospital's guidelines.

Delivery of the Placenta

24. Check for uterine size, shape, and firmness.

   The uterus must contract to expel the placenta and to control bleeding.
   Signs of placental separation are as follows:

   - A gush of blood
   - Lengthening of the cord
   - A change in the shape of the uterus from oval to globular

25. Control the delivery of the placenta by keeping a gentle, steady, downward traction on the cord as the other hand supports the uterine fundus. The mother can assist by bearing down when she feels a contraction.

   Tugging on the cord or vigorous rubbing of the uterus can cause problems and must not be done.
   Carefully inspect the placenta for signs of missing pieces or abnormalities. Count the number of vessels in the cord: There should be three (two arteries and one vein).

26. Observe the amount and color of the bleeding and the tone of the uterus.

   If the uterus feels soft, it can be stimulated to contract by massaging the fundus (the top of the uterus) or by having the baby breastfeed.

27. Inspect for lacerations.

   Gently inspect the perineum and labia for bleeding or tears in need of repair by the primary care provider. A sterile pad can be applied to provide pressure to control bleeding of a perineal or labial laceration.

28. Facilitate bonding.

   Families need time to inspect, hold, and "take in" the newborn. Immediately after birth, as soon as the mother and baby have settled down, the family must be provided private time to begin to "attach."

You will need to attend a skill session(s) to practice this skill with the help of your preceptor. Mastery of the skill is achieved when you can demonstrate techniques of delivering a baby, including the following:

- Taking preparatory steps
- Positioning the woman
- Following aseptic skin preparation
- Using sterile gloves and drapes
- Flexing and controlling the delivery of the head
- Guiding the delivery of the baby's body
- Checking for a nuchal cord
- Cutting the umbilical cord
- Delivering the placenta
- Inspecting the placenta and cord

REFERENCES

1. Glantz, J. C., & Woods, J. R. (1999). Significance of amniotic fluid meconium. In R. K. Creasy & R. Resnick (Eds.), *Maternal-fetal medicine* (4th ed., pp. 393–403). Philadelphia: WB Saunders.
2. American College of Obstetricians and Gynecologists. (1998). ACOG practice patterns: Shoulder dystocia. Number 7, October, 1997. *International Journal of Gynecology and Obstetrics, 60*(3), 306–313.

3. Hall, S. P. (1997). The nurse's role in the identification of risks and treatment of shoulder dystocia. *Journal of Obstetrics, Gynecologic and Neonatal Nursing, 26*(1), 25–32.

SUGGESTED READINGS

Hall, S. P. (1997). The nurse's role in the identification of risks and treatment of shoulder dystocia. *Journal of Obstetrics, Gynecologic and Neonatal Nursing, 26*(1), 25–32.

Jennings, B. (1979). Emergency delivery: How to attend to one safely. *American Journal of Maternal-Child Nursing, 4*(3), 148–153.

Oxorn, H. (1986). *Oxorn-Foote human labor & birth* (5th ed.). New York: Appleton-Century-Crofts.

Reeder, S. J., Martin, L. L., & Koneak-Griffin, D. (1997). *Maternity nursing: Family, newborn, and women's health care* (18th ed.) Philadelphia: Lippincott-Raven.

Simpson, K. R., & Knox, G. E. (2001). Fundal pressure during second stage of labor clinical perspectives and risk management issues. *American Journal of Maternal Child Nursing, 26*(2), 64–71.

MODULE 15

Assessment of the Newborn and Newly Delivered Mother

ANN MOGABGAB WEATHERSBY

Initial Assessment of the Newborn

As you complete Part 1 of this module, you will learn:

1. Normal signs of newborn adaptation to extrauterine life
2. Methods to assist the newborn in normal adaptation
3. Methods to evaluate newborn adaptation: Apgar scoring and umbilical cord blood analysis
4. The limitations of these evaluation methods
5. Preparations to be made before delivery of an infant requiring assistance with adaptation
6. Actions that must be taken when an infant requires resuscitation
7. Proper techniques for use when obtaining specimens for cord blood analysis

When you have completed Part 1 of this module, you should be able to recall the meaning of the following terms. You should also be able to use the terms when consulting with other health professionals. The terms are defined in this module or in the glossary at the end of this book.

Apgar score   neonatal resuscitation
asphyxia   newly born
hypopharynx   vagal stimulation

The birth of a baby is a life-changing event for a family, a change that has been anticipated for months or years. The dreams for this new life become reality as parents and family greet the baby and start the process of welcoming a new family member. Family roles shift: A mother becomes a grandmother; the baby becomes the older brother. Two families now have a bond in this new life. Families make this transition in many different ways, sometimes due to cultural conventions, family traditions, or personal decisions. It is a special joy for perinatal nurses to be able to witness this birth of family.

The physical care of the mother is an important part of the role of the perinatal nurse. This chapter contains information to guide the nurse in safe and appropriate care of the newborn and mother. However, it is also important for the nurse to recognize that much more is occurring than these physical changes. Being sensitive to the needs of the woman and her family during the early hours after birth is as important as providing physical care. The nurse has the opportunity to provide care to the whole woman, care that includes the physical and psychosocial, care that considers all aspects of the miracle of birth.

Assessment of the Newborn

■ What are the normal responses of the newborn to extrauterine life?[1-3]

With birth and the clamping of the umbilical cord, a sequence of events occurs that begins the adaptation of the newborn infant to life outside the womb. The term *newly born* is sometimes used to refer to the infant during this brief period of the first minutes to hours after birth. As the newborn takes the first breaths, the lungs change from fluid filled to air filled. It is thought that newborn respirations are triggered by a combination of factors. After the baby passes through the birth canal, the pressure on the newborn thorax is released and a passive recoil of the chest allows intake of air. Other factors that affect these first respirations include lowered oxygenation of the fetus as a result of occlusion of the cord during birth, clamping of the cord after delivery, and the drop in temperature from the warm uterine environment to the cooler birth room. Circulation begins the transition from the blood flow patterns of the fetus to the blood flow of the newborn. The newborn also begins to regulate temperature. These changes begin in the immediate newborn period, although not without obvious effort on the part of the infant.

An infant responding normally to extrauterine life will take initial breaths and have a lusty cry, maintain heart rate in the normal (greater than 100 bpm) range, and show good tone and normal reflexes. With adequate respirations and circulation, color will gradually change from dusky blue/pink immediately after birth to the overall pink of body and extremities.

■ How can the nurse assist the infant in adaptation to the extrauterine environment?[3-5]

Infants showing a normal response to the extrauterine environment can remain with their mother to receive routine care. Care of the mother–infant couplet in the first hours after birth is best provided by the mother/baby nurse. The initial status and needs of both the mother and the newborn can be evaluated by this specially trained nurse.

Assisting the newborn with transition to life outside the womb begins with preventing heat loss. The infant is thoroughly dried with warm blankets, placed skin to skin with the mother, and covered with another warm dry blanket. Covering the head with a cap can also decrease heat loss because the head is a major source of heat loss. This drying of the infant also stimulates the infant to establish spontaneous respirations.

The newborn may need assistance with clearing secretions from the airway. Positioning him or her in a side-lying position may help. Secretions can be wiped from the mouth and nose. If suctioning is necessary, the mouth should be suctioned first, then the nose, with a bulb syringe or suction catheter. Vigorous suctioning must be avoided because this can lead to laryngeal spasms and vagal bradycardia.

■ What are the methods used to evaluate the adaptation of the newly born?[5-8]

The newborn infant is initially evaluated for heart rate, cry or respirations, movement of extremities, and color. A quick method for this evaluation, called the Apgar score, was devised in 1952 by Virginia Apgar. The purpose of this scoring is to identify an infant who needs assistance with the adaptation to extrauterine environment. Using this scoring system, scores are determined as follows: heart rate is based on the rate being absent or above or below 100 bpm, and respiration is evaluated as absent, slow, or good respirations or crying activity. The muscle tone of the infant is also evaluated and is rated from flaccid to active motion. Reflexes can be evaluated by a tap on the sole of the foot or by the infant response to a catheter in the nostril, and the infant response can range from no response to cry, cough, or sneeze. The infant color is assessed and can range from blue or pale to completely pink. The components of the score are listed in Table 15.1 and are evaluated at 1 minute and 5 minutes after birth.

TABLE 15.1 Criteria for Apgar Scoring			
SIGN	**SCORE 0**	**SCORE 1**	**SCORE 2**
Heart rate	Not detectable	Below 100	Above 100
Respiratory effort	Absent	Slow, irregular	Good, crying
Muscle tone	Flaccid	Some extremity flexion	Active motion
Reflex irritability			
–Response to tap on sole of foot	No response	Grimace	Grimace
–Response to catheter in nostril (after oropharynx is cleared)	No response	Cry	Cough or sneeze
Color	Blue, pale	Body pink, blue extremities	Completely pink

Reprinted with permission from Apgar, V. (1953, July/August). A proposal for a new method of evaluation of the newborn infant. Current Researches in Anesthesia and Analgesia, 32(4), 260–267.

Evaluation of the newly born infant's cord blood gases is another method to evaluate the newborn's need for assistance with adaptation.

Apgar Score

■ What is the significance of an Apgar score?[3,7,8]

It can be argued that the Apgar scoring system is no longer of clinical significance. Practitioners of newborn care are trained in neonatal resuscitation following the American Academy of Pediatrics (AAP) guidelines. These guidelines recommend assessment of the infant at birth and institution of any needed resuscitation. The delay of resuscitation until a 1-minute Apgar score is obtained is not an appropriate use of the scoring system.

However, the Apgar score continues to be used and can be helpful in the initial evaluation of the newborn's need for further assistance with adaptation and in the evaluation of the newborn's response to resuscitation. Apgar scores may also be useful in resuscitations if continued at 5-minute intervals until the infant has stabilized.

Broad categories of scores that may indicate infant adaptation have been considered:

- **7 to 10**—May indicate adequate adaptation; no assistance is usually needed
- **4 to 6**—May indicate need for some resuscitation
- **0 to 3**—Usually indicates that resuscitation is needed immediately

Even with the guidance of these categories, it is important to consider each infant's condition and needs for assistance with adaptation.

Apgar scoring is most reliable when done by trained personnel and by someone who is giving complete attention to the newborn.

REMEMBER: The Apgar score is a clinical evaluation of the need for newborn resuscitation. It does not determine newborn hypoxia, acidosis, or neurologic impairment, nor does it predict long-term outcome.

■ What are some factors that can cause variations in Apgar scores?[3,6,8]

Several factors can cause variations in Apgar scores and may not indicate a need for resuscitation. An overall clinical evaluation is important in these situations when considering the care of the infant. Some of these factors include the following:

- **Gestational age**—The standard Apgar goal of 10 points might not be an appropriate gauge of fetal well-being for babies of less than 31 to 34 weeks' gestation. These infants often lack the tone of a term infant and the ability to respond appropriately when reflex irritability is tested.

- **Intubation and cord visualization**—Meconium-stained amniotic fluid may indicate the need for immediate intubation and suctioning of the hypopharynx and trachea. Intubation often produces stimulation of the vagus nerve and subsequent temporary lowering of the heart rate. Babies usually recover from this intervention spontaneously, but this temporary slowing of the heart rate can affect Apgar scoring.
- **Congenital defects**—Babies with congenital defects of the heart or neuromuscular or cerebral malformations may have Apgar scores that do not reflect a need for resuscitation. These infants need further evaluation.
- **Infection**—Infection in the newborn may affect tone, color, and reflexes.

Umbilical Cord Gas Values

■ **How are newborn umbilical cord gas values used to evaluate the newborn?**[9,10]

Umbilical cord blood sampling is a useful addition to Apgar scoring in the evaluation of the fetus' condition at the time of birth. Umbilical cord blood gas sampling is a method used to determine the oxygenation and acid-base status of the fetus at birth and the functioning of the placenta. *The arterial values reflect fetal conditions; venous values reflect placental function.*

REMEMBER: Umbilical arteries carry blood from the fetus to the placenta, and the umbilical vein carries oxygenated blood to the fetus.

The pH value is normal or abnormal. A low pH value indicates acidemia of the fetus, and this acidemia is then further evaluated. Gases are evaluated for the cause of the acidemia and can be classified as respiratory, metabolic, or mixed in origin.

■ **Can Apgar scores and cord blood gases identify a newborn with perinatal asphyxia?**[3,6-8]

The AAP and the American College of Obstetricians and Gynecologists (ACOG) have recommended that the term *asphyxia* be applied only to infants who have all of the following conditions:

- Metabolic or mixed acidemia with a pH value less than 7.0
- An Apgar score of 0 to 3 for longer than 5 minutes
- Neonatal neurologic manifestations such as seizures, coma, or poor tone and multisystem organ dysfunction

■ **Are cord gas values obtained for all infants?**[9]

Some physicians and midwives sample cord blood gases at every delivery. For the normal healthy newborn, little information of clinical value is obtained with this practice. Other practitioners clamp and reserve a segment of cord at every delivery and obtain gas analysis if the infant has low Apgar scores or any signs of distress. Many practitioners routinely obtain gases in high-risk pregnancies or complicated deliveries. It is important to understand the expectations of the physician or midwife before delivery in order to prepare for cord gas testing. The Skill Unit at the end of this section will help you learn the technique for cord blood sampling.

■ **What are normal blood gas values for healthy term babies?**[9,10]

Table 15.2 shows a range for normal cord blood gas values for healthy term babies. Other investigators have found a wide range of values to be normal. In general, an umbilical artery pH of 7.10 or greater can be considered normal and is associated with normal Apgar scores and vigorous newborns.

■ **If the cord gas shows acidemia, what else is evaluated?**[10]

The cord gases should be further evaluated for the type of acidemia that has occurred. Table 15.3 shows the classifications of acidemia.

- **Respiratory acidosis** is associated with insults to the fetus that are of short duration. The fetus is able to continue to compensate for these insults with normal physiologic responses. Examples are tight nuchal cords or other causes of cord compression that may occur just before delivery. With immediate and appropriate resuscitation, these infants generally make rapid adaptations to extrauterine life.

TABLE 15.2 Normal Umbilical Cord Blood pH and Blood Gas Values in Term Newborns (Mean ± One Standard Deviation)

VALUE	YEOMANS* (n = 146)	RAMIN* (n = 1,292)	RILEY† (n = 3,522)
Arterial blood			
pH	7.28 (0.05)	7.28 (0.07)	7.27 (0.069)
Pco₂ (mm Hg)	49.2 (8.4)	49.9 (14.2)	50.3 (11.1)
HCO₃⁻ (meq/L)	22.3 (2.5)	23.1 (2.8)	22.0 (3.6)
Base excess (meq/L)	—‡	−3.6 (2.8)	−2.7 (2.8)
Venous blood			
pH	7.35 (0.05)	—	7.34 (0.063)
Pco₂ (mm Hg)	38.2 (5.6)	—	40.7 (7.9)
HCO₃⁻ (meq/L)	20.4 (4.1)	—	21.4 (2.5)
Base excess (meq/L)	—‡	—	−2.4 (2)

*Data are from infants of selected patients with uncomplicated vaginal deliveries.

†Data are from infants of unselected patients with vaginal deliveries.

‡Data were not obtained.

Ramin SM, Gilstrap LC III, Leveno KJ, Burris J, Little BB. Umbilical artery acid–base status in the preterm infant. Obstet Gynecol 1989;74:256–258

Riley RJ, Johnson JWC. Collecting and analyzing cord blood gases. Clin Obstet Gynecol 1993;36:13–23

Yeomans ER, Hauth JC, Gilstrap LC III, Strickland DM. Umbilical cord pH, Pco₂ and bicarbonate following uncomplicated term vaginal deliveries. Am J Obstet Gynecol 1985;151:798–800

TABLE 15.3 Normal Umbilical Artery Blood pH and Blood Gas Values in Premature Infants (Mean ± One Standard Deviation)

VALUE FOR ARTERIAL BLOOD	RAMIN* (n = 77)	DICKINSON† (n = 949)	RILEY† (n = 1,015)
pH	7.29 (0.07)	7.27 (0.07)	7.28 (0.089)
Pco₂ (mm Hg)	49.2 (9.0)	51.6 (9.4)	50.2 (12.3)
HCO₃⁻ (meq/L)	23.0 (3.5)	23.9 (2.1)	22.4 (3.5)
Base excess (meq/L)	−3.3 (2.4)	−3.0 (2.5)	−2.5 (3)

*Data are from infants of selected patients with uncomplicated vaginal deliveries.

†Data are from infants of unselected patients with vaginal deliveries.

Dickinson JE, Eriksen NL, Meyer BA, Parisi VM. The effect of preterm birth on umbilical cord blood gases. Obstet Gynecol 1992;79:575–578

Ramin SM, Gilstrap LC III, Leveno KJ, Burris J, Little BB. Umbilical artery acid–base status in the preterm infant. Obstet Gynecol 1989;74:256–258

Riley RJ, Johnson JWC. Collecting and analyzing cord blood gases. Clin Obstet Gynecol 1993;36:13–23

- Infants with **metabolic or mixed acidosis** generally have had a more profound or longer-lasting insult that may include a poor prenatal environment. These infants require more intensive resuscitation and careful neonatal follow-up.

Care of Infants Requiring Resuscitation at Delivery

■ What are the preparations to be made before delivery of an infant requiring assistance with adaptation?[3,5]

Risk factors can identify many infants who may require resuscitation. For instance, the delivery of a preterm infant, an infant with meconium-stained amniotic fluid, or an infant with a nonreassuring fetal heart rate tracing may have a need for resuscitation at delivery. Maternal conditions that may indicate the need for resuscitation of the newborn include diabetes, chronic hypertension or preeclampsia, chorioamnionitis, or other conditions that can affect placental perfusion.

However, it is impossible to completely predict all infants who will need resuscitation. For this reason, *a person trained to begin neonatal resuscitation should be present at every delivery*. Individuals trained to continue resuscitations should be immediately available for all deliveries and present for high-risk situations.

Programs are available to train and certify personnel in neonatal resuscitation. Nurses who work in antepartal units, labor and delivery units, newborn nurseries, and postpartum or mother–baby units need training in neonatal resuscitation, much like the routinely required certification in adult cardiopulmonary resuscitation.

Each birth room needs to be stocked with the equipment, supplies, and medications for a complete resuscitation. The AAP neonatal resuscitation program is an excellent resource for guidelines for training personnel and supplying units.

■ What actions are required when an infant requires resuscitation?[3,5]

Newborn infants who do not respond normally to the extrauterine environment are in need of further assessment:

- Take the infant to a radiant warmer, place the infant supine, and thoroughly dry the infant to stimulate respirations and reduce cold stress. Remove all wet towels or blankets from the infant.
- Suction the infant, if necessary. Remember to suction the mouth first, then the nose.
- Assess the infant according to the resuscitation triad: respiration, heart rate, and color. Assessment will determine whether resuscitation is needed. Initiate those techniques in which you are skilled and obtain necessary help for other procedures.
- Remember to keep the mother and other family members informed of what is occurring, why it is occurring, and what is being done. Parents usually respond well to accurate information given in a timely manner.
- Documentation of newborn status and adaptation to the extrauterine environment is also a necessary component of the care of the newborn. Apgar scoring, blood gases, any need for resuscitation, and actions taken are to be documented.

Procedure for Obtaining Umbilical Cord Blood Sample
SKILL UNIT 1

This section details how to collect umbilical cord blood samples in a manner that achieves the most accurate results. Study this section and then attend a skill practice and demonstration session scheduled by your preceptor. You will need to demonstrate the procedure for collecting the specimen(s). The steps of the examination are listed at the end of this unit.

REMEMBER: Check with the procedures at your institution for recommendations. At some institutions, cord segments are transported rapidly to the laboratory and the lab technician will draw the sample. Also determine whether both arterial and venous samples are desired.

ACTIONS	REMARKS
1. Collect supplies: • Heparin 1,000 U/mL • Two 3-mL syringes with 22- or 23-gauge needles and caps • Labels and lab slips as needed • Gloves	Remember to use universal precautions when handling blood products. Prepare labels and requisition slips before delivery. Prepare one label marked *venous sample* and one label marked *arterial sample.*
2. Prepare syringes for sampling: Flush syringes with heparin solution and eject heparin and air from syringes. Recap.	The goal is to coat the syringe with heparin to prevent clotting of the specimen.
3. Receive segment of cord for sampling.	The physician or midwife will double-clamp a 6- to 8-inch segment of cord immediately after delivery and hand it to you for sampling.
4. Obtain samples: With the bevel of the needle up, insert the needle into the smaller and darker artery and withdraw 1 to 2 mL (Fig. 15.1). Remove air and recap the needle using the one-handed recap procedure or a hemostat to hold the needle cap. Repeat the procedure to obtain a specimen from the larger vein.	The venous specimen will be pinker than the darker arterial specimen. It is important to recap the needle using techniques to prevent needlestick injuries.
5. Send the labeled specimens with the appropriate requisitions to the lab.	Cord segments and heparinized samples are stable for at least 30 to 60 minutes at room temperature. Sample and transport as soon as possible.

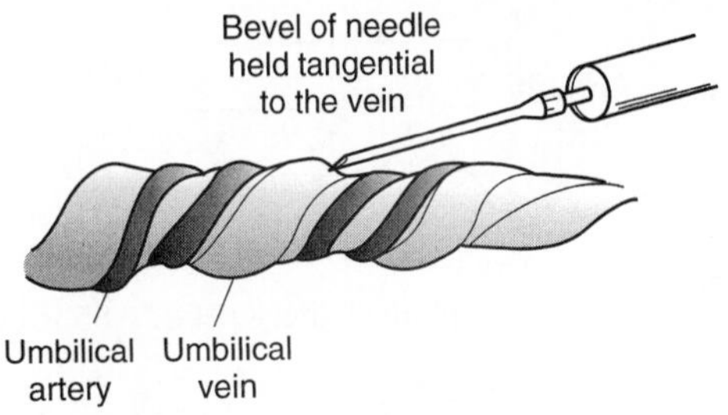

Bevel of needle held tangential to the vein

Umbilical artery   Umbilical vein

FIGURE 15.1

You will need to attend a skill session to practice this skill with the help of your preceptor. Mastery of this skill is achieved when you can do the following:

- Assemble all necessary equipment for the procedure
- Differentiate the arteries and vein in an umbilical cord
- Demonstrate collection and labeling of 0.3 to 3.0 mL of venous and arterial blood sample using heparinized syringes

PRACTICE/REVIEW QUESTIONS

After reviewing Part 1, answer the following questions.

1. What is the 1-minute Apgar score for the baby described below?_____

   Heart rate: 126 bpm

   Respiratory effort: Crying

   Muscle tone: Active

   Reflex irritability: Grimace

   Color: Blue extremities

2. Do you anticipate that this baby will require resuscitation?

   A. Yes

   B. No

3. What is the 1-minute Apgar score for the baby described below? _____

   Heart rate: 96 bpm

   Respiratory effort: Irregular

   Muscle tone: Flaccid

   Reflex irritability: No response

   Color: Blue

4. Do you anticipate that this baby will require resuscitation?

   A. Yes

   B. No

5. Which factor is most likely to cause a low Apgar score?

   A. A fall in maternal body temperature

   B. Visualization and suctioning of the infant's vocal cords

   C. Infant birth weight of more than 8 pounds

   D. An infant born at 41 weeks' gestation

6. List the steps of a recommended procedure for collection of umbilical cord blood gas samples.

   a. _____

   b. _____

   c. _____

   d. _____

   e. _____

7. An umbilical artery pH of 6.85 is considered abnormal.

   A. True

   B. False

8. Would you anticipate that an infant with a pH of 6.85 would need assistance with adaptation to extrauterine life?

   A. Yes

   B. No

PRACTICE/REVIEW ANSWER KEY

1. 8

2. B

3. 2

4. A

5. B

6. a. Collect supplies.
   b. Prepare syringes.
   c. Receive cord segment.
   d. Obtain samples.
   e. Send labeled samples.

7. A

8. A

Assessment of the Newly Delivered Mother

Pain Reassessment
Due at _____
50062

As you complete Part 2 of this module, you will learn:

1. Components and expected findings of the physical assessment of a newly delivered mother
2. Variations from normal findings during the early postpartum period and familiarity with common interventions
3. Nursing interventions that promote parent–infant attachment
4. Techniques to assist the mother with the initiation of breastfeeding in the immediate postpartum period
5. Necessary interventions for women with recovery complicated by surgery, anesthesia, infection, or pregnancy-related hypertension
6. Techniques to assist parents who have experienced a birth with neonatal complications
7. Ongoing needs of the newly delivered mother during postpartum hospitalization
8. General guidelines for discharge of mother and infant

When you have completed Part 2 of this module, you should be able to recall the meaning of the following terms. You should also be able to use the terms when consulting with other health professionals. The terms are defined in this module or in the glossary at the end of this book.

atony	lochia
dermatome	nipple confusion
eclampsia	rubra
en face	tubal ligation
hematoma	

Postpartum Assessment of the Mother

> ■ **What are the components and expected findings of the physical assessment of a newly delivered mother?**[2–4]

The period following delivery of the placenta and continuing until maternal stabilization—the immediate postpartum period—is a time of rapid physiologic change that requires careful monitoring by the nurse. Although women can be cared for in a variety of settings (e.g., traditional recovery room; labor, delivery, recovery room [LDR]; labor, delivery, recovery, and postpartum room [LDRP]), components of care are unchanged.

To care for a newly delivered mother's postpartum needs, the nurse must know both the prenatal and intrapartum history. Although assessments and interventions begin immediately postpartum, an orderly, ongoing, and complete assessment is needed during the first postpartum hour.

Postpartum education is a component of care. Explanation of the findings of assessments and needed interventions by the nurse to the mother and support person continues the educational process begun antepartally.

General Assessment

Note the overall appearance of the mother, including skin color, motor activity, facial expression, speech, manner, mood, state of awareness, and interactions with others.

Vital Signs

- **Blood pressure**—Monitor at least every 15 minutes for the first hour. Findings should return to prelabor values.
- **Pulse**—Monitor every 15 minutes for the first hour. Postpartum pulse rates may be lower than labor values.
- **Respirations**—Monitor every 15 minutes for the first hour. Findings should return to prelabor values.
- **Temperature**—Monitor at least once during the initial postpartum hour. Temperature should be in normal range (less than 100.4°F).

Uterus

Evaluation of the uterus includes assessment of fundal height and uterine tone. This evaluation is done with the vital sign evaluation, usually at least every 15 minutes, or more frequently as indicated by findings.

Procedure for Evaluation of Fundal Height

Starting well above the umbilicus, palpate firmly with the flat of the fingers and hand, midline in the abdomen, until the fundus of the uterus is felt. It might be helpful to cup the uterus with the hand to clearly outline its location and size. The fundal height is measured in relation to the umbilicus and is calculated in fingerbreadths above the umbilicus (e.g., 2 fingerbreadths below the umbilicus).

Normal Findings

In the immediate postpartum period, the fundus should be found midline in the abdomen and at about the level of the umbilicus. Figure 15.2 indicates expected fundal height measurements during the postpartum period.

Procedure for Evaluation of Uterine Tone

After assessing fundal height, palpate the tone of the uterus. A boggy uterus feels very soft and is often difficult to find.

Normal Findings

The uterus should be firm and midline.

Lochia

Procedure for Assessment

Observe **lochia** (vaginal bleeding) to identify the amount, color, and presence of any clots. Evaluate peripad for amount of saturation.

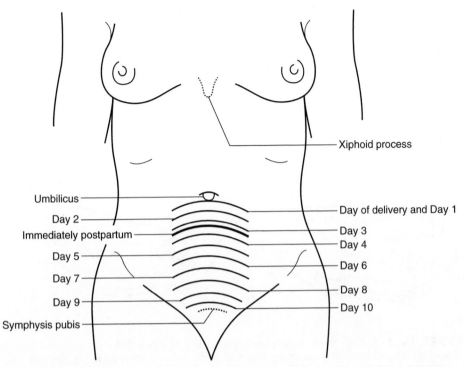

FIGURE 15.2 Fundal height and uterine involution. (Adapted with permission from Varney, H. [1997]. *Varney's midwifery* [3rd ed., p. 624]. Boston: Jones and Bartlett.)

Normal Findings

Lochia should be red (**rubra**) and moderate in flow during the first hour. Flow should not exceed the saturation of two peripads in the first hour.

Bladder

Procedure for Assessment

Gently palpate the lower abdominal area just above the symphysis pubis to palpate for bladder fullness or tenderness.

Normal Findings

The bladder should not be palpable.

Perineum

Procedure for Assessment

With adequate lighting and exposure, evaluate for edema and signs of hematoma (e.g., a discolored or bruised and edematous area). If an episiotomy or laceration repair has been performed, observe for intact stitches.

Normal Findings

The perineum should be pink, without signs of bruising or findings of considerable edema. Inspection of an episiotomy or laceration repair should reveal approximated tissues with little edema.

Breasts

Procedure for Assessment

Inspect the nipples of mother planning to breastfeed.

Normal Findings

Nipples may be erect, flat, or inverted (Fig. 15.3).

585

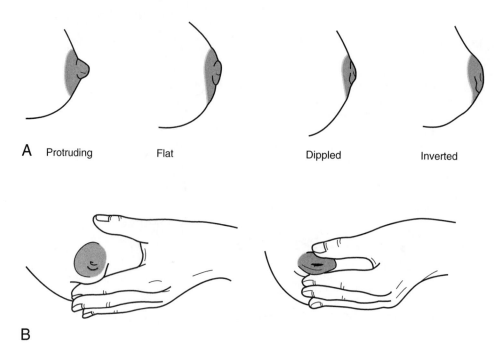

A   Protruding   Flat   Dippled   Inverted

B

FIGURE 15.3 **A.** Nipple shapes. **B.** *Left:* The mother can help the baby to latch on to an inverted nipple if she places her thumb above the areola and her fingers below and pushes the breast against her chest wall. *Right:* The mother should avoid squeezing her thumb and fingers together. The nipple might invert further. (Adapted from Huggins, K. [1990]. *The nursing mother's companion* [Rev. ed., pp. 29, 65]. Boston: Harvard Common Press.)

Variations From Normal Findings

> ■ **What are some variations from these normal findings in the postpartum period and how are they managed?**[2–4]

Findings of variations from normal on postpartum assessments require early interventions to prevent potentially serious consequences.

Vital Signs

Elevated Blood Pressure
Intervention
Validate the reading by retaking the blood pressure. Notify the physician or midwife of readings of 140/90 mm Hg or above or an elevation of 30 systolic or 15 diastolic above early pregnancy levels. Assess the patient for pain and provide pain relief as indicated.

Elevated blood pressure in the postpartum period can be a sign of pregnancy-related hypertension and preeclampsia. Patients diagnosed with pregnancy-related hypertension require vigilant monitoring in the early postpartum period.

Decreased Blood Pressure
Intervention
Validate readings by retaking blood pressure. Assess for increased lochia flow. Notify the physician of midwife if blood pressure does not stabilize or is accompanied by excessive flow of lochia or signs of shock.

Elevated Temperature
Intervention
Abnormal values must be evaluated to determine their cause. Dehydration after a lengthy labor with inadequate fluid intake is a common cause of early postpartum fever. Women who have had epidural anesthesia may have fever unrelated to infection. Notify the physician or midwife and infant care practitioner if maternal temperature is greater than 100.4°F.

Uterus

Increased Fundal Height

A fundus that is higher than 2 fingerbreadths above the umbilicus might indicate a distended bladder or a uterus that is filled with blood clots. After delivery of a large infant, the fundal height can be slightly elevated, and this may be a normal finding.

Intervention

Assist the mother to empty her bladder. Catheterize only if the mother is unable to void. Reevaluate the fundal height. Massage the fundus in an attempt to expel any retained blood clots. Report increased fundal height that does not respond to these measures.

Decreased Uterine Tone

Some clinical situations that can predispose a newly delivered woman to uterine **atony** (decreased muscle tone of the uterus) are as follows:

- Prolonged labor
- Oxytocin induction/augmentation of labor
- Magnesium sulfate therapy or use of tocolytics for labor suppression
- Large infant or multiple gestation
- Cesarean section under general anesthesia (halogenated anesthetics)

> REMEMBER: In most cases, postpartum hemorrhage related to uterine atony cannot be predicted before delivery. Every newly delivered mother needs careful monitoring.

Interventions

The finding of a boggy uterus requires the nurse to massage the uterus to prevent potentially profuse bleeding from the large maternal sinuses at the placental site. Explain the procedure to the woman and ask her to relax her abdominal muscles. To massage the uterus, place one hand midline on the abdomen near the umbilicus and begin massaging the area. The other hand should be placed just above the symphysis pubis to stabilize the uterus, as shown in Figure 15.4. Moderate massage usually stimulates the relaxed uterus to contract. If uterine massage does not result in a firm uterus, notify the primary care provider. Often, 10 to 20 units of oxytocin is ordered by the physician or midwife to be added to 1,000 mL of intravenous (IV) fluids (or given intramuscularly) to maintain a firmly contracted uterus. For many practitioners, this is a routine part of postpartum management. In addition, methylergonovine or 15-methylprostaglandin F_{2a} (a prostaglandin) may be ordered to ensure uterine contraction and prevent hemorrhage.

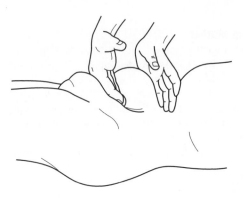

FIGURE 15.4 Placement of the hands for uterine massage.

Lochia

Increased Flow of Lochia

The most common cause of increased vaginal bleeding in the immediate postpartum period is uterine atony. Other causes that must be considered are retained placental fragments and bleeding from lacerations.

Intervention

If excessive lochia flow is identified, massage the fundus until firm. Notify the physician or midwife if bleeding becomes heavy, if a pad is saturated within 15 minutes, or if large clots are expressed. Anticipate the need for an IV line, if not already available. Monitor vital signs, including blood pressure and pulse. Remember that in the postpartum period, significant blood loss can occur without a decrease in blood pressure. Medications, as discussed in the section on decreased uterine tone, may be ordered. If bleeding continues despite a firm uterus, notify the physician or midwife. Assessment of the perineum, vagina, and cervix for lacerations or evaluation of the patient for retained placental fragments may be necessary.

Bladder

Distended Bladder or Inability of Patient to Void

Interventions

The sensation of needing to void might be decreased in the postpartum woman as a result of pressure on the bladder during labor and birth or because of the continued effects of regional (epidural or spinal) anesthesia. The bladder may become distended from IV fluids administered during labor or from the diuresis that normally occurs postpartum. A distended bladder can interfere with uterine contractility and lead to uterine atony and excessive vaginal bleeding. Many women are able to void when assisted to the bathroom, so this should be attempted before catheterization if there are no contraindications to ambulation. Avoid allowing the bladder to become overdistended, which can lead to loss of muscle tone and continued difficulty with voiding. Catheterization may become necessary. Remember that any catheterization increases the woman's risk for urinary tract infection.

Perineum

Perineal Edema or Hematoma Formation

Intervention

For all newly delivered women, perineal care with warm water is comforting, promotes healing, and allows good visualization of the area. An ice pack to the perineum during the first 24 hours is recommended after episiotomies or repaired lacerations or if edema is present. After 24 hours, the use of warm, moist heat in the form of a sitz bath facilitates healing and reduces discomfort. Nonsteroidal anti-inflammatory drugs may be ordered by the physician or midwife to reduce the inflammatory response and promote healing. Analgesics may be required. After initial treatment with ice, sitz baths may be ordered.

Notify the physician or midwife of excessive perineal edema or symptoms of hematoma formation. Carefully document the size and location of affected area for comparison during resolution. Occasionally, hematomas must be surgically drained. Observe carefully for signs of distended bladder that may occur if edema is extensive and the patient is unable to void.

Breasts

Flat or Inverted Nipples in the Breastfeeding Mother

Flat nipples that cannot be made to protrude when gently squeezed just behind the nipple can cause difficulty with the infant latching onto the breast. A truly inverted nipple will invert further when this pinch test is attempted.

Intervention

Breast shells should be worn by the mother to place pressure on the areola and encourage the nipple to protrude (Fig. 15.5). Shells are recommended during the last trimester of pregnancy but can be used postpartum if the nipple problem is not identified until after delivery. A manual or electric breast pump can also be used immediately before nursing to attempt to make the nipples easier for the infant to grasp.

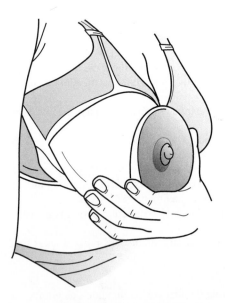

FIGURE 15.5 Breast shells may improve the nipple shape. (Adapted from Huggins, K. [1990]. *The nursing mother's companion* [Rev. ed., p. 30]. Boston: Harvard Common Press.)

Role of the Nurse in Postpartum Care

Promoting Bonding

■ **What can the nurse do to promote infant attachment?**[3,4]

The bond between parents and their infant begins during pregnancy and continues to develop during infancy. Attachments to other family members also develop with the birth. All infants need this nurturing bond with others to thrive.

As parents get to know their newborn, certain behaviors typically emerge. A parent often first touches the newborn with fingertips only and slowly progresses to use of the entire hand to caress the infant. The mother or father will hold the baby so that the infant's face is directly in front of the parent's face, the **en face** position, at a distance of about 10 to 12 inches, the distance at which the newborn can most clearly see. The parent will also typically talk to the newborn in a higher pitch than normal conversation, a pitch that elicits a response from the newborn.

The nurse can promote this attachment to the infant in simple ways. Parents and family need access to their infant. Well newborns should remain in the mother's room. Many hospitals encourage this practice by assigning one nurse to both mother and infant and organizing care for both in the mother's room. If an infant must be cared for in the nursery, it is important that policy allows either parent to visit at any time and to call as needed.

Parents need opportunities to get to know their infant and to learn to feel confident in caring for the infant's needs. The nurse can arrange these opportunities and give positive reinforcement. For example, the father gains confidence and learns much more about his new infant if he is assisted in changing the baby's diaper than if the expert nurse does the job.

It is important for the nurse to observe the interactions between parents and infant during the postpartum stay and to notify pediatric and obstetric care providers of observed difficulties with attachment.

Breastfeeding

■ **How can the nurse assist the mother in initiating breastfeeding in the immediate postpartum period?**[11,12]

Very few conditions exist that would contraindicate a mother's choice to breastfeed. Contraindications noted by AAP and ACOG in the Guidelines for Perinatal Care are as follows:

- Active tuberculosis in the mother before she has received adequate therapy
- Primary maternal infection with cytomegalovirus during the acute phase of the disease
- HBsAg-positive status (until the hepatitis B immune globulin and vaccine are given to the infant)

- HIV-positive status
- Active herpes infections in the breast area

The decision to breastfeed is often made early in the prenatal period. A discussion of the value of breastfeeding with the physician or midwife and an examination of the breasts to identify inverted nipples or other breast problems that might interfere with breastfeeding is an important part of prenatal education.

Initiation of breastfeeding during the first hour of the infant's life and frequent early nursing is associated with fewer problems with lactation.

A mother should be taught that the use of any medications while breastfeeding should be discussed with her physician, midwife, or primary care practitioner.

Artificial nipples (e.g., bottles, pacifiers) should be avoided during the early postpartum period to prevent the problem of nipple confusion. **Nipple confusion** is a term describing the difficulty some infants display in learning to breastfeed after having been fed by bottle.

Routine supplementation with formula or water in the early postpartum period is unnecessary and can interfere with successful lactation.

Breastfeeding is a learned activity for both the mother and infant. This process takes time and assistance from knowledgeable care providers.

Assessments/Interventions for Breastfeeding

As soon as possible after birth and, if possible, during the first postpartum hour, determine the readiness of the mother and infant to breastfeed. During this first hour, the infant is typically in the quiet/alert state and is receptive to breastfeeding.

Assist the mother to a comfortable position. Sitting in an almost upright position is often a position that is good for early nursings. The mother can see her infant, and the nurse can easily observe the nursing couple. Use pillows to position the mother and infant comfortably. The infant should be positioned so that the infant's body faces the mother's body and the infant's head is in a straight line with his or her own body (Fig. 15.6). The cradle hold, the cross cradle hold, and the football hold are all good positions for early nursings.

Assist the mother to position the infant's body to face the mother's body.

Show the mother how to grasp the breast with four fingers below and the thumb above.

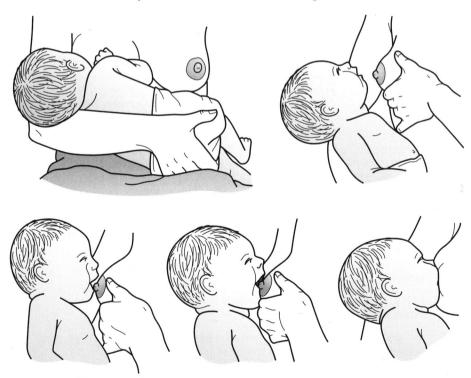

Instruct the mother to touch the nipple to the infant's lower lip.

When the infant's mouth opens wide, instruct the mother to pull the baby in to latch on.

FIGURE 15.6 Positioning for breastfeeding. (Adapted from Huggins, K. [1990]. *The nursing mother's companion* [Rev. ed., p. 43]. Boston: Harvard Common Press.)

Have the mother gently stroke the infant's lower lip until the infant opens the mouth wide. While the infant's mouth is wide open, instruct the mother to quickly move the infant toward the breast. The mother can cup her breast with her hand to guide the breast, grasping the breast with four fingers below and the thumb above the breast (see Fig. 15.6). Fingers need to be kept well back from the areola (i.e., the pigmented area of the breast that surround the nipple).

The infant should draw 0.5 to 1 inch of the areola into the mouth. At this first feeding, allow the infant to nurse on one breast for as long as the baby continues to actively nurse, then assist the mother to position the infant at the opposite breast. The infant may or may not vigorously nurse both breasts at this first feeding. Remind the mother to begin nursing with this second breast at the next feeding. Allow the infant to learn to nurse during this early feeding. Duration of the feeding is not as important as is the stimulation of the breasts and the learning process.

Teach the mother to break the infant's suction by inserting the tip of her finger into the corner of the infant's mouth when feeding is completed.

Encourage the mother to nurse frequently during the hospital stay. Have her offer the breast every 2 to 3 hours and teach her the cues that the infant is waking and getting ready to feed. It is easier to learn to nurse a calm infant who is not crying with hunger.

Some infants do not readily nurse for several feedings. Explain to the mother that this is normal and that her baby is also tired from birth. Most infants will nurse vigorously by 12 to 24 hours after birth. Continued difficulties should be referred to a lactation consultant or care provider experienced in lactation assistance. It is important that infants are feeding well before discharge from the hospital and that mothers know how to get assistance if needed.

Cesarean Birth

After a cesarean delivery, the woman should be cared for in a postanesthesia recovery room or an appropriately equipped LDRP room. Standards for care of this patient are no different from standards for any patient recovering from major surgery and anesthesia.

Routine separation of mother and infant is not necessary unless warranted by the condition of either the mother or the baby.

Assessments and interventions for the postpartum mother also apply after a cesarean delivery.

■ **What special assessments or interventions are needed for the woman who has undergone cesarean birth?**[3,4]

Assessment of Recovery From Regional Anesthesia
Procedure for Assessment

As a component of the assessment of recovery from anesthesia, it is important for the nurse to know the type of anesthesia used and the specific medication. Length of action of the different anesthetics will affect the recovery period.

For women who have received spinal or epidural anesthesia, the spinal level needs to be evaluated. A dermatome chart is helpful in this evaluation (Fig. 15.7). The chart is used to identify areas of the skin that correspond to the area of innervation in the spine. Assessment of the spinal level of the anesthesia may be performed by using an alcohol pad to touch the abdomen until sensation is identified by the woman. The level at which sensation is felt corresponds to the spinal level. As anesthesia wears off, the spinal level decreases. Ability to move the legs and sensation in the legs also indicates that the level of anesthesia is diminishing.

Interventions

While under the effect of a regional anesthetic, the newly delivered woman will not have the sensation of a full bladder, so the nurse must carefully evaluate the bladder for distention. Careful attention to positioning of the lower extremities to prevent injury is also important. Ambulation should not be attempted until full control of the legs returns. Even after motor control has returned, sensation in the lower body can be lessened. The temperature of the bath water must be monitored to prevent burns.

Assessment of Recovery From General Anesthesia
Procedure for Assessment

Recovery from general anesthesia occurs in a specially equipped recovery area so that the vital signs and respiratory status of the woman can be monitored closely. Nurses working in postanesthesia recovery rooms receive specialized training in monitoring of these patients. In labor and delivery units, nurses receive this training or are assisted by anesthesia personnel.

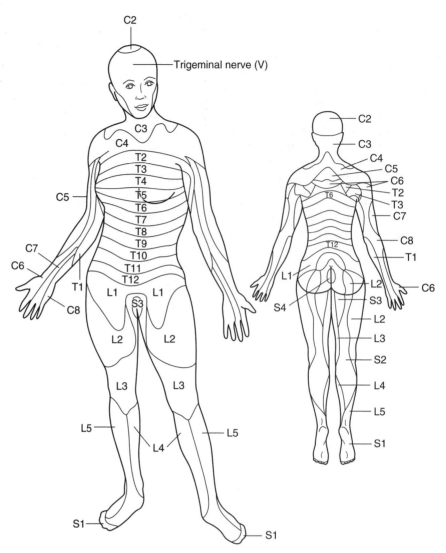

FIGURE 15.7 Segmental dermatome distribution of spinal nerves. C, cervical segments; L, lumbar segments; S, sacral segments; T, thoracic segments. (Adapted with permission from Thibodeau, G. [1987]. *Anatomy and physiology* [p. 71]. St. Louis: Mosby.)

Care of the Incision
Procedure for Assessment
Assess the status of the incision by evaluating the abdominal dressing.
Normal Findings
The dressing should be dry and intact, with no signs of bleeding or drainage. Note this finding in the chart.
Interventions
If any drainage is noted, chart the size and description of the drainage. (For example, "A 5-cm area of dark red drainage is noted on the left lower margin of the abdominal dressing.") Continue to inspect the dressing and notify the primary care provider of increased drainage.

Management of Pain
Assessments
As anesthesia wears off during the early postpartum period, the patient might report pain or request pain medication. It is important for the nurse to know which medications the patient received during surgery and which medications the physician has ordered for the postpartum period. Some patients might have received spinal or epidural narcotics that will decrease pain during the postpartum period. Remember to adequately assess the report of pain, including perception of severity and location.

Normal Findings

Pain and/or discomfort are normal findings immediately after surgery, but a goal of care is to reduce the severity of the pain.

Interventions

Medicate the postpartum cesarean-delivered mother as needed to achieve comfort. An adequately medicated person will have fewer complications related to immobility than a person in pain and will also recover more quickly from surgery. Comfort measures, such as positioning and massage techniques, should not be forgotten as means of decreasing discomfort.

Evaluation of Fluid Status

Assessments

The cesarean-delivered mother will have an IV line and a Foley catheter. The rate of the IV infusion and the fluid infused will be ordered by the physician and should be monitored. During the early postpartum period, oxytocin is often added to the infusion.

The catheter drainage bag should be emptied on admission to the recovery area and again after 1 hour to determine the initial hourly output. Until the catheter is removed, the output should be monitored at least every shift, or more frequently as ordered by the physician.

Normal Findings

The IV site should be free of signs of inflammation or edema, and the fluids should infuse freely. The urine should be amber or straw-colored and measure at least 30 mL per hour.

Interventions

Maintain the IV infusion as ordered by the physician. Unless excessive blood loss has occurred, the rate of the infusion is typically 125 or 150 mL per hour. Notify the primary care provider if urine output is less than 30 mL per hour or if it is blood-tinged after the first hour postpartum.

Sterilization

■ **What is the role of the nurse in postpartum sterilization?**[13]

The decision for postpartum sterilization is most appropriately made during the antepartum period and includes the process of informed consent. Informed consent is obtained by the physician and includes information that the patient can understand about the risks and benefits of a procedure and any alternatives to the procedure. The woman is allowed the opportunity to ask questions and then make her decision. A permit for the procedure is the documentation of this process of education, decision, and consent.

Tubal ligation (the interruption of the course of the fallopian tube) may be performed in the immediate postpartum period if a regional anesthetic has been used for the delivery and if the condition of the mother and infant is satisfactory. If an anesthetic must be initiated for the surgery, the anesthesia care provider will consider the risks and benefits of the timing of this procedure. Some providers postpone tubal ligation for several hours and request that the patient be given nothing by mouth during this period.

Assessments

Preoperative assessments include a review of the permit and evaluation of the woman's status in the immediate postpartum period. Vital signs, fundal height, and lochia flow are evaluated. Allow the woman the opportunity to ask questions about the procedure.

Postoperative Assessments

Refer to the assessments of a woman recovering from cesarean delivery. The incision is smaller, and pain is typically less severe. Often, women report pain localized to the right side of the abdomen after tubal surgery. A catheter in the bladder is not used for tubal sterilization.

Interventions

The anesthesia care provider or obstetrician might order preoperative medications. It is important to notify the care provider of any variations from the normal postpartum assessments of the mother or any problems of the newborn before tubal ligation is performed. Postoperative interventions are also similar to care after a cesarean delivery. Pain can usually be managed with oral medications.

Obstetric, Medical, or Surgical Complications

> ■ **What are the components of the recovery care for a woman with puerperal infection or with preeclampsia?[2-4]**

Women with obstetric, medical, or surgical complications need careful monitoring in the early postpartum period. *Puerperal infection* is a term used to describe any bacterial infection of the genital tract in the postpartum period. The pediatric care practitioner needs to be notified of infections in the mother, although mothers and infants are not routinely separated. The cure for preeclampsia is delivery. Usually, a woman rapidly improves after the birth; however, the risk for eclampsia (seizure activity in a preeclamptic woman) continues, especially in the first 24 hours.

Assessment of the Woman With a Genital Tract Infection

Infection during the birth process is most commonly chorioamnionitis, an infection of the fetal membranes that begins to resolve after delivery. Postpartum infections can include endometritis (an infection of the uterus) or a urinary tract infection. Prolonged rupture of the membranes, multiple vaginal examinations, and catheterization of the bladder are all risk factors for infection.

The vital signs of the newly delivered mother must be evaluated. An oral temperature of greater than 100.4°F is considered fever and should be reported to the physician or midwife. A single elevation of temperature may be related to dehydration but needs to be followed closely with additional temperature readings. Other signs of infection can include a tender uterus or the typical signs of cystitis, burning or pain with urination or suprapubic pain.

Interventions

The physician or midwife will consider the cause of the fever and, if infection is suspected, may order antibiotics. Fluids may also be ordered, either intravenously or by mouth. In addition, medication may be ordered to reduce fever. Monitoring of the course of the infection by evaluation of the temperature is important to determine the effectiveness of treatment.

Assessment of the Woman With Preeclampsia

Women with preeclampsia need careful assessment and monitoring of vital signs, especially blood pressure, and evaluation of reflexes in the early postpartum period. Reports of headache and visual changes by the mother are also important to consider in the overall assessment of recovery. Urinary output needs careful assessment. Less than 30 mL per hour is an abnormal finding.

Interventions

Blood pressure evaluation is important for these women. The physician or midwife will define parameters of blood pressure readings that are acceptable for this patient and those that require notification of the provider.

> Refer to the chapter on hypertensive disorders of pregnancy for a more complete description of preeclampsia and the necessary assessments and interventions.

Perinatal Loss and Newborn Illness

> ■ **How can the nurse assist parents who experience a perinatal loss or parents of an ill newborn?[13,14]**

The delivery of a stillborn infant or the birth of a newborn who requires the special care nursery is an event that produces enormous stresses for the new mother and her family. The perinatal nurse is often the person in the hospital setting who has contact with a family that has experienced a perinatal loss or the delivery of a sick newborn. In this role, the nurse must function as a patient care provider, a support person during the grief process, a patient advocate, and a facilitator and coordinator of care. See Appendix C for key elements about effective pain management for the dying newborn.

> ■ **What can help the parents who experience a stillbirth or the death of a newborn?[14,15]**

Many hospitals have developed programs to help care providers deal with the issues of perinatal loss and have instituted procedures to assist parents with the grief process through coordination of services and ongoing sensitive care.

Immediately after the delivery of a stillborn infant, both parents are in the shock phase of grief. The mother is concerned with her own personal health and safety, as after any delivery. Questions relating to the reason for the death will arise and are often difficult or impossible to answer. The nurse's role during this initial phase is both to provide physical care for the mother and to assist with the process of grief.

To begin to grieve for the infant lost, it is necessary for the parents to create memories of the child. Parents should be offered time to hold and touch the infant. The nurse can wrap the infant in a blanket and remain with the family, if needed or requested, to answer questions. It is common for parents to remark on the gender of the child, the perfection of hands or feet, and family resemblance—in effect, to claim the child as their own. Photographs can be taken, identification bracelets made, footprints and certificates prepared, and all of these offered to the family. Sometimes parents will initially refuse such mementos but then ask for them weeks or months later. Naming the child is another activity that assists parents with this process of claiming the child who has died.

The nurse has ongoing responsibilities in coordinating care for this mother and her family. Decisions about location of the postpartum stay, notification of hospital staff that will be in contact with the mother, and notification of support services (e.g., social services, clergy) are tasks for the nurse. It is important for all care providers to be aware of the family's loss.

Finally, perinatal nurses must consider their own feelings related to the loss. Just as parents search for the answers to why the loss occurred, so do the care providers. It is also common for nurses to avoid the family because of the uncertainty of how to help or feelings that medical care has failed this family. The belief that every pregnancy should have the outcome of a healthy infant is a common belief, but not a realistic one. Nurses need to examine their role in good outcomes, while accepting the fact that poor outcomes cannot always be prevented. A hospital with a carefully considered plan for assisting families with perinatal loss will also consider these needs of the care providers.

■ How can the nurse help the parents of an ill newborn?[14,15]

Many of the suggestions for the care of parents who have experienced a perinatal loss are appropriate for parents of an ill newborn. These parents have lost their dream of a healthy infant. The nurse can expect the family to exhibit signs of the grief process.

As soon as possible, considering the condition of the mother and the infant, it is important for the parents to visit the newborn. Intensive care nurseries can be frightening for parents, and a nurse should be available to the parents to explain equipment, answer questions, and encourage interaction with the infant.

If the mother is discharged from the hospital before the infant, parents should be given the telephone number of the nursery and instructions to call or visit frequently. Some newborn intensive care units have programs to contact parents at frequent intervals to provide information on the infant's condition.

Care of the Mother During Postpartum Hospitalization

■ What are the mother's ongoing needs during postpartum hospitalization?[3,4]

The period of postpartum hospitalization can be as brief as a few hours but is commonly at least a 24-hour stay. Women remain in the hospital during that time when intensive postpartum care is required and return to their home environment to recover completely. During the hospital stay, the newly delivered mother is often expected both to recover physically and also to demonstrate the capability to care for herself and her newborn. Rubin's identified periods of the postpartum, *taking in* and *taking on,* identify maternal readiness for self-care and infant care. During *taking in,* the mother is more passive and focuses primarily on her physical needs. In the *taking on* period, the mother begins to assume the care of herself and her infant. The mother is commonly discharged during the taking in period or the early taking on period and is not ready for assuming total care of herself or her infant. The family will need to understand the new mother's need for help with her care and the infant's care during this early phase of the postpartum period.

The educational needs of the new family have always been a concern and the responsibility of the postpartum and nursery nurse. As postpartum stays have become brief, opportunities for education have also decreased. New research supports the need for thorough prenatal education in postpartum and newborn care. In the early postpartum period, the newly delivered mother is only able to assimilate information that is reinforcement or review of that previously learned. Topics of education that are important for reinforcement of previous teaching include physical care of the mother, physical care of the infant, warning signs of problems of both infant and mother, infant nutrition, family adjustments, birth control, and needs for continued care. A simple technique that is effective for education of the new family is for the nurse to explain the care given as it is being provided. The woman has an immediate opportunity to ask questions.

The physical needs of mother and baby during the hospital stay include the needs of the mother for rest and nourishment. The nurse will be evaluating the continued recovery from delivery and monitoring the return to the prepregnant state. Variations from normal assessments should be discussed with the physician or midwife before discharge. Infant needs are similar and include the need for the establishment of nourishment. Whether the infant is breastfed or bottle-fed, patterns of feeding need to be observed by the nurse and assistance provided to the parents.

> ■ **How can the postpartum nurse begin to prepare the mother for the transition to care at home?**[3,4]

A well-organized and coordinated system of maternity care is needed to ensure that mothers and infants receive the follow-up care necessary to meet the needs of the early postpartum period. Health care systems are responding to these needs for follow-up care in a variety of ways. Home visits by specially trained home health nurses, sometimes called perinatal community nurses, are available for some women. Follow-up phone interviews to identify problems is another method used by care systems.

Every mother, before discharge, needs to know how she can obtain further care for herself and her newborn. Schedules for needed follow-up visits for mother and infant are important. Written lists of emergency phone numbers are also helpful. This information needs to be discussed with the new family and should also be provided in writing.

PRACTICE/REVIEW QUESTIONS

After reviewing Part 2, answer the following questions.

1. It is not unusual to be unable to palpate the uterus immediately after delivery. During this time, the uterus is often boggy and difficult to locate.

   A. True

   B. False

2. A distended bladder is suspected if the fundal height is above the umbilicus and deviated to the right of the midline.

   A. True

   B. False

3. During the first postpartum hour, the vital signs should be evaluated at least every 15 minutes.

   A. True

   B. False

4. Excessive edema of the perineum should be reported to the physician or midwife.

   A. True

   B. False

5. It is not uncommon for the newly delivered woman to have brisk vaginal bleeding during the first postpartum hour.

   A. True

   B. False

6. A newly delivered mother must be separated from her ill infant. The nurse can facilitate attachment by:

   A. Arranging a visit to the nursery as soon as the mother is physically able

   B. Reassuring the woman that her infant is being well cared for by the nursery nurses

   C. Explaining to the woman that bonding with the infant can wait until the infant is well

7. A woman is concerned that her infant did not vigorously nurse at the first feeding and may be hungry. You tell the woman:

   A. She might have to supplement breastfeeding with formula until the infant begins to nurse more effectively

   B. Newborns are learning to nurse at the first feeding and will learn with time; colostrum will meet the newborn's nutritional needs

   C. You will let the pediatrician know about the problem

8. A mother who is breastfeeding should be taught to check with her physician, midwife, or primary care provider before taking any medications.

   A. True

   B. False

9. Breast shells should be worn if the woman who is breastfeeding has inverted nipples.

   A. True

   B. False

10. Fewer problems with breastfeeding occur if the infant nurses during the first hour of life.

    A. True

    B. False

11. Informed consent for sterilization includes:

    A. Information on the risks of the procedure

    B. Reasons to have the surgery done

    C. Alternatives to the surgery

    D. A decision by the woman to have the surgery done

    E. All of these

12. Immediately after a cesarean delivery, the newly delivered mother:

    A. Can return to her postpartum room

    B. Should be cared for in a recovery room or an appropriately equipped LDR/P room

13. A family experiencing a perinatal loss will:

    A. Experience the grief process

    B. Have no special needs during the postpartum

    C. Request early discharge

14. Parents of an ill newborn require assistance with the grief process.

    A. True

    B. False

15. Postpartum education for the new family should include:

A. Infant care

B. Care of the new mother

C. Infant feeding

D. Contraception

E. A, B, and C

F. All of these

PRACTICE/REVIEW ANSWER KEY

1. B (Immediately after delivery, the uterus should be firm and easily palpable in the midline.)

2. A

3. A

4. A

5. B

6. A

7. B

8. A

9. A

10. A

11. E

12. B

13. A

14. A

15. F

REFERENCES

1. Auerbach, K. (2000, May/June). Evidence-based care and the breastfeeding couple: Key concerns. *Journal of Midwifery and Women's Health, 45*(3), 205–211.
2. Blackburn, S., & Loper, D. (1992). *Maternal, fetal, and neonatal physiology: A clinical perspective.* Philadelphia: WB Saunders.
3. Simpson, K. R., & Creehan, P. (2001). *Perinatal nursing* (2nd ed.). Philadelphia: Lippincott.
4. Mattson, S., & Smith, J. (Eds.). (1999, September). *AWHONN core curriculum for maternal-newborn nursing* (2nd ed.). Philadelphia: WB Saunders.
5. Niermeyer, S., Kattwinkel, J., Van Reempts, P., Nadkarni, V., Phillips, B., Zideman, D., Azzopardi, D., Berg, R., Boyle, D., Boyle, R., Burchfield, D., Carlo, W., Chameides, L., Denson, S., Fallat, M., Gerardi, M., Gunn, A., Hazinski, M. F., Keenan, W., Knaebel, S., Milner, A., Perlman, J., Saugstad, O. D., Schleien, C., Solimano, A., Speer, M., Toce, S., Wiswell, T., & Zaritsky, A. (2000, September). International Guidelines for Neonatal Resuscitation: An excerpt from the Guidelines 2000 for Cardiopulmonary Resuscitation and Emergency Cardiovascular Care—International Consensus on Science. *Pediatrics, 106*(3), E29.

6. ACOG Committee Opinion No. 174138. (1996, July). *Use and abuse of the Apgar score.* Washington, DC: American College of Obstetricians and Gynecologists.

7. Apgar, V. (1953, July/August). A proposal for a new method of evaluation of the newborn infant. *Current Researches in Anesthesia and Analgesia, 32*(4), 260–267.

8. American Academy of Pediatrics. (1996, July). Policy statement. *Journal of Pediatrics, 98*(1), 141–142.

9. ACOG Committee Opinion No. 138. (1994, April). *Utility of umbilical cord blood acid-base assessment.* Washington, DC: American College of Obstetricians and Gynecologists.

10. ACOG Technical Bulletin No. 216. (1995, November). *Umbilical artery blood acid-base analysis.* Washington, DC: American College of Obstetricians and Gynecologists.

11. Lawrence, R. A. (1998). *Breastfeeding—A guide for the medical profession* (5th ed.). St. Louis: Mosby.

12. American Academy of Pediatrics, American College of Obstetricians and Gynecologists. (1997). *Guidelines for perinatal care.* (4th ed., pp. 279–293). Elk Grove, IL; and Washington, DC: Authors.

13. ACOG Committee Opinion No. 105. (1992, March). *Postpartum tubal sterilization.* Washington, DC: American College of Obstetricians and Gynecologists.

14. Rybarik, F., & Bond, C. (2000, April). Conversations with a colleague: Documenting a neonate's death. *AWHONN Lifelines, 4*(2), 27–28.

15. Wolf-Gabor, S. (2000, April). Reflections of women's health: Individuality of grief. *AWHONN Lifelines, 4*(2), 72–73.

SUGGESTED READINGS

ACOG Technical Bulletin No. 225. (1996, July). *Obstetric analgesia and anesthesia.* Washington, DC: American College of Obstetricians and Gynecologists.

ACOG Technical Bulletin No. 243. (1998, January). *Postpartum hemorrhage.* Washington, DC: American College of Obstetricians and Gynecologists.

AWHONN Position Statement. (1999, June). *Issue: Breastfeeding.* Washington, DC: The Association of Women's Health, Obstetric and Neonatal Nurses.

AWHONN Position Statement. (1999, June). Issue: *The role of the nurse in the promotion of breastfeeding.* Washington, DC: The Association of Women's Health, Obstetric and Neonatal Nurses.

Donnelly, A., Snowden, H. M., Renfrew, M. J., & Woolridge, M. W. (2000). Commercial hospital discharge packs for breastfeeding women. *Cochrane Database System Review,* (2), CD002075.

Cunningham, F. G., MacDonald, P. C., Gant, N. F. Leveno, K., Gilstrap, L. C., III, Hankins, G. V. D., & Clark, S. L. (Eds.) (1997). *Williams obstetrics* (20th ed.). Norwalk, CT: Appleton & Lange.

Ferguson, S., & Englehard, C. L. (2000, February). Short stay: The art of legislating quality and economy. *AWHONN Lifelines, 4*(1), 27–28.

Malkin, J. D., Garber, S., Broder, M. S., & Keeler, E. (2000, August). Infant mortality and early postpartum discharge. *Obstetrics and Gynecology, 96*(2), 183–188.

Martell, L. K. (2000, January/February). The hospital experience and the postpartum experience: A historical analysis. *Journal of Obstetric, Gynecologic, and Neonatal Nursing, 29*(1), 65–72.

Mohrbacher, N., & Stock, B. A. (1997). *La Leche League International: The breastfeeding answer book* (Rev. ed.). Schaumburg, IL: La Leche League International.

Murray, M. (1997). *Antepartal and Intrapartal fetal monitoring* (2nd ed.). Albuquerque: Learning Resources International, Inc.

Renfrew, M. J., Lang, S., Martin, L., & Woolridge, M. W. (2000). Feeding schedules in hospitals for newborn infants. *Cochrane Database System Review,* (2), CD000090.

Ruchala, P. (2000, May/June). Teaching new mothers: Priorities of nurses and postpartum women. *Journal of Obstetric, Gynecologic, and Neonatal Nursing, 29*(3), 265–273.

Thorp, J. A., & Rushing, R. S. (1999, December). Umbilical cord blood gas analysis. *Obstetrics & Gynecologic Clinics of North America, 26*(4) 695–709.

Urbanski, P. (2000, June). Getting the *go ahead:* Helping patients understand informed consent. *AWHONN Lifelines, 4*(3), 45–49.

A RESOURCE OF NOTE

Kattwinkel, J., Cook, L.J., Hurt, H., Nowacek, G. A., Short, S. G., & Crosby, W. M. (2001). *Perinatal Continuing Education Program: Book I: Maternal fetal evaluation and immediate newborn care; Book II: Maternal and fetal care; Book III: Neonatal care; Book IV: Specialized newborn care.* (Contact Lynn J. Cook, RNC, MPH, Perinatal Continuing Education Program [PCEP], Department of Pediatrics, University of Virginia Health System, Charlottesville, VA 22908 or www.pcep.org.)

M O D U L E 16

Informed Consent and Documentation

MARCELLA T. HICKEY

*Informed Consent and
Documentation*

As you complete Part 1 of this module, you will learn:

1. Components of informed consent
2. Circumstances that require consent
3. When informed consent is not necessary
4. Who may give consent for the treatment of an adult
5. When nurses are responsible for obtaining the patient's consent
6. Protocol requirements for nurses when physicians delegate responsibility for obtaining informed consent

When you have completed Part 1 of this module, you should be able to recall the meaning of the following terms. You should also be able to use the terms when consulting with other health professionals. The terms are defined in this module or in the glossary at the end of this book.

capacity	information
collusion	informed consent
conservator	therapeutic privilege
emancipated	voluntariness
fraud	

Components of Informed Consent

One of the many legal issues affecting medical and nursing practice today is that of informed consent. Legally, professionals are required to obtain the patient's permission for procedures and treatments. It is crucial to understand the necessary content, applicability, and the professional nurse's role and responsibility in this area.

■ What are the components of informed consent?

There are three components of informed consent: capacity, information, and voluntariness. **Capacity** refers to the individual's age and competence. Eighteen is recognized as the legal age in most states. In some states, younger persons are considered **emancipated** if they (a) marry, (b) become a parent, (c) are economically independent, or (d) live in a separate setting from their parents. *Competence* refers to the individual's ability to make choices and understand the expected outcomes of a particular choice.[1]

Information refers to the content of the explanation given to the patient. Four standards are applied by the courts to this portion of a consent.[2]

1. The **professional standard** requires the practitioner to provide the information considered reasonable in the professional community. In other words, *information* is defined as what most professionals would tell most their patients in similar circumstances.
2. The **reasonable patient standard** requires that risk factors and expected outcomes be presented as they relate to the individual.
3. The **subjective patient standard** is one held in a small number of states. It requires a patient be provided information about potential risks as they relate to the patient's lifestyle.[3]
4. The **informed refusal** means the patient has received information about the risks of not consenting to treatments or diagnostic testing and yet refuses treatment or testing.[3]

The information should include the following:

- The nature of the individual's condition
- The purpose of the treatment
- Expected outcomes
- Major risks
- Reasonable alternatives
- Possible consequences of refusing treatment

Voluntariness refers to the circumstances surrounding the individual giving consent. If force, fraud, duress, or collusion is present, the consent is invalid. Remember that an individual can withdraw consent for a particular procedure. Withdrawal can be given verbally, in writing, or by gesture (e.g., shaking head "no," withdrawing arm from nurse's hand). The procedure should be discontinued as soon as safely possible.[2] Extenuating circumstances in a life-threatening situation can negate the patient's refusal of treatment.

> A lawsuit can be filed if it can be proved that the patient did not consent to a procedure or was poorly informed about it by the professional.

> REMEMBER: A positive outcome of a procedure does not protect you, the professional, from a lawsuit.

> IMPORTANT CONCERNS: Barriers of language, hearing impairment, and visual impairment must be addressed through interpreters and the use of available technology and services to assist the hearing and visually impaired.[4]

■ Under what circumstances should consent be obtained?

Many professionals believe that consent must be obtained only for major interventions (e.g., surgery, chemotherapy). This is incorrect. A written format is not necessary for every contact, but the components of informed consent must be present. The patient can give consent verbally or by actions that imply consent (e.g., extending an arm for you to draw blood).

> Consent must be obtained whenever the patient is going to be touched by a care provider. Your failure to obtain consent constitutes battery.

■ When is it unnecessary to obtain the individual's informed consent for a procedure?

It is not absolutely necessary to obtain consent when delay will cause the patient's death or seriously jeopardize the patient's health. When obtaining complete information might cause the patient's physical or mental status to degenerate, the physician can use **therapeutic privilege** to obtain a consent. This must be used with caution, and the rationale for withholding information must be documented.[3]

■ Under what circumstances may another individual give consent for treatment of an adult?

When an adult is mentally ill, retarded, comatose, or senile, a legal guardian, conservator, patient's attorney, or court may provide consent; these are the only sources for such consent. Family members do not automatically have the right to give consent. The court can overrule a competent adult's decision about a treatment. This is done when the state's interest of preservation of life is counter to the patient's wishes.[2]

NOTE: The preservation of life concept is the basis for many court decisions involving the fetus and/or newborn after the age of viability has been achieved.

EXAMPLE: A patient who refuses a cesarean section when the fetus is at term and a placenta previa is evident.

■ Who should obtain consent for treatment or a procedure?

- Nurses are responsible for obtaining consent for nursing procedures.
- Nurses in an expanded practice role are responsible for obtaining consents for procedures they order or perform.
- Physicians are responsible for obtaining consent for medical procedures or treatment.

In some settings, the physician might delegate the task of obtaining consent for specific procedures to nursing personnel. **THE PROTOCOLS FOR OBTAINING CONSENT IN THESE CASES MUST BE SPECIFICALLY WRITTEN FOR THE PROCEDURE, AND APPROVED, AND SIGNED BY MEDICAL AND NURSING ADMINISTRATION.** If the patient questions the information provided or refuses to sign the consent, you must not only refrain from trying to persuade the patient but are obligated to inform the attending physician of the patient's inquiries and/or refusal to sign. *Only* the physician is the person legally qualified and responsible for providing additional information or answering the patient's questions about the treatment.[1,2]

> COMPREHENSIVE PROTOCOLS THAT ADDRESS NURSING RESPINSIBILITY IN PROCEDURES SUCH AS PITOCIN INDUCTION/AUGMENTATION, TOCOLYSIS, AND ANTIHYPERTENSIVE THERAPY FOR THE PREECLEMPTIC PATIENT SHOULD BE DEVELOPED AT EACH INSTITUTION. THESE PROTOCOLS NEED TO INCLUDE CRITERIA FOR PATIENT SELECTION, RESPONSIBILITY FOR OBTAINING CONSENT, INFORMATION TO BE COVERED IN THE INFORMED CONSENT, DRUG PREPARATION AND ADMINISTRATION GUIDELINES, PATIENT MONITORING GUIDELINES, POTENTIAL SIDE EFFECTS, AND THERAPEUTIC GOALS.

PRACTICE/REVIEW QUESTIONS

After reviewing Part 1, answer the following questions.

1. List the three components of the informed consent.

   a. _____

   b. _____

   c. _____

2. List four circumstances that are considered in determining emancipation of a minor.

   a. _____

   b. _____

   c. _____

   d. _____

3. What four standards are applied to information provided to the patient? Describe the meaning of each standard.

   a. _____
   _____

   b. _____
   _____

   c. _____
   _____

   d. _____
   _____

4. List the type of information that should be included when obtaining informed consent.

   a. _____

   b. _____

   c. _____

   d. _____

   e. _____

   f. _____

5. When must the patient's consent be obtained?

   _____
   _____
   _____

6. What circumstance overrules the need for an informed consent?

   _____
   _____

7. Who may give consent for treatment when an adult is mentally ill?

   _____

8. Under what circumstances are nurses clearly responsible for obtaining a patient's consent?

   a. _____

   b. _____

9. Who is responsible for obtaining consents for medical procedures or treatments?

   _____

10. Under what circumstances may nurses obtain consent for medical procedures or treatment?

_____

_____

_____

11. List essential elements to be included when developing nursing protocols for a given procedure.

a. _____

b. _____

c. _____

d. _____

e. _____

f. _____

g. _____

PRACTICE/REVIEW ANSWER KEY

1. a. Capacity
   b. Information
   c. Voluntariness

2. a. Marriage
   b. Parenthood
   c. Economic independence
   d. Living in another setting

3. a. Professional standard—The practitioner provides the information considered reasonable in the professional community.
   b. Reasonable patient standard—The practitioner explains risk factors, expected outcomes, and alternatives as they relate to a reasonable person.
   c. Subjective patient standard—The practitioner provides information about risks as they relate to the patient's lifestyle.
   d. Informed refusal—The patient has received information about the risk of not consenting to treatment or diagnostic testing and yet refuses treatment or testing.

4. a. The nature of the individual's consideration
   b. The purpose of the treatment
   c. Expected outcomes
   d. Major risks
   e. Reasonable alternatives
   f. Possible outcomes of refusing treatment

5. Consent must be obtained whenever the patient is going to be touched by the care provider. This does not always mean written consent, but the components of informed consent must be present.

6. When delay will cause death or serious jeopardy to the patient's health.

7. Only a legal guardian, conservator, the patient's attorney, or a court

8. a. Before instituting a nursing procedure
   b. Before nurses in an expanded practice role order or perform procedures

9. The physician

10. Nurses can obtain consent for medical treatments or procedures only when a specific protocol delegates the authority to nursing personnel. The protocol must be written for a particular treatment or procedure, and it must be approved and signed by medical and nursing administrators.

11. a. Criteria for patient selection
    b. Who is responsible for obtaining the informed consent
    c. Information to be covered in obtaining the informed consent
    d. Drug preparation and administration guidelines
    e. Patient monitoring guidelines
    f. Potential side effects
    g. Therapeutic goals

Documentation

As you complete Part 2 of this module, you will learn:

1. The functions of the chart
2. The relationship that exists between national standards of nursing practice and documentation of care
3. Information that must be documented in the chart by nurses during care of the woman in the intrapartum period
4. The general guidelines for documentation in a chart
5. Guidelines for countersigning notes
6. Guidelines for documenting verbal orders
7. Guidelines for telephone triage
8. Why malpractice suits are a nursing concern

When you have completed Part 2 of this module, you should be able to recall the meaning of the following terms. You should also be able to use the terms when consulting with other health professionals. The terms are defined in this module or in the glossary at the end of this book.

addendum

documentation

malpractice

standard of practice

Guidelines for Documentation of Care

The following demonstrates how a professional nurse documents the provision of nursing care that meets the current national standards for nursing practice. One of the responsibilities of a professional group is to develop the standards that define and measure the practice of its members. In the area of intrapartum care, the Association of Women's Health, Obstetric and Neonatal Nurses (AWHONN) has developed the standards for nursing practice.[5] One of the standards requires the documentation of the care provided for each patient. **Documentation** refers to accurate recording on the appropriate chart forms, observations, assessments, nursing actions, and outcomes. These documents serve as a legal record of the professional nursing care provided for each patient.[1,6]

■ What are the functions of the chart?[1,2]

The chart may be a written or computerized record and serves the following purposes:

- Provides an ongoing written record of the patient's status, the care provided, and the outcomes of the interventions
- Documents that appropriate standards of care were implemented by a qualified professional
- Provides a permanent legal record of the patient's course while in the health care system
- Serves as a means of communication from one care provider to another
- Can be used for reimbursement purposes
- Can be a source for research data or problems

> **According to existing law and court decisions, appropriate care was not provided if it was not recorded in the chart.**

Components of the Nursing Portion of the Chart

■ In the intrapartum setting, what should be documented in the nursing portion of the chart?

From the time of admission until discharge from the unit, chart documentation should cite information on the woman and fetus, which includes the following:

- The nurse's assessment
- Interventions
- Outcomes of care

Specifically, you must take a history, do a review of systems, and perform a physical examination that meets the standards of practice as outlined by AWHONN and that incorporates hospital policies and procedures for the unit.

1. **Presenting complaint in the patient's words**
2. **History**
   Family history: genetic and congenital abnormalities, mental retardation, metabolic problems, multiple births
   Past medical history: allergies, diabetes, hypertension, herpes, HIV, exposure to tuberculosis, recent exposure to chickenpox
   Previous obstetric history:
   > Gravida _____
   > Term _____
   > Premature _____
   > Abortion _____
   >> (Spontaneous) _____
   >> (Termination) _____
   > Living _____
   Type of delivery, newborn weight, problems, gynecologic surgery or infections (group B streptococcus, herpes simplex)

Social history: smoking, alcohol intake, support person for labor, labor preparation classes

Course of this pregnancy: last menstrual period; expected date of confinement; weight gain; infections; gestational diabetes; hypertension; vaginal bleeding; results of ultrasound examinations, nonstress test, contraction stress test, amniocentesis, and laboratory studies; blood type; Rh status; antibody status; serology titer; rubella titer; hemoglobin/hematocrit; triple screen; HIV testing; and culture results for chlamydia, gonorrhea, and group B streptococcus

Current history: onset of uterine contractions, frequency, duration, quality; vaginal discharge; bleeding consistency and amount; status of membranes, intact, rupture time, color of fluid; fetal activity; oral intake of liquid, solids, time; current medications (including over-the-counter preparations, herbs, and illicit drugs) with dosage and time last taken; any concurrent symptoms of visual disturbance, headache, or dysuria; timing of last bowel movement and voiding

Care provider: name, title, date and time of notification and by whom

Infant care plans: feeding, breast/bottle; nursery care, rooming in; care provider; adoption plans

3. **Review of systems:** notation of any loss of function; presence of prosthesis, dentures, glasses, contact lenses
4. **Physical examination**

- Height
- Weight
- Blood pressure
- Pulse, respirations
- Temperature
- Uterine contraction, frequency, intensity, duration, and relaxation
- Deep tendon reflexes
- Urine dipstick results

In some settings, head, eyes, ears, nose, throat, breast, heart and lungs, abdomen (general), and extremities may be examined by other care providers according to unit policies. However, the nurse must be aware of the findings and their impact on the nursing assessment and care plan.

Fetal assessment includes fundal height, estimated weight, heart rate (includes baseline, accelerations, and periodic changes), position, and presentation.

Pelvic examination includes effacement, dilatation, station, presentation, condition of membranes, and if present, amniotic fluid amount, color, odor; results of Nitrazine or fern tests; and the collection of cultures when appropriate.

Your continuous evaluation of the patient must include evaluation of both maternal and fetal well-being. The record should reflect why nursing procedures and interventions were instituted and what the maternal and fetal responses were to them. When the care provider is notified of a deviation from normal, his or her response is to be noted in the record.[1,6]

When a standard of care is not met, or a medication or procedure is withheld, the reason for this action must be recorded.

You must develop the skills needed for clear documentation when you are in a stable situation. Then when an emergency situation occurs, you will be able to record the situation accurately.

General Guidelines for Chart Documentation[1]

- Record only factual information.
- Make entries legible.
- Use only standard abbreviations.
- Include the date, time, and your (the recorder's) name and title.
- To correct an error, draw a line through the incorrect information, write "error" above it, write the date and time, and initial the entry. *The accurate information is entered as an* **addendum.**

- Enter an addendum at the next available space on the chart form. Use the current date and time for the new entry. The content can be referenced to the previous material.
- *When there is a delay in entering chart information, write the phrase "late entry" at the beginning of the note. Enter the note at the next available space on the chart form. Use the current date and time for the entry.* Explain the delay in recording the information and cross-reference it to the area of the record where it should have appeared in chronologic order.
- Never make entries for another person in the labor and delivery setting.
- An addendum made after the record is requested for legal action is suspect.
- *Legally, if it is not recorded, it was not observed, acted on, or evaluated by the care provider.*
- If necessary, the record you create today is the one you go into court with in the future.

Guidelines for Electronic Charting

Brent provides some guidelines for the use of electronic medical record and electronic medical charting[1]:

- Never share your access code or password for the system.
- Only access information as part of your job function.
- Do not ignore computer alerts about data entry or missing data.
- Use correct procedures for adding late entry information to a record.
- Take care to use your correct code and the patient's personal code.
- Attend in-services and use information provided about changes in the system.

Guidelines for Specific Communication Problems

Countersigning Notes

When policies of an institution require the professional nurse to countersign or sign off for other personnel, consider the following:

- Countersigning means that you reviewed the entry and consider it accurate.
- It also means that you approved the care provided by the other person.
- Make sure the note indicates who provided the care.[2]

Verbal Orders

Verbal orders are legitimate, and most institutions have policies governing time frames for the practitioner cosigning the order (e.g., verbal orders for medications must be cosigned within 24 hours). When taking a verbal order, restate the order, including the patient's name, and ask for confirmation. In charting the order, indicate "repeated and confirmed."[2]

Telephone Triage

Telephone calls from patients are becoming an everyday occurrence in today's health care world. These calls are a potential source of legal problems in two ways. First, an unqualified person might be providing health care information to the patient. Second, documentation of the interaction might be incomplete. Cady provides useful information about **establishing a telephone triage protocol.**[7] The protocol includes the following:

- What information should be obtained about the problem
- Who will handle the calls: nurse, practitioner, or physician
- What problems require an immediate visit
- Where the patient will be seen
- The documentation required for each telephone contact

> Cady identifies bleeding in pregnancy, ruling out labor, abdominal pain, headache, fetal activity concerns, persistent nausea and vomiting, vaginal discharge, and breast complaints as clinical problems appropriate for development of telephone protocols.[7]

Appropriate documentation for telephone triage will reflect the following:

- Date and time of contact
- The name of the caller (e.g., "patient Mary Smith" or "Joe Smith, husband of patient, Mary Smith")
- The care provider or practice name that manages the patient's care
- The reason for the call in the caller's words
- Pertinent information about the problem (e.g., signs/symptoms, onset, duration, frequency; actions that alleviate or increase them)
- Significant background information (e.g., prior history, chronic problems, allergies, current medications)
- Conclusions reached about the problem and its urgency
- Instructions given to the individual, including when to seek additional evaluation and care
- The person's response to instructions

It is critical to document the person's response to the instructions. A documented refusal to comply when there is an adverse outcome demonstrates the individual's contributory negligence to the situation. Also, a patient who requests a visit should be directed to the most expedient source of evaluation.

Malpractice

■ Why should nurses be more concerned about malpractice?

The current **standards of practice** publicized by national professional nursing organizations hold the nurse accountable for nursing practice. These are the standards that the legal profession and courts use in malpractice cases. Therefore, a nurse can be sued for negligence and **malpractice.**

■ What are malpractice and negligence?

Rostant and Cady provide the following definitions[8]:

> "Malpractice: Professional misconduct, improper discharge of professional duties, or a failure to meet the standard of care of a professional that results in harm to another."

> "Negligence: Failure to act as an ordinary prudent person; conduct contrary to that of a reasonable person under specific circumstances."

Areas of Nursing Management Cited in Legal Cases Involving Nurses[6,9–11]

- Incomplete documentation of initial evaluation of patient and fetus
- Medication errors
- Violations of the standards for nursing observations of the woman and fetus (e.g., ongoing documentation of vital signs, the progress of labor, response to procedures, and fetal well-being)
- Improper use of equipment
- Failure to notify the appropriate professional when maternal or fetal status falls outside normal parameters
- Failure to follow physician orders, hospital policies, and hospital procedures
- Failure to recognize and respond appropriately in situations of fetal distress
- Failure to intervene appropriately in the presence of negligence on the part of the providers

What to Do If You Are Called to Testify

In-depth information about depositions or testifying in a malpractice suit is beyond the scope of this book. However, some broad guidelines are as follows[12]:

- Notify your malpractice insurance carrier.
- Engage your own counsel.
- Know the patient's record inside and out.

- Review the institution's policy and procedure manual for the year in which the incident occurred.
- Have a current curriculum vitae documenting your continuing education.
- Do not discuss the suit with anyone other than your counsel.

PRACTICE/REVIEW QUESTIONS

After reviewing Part 2, answer the following questions.

1. State at least three important functions of the chart from a legal standpoint.

    a. _____

    b. _____

    c. _____

2. In general, what are the nurse's responsibilities for documentation in the chart?

    _____

    _____

3. When medications or procedures are withheld, what action should the nurse take?

    _____

    _____

4. How should an error in charting be corrected?

    _____

    _____

5. What three circumstances should be present when a professional nurse countersigns another person's notes?

    a. _____

    b. _____

    c. _____

6. State the precautions to be taken when accepting a verbal order.

    a. _____

    b. _____

    c. _____

7. In handling a telephone triage, what information is needed about the current problem?

    a. _____

    b. _____

8. List items to review in preparation for giving a deposition or testimony.

    a. _____

    b. _____

9. What criteria will be used to judge a nurse's practice?

    _____

    _____

10. List four of the areas of nursing management that are most often cited in legal actions.

a. _____

b. _____

c. _____

d. _____

PRACTICE/REVIEW ANSWER KEY

1. Any three of the following:
   a. Provides an ongoing written record of the patient's status, care provided, and the outcomes of the interventions
   b. Documents that appropriate standards of care were implemented by a qualified professional
   c. Provides a permanent legal record of the patient's course while in the health care system
   d. Serves as a means of communication from one care provider to another

2. Nurse's assessments, interventions, and the outcomes of care for the woman and the fetus

3. Document in the chart the reasons that the medication or procedure was not administered.

4. Draw a line through the incorrect information, write "error" above it, write the date and time, and initial the entry. The accurate information is entered as an addendum.

5. a. It is a requirement of the institution's policies and procedures.
   b. The nurse has reviewed the content of the note.
   c. The nurse approves the care provided to the patient.

6. a. Restate the order, including the patient's name.
   b. Ask for confirmation.
   c. Chart "repeated and confirmed."

7. a. Signs/symptoms, onset, duration, and frequency
   b. Actions that alleviate or increase the signs and symptoms

8. a. The patient's chart
   b. Policy and procedure manual enforced at the time of the incident

9. Current national standards as developed by national professional organizations such as AWHONN

10. Any four of the following:
    a. Incomplete documentation
    b. Medication errors
    c. Violation of national standards of practice
    d. Improper use of equipment
    e. Failure to notify the appropriate professionals when maternal or fetal status falls outside normal parameters
    f. Failure to follow physician orders, hospital policies, and hospital procedures
    g. Failure to recognize and respond to cases of fetal distress
    h. Failure to intervene appropriately in the presence of negligence on the part of the providers

REFERENCES

1. Brent, N. J. (1997). *Nurses and the law: A guide to principles and applications* (pp. 65–84, 237–268). Philadelphia: WB Saunders.
2. Trandel-Korenchuk, D. M., & Trandel-Korenchuk, K. M. (1997). *Nursing and the law.* (5th ed., pp. 166–173, 184). Philadelphia: Lippincott.
3. Guido, G. W. (1997). *Legal issues in nursing* (2nd ed., pp. 113–147). Stamford, CT: Appleton & Lange.
4. Harris, C., Curtis, C., & Copeland, P. (1999). Informed consent. In D. M. Rostant & R. F. Cady (Eds.), *Liability issues in perinatal nursing* (2nd ed., pp. 187–200). Philadelphia: Lippincott.
5. Association of Women's Health, Obstetric and Neonatal Nurses. (1998). *Standards and guidelines for professional nursing practice in the care of women and newborns* (5th ed., pp. 1–43). Washington, DC: Author.
6. Drummond, S. (1999). Assessment of the patient in labor. In D. M. Rostant & R. F. Cady (Eds.), *Liability issues in perinatal nursing* (2nd ed., pp. 89–103). Philadelphia: Lippincott.
7. Cady, R. F. (1999). Telephone triage and the office nurse. In D. M. Rostant & R. F. Cady (Eds.), *Liability issues in perinatal nursing* (2nd ed., pp. 149–155). Philadelphia: Lippincott.
8. Rostant, D. M., & Cady, R. F. (Eds.). (1999). *Liability issues in perinatal nursing* (2nd ed., p. 328). Philadelphia: Lippincott.
9. King-Urbanski, T., & Cady, R. F. (1999). Documentation. In D. M. Rostant & R. F. Cady (Eds.), *Liability issues in perinatal nursing* (2nd ed., pp. 225–241). Philadelphia: Lippincott.
10. Rostant, D. M., & Murray, M. L. (1999). Fetal heart rate monitoring and implementation. In D. M. Rostant & R. F. Cady (Eds.), *Liability issues in perinatal nursing* (2nd ed., pp. 105–117). Philadelphia: Lippincott.
11. Solomon, D., & Cady, R. F. (1999). Professional negligence and nursing malpractice. In D. M. Rostant & R. F. Cady (Eds.), *Liability issues in perinatal nursing* (2nd ed., pp. 41–49). Philadelphia: Lippincott.
12. Kuhlman, C. (1990). Surviving a malpractice suit: Personal experience and general information. *Journal of Nurse-Midwifery, 35*(3), 166–171.

SUGGESTED READINGS

Fiesta, J. (1994). *20 Legal pitfalls of nurses to avoid* (2nd ed.). Albany, NY: Delmar.
Nielsen, P. E., Thomson, B. A., Jackson, R. B., Kosman, K., & Kiley, K. C. (2000). Standard obstetric record charting system: Evaluation of a new electronic medical record. *Obstetrics and Gynecology, 96*(6), 1003–1008.
Phelan, J. P. (1998). Ambulatory obstetrical care: Strategies to reduce telephone liability. *Clinical Obstetrics and Gynecology, 41*(3), 640–646.
Robinson, D. L., Anderson, M. M., & Erpenbeck, P. M. (1997). Telephone advice: New solutions for old problems. *Nurse Practitioner, 22*(3), 179–192.

MODULE 17

Maternal Transport

E. JEAN MARTIN

As you complete this module, you will learn:

1. Advantages and disadvantages of maternal transport
2. Recommendations for the optimal time for maternal transport
3. What constitutes a high-risk maternal transport
4. Who should be involved in making the decision for maternal transport and a suggested process for implementing the referral
5. Levels of skilled personnel who might accompany the mother during transplant
6. Contraindications to maternal transport
7. Conditions warranting consultation and/or transport of the pregnant woman from a Level I or Level II community hospital to a high-risk Level III regional center
8. Responsibilities of referring and receiving centers
9. Appropriate documentation and records that should accompany a maternal transport patient
10. Nursing interventions designed to assist the mother and family through the transfer process at both the referring and receiving hospitals
11. Basic equipment needed for maternal transport
12. Specific liability issues related to transport
13. About a program to which hospitals involved in medical transport may voluntarily apply; the program provides evaluation of compliance with accreditation standards

When you have completed this module, you should be able to recall the meaning of the following terms. You should also be able to use the terms when consulting with other health professionals. The terms are defined in this module or in the glossary at the end of this book.

inborn neonate

morbidity

mortality

outborn neonate

Determining the Need for Maternal Transport

■ What is maternal transport?

An essential component of any perinatal care system is the capability of providing interhospital transport of pregnant women and neonates.[1] *Maternal transport* refers to the process of transferring the pregnant woman under the supervision of skilled medical personnel from a Level I or Level II institution (referring hospitals) to a Level III institution (receiving hospital). Each situation is considered individually. The transfer can be accomplished by private vehicle, ambulance, rotary-wing aircraft (helicopter), or fixed-wing aircraft. The decision regarding the type of vehicle depends on the condition of the pregnant woman and fetus as well as distance. It is a decision that should be shared jointly by the referring care provider and flight nurse or receiving physician.

Advantages to Maternal Transport

During recent years, the transport of the premature or sick newborn to intensive care units of regional centers after birth has become widely accepted. These babies are often referred to as **outborn neonates,** in distinction to those born within the referral hospital (i.e., **inborn neonates**). The survival rates and quality of life for the high-risk neonate have improved significantly. However, documentation and research over the past 15 years have shown that there are further improved outcomes, including long-term sequelae for high-risk neonates transported before delivery. Transport of the neonate involves not only the availability of a local neonatal intensive care unit but also the complication risk during transport, the need for highly skilled personnel and specialized equipment, and the expense of the transport. In utero transport of selected risk pregnancies is strongly recommended. The outcome of an outborn neonate with major medical or surgical problems (which includes extreme prematurity) remains worse than that for an inborn infant. When possible the primary emphasis should always be on prenatal diagnosis and subsequent maternal transfer. Even with advanced training and technologies, mothers usually make the best transport incubator.[2] Transport within regionalized perinatal care networks allows for benefits of high-technology maternity and fetal/neonatal care and services, while presumably reducing costs and decreasing duplication of services within a region.

Advantages include several considerations:

- If the baby is transferred in utero, the need for sophisticated equipment and the risk of neonatal problems during transport are reduced. Advanced testing and treatment at the center enables a more accurate assessment of when and how to deliver the baby. Advanced therapeutic techniques can be provided for the high-risk mother.
- If an ill or severely preterm baby is delivered, immediate steps can be taken to stabilize and treat the newborn without losing precious time during transport.
- The hospital stay of the mother and her newborn tends to be shorter, resulting in a reduction of hospital costs.
- Finally, maternal transport ensures that the mother and baby are together during the first few days after birth. This provides the opportunity for the mother and baby to become acquainted and attached to each other in the unique process of bonding.

Disadvantages of Maternal Transport

Probably the greatest concern in transferring the undelivered mother to the regional center is the physical separation from her family and friends. Because of this, it is important that a family member accompany the mother or follow in a car, if possible, at the time of transport.

> The referring nursing staff and flight nurse must help reduce the disruption and stress for the pregnant woman and her family during transfer. Create a quiet private place to explain to the expectant woman and her family why the transfer is necessary and exactly how it is going to take place. Stress any positive aspect of the clinical situation (e.g., the baby is doing well presently).

The rate of admissions to neonatal intensive care units increases with a maternal transport system. A great percentage of these babies have extremely low birth weights. In the past, these babies did not survive. They require special care, which is met in tertiary care centers that have established maternal–fetal medicine programs. Administrative and fiscal considerations may necessitate a commitment of additional resources for such a program.[3]

Timing of Maternal Transport

■ When is the best time to transport the mother?

Transport of the undelivered mother to a regional center should be considered in the following situations:

- It is anticipated that the infant might require intensive care not available at the referring hospital.
- The obstetric, medical, or surgical needs of the mother require diagnosis, treatment, and care using highly specialized equipment, skills, and staff not available at the referring hospital.

When possible, referral should be made while the mother and fetus are in a stable condition and delivery is not expected during the immediate 24-hour period. This presents a low risk for transferring the mother and fetus. It is optimum, of course, to refer early enough to allow beginning assessment and treatment at the receiving hospital, thus preventing a crisis situation for either mother or fetus when they reach the receiving hospital.

High-reliability perinatal units* promote clinical practices based on nationally recognized guidelines and espouse a team philosophy of "safety first." One feature of such perinatal units is that "patients are transferred in a timely and reliable way" to facilities that can care for all potential problems rather then operating on the hope "that the disaster will not occur."[4]

Transfer of patients in early labor is recommended in the following circumstances:

- Time for transport will take less than 2 hours.
- The mother's condition is stable.
- Delivery is not anticipated for 4 to 6 hours.
- A professional attendant, such as a flight nurse, physician, or an experienced emergency medical technician, can accompany the mother.

High-risk transport situations include the following:

- The mother's condition is unstable.
- Time of delivery is unpredictable.

In high-risk transport situations, the decision as to whether the mother is stable enough for transport and who should accompany the mother should be made by the perinatal specialist and transport team experienced in such decision making.

In either of these high-risk situations, the mother must be accompanied by the following:

- Skilled medical attendant, such as an obstetrician or a certified nurse-midwife
- Nurse or neonatologist with the skill and experience to manage resuscitation and care of the newborn

---

NOTE: *Maternal transport might be contraindicated in women who are too unstable at the time of the transport request. For example, a mother in premature labor who is dilated beyond 5 cm should be evaluated carefully. Decisions depend on the makeup of the transport team, distance, and time. Safety of the mother and the fetus are the primary considerations.*

Other contraindications can include women with the following:

- Actively bleeding placenta previa
- Abruptio placentae
- Unstable fetal condition

*Behavioral scientists define *high-reliability organizations* as those with "the ability to operate technologically complex systems essentially without error over long periods."[4]

> Many times, the transport team will need to make critical decisions before leaving the referring hospital.

REMEMBER: *Critical factors in successful maternal transport are appropriate treatment of the mother before transport and attendance by skilled personnel.*

Conditions Requiring Transport to a Regional Center

■ What conditions in the mother require referral to a regional center?

The majority of maternal transports will be carried out because of concern for a potentially compromised fetus. Prematurity remains the predominant cause of neonatal morbidity and mortality. Although premature infants represent less than 10% of all deliveries, this group constitutes approximately 75% of neonatal mortalities. Statistics from selected regional centers indicates uniformly better outcomes for in utero fetal transport (i.e., the mortality risk for fetuses transported in utero is approximately half that of neonates transported after delivery).

The following conditions usually require that the mother be transported to a regional center for high-risk care.[5,6]

Obstetric Complications

- **Preterm premature rupture of membranes occurring before 34 weeks' gestation or with a fetus estimated to weigh less than 2,000 g**

Maternal risks with preterm premature rupture of membranes:

- Infection
- Abruptio placentae (occurs in approximately 5% of these women)

Fetal/neonatal risks with preterm premature rupture of membranes:

- Infection
- Prematurity
- Pulmonary immaturity
- Cord prolapse

Management varies with gestational age. A vaginal culture for group B streptococcus (GBS) should be obtained using a *sterile* cotton-tipped applicator on women when presenting with preterm premature rupture of membranes. Infection with GBS is responsible for serious neonatal morbidity and mortality.[7,8] See Appendix A for GBS discussion.

- Any condition in which the probability exists for the delivery of an infant less than 34 weeks' gestation or weighing less than 2,000 g, such as the following:
  - Severe preeclampsia or other hypertensive complications
  - Certain anticipated multiple births
  - Poorly controlled or severe diabetes mellitus
  - Severe intrauterine growth restriction
  - Some women with third trimester bleeding
  - Rh isoimmunization
  - Severe oligohydramnios

Medical Complications

- Infections that are likely to result in premature birth
- Severe organic heart disease
- Renal disease with deteriorating function or increasing hypertension
- Drug overdose
- Some women with carcinoma

Surgical Complications
- Trauma requiring intensive care or surgery beyond the capabilities of local facilities or where the procedure can result in the onset of premature labor
- Acute abdominal emergencies at less than 34 weeks' gestation or with a fetus estimated to weigh less than 2,000 g
- Thoracic emergencies requiring intensive care or surgical correction

Fetal Complications
- Fetal congenital anomalies diagnosed by ultrasound can dictate the need for maternal transport

NOTE: Transfer from a Level II institution is appropriate for the following:
- *Any fetus anticipated to require long-term ventilation support after birth.*
- *Any fetus anticipated to require neonatal care at less than 30 to 34 weeks' gestation (This will depend on the skilled personnel and advanced technology of the institution.[14])*

Other Considerations
After birth, many babies are cyanotic, often peripherally. Typically, cyanotic babies have the following characteristics[9]:

- Are premature, have experienced a difficult delivery or injested meconium, or had premature rupture of membranes
- Are in marked respiratory distress
- Have radiographic evidence of lung disease
- Have elevated PCO_2 levels
- Have PO_2 increases with 100% oxygen

On the other hand, a baby experiencing a cardiac abnormality usually has the following characteristics[9]:

- Is term
- Has had a normal delivery
- Has little respiratory distress
- Has cyanosis, which is central and disproportionate to distress; tongue and mucous membranes are blue
- Has no radiologic evidence of lung disease

When born with cyanotic congenital heart disease in a Level I or Level II hospital, a baby should be transported by a neonatal transport team immediately because he or she is only going to get worse. Most babies should be referred to a major pediatric cardiac unit. Most require surgical treatment.[5] **IT IS FAR BETTER TO ANTICIPATE THIS NEED WHEN POSSIBLE AND TRANSPORT THE MOTHER BEFORE DELIVERY.**

Glucocorticoid Therapy for Fetal Maturation
Preterm delivery continues to be a major cause of illness and death in infants. In March 1994, the National Institutes of Health (NIH) sponsored a consensus Development Conference on the Effect of Corticosteroids for Fetal Maturation on Perinatal Outcomes.[10] The consensus panel concluded that *giving a single course of corticosteroids* to pregnant women at risk for preterm delivery reduces the risk of death, respiratory distress syndrome (RDS), and intraventricular hemorrhage in their preterm infants. Such therapy brought about a significant and clear decrease in RDS in infants born between 29 and 34 weeks' gestation. For infants born between 24 and 28 weeks' gestation, only the severity of the disease was decreased, not the incidence.[11]

Antenatal glucocorticoid therapy promotes fetal lung maturation. Clinical studies reveal that glucocorticoids can accelerate lung maturation in immature fetuses. Administration of glucocorticoids (corticosteroids) such as betamethasone or dexamethasone to pregnant women 24 to 48 hours before delivery has been shown to stimulate surfactant production. Fetal lung alveoli remain expanded because of decreased surface tension within the alveoli.

Based on scientific studies, both prenatal glucocorticoids (betamethasone or dexamethasone) and postnatal surfactant therapy are effective in preventing RDS. Studies also demonstrate that combination therapy is often better than either treatment alone.

Recently, widespread practice in the United States and other countries is to use repeat courses of antenatal corticosteroids (e.g., weekly dosages, occasional dosages, or rescue [single-course steroids] therapy).[11] The NIH recently called a conference to present research on repeat courses of antenatal corticosteroid therapy. The conclusion was that "data from currently available studies assessing benefits and risks are inadequate to argue for or against the use of repeat or rescue courses of antenatal corticosteroids for fetal maturation."[11]

Clinical recommendations are as follows[11]:

- All pregnant women between 24 and 34 weeks' gestation who are at risk for preterm delivery within 7 days should be considered for antenatal treatment with a single course of corticosteroids. Optimal benefit from such therapy lasts 7 days.
- Treatment consists of two doses of 12 mg of **betamethasone** given intramuscularly 24 hours apart **OR** four doses of 6 mg of **dexamethasone** given intramuscularly 12 hours apart, as recommended by the consensus panel in 1994. There is no proof of efficacy for any other regimen.
- Because of insufficient scientific data from randomized clinical trials regarding efficacy and safety, repeat courses of corticosteroids should not be used routinely. In general, this should be reserved for patients enrolled in randomized controlled trials.

Fetal Echocardiography

The use of fetal echocardiography is currently evolving and requires extensive experience by the diagnostician to accurately diagnose some congenital cardiac abnormalities. A diagnosis by an inexperienced individual can be wrong or incomplete. When a cardiac abnormality is suspected in utero in a facility other than a tertiary care center, maternal transport is indicated.[9]

Responsibilities of the Referring and Receiving Centers

■ **What steps should be taken by the referring physician and hospital in initiating the transport?**

The decision to transport the pregnant or laboring woman should be made jointly by her physician and the physician to whom the referral is being made. The situation should be discussed with the mother and/or her family. The following guidelines for the organization of the transport are divided into referring center responsibilities and receiving center responsibilities.[12]

Referring Center Responsibilities
- The referring care provider confers with the receiving physician by phone. This should assist the receiving physician in developing a treatment plan to maintain stabilization of the patient. It is the referring center's responsibility to follow COBRA/EMTALA guidelines.[a]
- An ambulance is the most appropriate vehicle for the majority of maternal transports. An alternative form of transportation should be agreed on by the referring and receiving physicians.
- The composition of the transport team should be a joint decision between the referring and receiving care providers based on the condition of the mother and/or fetus.
- If transport is by ambulance without a transport team or by private car, the referring center and physician are responsible for the patient before and during transport until she is received at the high-risk regional center.
- *An up-to-date copy of the mother's prenatal record, hospital chart, laboratory data, and the mother's signed consent form are sent with her.*
- The mother is transported from the obstetric unit of the referring center or physician's office to the obstetric unit of the receiving hospital. This reduces the risk of unnecessary delays in the emergency room or admitting office.

NOTE: *A member of the mother's family should be encouraged to accompany her. If the mother requires care by the ambulance attendants, the family member may sit with the ambulance driver or follow in a car.*

[a]COBRA/EMTALA Statute: 42 USC 1395 federal regulation relating to the transfer and medical treatment of women in labor. Circumstances are delineated under which an individual may be transferred to another medical care facility, including the steps to be taken for stabilization and treatment before transfer.[12]

■ **What steps should be taken by the receiving physician and hospital in accepting the transport?**

Receiving Center Responsibilities

- The receiving physician is responsible for accepting the referring care provider's request for transport and for making preparations to receive the transport.
- Shared responsibility for the patient by the receiving physician and the referring provider begins on initial consultation and acceptance for the transfer. Full responsibility begins with admission to the receiving center.
- Every patient accepted by transport from a referring hospital should be seen by a physician within 30 minutes of arrival.
- Communication with the referring care provider should occur following admission.
- If the patient is discharged undelivered, communication should occur before the discharge.
- A discharge summary of both mother and baby should be sent to the referring physician.
- The mother should return to the care of the referring care provider as soon as possible. Separation of mother and infant should be avoided when possible.
- If the mother needs to be referred to the receiving center or physician again, the referral process begins again with a physician-to-physician phone call.

REMEMBER: *Adequate documentation of the mother's health status is essential for developing a treatment plan at the receiving center. Send all available medical records and complete prenatal records, including any ultrasonography reports and laboratory test results.*

Nursing Care in Maternal Transport

■ **How can the nurse assist the mother and her family through the transfer process?**

The process of being transferred from one hospital to another increases the mother's and family's awareness of the medical problems accompanying the pregnancy. At the same time, geographically distancing mothers and members of her family reduces the opportunity for mutual support. Coping abilities of both parties can suffer. It is important that communication between mother and father or other family members be facilitated throughout the stay at the high-risk center. Many transport teams have printed information for the mother and family that can be helpful.

Nursing Interventions Throughout the Stay at the Referring Hospital[13]

These interventions are aimed at preparing the family for the transport.

- Ensure that the woman and her family understand the reasons for the transfer. **Ask the woman to say why she is being transported.** *This is important.*
- Inform the family about the regional hospital to which the transfer is being made. Information should include the following:
  - The name of the physician and a primary nurse at the regional hospital (sometimes this is unknown)
  - The type of care given at the regional hospital (teaching facility or private hospital)
  - How the mother will be transported (e.g., ambulance, helicopter)
  - How long the trip will take
  - When the trip is to occur
  - Who will accompany her (check with the transport team to see if someone is allowed)
  - Hospital unit policies, including visiting hours and telephone numbers
  - How family members can travel to the regional hospital by car or mass transportation
  - Cost of transport and whether covered by insurance
- Encourage the mother to discuss her fears and concerns with you.

Nursing Interventions at the Receiving Hospital[13]

Patients/families under great stress have difficulty dealing with more than a few people. Ideally, one nurse should be assigned initially to assist the mother and her family.

- Welcome the woman and her family while orienting them to the unit.
- Review unit policies and encourage the mother's support person to visit as appropriate.
- Facilitate telephone communication with family members as appropriate.
- Promote prebirth bonding of the mother and family to the fetus by discussing the fetus' unique characteristics, such as activity levels and times of quiet.

> Have the neonatal nurse practitioner or neonatologist speak to the mother and family members regarding their concerns for the premature infant.

> Parents need to be assisted to identify the fetus as a developing individual—a part of the family—even with a fetus who is greatly compromised during the pregnancy.

- After the infant's birth, promote parent–infant interaction at whatever level is appropriate. If the infant is in a neonatal intensive care unit (NICU), do the following:
  –Encourage parental visits.
  –Have the NICU nurse report to or write down information about the infant's progress.
  –Involve parents, when possible, with decisions about their baby's care.
  –Provide opportunities for parents to care for their baby at whatever level appropriate.
- Allow the mother and family to discuss their fears, concerns, and anxieties.
- Provide the family with some privacy during visits.
- Assist the family to contact the appropriate support services (e.g., social service, clergy, psychologists, parent groups).
- Facilitate continuity of care for infant and parents if the infant is transferred back to the referring hospital for final recovery closer to the parent's home.

Ensuring Safe Transport

■ What basic equipment is needed for maternal transport?

Most ambulances have basic life support (BLS) equipment adequate for the majority of maternal transports. The referring physician should be familiar with the availability of BLS and advanced life support (ALS) ambulances in the area. Equipment should also be available for anticipated complications such as delivery, seizure, and hemorrhage. The Tennessee Perinatal Care System *Guidelines for Transportation*[12] lists additional equipment that may be necessary:

- Fetoscope/Doppler
- Reflex hammer
- Infusion pump
- Medications
  –Pitocin
  –Methergine
  –Magnesium sulfate
  –Calcium gluconate
  –Tocolytic agent
- Oxygen masks (premature and newborn size)
- Infant positive-pressure bag and mask
- Suction catheter (10 Fr)

> When preterm labor is a risk during transport, a birth kit from the referring hospital should be included—that is, suction catheters, suction bulbs, blankets, and a hat for the newborn.[14]

Organization and maintenance of additional transport equipment is the responsibility of the transport team.

> In transporting a high-risk laboring mother who has the possibility of delivery before reaching the referral hospital, a *transport incubator* should be part of the equipment.

An incubator must be capable of the following:

- Providing a stable, adjustable heat source
- Providing constant and adjustable oxygen

- Providing good visibility of the infant
- Being easily transported
- Providing easy access to the infant for care and treatment
- Operating on DC sources of electric power while in transport and AC sources for hospital use

NOTE: In all transport situations, the mother should be encouraged to avoid positions that compromise maternal blood flow. Keep the mother in a high semi-Fowler's or left side-lying position. This displaces the gravid uterus off the vena cava, preventing compromised maternal circulation.

It is recommended that all women have at least two infusion lines established because of difficulty starting an intravenous line during transport.[14]

An important step in the transfer preparation is to change any bottle of intravenous fluid just before transport. Even with excellent communication between medical personnel, a bottle of intravenous fluid can be mislabeled, resulting in a drug or dose being administered that is different from that stated.[15]

Oxygen administration is advised in any clinical situation for which there is concern about potential fetal distress.

Specific Liability Issues Related to Transport[16]

Every nurse and provider involved in transport should be keenly aware of liability issues. Such sensitivity may serve to sharpen all facets of clinical practice to the benefit of both the patient and health care personnel.

Specific liability issues include the following:

- Use of treatment protocols or algorithms
- Lack of informed consent
- Failure to stabilize before transport
- Failure to diagnose or delay in diagnosing a problem more significant than what was relayed by the transferring hospital
- Equipment issues
- Delay in treatment or transfer
- Actual error (e.g., wrong drug or dose)
- When does liability transfer from the referring facility to the receiving facility?

The Commission of Accreditation of Medical Transport Systems (CAMTS) offers a program of voluntary evaluation of compliance with accreditation standards. This provides professionals involved with air medical and ground transport systems to improve services and can serve as a marker of excellence for federal, state, and local agencies, as well as to the public.[17] See "Resources of Note" for further information.

PRACTICE/REVIEW QUESTIONS
After reviewing this module, answer the following questions.

1. What is the primary advantage of transporting the high-risk mother to a regional center before the baby is born? _____

2. What is the primary disadvantage of transporting the high-risk mother to a regional center?

   _____

   _____

3. Describe a *low-risk* maternal transport situation.

   _____

   _____

   _____

4. Under what conditions should the *high-risk* woman in *early* labor be transported?

   a. _____

   b. _____

   c. _____

   d. _____

5. Describe a *high-risk* maternal transport situation.

   _____

   _____

   _____

6. The obstetric complications necessitating high-risk care involve conditions occurring be-

   fore _____ weeks' gestation or an estimated birth weight below _____ g.

7. List several *obstetric complications* that require high-risk care and therefore maternal transport from community hospitals in some cases.

   a. _____

   b. _____

   c. _____

   d. _____

   e. _____

8. Briefly list *medical* and *surgical complications* necessitating high-risk care.
   Medical Complications

   a. _____

   b. _____

   c. _____

   d. _____

   e. _____

   Surgical Complications

   a. _____

   b. _____

   c. _____

9. What fetal situations necessitate the transfer of a mother from a Level II to a Level III institution?

   a. _____

   _____

   b. _____

   _____

10. Babies often experience cyanosis after birth, often peripherally. List three characteristics of cyanotic babies, who are generally not experiencing a cardiac abnormality.

   a. _____

   b. _____

   c. _____

11. A baby with a cyanotic congenital heart abnormality needs to be kept at the Level I or Level II hospital until he or she is stabilized. After stabilization, the baby may be transferred.

    A. True

    B. False

12. Cyanosis of mucous membranes and the tongue in a term baby who has no radiologic evidence of lung disease is suspicious for:

    A. Cardiac abnormality

    B. Peripheral cyanosis, common in many babies

13. Current recommendations from the NIH (2000) advise antenatal treatment for all pregnant women between _____ weeks' gestation and _____ weeks' gestation who are at risk for preterm delivery within _____ days and that they be considered for treatment with a single course of corticosteroids.

14. Corticosteroid therapy (e.g., betamethasone, dexamethasone) brings about a significant decrease in RDS in infants born between 29 and 34 weeks' gestation.

    A. True

    B. False

15. A *single course* of treatment with *betamethasone* consists of _____ doses of _____ mg given intramuscularly _____ hours apart.

16. A single course of treatment with *dexamethasone* consists of _____ doses of _____ mg given intramuscularly _____ hours apart.

17. The referring physician must initiate the transport by contacting the receiving physician.

    A. True

    B. False

18. A health professional should always accompany the mother during transport.

    A. True

    B. False

19. The mother's record and laboratory data should be sent to the high-risk center by mail.

    A. True

    B. False

20. The mother should be taken to the emergency room of the receiving hospital.

    A. True

    B. False

21. A discharge summary sheet should be sent to the referring care provider.

    A. True

    B. False

22. A woman who is a gravida 3, para 2, is at a Level I hospital in her thirty-fourth week of pregnancy. She is dilated 4 cm, and her preterm labor is complicated by severe preeclampsia. The receiving and referring physicians have agreed on maternal transport by helicopter to the high-risk regional center, which is 40 miles away. Who is the most appropriate member of the health team to accompany the patient? _____

    Why? _____

23. List eight nursing interventions that the nurse at the referring hospital can do to assist the mother and her family in the transfer to the high-risk regional center.

    a. _____

    b. _____

    c. _____

    d. _____

    e. _____

    f. _____

    g. _____

    h. _____

24. List eight nursing interventions designed to assist the mother in adjusting to the high-risk regional center after transfer.

    a. _____

    b. _____

    c. _____

    d. _____

    e. _____

    f. _____

    g. _____

    h. _____

25. List five specific liability issues related to transport.

    a. _____

    b. _____

    c. _____

    d. _____

    e. _____

PRACTICE/REVIEW ANSWER KEY

1. Survival rates and quality of life (long-term sequelae) for the high-risk neonate are improved.

2. The mother is separated from friends and family.

3. The low-risk transport situation is one in which the mother and fetus are in a stable condition and delivery is not expected during the immediate 24-hour period.

4. a. Transport will take less than 2 hours.
   b. The mother's condition is stable.
   c. Delivery is not anticipated for 4 to 6 hours.
   d. An experienced health professional can accompany the mother.

5. The high-risk transport situation is one in which the mother's or fetus' condition is unstable (e.g., actively bleeding with a placenta previa or in active labor and dilated 5 cm or beyond) and the time of delivery is unpredictable.

6. 34; 2,000

7. Answers should include:
   a. Premature rupture of membranes before 34 weeks' gestation or with a fetus thought to weigh less than 2,000 g
   b. Premature labor before 34 weeks' gestation
   c. Conditions in which the infant might deliver before 34 weeks' gestation or weigh less than 2,000 g (e.g., severe preeclampsia or hypertensive disorder, multiple gestation, poorly controlled or severe diabetes mellitus, intrauterine growth restriction with signs of fetal distress, bleeding in the third trimester, Rh isoimmunization, severe oligohydramnios)

8. *Medical Complications:*
   a. Infections that can result in premature birth
   b. Severe heart disease
   c. Renal disease with deteriorating function or increasing hypertension
   d. Drug overdose
   e. Some patients with carcinoma
   Surgical Complications:
   a. Trauma that requires care or surgery beyond what the local hospital can provide
   b. Acute abdominal problems at less than 34 weeks' gestation or a baby weighing less than 2,000 g
   c. Thoracic emergencies

9. a. Any fetus anticipated to require long-term ventilation support after birth
   b. Any fetus anticipated to require neonatal care at less than 30 to 34 week's gestation (This will depend on the skilled personnel and advanced technology of the institution.)

10. Any three of the following:
    a. Are premature, had a difficult delivery, experienced meconium passages in utero, had premature rupture of membranes
    b. Are in marked respiratory distress
    c. Have radiologic evidence of lung disease
    d. Have an elevated P_{CO_2} level
    e. Have P_{O_2} increases with 100% oxygen

11. B (The infant is going to get worse with time.)

12. A

13. 24; 34; 7

14. A

15. 2; 12; 24

16. 4; 6; 12

17. A

18. B (This depends on the circumstances under which the mother is being transported. Occasionally, a private car may be used, in which case the health professional would not accompany the mother.)

19. B

20. B

21. A

22. A physician
    This represents a high-risk maternal transport.

23. Any eight of the following:
    a. Ensure that the woman and her family understand the reasons for the transfer.
    b. Inform the family about the regional hospital to which the mother is being transferred.
    c. Give the names of the physician and a primary nurse at the regional center.
    d. Discuss the type of care given.
    e. Tell the mother how she will be transported and how long the trip will take.
    f. Tell her when the trip is to occur and who will be accompanying her.
    g. Familiarize her with the hospital unit policies, including visiting hours and telephone numbers.
    h. Discuss how family members can get to the regional center and where they might be able to stay.
    i. Allow the mother to discuss her fears and concerns with you.

24. Any eight of the following:
    a. Welcome the woman and her family while orienting them to the unit.
    b. Review unit policies and promote visiting of the mother's support person as appropriate to her level of illness.
    c. Facilitate telephone communication with family members as appropriate.
    d. Promote prebirth bonding of the mother and family to the fetus by discussing the fetus' unique characteristics, such as activity levels and times of quiet.
    e. Promote parent–infant interaction at whatever level is possible and appropriate.
    f. Encourage the mother and family to discuss their fears, concerns, and anxieties.
    g. Provide the family with some privacy during visits.
    h. Assist the family to contact appropriate support services (e.g., social service, clergy, psychologists, parent groups).
    i. Facilitate continuity of care for infant and parents if the infant is transferred back to the referring hospital for final recovery.

25. Any five of the following:
    a. Use of treatment protocols or algorithms
    b. Lack of informed consent
    c. Failure to stabilize
    d. Failure to diagnose or delay in diagnosing a problem more significant than what was relayed by the transferring hospital
    e. Equipment issues
    f. Delay in treatment or transfer
    g. Actual error (e.g., wrong drug or dose)
    h. When does liability transfer from the referring facility to the receiving facility

REFERENCES

1. American Academy of Pediatrics and the American College of Obstetricians and Gynecologists. (1997). Interhospital care of the perinatal patient. In *Guidelines for perinatal care* (4th ed., pp. 51–63). Washington, DC: Author.
2. Ohning, B. L., & Driggers, K. P. (2001, May). Transport of the critically ill newborn. *EMedicine Journal, 2*(5). Available at: www.emedicine.com/ped/topic2730.htm
3. Cowett, R. M., Coustan, D. R., & Oh, W. (1986). Effects of maternal transport on admission patterns at a tertiary care center. *American Journal of Obstetrics and Gynecology, 154*(5), 1098–1100.
4. Knox, G. E., Simpson, K. R., & Garite, T. J. (1999). Highly reliable perinatal units: An approach to the prevention of patient injury and medical malpractice claims. *Journal of Healthcare Risk Management, 19*(2), 24–27.
5. Rehm, N. E. (1987). Indications for maternal transport—The Utah experience. In D. M. Coulter (Ed.), *Current concepts in transport: Neonatal, maternal, administrative* (3rd ed., pp. 297–298). Salt Lake City: Perinatal Transport Service, University of Utah Medical Center.

6. Strobino, D. M., Frank, R., Oberdorf, M. A., Shachtman, Kim, Y. J., Callan, N., & Nagey, D. (1993). Development of an index of maternal transport. *Medical Decisions Making, 13*(1), 64–73.

7. Centers for Disease Control and Prevention. (1996). Prevention of perinatal group B streptococcal disease: A public health perspective. *MMWR Morbidity and Mortality Weekly Report, 45*(RR-7), 1–24.

8. American College of Obstetricians and Gynecologists. (1996). Prevention of early-onset group B streptococcal disease in newborns. *Committee Opinion, 173,* 1–8.

9. Orsmond, G. S. (1995). Management of cyanotic heart disease. In M. S. Trautman (Ed.), *Current concepts in transport. Neonatal syllabus* (7th ed., pp. 16–20). Salt Lake City: University of Utah.

10. National Institutes of Health. (1994, February 28–March 2). Effect of corticosteroids for fetal maturation on perinatal outcomes. *NIH Consensus Statement, 12*(2), 1–24.

11. National Institutes of Health. (2001, September 5). Antenatal corticosteroids revisited: Repeat courses. *NIH Consensus Statement Online 2000, 17*(2), 1–10.

12. Tennessee Perinatal Care System. (2001). *Guidelines for transportation* (4th ed.). Tennessee Department of Health. Maternal and Child Health. Prepared by the Subcommittee on Perinatal Transportation of the Perinatal Advisory Committee, 6–7; Appendix IX. Nashville.

13. Davis, D. H., & Hawkins, J. W. (1985). High-risk maternal and neonatal transport: Psychosocial implications for practice. *Dimensions of Critical Care Nursing, 4*(6), 373–379.

14. Simpson, K. R., & Creehan, P. A. (Eds.). (2001). *Perinatal nursing* (2nd ed., p. 275). Philadelphia: Lippincott.

15. Dennis, L. G. (1989). Stabilization and management of the pregnant patient prior to transport. In M. G. MacDonald & M. K. Miller (Eds.), *Emergency transport of the perinatal patient.* Boston: Little, Brown.

16. Youngberg, B. (2001). Liability issues every transport nurse should consider. In *Current concepts in transport (syllabus).* Annual Conference, February 28–March 3.

17. Commission on Accreditation of Medical Transport Systems. (1999). *Accreditation standards of the Commission on Accreditation of Medical Transport Systems. Mission statement.* Anderson, SC: Author.

SUGGESTED READINGS

National Institutes of Health. (2001, September 5). Antenatal corticosteroids revisited: Repeat courses. *NIH Consensus Statement Online 2000, 17*(2), 1–10.

American Academy of Pediatrics and the American College of Obstetricians and Gynecologists. (1997). Interhospital care of the perinatal patient. In *Guidelines for perinatal care* (4th ed.). Washington, DC: Author. (Addresses: American Academy of Pediatrics, 141 Northwest Point Boulevard, P.O. Box 927, Elk Grove Village, IL 60009-0927; American College of Obstetricians and Gynecologists, 409 12th Street, SW, P.O. Box 96920, Washington, DC 20090-6920.)

RESOURCES OF NOTE

Commission on Accreditation of Medical Transport Systems. (1999). *Accreditation standards of the Commission on Accreditation of Medical Transport Systems. Mission statement.* Anderson, SC: Author.

Conference. (Annual). *Current concepts in transport (neonatal, pediatric).* Sponsored by the Pediatric Education by the Pediatric Education Services at Primary Children's Medical Center, University of Utah, School of Medicine, Salt Lake City, Education Department. Phone: 801-588-4060.

Tennessee Perinatal Care System. (2001). *Guidelines for transportation* (4th ed.). Subcommittee on Perinatal Transportation of the Perinatal Advisory Committee. Tennessee Department of Health, Maternal and Child Health. Address: 425 5th Avenue North, 5th Floor, Cordell Hull Building, Nashville, TN 37247-4701.

ABO incompatibility a lack of compatibility between two groups of blood cells having different antigens because of the presence of one of the type antigens (A, B, or both) and its absence in the other

abruptio placentae premature separation of a normally implanted placenta; the separation can be partial or complete

accelerations, fetal see **fetal accelerations**

acidemia buildup of acid in the blood

acidosis condition in which there is a disturbance in the acid-base balance of the body, resulting in an accumulation of acids or an excessive loss of bicarbonate

active immunity an immunity to a disease resulting from the development within the body of substances that render a person immune; this could result from having the disease or by the injection of an organism or products of an organism

addendum statements added to the chart after the original documentation of an event; may contain additional facts about the situation or correct misinformation in the first entry

agonist chemical substances that exert a quieting effect on smooth muscle by interacting with specific areas on the surface of the cells; some agonists are referred to as beta-mimetic or beta-adrenergic substances

AIDS acquired immunodeficiency syndrome

algorithm a logical progression that, for example, outlines sequential steps to be taken in the diagnosis and management of a disease

alpha-fetoprotein (AFP) test determination of fetal antigen levels during pregnancy; elevated levels in amniotic fluid are associated with neural tube defects, and low levels may be associated with Down's syndrome

ALT alanine aminotransferase; an enzyme that contributes to protein metabolism; specifically, it catalyzes the reversible transfer of an amino group from glutamic acid to pyruvic acid to form alanine; the old term for this enzyme was *serum glutamic-pyruvic transaminase* (SGPT); this enzyme is present in the liver; during viral hepatitis and in cases of hepatocellular necrosis, marked elevations are seen

amniocentesis puncturing the amniotic sac using a needle so that amniotic fluid can be obtained for testing

amniotic phosphatidylglycerol (PG) a class of compounds found in amniotic fluid that can be analyzed to determine fetal pulmonary maturity

amniotomy puncturing the amniotic sac, allowing amniotic fluid to escape; this is sometimes done during active labor

anoxia deficiency of oxygen; *see also* **hypoxia**

antibody protein substances developed in response to the presence of an antigen; antibodies, which the body produces to inhibit or destroy the antigen, are part of the body's defense against foreign substances such as bacteria and viruses

antigen a substance that, when introduced into a host, is capable of producing antibodies; an antigen can be introduced into the host body, or it can be formed within the body; bacteria and viruses are examples of antigens

antiretroviral therapy treatment with drugs designed to prevent the HIV virus from replicating in HIV-infected persons

arborization fernlike appearance

ARC AIDS-related complex, which is a milder form of the immune deficiency causing a disease process

asphyxia decrease in the body's oxygen along with an increase in the carbon dioxide content caused by interference with respiration

AST aspartate aminotransferase; an enzyme that contributes to protein metabolism; specifically, it is important in the biosynthesis of amino acids because it catalyzes the reversible transfer of an amino group between glutamic and aspartic acid; the old term for this enzyme was *serum glutamic-oxaloacetic transaminase* (SGOT); when cell damage occurs (e.g., in the liver), AST is released into the tissues and bloodstream

atypical variable decelerations decelerations that possess characteristics that indicate fetal hypoxia

augmentation increasing contractions by chemical stimulation to help labor progress

average variability change of 5 to 15 bpm in the baseline fetal heart rate, which serves as an indication of a healthy fetus; *see also* **variability**

AZT azidothymide (chemical name), ZVD (zidovudine, generic name), and Retrovir (brand name); a nucleoside analog reverse transcriptase inhibitor drug commonly used to treat HIV infection; special precautions are recommended for dentistry

ballottement a sign that can be determined during abdominal examination of the pregnant woman; when the fingers tap lightly over a fetal part, it will "bounce" back under the fingers; this sign can also be felt during a vaginal examination

baroreceptors specialized tissue located in the carotid arch and aortic sinus; cells in these areas are sensitive to stretching of surrounding tissues caused by increased blood pressure; when pressure is increased, these areas communicate this change to the brain, which responds by reducing the heart rate and cardiac output in an attempt to reduce blood pressure

base deficit (BD) the amount of bases used by the body in an attempt to normalize a reduced pH (neutralize the acid); illustrates the degree of change in the bicarbonate concentration of the body

baseline fetal heart rate fetal heart rate occurring between contractions, usually between 120 and 160 bpm

baseline uterine tonus amount of tone in the uterus between contractions, usually between 5 and 15 mm Hg; can be measured only by an intrauterine pressure catheter

beta-adrenergic receptors specific sites on smooth muscle cells (e.g., the cells of the myometrium) where chemicals (agonists) can couple to produce a chemical reaction

beta-mimetic drugs unique chemical substances that are able to bind to beta-receptor sites on smooth muscle cells, causing a depressant or relaxing effect on the contracting ability of that cell; such cells are found in the myometrium of the uterus; beta-mimetic drugs belong to a group of chemicals called agonists

biparietal diameter (BPD) the largest transverse diameter of the fetal head; measures the distance between the parietal bones

bradycardia, fetal see **fetal bradycardia**

capacity the age and competence of an individual required for giving informed consent

caput succedaneum a swelling produced on the presenting part of the fetal head during labor; can be mistaken for the bag of waters

carrier an individual who is capable of transmitting a disease to another person; many times, carriers are not sick and have no idea that they are capable of spreading the disease

catecholamines a group of chemicals that mediate physiologic and metabolic responses associated with sympathetic nervous system functioning

cephalopelvic disproportion (CPD) a condition that develops when the infant's head is of size, shape, or position that it cannot pass through the mother's pelvis

cervix the "neck," or lowest part, of the uterus that extends into the vagina; during labor, the cervix dilates, allowing the fetus to pass through it

chemoreceptors specialized tissue, located in the aortic and carotid bodies and in the medulla, that are sensitive to decreases in oxygen, carbon dioxide content, and pH in the blood; they recognize these changes, initiating responses that assist the body in compensating for these problems

chorioamnionitis an infection of one of the membranes forming the amniotic sac, which holds the fetus during the pregnancy

cleft palate a congenital defect in which an opening is left in the roof of the mouth (the palate); during fetal development, this area fails to close and a communicating passageway between the mouth and nasal cavities is left

clonus the spasmodic alteration of contraction and relaxation of a foot or hand

collusion a secret agreement or cooperation between or among individuals for illegal or deceitful actions

conduction anesthesia (regional anesthesia) a form of anesthesia that is given centrally (i.e., in the spinal canal) or peripherally (i.e., in the skin) to block pain impulses without causing a loss of consciousness

confirmatory test a highly specific test designed to confirm the results of an earlier screening test

conservator a person appointed by a court to manage the personal and legal affairs of an incompetent adult

contraction(s) a shortening or tightening of a muscle; often used to describe the activity of the uterus that brings about dilatation of the cervix and descent of the fetus during labor

cytokines substances produced by the immune system in response to infection; also, recent findings indicate that cytokines (e.g., interlukin-1β) seem to play a role in labor initiation

decelerations see **early deceleration, late deceleration, variable deceleration**

decreased variability a change in fetal heart rate of less than 5 bpm; regarded as a sign of fetal distress if benign causes such as drugs or fetal sleep are not responsible; see also **variability**

dermatome the area of skin supplied with afferent nerve fibers by a single posterior spinal root

diabetogenic producing diabetes symptoms

dipping when the presenting part has descended into the false pelvis but is not through the pelvic inlet

direct fetal monitoring see **internal fetal monitoring**

disseminated intravascular coagulation (DIC) a grave disorder in blood clotting resulting from the overstimulation of the body's clotting processes; initially, generalized intravascular clotting occurs, succeeded by a deficiency in clotting factors and subsequent hemorrhaging; signs of hemorrhage may appear beneath the skin or mucous membranes, as evidenced by ecchymosis or petechiae

dizygotic pertaining to or derived from two separate zygotes (fertilized ova), as in a twin gestation resulting from two different fertilized ova

Down's syndrome a congenital condition accompanied by moderate to severe mental retardation

dysmature a condition in which the fetus or newborn is abnormally small or large for its gestational age; implies failure to achieve maturity in structure or function

dysrhythmia an irregularity in the heart rate that can be a result of an electrical abnormality, congenital anomaly, or injury; can be a transient and benign problem or a continuous and serious condition; most fetal dysrhythmias are benign

dystocia abnormal labor as seen in very slow cervical dilatation or fetal descent or a complete halt in progress, which can be due to maternal or fetal conditions

early decelerations a transitory decrease in fetal heart rate caused by head compression, which stimulates the vagus nerve to decrease heart rate

eclampsia a pregnancy-related hypertensive disease accompanied by hypertension, proteinuria, edema, tonic and clonic convulsions, and coma; can occur during pregnancy or shortly after delivery

EIA an enzyme immunoassay test for HIV infection; has 99% sensitivity when performed under optimal laboratory conditions on serum specimens from persons infected for 12 weeks or more (formerly called **ELISA**)

emancipated released from parental care and responsibility; freed from the power of another individual

embolism obstruction of a blood vessel by foreign substances or a blood clot (as in erythroblastosis fetalis)

endemic a disease that is indigenous to a geographic area or population

endothelium the layer of epithelial cells that lines the cavities of the heart and of the blood and lymph vessels

en face face to face

Engerix-B a currently licensed hepatitis B vaccine that is the result of genetic engineering; the usual schedule of doses is at birth, and then at 1 and 6 months of age; may be given in an alternate four-dose schedule at birth, 1, 2, and 12 months; a recent CDC advisory also recommends administration before 2 months of age, at 2 to 4 months, and at 6 to 18 months

enteric precautions procedures followed in the care of certain patients that are intended to reduce the risk of contamination of personnel or other patients from potentially infected intestinal waste

epigastric pain pain occurring in the right upper quadrant of the abdomen and that is the result of hepatic edema and hemorrhages in the liver capsule

epinephrine a substance produced by the adrenal medulla gland predominantly; it is produced synthetically and is used therapeutically as a vasoconstrictor, cardiac stimulant, and bronchiole relaxant

erythroblastosis a condition of hemolytic disease of the newborn characterized by anemia, jaundice, and enlargement of the liver and spleen

esophageal atresia a closure or absence of the esophagus

euglycemia a normal level of glucose in the blood

external fetal monitoring—also called indirect or noninvasive fetal monitoring; this method involves the use of an ultrasonic transducer and tocodynamometer to monitor fetal heart tones and contractions, respectively; these are held in place by belts

fetal accelerations transitory increase in fetal heart rate associated with uterine contractions; not associated with fetal distress

fetal anencephaly a condition in the fetus in which there is an absence of the brain and spinal cord

fetal attitude relation of fetal parts to each other; the basic attitudes are flexion and extension; for example, when the baby's head is bent toward its chest, the head is in an attitude of flexion

fetal bradycardia decrease in the baseline fetal heart rate to less than 110 bpm

fetal hydrocephaly a condition in the fetus in which there is an increased accumulation of cerebrospinal fluid within the ventricles of the fetus' brain; this leads to rapid head growth; it is a result of interference with normal circulation and absorption of the fluid

fetal karyotype the chromosomal contents found in the cell nucleus of the fetus

fetal lie relationship of the body of the fetus to the body of the mother; fetal lies are longitudinal or transverse; in a longitudinal lie, the fetal body from head to toe is parallel to the length of the mother; in a transverse lie, the fetal body lies at right angles to the mother's body

fetal monitoring type of electronic monitoring in which information about the fetal heart rate and the laboring woman's contraction pattern is continually assessed; *see also* **external fetal monitoring**

fetal presentation within the uterus, the lowest part of the fetus that comes first, either the head, buttocks, or rarely, the shoulders

fetal reserve the amount of oxygen provided to the fetus above that which is needed; it is the oxygen supplied minus the oxygen needed

fetal tachycardia increase in the baseline fetal heart rate to greater than 160 bpm

floating when the presenting part is entirely out of the pelvis and can be moved by the examiner

fontanelle spaces where the sutures of the skull bones meet; "soft spots" on the baby's head

fraud the intentional deception of an individual to gain that person's cooperation in surrendering their property or legal rights

fulminant occurring with great rapidity

gluconeogenesis the synthesis of glucose from noncarbohydrate sources, such as amino acids and glycerol; occurs primarily with the liver and kidneys when carbohydrate supply is low

glycogenolysis the splitting up of glycogen in the liver, which yields glucose

grandmultipara a woman who has had five or more live births

HAART highly active antiretroviral therapy; a combination of antiretroviral medications that work well against HIV

HBIG hepatitis B immune globulin; this substance supplies antibodies needed to provide immediate protection against hepatitis B

HBV hepatitis B virus

helix electrode spiral electrode attached directly to the presenting part of the fetus; determines the fetal heart rate by counting R waves in the fetal ECG; this results in a tracing that allows variability to be assessed; is part of the internal monitoring system

hematoma a tumor or swelling that contains blood

hepatocellular carcinoma (HPC) cancer of the liver

Heptavax B plasma-derived hepatitis B vaccine that is no longer produced in the United States

herpes virus type 1 a serologic subtype of the herpesvirus strain that primarily infects nongenital areas of the body, mainly mucocutaneous tissue of the mouth; however, HSV-1 can cause genital herpes infections as well

herpes virus type 2 a virus that causes infections in the genital organs; it is the second most common venereal disease; when it occurs in the pregnant woman, it has been associated with spontaneous abortion, stillbirths, congenital malformations, and serious infections in the neonate

HIV the human immunodeficiency virus that causes AIDS

  HIV-1 One of five known retroviruses; discovered in 1984 and once called human T-cell lymphotrophic virus type III

  HIV-2 One of five known retroviruses; discovered in 1986 and once called human T-cell lymphotrophic virus type IV

HIV DNA PCR the preferred virologic method for diagnosing HIV infection in infants

HIV infection the acquiring of HIV in the blood and other body fluids and tissues; the individual may have no symptoms whatsoever

HIV RNA test also called viral load or just RNA; a blood test that measures the amount of HIV virus in a person's blood plasma

horizontal transmission transmission of microscopic organisms (e.g., viruses) from one sexual partner to another

HTLV-III a retrovirus known as human T-cell lymphotropic virus type III; this is simply a more specific name for HIV-1

hyaline membrane disease a disease of preterm infants that results in poor lung expansion and therefore respiratory difficulties; often referred to as respiratory distress syndrome

hydatidiform mole the result of a degeneration of the early developing placenta; multiple grape-like cysts develop, along with rapid growth of the uterus and bleeding

hydralazine (Apresoline) an arterial vasodilator used as an antihypertensive agent in the treatment of severe preeclampsia

hydramnios presence of excessive amounts of amniotic fluid (2,000 mL or greater) in the uterus

hyperbilirubinemia excessive amounts of bilirubin in the blood; prenatal conditions in the mother such as diabetes, infections, drug ingestion, and blood incompatibility between mother and fetus can predispose the newborn to hyperbilirubinemia; certain neonatal conditions such as obstruction of the biliary duct or the lower bowel can also predispose the newborn to this condition; treatment to lower and stabilize bilirubin levels is necessary because excessive levels can lead to brain damage

hypertonic uterus labor contractions that last longer than 90 seconds; caused by overstimulation of the uterus

hyperventilation increased inspiration and expiration of air as a result of rapid or deep breathing, which leads to the reduction of carbon dioxide in the blood; symptoms include dizziness, light-headedness, and tingling in the fingers and around the mouth

hypocalcemia abnormally low levels of calcium in the blood

hypoglycemia abnormally low levels of glucose in the blood

hypothermia having a body temperature below normal

hypoxemia decreased oxygen content in the blood

hypoxia insufficient availability of oxygen to meet the body's metabolic needs

iatrogenic caused by treatment or diagnostic procedures

idiosyncratic an abnormal susceptibility to an agent, such as a drug, which is peculiar or unique to the individual

IgM immunoglobulin M; special proteins produced by the lymphatic system against foreign substances shortly after their invasion; they are larger in size than IgG molecules and incapable of crossing the placenta to any great extent; blood levels rise within days of an infection and fall to a nondetectable level within a few months

ileus an intestinal obstruction

immunization becoming immune or the process of rendering a patient immune

immunogenicity the capability to stimulate the formation of antibodies

increased variability a change in fetal heart rate of greater than 25 bpm; *see also* **variability**

indirect fetal monitoring see **external fetal monitoring**

induction artificially starting labor and ensuring ongoing labor, usually through oxytocin administration

internal fetal monitoring also called direct and invasive fetal monitoring; type of electronic monitoring in which the fetal heart rate is monitored by the use of a helix electrode and the laboring woman's contraction pattern is monitored by the use of an intrauterine pressure catheter

intrauterine pressure catheter catheter inserted into the uterine cavity alongside the presenting part of the fetus, allowing baseline uterine tonus and contraction intensity to be assessed; is part of the internal monitoring system

invasive fetal monitoring see **internal fetal monitoring**

ISG immune serum globulin; this substance contains proteins capable of acting as antibodies and thus potentially confers some passive immunity to the individual receiving it

ketosis an excess of ketone bodies in the blood; in uncontrolled diabetes mellitus, there is a great increase in fatty acid metabolism and impaired or absent carbohydrate metabolism, resulting in the increased production of ketone bodies

late deceleration transitory decrease in fetal heart rate caused by uteroplacental insufficiency and associated with fetal distress

lecithin:sphingomyelin ratio (L/S ratio) a complex and fairly lengthy test used to assess lung maturity in the fetus; a ratio of 2.0 or greater usually indicates mature lungs

lithotomy a position in which the woman lies on her back with her thighs drawn up toward her chest, her knees flexed, and her legs extended out to the side

lochia the discharge of blood, mucus, and tissue from the uterus during the postdelivery period

long-term variability rhythmic fluctuations around the fetal heart rate baseline, determined when using an internal or external fetal monitor; *see also* **variability**

L/S ratio See **lecithin:sphingomyelin ratio**

macrosomia large body size, including enlargement of organs such as the liver and spleen

malpractice the failure of a professional person to act in accordance with current accepted professional standards or failure to foresee possibilities and consequences that a professional person, having the necessary skills and training to act professionally, should foresee no matter what the motivation

meconium dark green or black material present in the large intestine of the near-term or term fetus; also the first stool passed by the newborn

mentum chin

microcephaly a congenital deformity in the fetus in which the head is abnormally small in relation to the body; mental retardation is often associated with this condition

midpelvis the most important plane of the pelvis because it has the least room

molding normal overlapping of skull bones of the baby so that the head will fit through the pelvis during labor

monozygotic pertaining to or derived from a single zygote (fertilized ovum), as in a twin gestation occurring from a single fertilization ovum

morbidity state of disease; cases of disease in relation to a specific group or population

mortality death rate; ratio of number of deaths to a specific group or population

multipara a woman who is in other than her first labor

multiple gestation pregnancy with more than one fetus; an example is twins

nasopharynx part of the pharynx situated above the soft palate (postnasal space)

necrotizing enterocolitis a serious illness involving necrotic lesions of the intestines; occurs primarily in preterm or low-birth-weight neonates

noninvasive fetal monitoring see **external fetal monitoring**

nosocomial describes infections that are hospital acquired, in contrast to community-acquired infections

nuchal cord the umbilical cord with one or more loops around the neck of the infant; commonly present and ordinarily does no harm

nullipara a woman in labor for the first time

nulliparous having never given birth to a child

occiput the back of the fetal skull, below and behind the posterior fontanelle

oligohydramnios abnormally small amount of amniotic fluid; an AFI of 5 cm or less

oliguria a severely decreased urinary output of less than 400 mL in 24 hours

opportunistic infection an infection developing in the host organism because of a lowered immune capability

oropharynx the central portion of the pharynx lying between the soft palate and upper portion of the epiglottis

oxytocin a hormone that stimulates the uterus to contract or a drug (Syntocinon or Pitocin) that imitates the natural hormone

oxytoxic having the effect of stimulating the uterus to contract

paracrine a type of hormone function in which the hormone synthesized and released from endocrine cells binds to receptors in nearby cells, affecting their function

parous having had at least one child, either alive or dead at birth

parturition the act or process of giving birth

passive immunity an immunity to a disease produced by injection of material containing the antibodies against a specific disease

pathogen a microorganism or substance capable of producing disease

pelvic planes imaginary flat surfaces passing across parts of the true pelvis at different levels; used to describe dimensions of various parts of the pelvis

perinatal the time between 20 weeks' gestational age and 28 days after birth

perinatal morbidity the frequency or rate of disease among fetuses or infants between 20 weeks' gestational age and 28 days after birth

perinatal mortality the death of a fetus or infant between 20 weeks' gestational age and 28 days after birth

periodic rate changes transient fetal heart rate changes associated with contractions; classified as accelerations or decelerations; *see also* **fetal accelerations** and **fetal decelerations**

placenta the spongy structure attached to the wall of the uterus throughout pregnancy through which nutrients and oxygen pass from the mother's blood to the fetus and through which waste products from the fetus pass into the mother's blood

placenta accreta a placenta abnormally adhered to the myometrium of the uterus

placenta battledore a placenta with the umbilical cord inserted at the edge

placenta circumvallate a placenta encircled with a dense, raised, white nodular ring

placenta previa abnormal implantation of the placenta in the lower uterine segment; classification of the type of previa is based on how close the placenta lies to the cervical opening (os): total, completely covers the os; partial, covers a portion of the os; marginal, is close to the os

plasma the fluid part of the blood

Po$_2$ the partial pressure of oxygen (quantity of O$_2$ in the blood)

Pco$_2$ the partial pressure of carbon dioxide (quantity of CO$_2$ in the blood)

postterm infant an infant with a gestational age of more than 42 weeks; the term *postmature* is also used

preeclampsia a disease occurring during pregnancy (after 20 weeks or during the first week after delivery) with the development of high blood pressure in addition to protein in the urine, edema, or both

prematurity has been used to describe the fetus or infant of less than 37 weeks' gestation; is now being suggested that this term be replaced by the word *preterm* in describing an infant of less than 37 weeks

preterm infant an infant with a gestational age of less than 37 weeks; the term *premature* is sometimes used

primigravida a woman who is pregnant for the first time

primipara a woman who has given birth to her first child, whether or not the child is living or was alive at birth

prodromal a time in which a symptom indicates the onset of a state (e.g., labor or a disease)

progesterone a hormone produced by the ovaries when a woman is not pregnant and by the placenta during pregnancy; it has many important functions, including preventing the uterus from contracting during pregnancy

proinsulin precursor of insulin

prolapsed cord a condition in which the umbilical cord slips down along the side of the fetal presenting part or comes ahead of the presenting part

proliferative retinopathy new blood vessel formation near the optic disk that can extend to growth in the vitreous chamber, rupture, and vitreous hemorrhage; in addition, fibrous tissue is generated and adheres to the posterior vitreous membrane and can lead to retinal detachment

prophylaxis observing procedures or steps to prevent a disease or harmful effect

prostaglandins a group of chemical substances (derivatives of fatty acids) present in many tissues; stimulate the uterus to contract

proteinuria presence in the urine of abnormally large quantities of protein, usually albumin; by definition, occurs with a reading of 2+ on a random urine specimen or when there is 500 mg of protein in a 24-hour specimen (less than 250 mg of protein per day is excreted in the healthy adult)

pyelonephritis inflammation of the kidney caused by an infective process

pyloric stenosis a condition found in the infant in which the opening from the stomach to the small intestines is narrowed so much that partially digested food cannot pass in a normal manner; a characteristic sign of this is highly forceful vomiting

Recombivax B a synthetic, genetically engineered vaccine for hepatitis B

relaxin a hormone secreted by the corpus luteum; acts on smooth muscle of the uterus to produce relaxation of muscle fibers

replication the process of duplicating or reproducing (e.g., replication of an exact copy of a polynucleotide strand of DNA or RNA)

restitute the movement of the newborn head once it is born wherein the neck untwists and the head turns approximately 45 degrees to resume its normal relationship with the shoulders, which are in an anteroposterior position at the pelvic outlet

retrovirus a unique virus form that contains an enzyme, reverse transcriptase, enabling it to synthesize DNA in the cells of a host; this DNA then enters the nucleus of that cell and becomes part of it; the viral DNA (genes) therefore becomes duplicated along with the host's cell genes, and new generations of cells are produced; these new generations contain the virus's genetic material

Rh incompatibility a lack of compatibility between two groups of blood cells having different antigens; caused by the presence of the Rh factor in one group and its absence in the other

scotomata the presence of specks or spots in the vision disturbing vision temporarily; this is suggestive of lesions in the retina or visual pathway

semi-Fowler's position a semisitting position in which the patient is positioned at approximately 45 degrees

sensitivity the probability that a test will be positive when infection or a specific condition is present

seroconversion the process of blood serum developing an antibody response to a specific antigen (e.g., a virus or bacteria)

seropositive producing a positive reaction to serologic tests

serous exudate an accumulation of a fluid, having the nature of serum, in a cavity or on a surface

serum that part of blood that remains after clotting has occurred

short-term variability irregular, beat-to-beat changes from the fetal heart rate baseline; determined when using a helix electrode and indicative of fetal reserve; *see also* **variability**

shoulder dystocia difficult delivery of the shoulders of the fetus

sinciput the brow or forehead of the fetus

sinusoidal pattern a baseline pattern that demonstrates a regular undulating pattern above and below the fetal heart baseline; can be a sign of severe fetal anemia or fetal asphyxia or may be the effect of certain medications

spaces used in conduction anesthesia the spinal cord is covered by three layers; the outermost layer is the dura, the middle layer is the arachnoid, and the inner layer is the pia

    arachnoid space the arachnoid space is between the middle and inner layer covering the spinal cord and contains the spinal fluid

    extradural space (epidural, peridural) a space found outside the outermost covering of the spinal cord into which chemicals may be injected for the purpose of inducing anesthesia

subdural space a space found between the outermost and the middle layer of the spinal cord

specificity the probability that a test will be negative when the infection or specific condition is not present

spina bifida a congenital defect in the walls of the spinal canal caused by lack of union between parts of the vertebrae; as a result, the membranes of the spinal cord are pushed through the opening, forming a tumor

standards of practice accepted published professional levels of care for which the individual professional is held accountable; the legal profession and courts use these in malpractice cases

steroids chemical compounds that make up, among other things, hormones found in humans; many drugs are composed of steroids

strip graph tracing produced on graph paper by the electronic fetal monitor; allows fetal heart rate and contraction patterns to be continually assessed

SUDS single-use diagnostic system; the only HIV-1 rapid test that is licensed by the Food and Drug Administration for use in the United States

surfactant a mixture of phospholipid (primarily lecithin and sphingomyelin) secreted by alveolar cells into the alveoli and respiratory air passages, which reduces the surface tension of pulmonary fluids and contributes to the elastic properties of pulmonary tissue

sutures spaces between the bones of the fetal skull, which are covered by membranes

tachycardia, fetal see **fetal tachycardia**

term infant an infant with a gestational age of 38 to 42 weeks

therapeutic privilege refers to withholding information about a treatment or medication when the individual's health would be significantly jeopardized by full disclosure of the information

thermoregulation the regulation of temperature, especially body temperature

thrombocytopenia an abnormal decrease in the number of blood platelets, usually caused by the destruction of erythroid tissue in bone marrow, which can be brought about by certain neoplastic diseases or an immune response to a drug; bleeding disorders are a consequence

thrombophlebitis inflammation of a vein; associated with the formation of a blood clot

tocodynamometer part of an external monitoring system that provides information about the laboring woman's contraction pattern by detecting changes in the shape of her abdominal wall directly above the uterine fundus

tocolytic an effect of quieting or inhibiting smooth muscle activity; the myometrium of the uterus is composed of smooth muscle

trophoblastic disease a disease resulting from degeneration in the early development of the placenta; a hydatidiform mole results

tubal sterilization an operative procedure using ligation, surgical closure, and/or cauterization to render the fallopian tubes incapable of sperm or ova transport

ultrasonic transducer part of the external monitoring system that monitors fetal heart rate by detecting movement within the fetal heart as the heart valves open and close; similar to sonar

uterine atony the loss of normal tone of the muscles of the uterus; results in relaxation of the muscles that normally control postpartum uterine bleeding

uterine dystocia abnormal labor or difficult labor

uterine tonus degree of muscle tone within the uterus; *see also* **baseline uterine tonus**

uteroplacental insufficiency compromised blood flow through the placenta that results in the fetus not receiving the amount of oxygen needed to withstand the stress of labor; *see* **late deceleration**

variability normal, irregular, beat-to-beat changes and fluctuations around the baseline fetal heart rate indicative of a mature fetal neurologic system and used as a measure of fetal reserve; *see also* **increased variability, decreased variability, average variability, long-term variability,** and **short-term variability**

variable deceleration transitory decrease in fetal heart rate caused by umbilical cord compression or occlusion; associated with fetal distress if the decelerations are severe and prolonged and there is a loss of variability

velamentous cord insertion the major vessels found in the cord separate in the membranes at a distance from the edge of the placenta where they are surrounded only by a fold of amnion

vertex the top of the skull between the anterior and posterior fontanelles

vertical transmission transmission of microscopic organisms (e.g., viruses) to the fetus and newborn either through breaks in the placental barrier during pregnancy or at the time of birth

vibroacoustic stimulation process of fetal stimulation using sound; objective is to elicit a fetal startle or movement that is then used to evaluate fetal status

viral replication the process of a virus reproducing itself

viremia (viremic) a state of having viruses in the blood

virulent very poisonous; infectious

voluntariness the circumstances surrounding an individual's giving consent

Western blot a supplemental laboratory test that detects specific antibodies to components of a virus; mainly used to validate repeatedly reactive enzyme immunoassays (EIA) or enzyme-linked immunoassays (ELISA) for HIV infection; is highly specific when strict criteria are used to interpret the results; when a repeatedly reactive EIA or ELISA and a positive Western blot test occur, it is highly predictive of HIV infection, even in a population with a low prevalence of infection

Sexually Transmitted Diseases: Overview, Perinatal Issues, and Management

Introduction

Sexually transmitted diseases (STDs) pose multiple threats in pregnancy. Maternal infection with an STD is often associated with spontaneous abortion, fetal anomalies, stillbirth, preterm labor, and low birth weight, as well as increased neonatal morbidity and mortality and long-term adverse health consequences in childhood.

Most of the diseases outlined in this appendix are defined as STDs. Although not currently categorized as such, bacterial vaginosis (BV), group B streptococcus (GBS) infection, and candidiasis (monilia) are included in this appendix because of the potential adverse perinatal events associated with them.

Infections with HIV, hepatitis B virus (HBV), hepatitis C virus (HCV), herpes simplex virus 1 and 2 (HSV-1 and HSV-2, respectively), and human papillomavirus (HPV) currently have no associated cures. With the exception of HBV infection, no vaccines exist to offer prevention or protection. During admission of the laboring woman, careful attention to her prenatal history, physical examination, and laboratory workup can identify the presence of an unresolved, untreated, or undertreated STD or the potential for such.

When such risk is diagnosed, therapies and preventive strategies for the birthing process and postpartum can be integrated into the mother's nursing and medical management. Newborn evaluation and appropriate therapy can be instituted immediately. The challenge is to identify the risk! Subsequent education during the postpartum period will affect the mother's understanding of the infection, self-care, and prevention. It is especially important that the mother appreciates any need for special newborn care, including early symptoms and the need for prompt medical attention.

Bacterial Vaginosis

Bacterial vaginosis (BV) is a condition in which normal hydrogen peroxide–producing lactobacillus predominant in the healthy vagina are replaced with anaerobic bacteria, mostly *Gardnerella vaginalis, Mobiluncus* species, and *Mycoplasma hominis.*

Although not considered a definitive STD, BV has epidemiologic elements consistent with those of an STD.

Epidemiology[1-5]

- The prevalence of BV in pregnant women is similar to that in the general population.[1]
- In the United States, BV is found in approximately 25% to 40% of African American women and in approximately 10% to 15% of Caucasian women.[2]
- BV is associated with spontaneous preterm birth, preterm rupture of membranes, infection of the chorion and amnion, and amniotic fluid infection.[1,4]
- The alteration in the vaginal environment (vaginal flora) in BV during pregnancy is associated with a 1.5- to 4.0-fold increased risk of preterm birth and approximately twice the likelihood of preterm labor. This may point to one reason for the higher rate of preterm births in African American women.[3]
- Research in pregnant and nonpregnant women suggests that BV in the lower genital tract is associated with an increased risk of infection in the upper genital tract; upper genital tract involvement may be one mechanism by which infection leads to inflammation, uterine contractions, and subsequent preterm labor.[2,3]
- Studies indicate that BV may be more associated with early preterm birth than with late preterm birth.[2]
- It is uncertain whether BV should be classified as an STD or whether it is simply a situation of abnormal microbial colonization.[2,5]

Clinical Features[2,5-7]

- The vagina harbors both Gram-positive and Gram-negative bacteria. However, only relatively few different types of bacteria are found in large numbers in the healthy vaginal environment. Lactobacilli are a dominant bacteria and contribute to the maintenance of a healthy vaginal environment with a pH of 3.8 to less than 4.5.
- The loss of normally occurring (endogenous) vaginal lactobacilli is important in the acquisition of BV. The loss of these lactobacilli correlates with a loss of vaginal acidity (pH greater than 4.5) seen in BV.[5]
- Hormonal changes (e.g., during menstruation and pregnancy) appear to play a significant role in stimulating lactobacilli loss.[5]
- Risk factors consistently associated with BV (and other STDs) include smoking (this may simply be a marker for sexual behavior, however), racial origin, contraceptive practice (oral contraceptive use), and sexual activity practice.[5]

- BV is seen somewhat more frequently in conjunction with other STDs and occurs more often in women who are sexually active than in women who are not.[2]
- Many women and their infants who harbor anaerobic bacteria such as *Gardnerella vaginalis, Mobiluncus* species, and *Mycoplasmas* never manifest any signs of infection or adverse outcomes.[2] Therefore, "colonization" and "disease" are seen as different entities with different consequences.
- BV is strongly associated with age greater than 25 years. This is contrary to most STDs, whose highest rates are almost always in women younger than 25.[5]
- The pathogenesis associated with BV (and other vaginal infections) is believed to result, in part, from enzymes and endotoxins that weaken the amniotic membrane, leading to bacterial penetration of the intrauterine environment and subsequent infection and labor stimulation.[5,6]
- Causal relationship between BV and infertility, pelvic inflammatory disease, miscarriage, postpartum endometritis, and other gynecologic conditions is unknown and under investigation.[5,7]

Perinatal Consequences[5,6,8]

- Forty percent of preterm births are associated with an etiology related to infection, but just how much of the infection incidence is related to BV is unknown.[5,6]
- Findings indicate that as many as 80% of early preterm births (24 to 28 weeks' gestation) are associated with intrauterine infection.[8]
- African American women experience a disproportionate incidence of preterm birth. BV and other vaginal infections and low birth weight account for 40% of those births.[5,8]
- Preterm birth and low birth weight are major contributors to infant mortality, as well as infant and early childhood morbidity.
- The presence of BV increases a woman's susceptibility to HIV infection.[5]

Screening/Diagnosis[1,9–12]

- A detailed gynecologic and obstetric history should accompany a workup for BV.
- Diagnosis is not difficult and is usually made according to Amsel criteria; that is, three of the following four elements must be present to make the diagnosis. The four criteria are (1) the presence of a thin homogeneous discharge (usually profuse and grayish white in color), (2) a vaginal pH of greater than 4.5, (3) a positive "whiff" test (fishy odor), and (4) the presence of "clue" cells under microscopic examination (called a "wet prep").
- Vaginal cultures are unreliable and are not used.
- Half of all woman who meet the current criteria for the diagnosis of BV are asymptomatic.
- Controversy exists regarding the value of treating asymptomatic nonpregnant women because of the low response rates and treatment side effects.[9]
- Currently, *universal* testing is not recommended for *nonpregnant* women because there is a high rate of recurrence, concern regarding microbial resistance development, and a lack of documentation of the effectiveness of prepregnancy detection/treatment for preterm birth prevention.[1]
- Many clinicians believe that routine screening for most STDs and BV is needed during early pregnancy, especially in high-risk populations.[10,11] Adverse outcomes with BV appear to be much more significant when infection is present before 20 weeks' gestation.
- The American College of Nurse-Midwives advocates BV testing for all women during the first prenatal visit. Testing should be a standard part of care for women who have a history of previous preterm birth, a diagnosed STD, or bleeding in the current pregnancy—regardless of whether symptoms are present or not.[1]
- The Centers for Disease Control and Prevention (CDC) recommends evaluation and treatment for women at high risk of adverse pregnancy outcomes in the second trimester and treatment of low-risk, symptomatic woman.[1,12]

Treatment[10,12]

- There is no consensus regarding the approach to the treatment of BV. The recommendations that follow are according 1998 CDC guidelines.
- Treatment regimens are as follows:
  - Metronidazole 250 mg orally, three doses daily for 5 to 7 days (This dosage is offered to minimize possible adverse fetal effects.)
  - Metronidazole 2 g as a single oral dose
  - Metronidazole 500 mg orally, twice daily for 5 days
  - Clindamycin 300 mg orally, twice daily for 7 days
  - Metronidazole vaginal gel 0.75%, one full application (5 g) intravaginally twice daily for 5 days
  - Clindamycin cream 2%, one full application (5 g) intravaginally at bedtime for 7 days

Note: Oral doses are preferred. Vaginal administration of drugs has less systemic efficacy for the treatment of upper genital infection. The CDC states that concerns regarding teratogenicity of metronidazole in humans have not been borne out in a recent meta-analysis (review of many studies conducted on the topic).

- Follow-up evaluation is as follows:
  - Retesting in nonpregnant women is currently not considered necessary.[12]
  - In pregnant women, especially high-risk pregnant women who are asymptomatic, follow-up testing is recommended 1 month after treatment is completed to ensure that therapy was successful. This may prevent adverse pregnancy outcomes.[12]

REFERENCES

1. ACNM Clinical Bulletins (1999). Clinical Bulletin No. 4—December 1998. Bacterial vaginosis in pregnancy. *Journal of Nurse-Midwifery, 44*(2), 129–134.
2. Goldenberg, R. L., Andrews, W. W., Yuan, A. C., Mackay, H. T., & St. Louis, M. E. (1997). Sexually transmitted diseases and adverse outcomes of pregnancy. *Clinics in Perinatology, 24*(1), 23–41.
3. Berkman, N. D., Thorp, J. M., Hartman, K. E., et al. (2000, December). *Management of preterm labor. Evidence Report/Technology Assessment No. 18* (Prepared by Research Triangle Institute under Contract No. 290-97-0011). AHRQ Publication No. 01-E021 (pp. 18–20). Rockville, MD: Agency for Healthcare Research and Quality.
4. Cunningham, F. G., Gant, N. F., Leveno, K. J., Gilstrap, L. C., Hauth, J. C., & Wenstrom, K. D. (Eds.). (2001). *Williams obstetrics* (21st ed., pp. 1485–1513). New York: McGraw-Hill.
5. Morris, M., Nicoll, A., Simms, I., Wilson, J., & Catchpole, M. (2001). Bacterial vaginosis: A public health view. *British Journal of Obstetrics and Gynecology, 108,* 439–450.
6. Hill, G. B. (1998). Preterm birth: Associates with genital and possibly oral microflora. *Annuals of Periodontology, 3*(1), 222–232.
7. Sweet, R. L. (2000). Gynecologic conditions and bacterial vaginosis: Implications for the non-pregnant patient. *Infectious Disease in Obstetrics and Gynecology, 8*(3–4), 184–190.
8. Goldenberg, R. L. (1998). Low birthweight in minority and high-risk women. Patient Outcomes Research Team final report. (Contract Number 290-92-0055) (pp. 16–20, 64–65). Rockville, MD: Agency for Health Care Policy and Research.
9. Schwebke, J. R. (2000). Asymptomatic bacterial vaginosis: Response to therapy. *American Journal of Obstetrics and Gynecology, 183*(6), 1434–1439.
10. Donders, G. G. (2000). Treatment of sexually transmitted bacterial diseases in pregnant women. *Drugs, 59*(3), 477–485.
11. Donders, G. G. (1999). Bacterial vaginosis during pregnancy: Screen or treat [Guest Editorial]. *European Journal of Obstetrics and Gynecology, 83,* 1–4.
12. Centers for Disease Control and Prevention. (1998). 1998 guidelines for treatment of sexually transmitted diseases. *MMWR Morbidity and Mortality Weekly Report, 47*(RR-1), 70–74.

Candidiasis Vaginalis (Monilia)

Candidal vulvovaginal infection is a common fungal infection usually caused by one of three *Candida* species: *C. albicans, C. glabrata,* or *C. tropicalis. C. albicans* is the causative agent in 80% to 90% of infections, but the other two species are increasingly being associated with infection.[1,2]

Epidemiology[2,3]

- Candidiasis is the second most common vaginal infection in women (BV being the most common).[2]
- Approximately 75% of women will have at least one infection in their lifetime, and approximately 45% will experience two or more episodes.[3]
- Epidemiologic data on the disease are incomplete. It is nonreportable, often self-treated or self-diagnosed without the benefit of microscopy or culture.

Clinical Features

- Symptoms include pruritus, vaginal discharge, vaginal soreness, vulvar burning, painful intercourse (dyspareunia), and painful urination (dysuria).
- Erythema in the vulvovaginal area; white, cheesy patches adhering to the vaginal walls; or a thin, watery discharge may be observed on inspection.
- It is generally not considered a sexually transmitted disease; however, it appears to be sexually associated because there is increased frequency of the infection at the time women become sexually active.
- Risk for acquiring vulvovaginal candidal infection is associated with uncontrolled diabetes, use of oral contraceptives containing high levels of estrogen, and antibiotic use.
- Candidal organisms are ubiquitous in nature and part of the microbial flora in humans. Pregnancy may predispose some women to candidiasis due to significant increases in estrogen, which alter glycogen content in the vagina. Although various species of *Candida* normally inhabit the vagina, any change in vaginal homeostasis may permit an overgrowth on fungi, resulting in infection.

Perinatal Consequences[4,5]

- Vulvovaginal candidiasis commonly occurs during pregnancy. The organism can be cultured from the vagina in approximately 25% of women nearing term.[4]
- Maternal vaginal infection does not appear to have any association with preterm birth.[4]
- *Candida* species may be transmitted to the newborn from the vagina during birth.
- The clinical manifestations in the newborn vary depending the on location and extent of the infection. Thrush is an infection of the buccal mucosa, gingiva, and tongue. *Candida* also can appear as a diaper dermatitis.[5]
- Newborns and especially infants with very low birth weight (VLBW) have qualitative and quantitative deficiencies in humoral and cellular immunity. This can allow *Candida* to penetrate lymphatics, blood vessels, and other tissues, resulting in disseminated infection.[5]

Screening/Diagnosis[3]

- Maternal diagnosis is most frequently done by microscopic examination of vaginal discharge to visualize the yeast and mycelia or pseudohyphae. Gram's stain and culture can also be done. *Note that a positive culture in the absence of symptoms should not lead to treatment.* As has been stated, *Candida* species are a part of many women's vaginal flora.[3]
- Newborn evaluation *of local infection* can be done by microscopic examination (wet prep) of the local site. Newborn disseminated *candidiasis* is diagnosed by blood culture.

Treatment

Maternal Treatment[1-3]

A number of over-the-counter (OTC) treatments are available to women and provide greater than 80% cure rates in women with uncomplicated infection. *Examples of OTC vaginal creams include the following:*

Butoconazole (Femstat) 2% cream, 5 g per vagina for 3 days
Clotrimazole (Gyne-Lotrimin, Mycelex) 1% cream, 5 g per vagina at bedtime for 7 to 14 days
Miconazole (Monostat), 2% cream, 5 g per vagina for 7 days

Examples of prescriptive regimens include the following:

Terconazole (Terazol) 0.4% cream, 5 g per vagina for 7 days
Terconazole, 80-mg suppository, 1 suppository per vagina at bedtime for 3 days
Oral medication: fluconazole (Diflucan) 150-mg oral tablet, 1 tablet only; contraindicated in pregnancy

Regimen for pregnancy includes the following antifungal agents:

Butoconazole
Clotrimazole
Miconazole
Terconazole

Newborn Treatment[5]

- Treatment varies with the location and extent of infection and the infant's age.
- *Thrush* is usually treated with nystatin (Mycostatin) suspension, 1 to 2 mL given orally four times each day for 5 to 10 days.
- *Candida diaper dermatitis* is treated with nystatin ointment three times a day for 7 to 10 days. Nystatin with a corticosteroid (mycology ointment) is used in severe cases.
- Systemic or disseminated candidal infection is treated with amphotericin B. This is the mainstay of therapy for the newborn infant and is well tolerated by the VLBW infant.

REFERENCES

1 Sobel J. D. (1997). Vaginitis. *The New England Journal of Medicine, 337*(26), 1896–1902.
2. Andrist L. C. (2001). Vaginal health and infections. *Journal of Obstetric, Gynecologic and Neonatal Nursing, 30*(3), 306–315.
3. Centers for Disease Control and Prevention. (1998). 1998 guidelines for treatment of sexually transmitted diseases. *MMWR Morbidity and Mortality Weekly Report, 47*(RR-1), 75–79.
4. Cunningham, F. G., Gant, N. F., Leveno, K. J., Gilstrap, L. C., Hauth, J. C., & Wenstrom, K. D. (Eds.). (2001). *Williams obstetrics* (21st ed., pp. 244, 700). New York: McGraw-Hill.
5. Edwards, M. S. (2002). The immune system: Part three. Fungal and protozoal infections. In A. A. Fanaroff & R. J. Martin (Eds.), *Neonatal-perinatal medicine: Diseases of the fetus and infant* (Vol. 2., 7th ed., pp. 745–748). St. Louis: Mosby.

Chlamydia

Chlamydia is a bacteria whose most common strains infect the mucosal epithelium (columnar or transitional) of the genital tract, causing infection of the cervix and, when untreated, infection of the upper genital tract.

Epidemiology[1-3]

- Chlamydia is the most common bacterial STD in the United States and is common in pregnant women. Infection in pregnancy can have serious maternal and newborn consequences.[1]
- From 3 to 4 million new cases are estimated to occur in the United States each year. The World Health Organization (WHO) reports that 90 million infections are detected annually worldwide. Infection is significantly underreported because of asymptomatic infection. Simple, cost-effective screening tests are not available.[2]
- The highest rates are seen in 15- to 19-year-old adolescents.
- Prevalence rates are higher among women of childbearing age in STD clinics; urban, inner-city poor women; and non-Caucasian women.
- Undiagnosed, untreated infection leads to pelvic inflammatory disease (PID), which is a major cause of infertility among women; estimates are that one third of infections result in PID. Ectopic pregnancy is another adverse outcome.
- Many infected men and women have no symptoms at all.
- Newborns can acquire the infection through vertical transmission during delivery.

- Despite effective therapy, approximately 155,000 infants are born to infected mothers annually.[3] Consequences are more damaging to the reproductive health of women than of men.[1] Untreated partners, noncompliance in treatment, reinfection, and lack of prenatal care all play a role.

Clinical Features[3]

- Risk factors are age younger than 25, the presence or history of other STDs, multiple sexual partners, and a new partner within 3 months.
- Epithelial tissues of the urethra, rectum, conjunctiva, and the nasopharynx are susceptible to infection.
- Infection of cervical epithelial tissue may extend to the endometrium, salpinx, and peritoneum (PID).
- Perinatal transmission may be transplacental (intrauterine) or through exposure to maternal secretions such as breast milk; however, transmission most commonly occurs through exposure to maternal blood and vaginal secretions at the time of delivery.
- This infection is often found concomitantly with gonorrhea.
- Recent research indicates a threefold to fivefold increased risk of acquiring HIV when chlamydia infection is present. As many as 70% of women may have no symptoms.
- Signs of local (cervical) infection are mucopurulent discharge and a friable cervix. Bleeding occurs when the cervix is touched (e.g., in obtaining a Pap smear or simply swabbing with a cotton-tipped applicator).

Perinatal Consequences[1,3–6]

- Approximately 50% of infants delivered vaginally of an infected mother will become infected.
- Among infected infants, as many as one third will develop conjunctivitis.
- Afebrile pneumonia in infants up to 3 months of age is often caused by maternally transmitted chlamydial infection. The infection often occurs weeks after hospital discharge.
- Effective prenatal screening and maternal treatment would prevent neonatal infection. However, reinfection during pregnancy is not uncommon, especially among adolescents and inner-city minority young women.
- Clinical studies indicate a role of recent chlamydial infections in pregnant women with adverse pregnancy outcomes such as premature and preterm labor and rupture of membranes.[5]
- Genitourinary infection at 24 weeks' gestation has been found to be associated with a twofold to threefold increased risk of subsequent preterm birth.[6]

Screening/Diagnosis[4]

- Diagnosis by culture is the most common current method, but DNA probes and polymerase chain reaction (PCR) techniques are evolving into less expensive and quicker tests.
- Universal prenatal screening is currently not considered cost effective.
- The CDC recommends the following[4]:
  –Screening all sexually active women younger than 20 years of age at least annually
  –Performing annual screening of women ages 20 and older who have one or more risk factors (new or multiple sex partner and lack of barrier contraception)
  –Testing all women with cervical infection and all pregnant women
- When screening/testing for chlamydia, one should also test for gonorrhea in susceptible adults and neonates.

Treatment

Maternal Treatment[3,4,7,8]

- Appropriate completed treatment prevents transmission to sex partners and to infants during birth.

NOTE: *Treatment of the infected individual and partner should be done at the same time. Both partners should abstain from intercourse until treatment is completed.*

- Treatment regimens are as follows[4]:
  –Azithromycin, 1 g orally in a single dose, ensures compliance.
  –*Other regimens for pregnant women include the following:*
     Erythromycin base, 500 mg orally four times a day for 7 days
     Amoxicillin, 500 mg orally three times a day for 7 days

NOTE: *Doxycycline and ofloxacin are contraindicated in pregnancy.*

- Treatment success is affected by key factors such as compliance, or rather noncompliance (failure to take all of the medication in the prescribed time, which can be done for many different reasons, including cost); tolerance of the medication itself; efficacy of the drug and choice; and partner treatment and compliance.
- A common problem in treatment during pregnancy is patient compliance in completing the treatment regimen. Erythromycin is tolerated poorly by many pregnant women primarily because of gastrointestinal side effects, including nausea, vomiting, cramps or pain, and diarrhea. Amoxicillin and clindamycin also have adverse side effects, but at lower occurrence rates. Azithromycin also can have mild to moderate side effects in some women.[7]
- Miller and Martin provide an excellent analysis of treatment issues and conclude that the best choices for treating chlamydial infections in pregnant women are amoxicillin or azithromycin.[7] Compliance issues, drug cost, treatment doses, and re-treatment rates were among several important elements considered.

Neonatal Treatment[8]

- The recommended regimen for ophthalmia neonatorum caused by *C. trachomatis* is as follows:
  - Erythromycin base, 50 mg/kg per day, orally divided into four doses daily for 10 to 14 days. Topical treatment is ineffective and not recommended. Preliminary data indicate that a short course of azithromycin treatment may be effective but is still under study.[8]

REFERENCES

1. Paavonen, J., & Eggert-Kruse, W. (1999). *Chlamydia trachomatis:* Impact on human reproduction. *Human Reproduction Update, 5*(5), 433–447.
2. Chlamydia in the United States. (2001, April). Available at: http://www.cdc.gov/nchstp/dstd/ Fact_Sheets/chlamydia_facts.htm.
3. Cunningham, F. G., Gant, N. F., Leveno, K. J., Gilstrap, L. C., Hauth, J. C., & Wenstrom, K. D. (Eds.). (2001). *Williams obstetrics* (21st ed., pp. 1485–1513). New York: McGraw-Hill.
4. Centers for Disease Control and Prevention. (1998). 1998 guidelines for treatment of sexually transmitted diseases. *MMWR Morbidity and Mortality Weekly Report, 47*(RR-1): 53–59.
5. Berkman, N. D., Thorp, J. M., Hartman, K. E., et al. (2000, December). *Management of preterm labor.* Evidence Report/Technology Assessment No. 18 (Prepared by Research Triangle Institute under Contract No. 290-97-0011). AHRQ Publication No. 01-E021 (pp. 18–20). Rockville: MD: Agency for Healthcare Research and Quality.
6. Andrews, W. W., Goldenberg, R. L., Mercer, B., Iams, J., Meis, P., Moawad, A., Das, A., Vandorsten, J. P., Caritis, S. N., Thurnau, G., Miodovnik, M., Roberts, J., & McNellis, D. (2000). The Preterm Prediction Study: Association of second-trimester genitourinary chlamydia infection with subsequent spontaneous preterm birth. *American Journal of Obstetrics and Gynecology, 183*(3), 662–668.
7. Miller, J. M., & Martin, D. H. (2000). Treatment of *Chlamydia trachomatis* infections in pregnant women. *Drugs, 60*(3), 597–605.
8. Edwards, M. S. (2002). Part two: Postnatal bacterial infections. In A. A. Fanaroff & R. J. Martin (Eds.), *Neonatal-perinatal medicine: Diseases of the fetus and infant* (Vol. 2., 7th ed., pp. 724–726). St. Louis: Mosby.

Gonorrhea

Gonorrhea is a bacterial infection of the mucous membranes of the genitourinary tract; it is caused by the bacterium *Neisseria gonorrhoeae.*

Epidemiology[1-3]

- The incidence of gonorrhea for 1998 was 133 cases per 100,000 population.[1]
- The disease is transmitted almost exclusively by sexual contact.[3]
- The presence of gonorrhea is a marker for the possibility of concomitant chlamydial infection.
- The prevalence during pregnancy may be as high as 7%.[2]
- Risk factors include adolescence, drug abuse, prostitution, and poverty, as well as being single or having other STDs.
- Adolescents experience some of the highest rates.
- Newborns may acquire the infection during delivery through an infected birth canal.
- Gonorrhea is the most common STD in sexually abused children.

Clinical Features[3,4]

- The risk of a woman being infected by an infected male partner is approximately 50% per episode of vaginal intercourse. The risk of a male being infected by an infected female is 20% per episode of vaginal intercourse.[3]
- Although rectal intercourse is an effective mode of transmission, oral-genital transmission is rare.
- Immunity is not conferred by infection.
- Most cases either resolve spontaneously or are treated and resolve within a few weeks.[3]
- Most infections are symptomatic, but asymptomatic infections do occur.
- Signs and symptoms are painful urination (dysuria), usually without frequency or urgency; purulent cervical discharge; bleeding upon swabbing the cervix; and cervical, uterine, or adnexal tenderness.
- Disseminated gonococcal infection results from gonococcal bacteremia and has been cited as occurring in 0.5% to 3% of infected individuals. In pregnant women, stillbirth and spontaneous abortion are risks.[3]

Perinatal Consequences[2,3]

- Gonococcal infection may result in adverse pregnancy outcomes in any of the trimesters. Preterm delivery, premature rupture of membranes, chorioamnionitis, and postpartum infection are associated with infection at the time of delivery.[2]
- Ophthalmia neonatorum is the most common form of gonorrhea in infants and occurs through vertical transmission from an infected mother during delivery. Without prompt treatment, blindness can occur as a result of corneal ulceration and perforation.
- Isolation of an infected infant is recommended until treatment has been in effect for 24 hours.[2]

Screening/Diagnosis[2,3]

- Laboratory diagnosis depends on identification of *N. gonorrhoeae* at an infected site.
- A screening test for gonorrhea is recommended at the first prenatal visit, and a repeat test should be done after 28 weeks' gestation in high-risk populations.[2]

- Repeat testing in the third trimester is recommended in any pregnant woman who tested positive at an earlier workup because reinfection is common.[2]
- Diagnosis is done by culture, Gram's stain, or detection of bacterial DNA genes.
- **Syphilis and chlamydia screening is strongly recommended in any individual who has tested positive for gonorrhea because these infections are commonly found concomitantly with gonorrheal infection.**

Treatment[2-4]

- For uncomplicated gonococcal infections during pregnancy, treatment consists of ceftriaxone, 125 mg intramuscularly (IM; single dose); **or** cefixime, 400 mg orally (single dose); **or** spectinomycin, 2 g IM (single dose).[2]
- Intrapartum prophylaxis for the newborn is instituted by the instillation of a 1% aqueous solution of silver nitrate into the conjunctiva soon after delivery. Topical application of erythromycin or tetracycline ointment can also be used.
- Treatment failures can occur.
- Both parents of an infected infant should be treated and screened for chlamydia.

REFERENCES

1. Centers for Disease Control and Prevention. (2000). Gonorrhea—United States, 1998. *MMWR Morbidity and Mortality Weekly Report, 49*(24),538–542.
2. Cunningham, F. G., Gant, N. F., Leveno, K. J., Gilstrap, L. C., Hauth, J. C., & Wenstrom, K. D. (Eds.). (2001). *Williams obstetrics* (21st ed., pp. 1485–1513). New York: McGraw-Hill.
3. Darville, T. (1999) Gonorrhea. *Pediatrics in Review, 20*(4), 125–128.
4. Centers for Disease Control and Prevention. (1998). 1998 guidelines for treatment of sexually transmitted diseases. *MMWR Morbidity and Mortality Weekly Report, 47*(RR-1): 59–70.

Group B Streptococcus Infection

Group B streptococcus (GBS) is a Gram-positive bacteria with several different serotypes. The organism occurs naturally in both men and women. Serotypes Ia, II, III, and V cause up to 90% of all cases in the United States. Serotype III is the most common cause of early-onset (first week of life) meningitis and late-onset (1 week to several months after birth) infection. It is a major cause of neonatal morbidity and mortality, although recent screening and treatment recommendations are beginning to bring about some reduction in incidence.[1,2]

Terminology

Colonization—The presence of microorganisms in an organ or tissue of the body with or without any pathology. The presence of the organism is determined by culture. A positive culture does not indicate infection but rather that the individual harbors or carries the organism without adverse consequences. For example, if the organism is obtained from surfaces such as skin, ears, or umbilical cord or from gastric contents in a healthy individual, exposure to the organism and colonization are documented. However, infection is not necessarily present.

Infection—The invasion by microorganisms of a body site that is normally considered sterile (e.g., bladder, amniotic fluid, blood, lungs, cerebrospinal fluid), causing disease by local cellular injury, secretion of toxins, and other pathologic mechanisms.

Invasive disease—High bacterial load affecting major body systems and inducing serious pathologic events, such as meningitis and respiratory distress.

NOTE: *GBS resides in the gastrointestinal tract of many individuals (men and women) without causing any complications. However, close approximation of the anus to the introitus and urethra facilitates colonization of the vagina and urinary tract with GBS. Antibiotic treatment sufficient to eliminate GBS in the gastrointestinal tract of a colonized individual is not possible. Treatment will eradicate the organism or, in instances of heavy colonization, lower the colony count, for locally colonized or infected sites such as the cervix, vagina, or bladder. Recolonization of those sites remains a possibility. GBS colonization of the maternal genital tract involves the most risk to the newborn because of exposure during the birth process. Medical management of the maternal carrier aims at reducing infection risks for both mother and neonate.*

Epidemiology[2-6]

- GBS is the most common cause of sepsis and meningitis in neonates and young infants, affecting 1% to 3% per 1,000 neonates.[4]
- Most neonatal infections occur in the first few days of life (early onset).
- Reinfection can occur in a small percentage of neonates, and often this is at a new site.
- The lower female genital tract, that is, the lower third of the vagina, the vaginal introitus, and the rectum, are the most common sites of colonization. The upper third of the vagina and cervix are less commonly colonized. The urethra can be colonized, leading to urinary tract involvement.[6]
- Colonization of the lower maternal genital tract can lead to chorioamnionitis, postpartum endometritis, and neonatal infection. Each year, approximately 50,000 women are diagnosed with GBS-associated chorioamnionitis or endometritis.[5,6]
- Although approximately 15% to 40% of pregnant women are estimated to be colonized with GBS, prevalence varies with populations and geographic location and from hospital to hospital (perhaps because of policies, or lack thereof, for intrapartum maternal treatment). Higher rates are found in African Americans and nonsmokers.[3]
- GBS is a common cause of bacteremia (urinary tract infection) in pregnant women. This can be asymptomatic in a small percentage of

women and can lead to pyelonephritis if untreated.
- It is the most common cause of intrapartal acute chorioamnionitis.

Clinical Features[3-6]

- Early-onset GBS infection is caused by vertical transmission whereby the organism invades the amniotic membranes and infects the fetus in utero. Many newborns are infected before birth.
- Although perhaps half of newborns are exposed to GBS when membranes rupture or during the birth process, only a small percentage (1% to 2%) will develop the *disease.*[3]
- Maternal risk factors associated with *early-onset newborn disease* include a positive vaginal/rectal culture, rupture of membranes 18 hours or more before delivery, delivery before 37 weeks' gestation, maternal fever, GBS-positive urine culture during pregnancy, and a history of having a GBS-infected newborn.[6]
- Maternal risk factors associated with *late-onset neonatal infection* are thought to be vertical transmission and hospital-acquired infection.[3,6]

NOTE: When a GBS-positive infant has been identified, isolation of the infant is not recommended. Outbreaks in nurseries do not occur.[3]

- Intrapartal risk factors for GBS infection include the following[5]:
  –Prolonged rupture of membranes of 12 hours or more
  –Premature rupture of membranes (i.e., at less than 37 weeks' gestation)
  –Greater than 6 vaginal examinations
  –Use of an intrauterine pressure catheter for more than 12 hours
  –History of a previous infant with GBS disease
  –Preterm labor
  –African American or Hispanic race
  –Age younger than 20 years

Perinatal Consequences[3,6]

- Colonization in women can lead to spontaneous abortion, sepsis, stillbirth, premature rupture of membranes, preterm birth, and postpartum endometritis.
- Most newborns who develop *early-onset invasive GBS disease* are term infants.
- Preterm infants are more susceptible to *early-onset infection.*
- Signs and symptoms of *early-onset infection* are seen within the first 24 hours of life (even within the first hour) and include septicemia, pneumonia, and meningitis. Respiratory distress is the most common sign. Infants may be lethargic, have labile temperatures, exhibit poor feeding, and have glucose intolerance.
- *Signs of severe infection include fetal asphyxia (indicating in utero infection), newborn hypotension, accelerating signs of respiratory distress, and persistent pulmonary hypertension. This requires immediate attention.*
- *Early-onset GBS infection* is associated with a high incidence of invasive disease. The mortality rate is estimated at 4.5% to 15%. Preterm infants can have mortality rates that are double those of term infants.[3]

Screening/Diagnosis on Which to Base Treatment[3,7-10]

The American College of Obstetricians and Gynecologists (ACOG), American Academy of Pediatrics (AAP), and CDC are in essential agreement with recommendations for GBS antenatal screening and the adoption of intrapartal risk factors as markers that identify the need for intrapartum antibiotic prophylaxis. Mullaney summarizes three different approaches using the various recommendations.[3]

1. **Culture-based approach**—Recommendations are that vaginal and rectal cultures be done at 35 to 37 weeks' gestation on all pregnant women. Cultures done earlier do not predict that colonization will be present at birth. All culture-positive women are treated in the intrapartum period.

NOTE: Women who have been previously identified as GBS positive (e.g., from an earlier pregnancy) do not need to be cultured because they are considered permanently GBS positive (carriers) and are candidates for intrapartum antibiotic prophylaxis.
NOTE: A GBS-positive urine culture in the prenatal period indicates heavy colonization and an increased risk for infection or invasive disease. This requires immediate antibiotic treatment.

2. **Risk factor–based approach**—Any woman with one or more of the following risk factors in the intrapartum period should be considered for antibiotic treatment.
   –A history of a previous newborn with invasive GBS infection
   –A history of GBS bacteriuria during the current pregnancy
   –Delivery predicted to occur before 37 weeks' gestation
   –Rupture of membranes for 18 hours or more
   –Presence of maternal fever of 38°C or higher
3. **Combined culture and risk factor approach**—When culture results are unknown in the intrapartum period, treat all women with a known risk factor.

Maternal Treatment[6,8,9]

- Intrapartal treatment is targeted for women documented as being GBS positive (by history or antenatal culture) or for women with intrapartal risk factors.
- Treatment must be completed at least 4 hours before the birth so that adequate antibiotic levels are reached in serum and amniotic fluid, thus reducing the risk of infant colonization.

NOTE: The antibiotics used in treatment (bactericidal) are known to rapidly reach effective levels in amniotic fluid. Therefore, treatment given less than 4 hours before birth is beneficial.

- Intrapartum chemoprophylaxis includes penicillin G with clindamycin, ampicillin, or erythromycin as alternatives for women with penicillin allergy. The following intravenous treatment protocols are summarized by James.[6]

    –No known allergies to penicillin:

Penicillin G	5 million units intravenously (IV) initially
	2.5 million units IV every 4 hours until birth
Ampicillin	2 g IV initially
	1 to 2 g every 4 hours until birth

    –Penicillin allergies:

Clindamycin	900 mg IV every 8 hours
Erythromycin	1 to 2 g IV every 6 hours
Cefoxitin	2 g IV 30 to 60 minutes preoperatively or every 6 to 8 hours
Cephalothin	1 to 2 g IV 30 to 60 minutes preoperatively or every 6 hours

- In women requiring a scheduled or emergency cesarean birth, intravenous administration of 2 g of cefazolin may be recommended. However, this is controversial because neonatal early-onset GBS disease is a low risk in women known to be GBS positive but who experience no labor, remain afebrile, and have intact membranes until birth.
- Any symptomatic newborn, whether term or preterm, should have a sepsis workup to rule out or identify the causative organism.

Neonatal Treatment[3,9,11]

- Current treatment recommendation for the newborn at risk is ampicillin with the addition of an aminoglycoside (usually gentamicin) while laboratory work is pending.[11]
- Antibiotics are discontinued after 48 hours of treatment if laboratory results are negative and invasive disease is not suspected.[11]
- Penicillin G (ampicillin is an option) is the preferred antibiotic when GBS infection is confirmed.
- *Prophylactic treatment is not recommended for an asymptomatic newborn born beyond 35 weeks' gestation whose mother has had at least one dose of intrapartum antibiotics 4 hours before delivery.*[9]
- Asymptomatic newborns born at or before 35 weeks' gestation should be evaluated with a complete blood count (CBC) and blood culture and should not be given antibiotics; careful observation during 48 hours of hospitalization is recommended.[9]
- Mullaney summarizes neonatal antibiotic dosing recommendations as follows[3]:

Treatment (Intravenous)	Commentary
Ampicillin, 150 to 450 mg/kg per day	Higher dosing until meningitis is ruled out
Penicillin G, 250,000 to 500,000 units/kg per day	Higher dosing until meningitis is ruled out
Gentamicin (or equivalent aminoglycoside), dosage depends on gestational and chronologic age	Continued until cerebrospinal fluid is sterile

NOTE: Intramuscular injections of aminoglycosides has variable absorption and is not the preferred route.[3]

REFERENCES

1. Centers for Disease Control and Prevention. (2000). Early-onset group B streptococcal disease: United States, 1998-1999. *MMWR Morbidity and Mortality Weekly Report, 49,* 793–796.
2. Share, L., Chaikin, S., Pomeranets, S., Kiwi, R., Jacobas, M., & Fanoraff, A. A (2001). Implementation of guidelines for preventing early onset group B streptococcal infection. *Seminars in Perinatology, 25*(2), 107–113.
3. Mullaney, D. M. (2001). Group B streptococcal infections in newborns. *Journal of Obstetric, Gynecology and Neonatal Nursing, 30*(6), 649–658.
4. Gilstrap, L. C., & Faro, A. (1997). *Group B streptococcus infection in pregnancy* (2nd ed., pp. 79–85). New York: John Wiley & Sons.
5. Baker, C. J. (1997). Group B streptococcal infections. *Clinics in Perinatology, 24*(1), 59–70.
6. James, D. C. (2001). Maternal screening and treatment for group B streptococcus. *Journal of Obstetric, Gynecologic and Neonatal Nursing, 30*(6), 659–666.
7. Centers for Disease Control and Prevention. (1996). Prevention of perinatal group B streptococcal disease: A public health perspective. *MMWR Morbidity and Mortality Weekly Report, 45*(RR-7), 1–24.
8. American College of Obstetricians and Gynecologists Committee on Obstetric Practice. (1996). *Prevention of early-onset group B streptococcal disease in newborns* (ACOG committee opinion NO. 173). Washington, DC: Author.
9. American Academy of Pediatrics Committee on Infectious Disease and Committee of Fetus and Newborn. (1997). Revised guidelines for prevention of early onset group B streptococcal (GBS) infection. *Pediatrics, 99*(3), 489–496.
10. Centers for Disease Control and Prevention. (1998). Adoption of hospital policies for prevention of perinatal group B streptococcal disease—United States, 1997. *Journal of the American Medical Association, 280*(11), 958–959.
11. American Academy of Pediatrics. (2000). Group B streptococcal infection. In L. K. Pickering (Ed.), *2000 Red Book: Report of the Committee on Infectious Diseases* (25th ed., pp. 537–544). Elk Grove Village, IL. Author.

Herpes Simplex Virus Infection

The herpes simplex virus (HSV) invades sensory or autonomic nervous system ganglia and is expressed as an infection of mucosal surfaces such as the oropharynx, cervix, and vulva. Acute infection (often asymptomatic) is followed by a remission period. It is essentially a chronic infection with frequent or rare exacerbations. Two types of the virus, HSV-1 and HSV-2, differ to some degree in biologic, biochemical, and antigenic properties. HSV-1 is generally associated with infection "above the waist," whereas HSV-2 is associated with genital and neonatal infections.[1,2]

Epidemiology[1-4]

- Genital herpes is the second most prevalent sexually transmitted viral infection in the world. Unfortunately, it is incurable, and at present, no effective vaccine exists.[3]
- Approximately 45 million people have been diagnosed with HSV-2. **However, most infected individuals are asymptomatic and have never been diagnosed.** The true prevalence rate is much greater than that reported.[1,4]
- Studies indicate that 30% of the female population in the United States has antibodies to HSV-2.[1]
- The virus can be transmitted through kissing and sexual activity, as well as during vaginal birth.
- An individual with herpes oral infection can transmit HSV-1 by means of oral sex to male or female genitalia.
- Approximately 1,500 to 2,000 newborns contract neonatal herpes annually.[1] The majority of genital and neonatal infections are caused by HSV-2.[1]
- More women are infected with HSV-2 than men.[1]
- Higher incidences occur in adolescents and young women (early twenties).[1]
- Risk factors are age, duration of sexual activity, race, previous genital infections, family income, and number of sexual partners.[1]

Clinical Features[1,5]

- Transmission of genital herpes is most often by individuals who are not aware they are carrying the virus.
- Neonatal infection and an increased risk of contracting HIV are serious consequences of infection. Genital ulcerative lesions are vulnerable to infection with other STDs (e.g., syphilis, HIV).[5]
- Lesions of HSV are often multiple, are quite painful, and have the appearance of wet blisters or crusted vesicles.
- Fever, malaise, inguinal lymphadenopathy, and dysuria are common, although they by no means always accompany an initial HSV-2 genital infection. Symptoms usually peak in 4 to 5 days and last 2 to 3 weeks.
- After an initial infection, recurrences can be frequent and triggered by menstruation, stress, trauma, and ultraviolet light rays (sun exposure).
- Over time, symptoms are usually less acute and frequency of outbreaks is reduced.
- Many individuals experience *prodromal symptoms* of tingling, burning, itching, tenderness, or a swelling sensation followed by the herpes outbreak of lesions in about 24 hours.[5]
- **Primary genital infection**[1] may by symptomatic or asymptomatic (subclinical). Clinical confirmation depends on the absence of **HSV-1** and **HSV-2** antibodies at the time the individual acquires the genital infection due to **HSV-1** or **HSV-2.**
  - –When systemic symptoms (malaise, fever, and myalgia) occur with herpetic infections, it is generally thought to be a primary infection reflecting a high viremic load.
  - –Without therapy, these lesions resolve in about 3 weeks.
  - –Shedding of the virus from the cervix occurs intermittently in infected women, regardless of whether symptoms are present. This shedding is increased for about 3 months following the healing of the primary genital **HSV-2** lesions.
- **Nonprimary first-episode genital HSV**[1] may be symptomatic or asymptomatic. This diagnostic designation is assigned when the development of genital **HSV-1** infection occurs in an individual who has preexisting **HSV-2** antibodies, indicating previous **HSV-2** infection. This same diagnostic clinical designation is assigned when the development of genital **HSV-2** occurs in an individual with preexisting **HSV-1** antibodies, indicating previous infection.
  - –Prior HSV-1 infection does not provide full protection from a first genital HSV-2 infection.
  - –Nonprimary first-episode infections usually do not have quite the severe clinical symptoms that characterize a symptomatic primary infection. It is believed that having preexisting HSV-1 antibodies offers partial protection when HSV-2 infection occurs.
- **Recurrent infection**[1] may be symptomatic or asymptomatic.
  - –Individual patient response varies widely in terms of frequency, severity, duration of symptoms, and amount of viral shedding.
  - –Usually, herpetic blisters or ulcers are confined to the genital region.
  - –Symptoms tend to be local, not systemic.
  - –**Shedding of the virus from the genital tract is intermittent, occurring in both symptomatic and asymptomatic individuals, and lasts an average of 1.5 days.** Viral quantity tends to be lower when no lesion is present, but a susceptible partner can be infected. This is what makes this STD so difficult to prevent.

Perinatal Consequences[1,2,5,6]

- Maternal-fetal (vertical) transmission appears to be related to gestational age. This is true for all three clinical designations: primary, nonprimary, and recurrent.
- The rate of vertical transmission is reduced in the presence of preexisting maternal HSV-2 antibodies. However, having HSV-1 antibodies does not appear to reduce vertical transmission.
- In clinical studies, vertical transmission rates at the time of vaginal delivery have been found to correlate with the type of maternal infection and probably is related to degree of viral load.

Primary:	50% transmission
Nonprimary:	33% transmission
Recurrent:	0% to 3% transmission

- Primary maternal genital infection in early pregnancy is associated with an increase in spontaneous abortion and in utero fetal infection. Fetal infection during the first 12 to 14 gestational weeks has been associated with anomalies such as microcephaly and aberrations in fetal eye development.
- Primary infection[2,5] in the second and third trimesters poses an increased risk for preterm delivery and the risk of HSV transmission to the newborn during vaginal delivery.

NOTE: When maternal infection is primary but asymptomatic, cervical shedding of the virus also incurs a risk of preterm delivery and possible HSV transmission to the newborn.

- Neonatal infections can develop as three different entities.[6]
  1. Localized to the skin, eye, or mouth
  2. Systemic, causing encephalitis with or without skin lesions
  3. Disseminated in organs such as the lungs, liver, adrenal glands, skin, or central nervous system (CNS)
- No neonatal mortality occurs when infection is localized to the skin, eyes, or mouth. Mortality is about 15% with CNS involvement and 57% with disseminated disease.
- Breastfeeding is contraindicated only if an obvious herpetic lesion is on the breast.

NOTE: The herpes virus is acquired by direct contact. Family members with oral lesions can infect the newborn by hand/mouth contact.

- Mothers with active lesions should be careful when handling their babies.

Screening/Diagnosis[1,2,6–9]

- Weekly late third trimester screening is **not** recommended for women with a history of herpes. Many, if not most, newborns develop HSV infection in the absence of a maternal history of the disease.
- The Pap and Tzank tests are not recommended as screening tests.
- Viral cell culture of suspicious lesions is the standard and most sensitive test: 95% for vesicles, 70% for ulcers, and 30% for crusts.[6] A Dacron swab is used to collect specimens. The vesicles should be scraped (unroofed) to sample the fluid within; moist ulcers and crusts are scraped well. Specimens are placed in viral transport media.[1]
- Serologic diagnosis of primary HSV-1 or HSV-2 has been done by documenting seroconversion from a negative to a positive antibody titer. Blood is analyzed immediately upon suspicion of HSV infection. Two to three weeks should pass before a second serology test is performed.[1,2,6]
- Clinicians and patients more recently have the benefit of laboratory tests approved by the U.S. Food and Drug Administration (FDA)—enzyme-linked immunosorbent assay (ELISA) or immunoblot formats—as well as FDA-approved point-of-care tests for accurately detecting HSV-2 antibodies. Until recently, sensitivity or specificity for HSV type testing produced limited accuracy. A number of companies market tests that can give misleading results.[7]
- Some experts suggest routine serologic screening of high-risk women who are in discordant relationships (one partner is seronegative and the other seropositive) to assist in identifying women at risk for cervical shedding at the time of delivery.[2] Sandhaus, referring to studies by Brown et al. and Garland, Lee, and Sacks, states that among women who are HSV seronegative in early pregnancy but whose partners are seropositive, 13% will have genital herpes at the time of labor.[2,8,9]

Treatment[1,2,4,5,10]

- The goal of management is to reduce or prevent neonatal risk of exposure to HSV during the later half of pregnancy and during delivery.
- Studies demonstrate that antiviral therapy (oral or parenteral) shortens the course of infection and the duration of viral shedding.
- The ACOG treatment recommendations are summarized as follows[1]:
  A. Based on limited or inconsistent scientific evidence (Level B)
     –Women with primary HSV during pregnancy should be treated with antiviral therapy.
     –Cesarean delivery should be performed on women with first-episode HSV who have active genital lesions at delivery.
     –For women at or beyond 26 weeks' gestation with a first episode of HSV occurring during the current pregnancy, antiviral therapy should be considered.
  B. Based on consensus and expert opinion primarily[1]:
     –Cesarean delivery should be performed on women with recurrent HSV infection who have active genital lesions or prodromal symptoms at delivery.
     –Expectant management of patients with preterm labor or preterm premature rupture of membranes and active HSV may be warranted.
     –For women at or beyond 36 weeks' gestation who are at risk for recurrent HSV, antiviral therapy also may be considered, although such therapy may not reduce the likelihood of cesarean delivery.
     –In women with no active lesions or prodromal symptoms during labor, cesarean delivery should not be performed on the basis of a history or recurrent disease.
  In addition, nongenital herpetic lesions (e.g., on the thigh or buttocks) should be covered with an occlusive dressing. The woman can then deliver vaginally.
- The CDC recommends using oral acyclovir (Class C) during pregnancy if a first episode of HSV infection occurs. The routine use of acyclovir by pregnant women with a history of recurrent HSV is not recommended.
- Two newer Class B antiherpetic drugs, famciclovir (Famvir) and valacyclovir (Valtrex), with their increased bioavailability, involve less frequent dosing to achieve the same therapeutic results as acyclovir. However, currently only acyclovir is FDA approved for use during pregnancy. The CDC has maintained a drug registry for women treated with acyclovir during pregnancy. To date, no increase in fetal abnormalities has been shown.[2,4,5]
- Vaccines are under research.

REFERENCES

1. American College of Obstetricians and Gynecologists. (1999). Management of herpes in pregnancy. ACOG Practice Bulletin Number 8. Washington, DC: Author.
2. Sandhous, S. (2001). Genital herpes in pregnant and nonpregnant women. *The Nurse Practitioner, 26*(4), 15–35.
3. Patrick, D. M., Dawar, M., Cook, D. A., Krajden, M., Ng, H. C., & Rekart, M. L. (2001). Antenatal seroprevalence of herpes simplex virus type 2 (HSV-2) in Canadian women. *Sexually Transmitted Diseases, 28*(7), 424–428.
4. Centers for Disease Control and Prevention. (1998). 1998 guidelines for treatment of sexually transmitted diseases. *MMWR Morbidity and Mortality Weekly Report, 47*(RR-1): 20–26.
5. Thomas, D. J. (2001). Sexually transmitted viral infections: Epidemiology and treatment. *Journal of Obstetric, Gynecologic, and Neonatal Nursing, 30*(3), 316–323.
6. Desselberger, U. (1998). Herpes simplex virus infection in pregnancy: Diagnosis and significance. *Intervirology, 41,* 185–190.
7. Ashley, R. L. (2001) Sorting out the new HSV type specific antibody tests. *Sexually Transmitted Infections, 77*(4), 232–237.
8. Brown, Z. A., Selke, S., Zeh, J., Kopelman, J., Maslow, A., & Ashley, R. L. (1997). The acquisition of herpes simplex virus during pregnancy. *The New England Journal of Medicine, 337,* 509–515.
9. Garland, S., Lee, T., & Sacks, S. (1999). Do antepartum herpes simplex virus cultures predict intrapartum shedding for pregnant women with recurrent disease? *Infections Diseases in Obstetrics and Gynecology, 7*(5), 230–236.
10. Braig, S., Luton, D., Sibony, O., Edlinger, C., Boissinot, C., Blot, P., & Oury, J. F. (2001). Acyclovir prophylaxis in late pregnancy prevents recurrent genital herpes and viral shedding. *European Journal of Obstetrics and Gynecology and Reproductive Biology, 96,* 55–58.

Human Papillomavirus Infection

Human papillomavirus (HPV) infection is an infection of the skin and mucous membranes of the anogenital tract; it is caused by one of many human papilloma viral types. Manifestations of the infection can be single or multiple raised warts, or *condylomata acuminata,* and occurs in both men and women.

Epidemiology[1-3]

- Genital HPV is the most prevalent STD in the United States, with more than 20 million Americans *currently* infected and an estimated 5.5 million more infected annually.[1,2]
- Studies repeatedly show high levels of infection in women, with the highest levels among young women.[2]
- Recent studies among the female college student population found that, on average, 14% become infected yearly.
- Fewer data are available on HPV among men; however, levels of current infection in men appear to be similar to those in women.[2] For both men and women, the infection is more common than current reporting reveals.
- Data on actual prevalence are difficult to gather because reporting of HPV is based on visible lesions and some testing measures (e.g., Pap smears and subsequent workup) but many patients have no symptoms and remain undiagnosed.
- More than 100 HPV types have been identified; more than 33 types are known to infect the genital tract. Certain types are strongly associated with cervical, penile, and anal cancer.[1-3]

Clinical Features[3-7]

- HPV infections are transmitted primarily by sexual contact with an infected partner. Lesions are highly contagious.
- Considerable evidence exists that HPV is the main infectious etiologic agent in the sexual transmission of a carcinogen, which can lead to cervical cancer.[5]
- Many of the risk factors that place a woman at risk for HPV infection also characterize risk factors for cervical cancer.[5]
- *Strong risk factors for cervical cancer and its precursors* include age at first intercourse (16 years or younger), a history of multiple sexual partners, a history of genital HPV infection or another STD, the presence of other genital tract neoplasia, and prior cervical tissue changes such as a squamous intraepithelial lesion. Additional risk factors include active or passive smoking, immunodeficiency (as in HIV infection), poor nutrition, and a current or past sexual partner with risk factors for STDs.[5]
- Nonsexual transmission may also occur; the virus has been detected on underwear, sex toys, tanning salon benches, and wet towels and has been cultured from gloves, instruments, and specula. The inability to culture HPV eliminates the possibility of documenting infectability.[4]
- The incubation period ranges from 3 weeks to 8 months, with an average of 3 months.
- Infection can by symptomatic or asymptomatic. In symptomatic cases, irritation, bleeding, pruritus, and often, fleshy, pink, warty raised lesions are present singularly or in clusters on affected areas, such as the surface of the perineum, introitus, vagina, cervix, and anus.
- The diagnostic spectrum of HPV infection ranges from clinically visible lesions to subclinical infection as seen by colposcopy to latent infection in which HPV DNA is diagnosed with tissue evaluation.
- Viral types 16, 18, 31, 33, 35, and 45 have a strong correlation with cervical dysplasia, high-grade squamous intraepithelial lesions, and invasive cancer,[3] as well as with types 51, 52, 56, 58, 59, and 68. Identification of these types can now be done.
- On Pap smear screening, the spectrum of abnormality may begin with atypia, progress to mild dysplasia to severe dysplasia or carcinoma in situ, and conclude with invasive cancer of the cervix.
- Studies comparing HPV prevalence and annual incidence rates for cervical cancer suggest that only up to 3% of HPV-positive women will go on to develop cervical cancer within 20 to 50 years; most women who are HPV positive at any one point in time are not at great risk.[6]
- Many HPV infections appear to be temporary and are probably cleared by an active cell-mediated immune response. However, reactivation to reinfection is possible.[7]
- Evidence suggests the following[5]:
  –Barrier methods of contraception lower the incidence of cervical neoplasia, probably because of lessened exposure to HPV.

–Exposure to cigarette smoking is associated with increased risk.

–Increased intake of micronutrients and other dietary factors such as carotenoids is associated with decreased risk.

–Education about risk factors for cervical cancer may lead to behavioral modification, resulting in diminished exposure.

Perinatal Consequences[3,8,9]

• Genital warts tend to grow more rapidly during pregnancy.

• Perinatal viral transmission of types 6 or 11 through aspiration of infected material during delivery can cause laryngeal papillomatosis (juvenile onset of recurrent respiratory papillomatosis [JORRP]) in infants and children. The rate of infection is unclear. Studies indicate higher incidence for children delivered vaginally compared with those delivered by means of cesarean section.[3] One estimated overall incidence of JORRP is 600 to 700 cases annually.[8]

• Although the transmission rate to the newborn's oropharynx may be high (Cunningham cites one study at 30%), it is significant to know that most of the infants cleared the virus in 5 weeks.[9] Thomas cites infection rates at 2% to 5% within the first 5 years of life. The lesions can develop in 2 to 3 months. Clinical signs are stridor, hoarseness, abnormal cry, cough, and respiratory distress.[3]

• Occasionally, clusters of condylomata acuminata on the perineum are so profuse that they interfere with vaginal delivery when performing an episiotomy is deemed necessary (the lesions tend to bleed profusely).[3]

Screening/Diagnosis[3,4,10–12]

• Screening and diagnostic methods have become more efficient and include the following:

–Direct visualization of condylomata and biopsy

NOTE: Although condylomata acuminata are easily seen on external surfaces with the naked eye, HPV disease on the cervix usually requires magnification (colposcopy) and the application of acetic acid for identification.

–Pap smear with directed biopsy

–HPV testing (FDA approved of Hybrid Capture II in 1999). The test has a consistently high sensitivity for the detection of CIN3 or cancer.

• Adding periodic HPV testing to the annual gynecologic examination has been proposed as an approach to identifying women who are at high risk for developing cervical cancer.

Treatment

Maternal Treatment[3,4,10–12]

• Genital HPV lesions may regress without treatment. It is not currently possible to predict who will have a spontaneous remission or when that could occur.[4] Regression rates for cervical intraepithelial neoplasia (CIN) are cited from composite data as analyzed by Östör.[10] He states that the approximate likelihood of regression of CIN1 is 60%, persistence is 30%, progression to CIN3 is 10%, and progression to invasive cancer is 1%. Corresponding approximations for CIN2 are 40%, 40%, 20%, and 5%, respectively. The likelihood of CIN3 regressing is 33%, and the likelihood of progressing to invasion is greater than 12%.[10] There may be no single "best" treatment, and for some patients a combination of treatments may be appropriate, depending on the site and extent of infection, response to treatment, and patient choice.[4] Resources and the expertise of the health care provider play a pivotal role.

• No evidence exists that treatments eradicate or affect the natural course of HPV infection. The goal of treatment for visible genital warts is simply removal.[3]

• Examination and treatment of partners is unnecessary as part of the woman's treatment plan. Recurrence from reinfection is not likely. Partner treatment should be based on that individual's choice and may often be related to psychosocial and emotional health.[3] If the patient is lesbian or bisexual, female partners should be treated.

• Treatment options include the following[3]:

–Topical medication such as podofilox (Condylox) solution or gel and imiquimod (Aldara) cream, which can be applied by the patient at home (Although clinical trials are under way, Condylox and Aldara are not yet approved for use in pregnancy.)

–Trichloroacetic acid (TCA) or bichloracetic acid (BCA)—commonly used but must be applied by a care provider

–Cryotherapy—freezing that destroys targeted tissue

–Laser vaporization—surgery using a high-intensity light

–LLETZ—large loop excision of the transformation zone: removal of tissue using a hot wire loop (also called LEEP)

• Trichloroacetic acid (TCA) and bichloroacetic acid (BCA) have been approved by the FDA for use during pregnancy.

• HPV vaccine research, including clinical trials, is in process under the auspices of the National Institutes of Health (NIH) and private companies. Although there is considerable optimism that vaccines can be developed, many more years of study will be needed.[11,12]

Newborn Treatment

• Both medical and surgical approaches may be used in treating laryngeal papillomatosis in the newborn.

REFERENCES

1. Centers for Disease Control and Prevention, Division of STD Prevention. (1999). *Prevention of genital HPV infection and sequelae: Report of an External Consultants' Meeting* (pp. 1–35). Atlanta: Department of Health and Human Services.

2. Centers for Disease Control and Prevention. (2001). *Tracking the hidden epidemics: Trends in STDs in the United States, 2000* (pp. 10–19). Atlanta: Author. Available at: http://www.cdc.gov/nchstp/dstd/disease-info.htm.

3. Thomas, D. J. (2001). Sexually transmitted viral infections: Epidemiology and treatment. *Journal of Obstetric, Gynecologic, and Neonatal Nursing, 30*(3), 316–323.

4. *Human papillomavirus (HPV) and cervical cancer.* (2001, March). AHRP Clinical Proceedings (pp. 1–32). Washington, DC: The Association of Reproductive Health Professionals.

5. National Cancer Institute. (2002). *Cervical cancer (PDQ"): Prevention summary of evidence; significance and evidence of benefits.* Available at: http://www.cancer.gov/cancer_infor...409fa2-ff12-41e7-9f5d-2911d566d242.

6. Bristow, R. E., & Montz, F. J. (1998). Human papillomavirus: Molecular biology and screening applications in cervical neoplasia—A primer for primary care physicians. *Primary Care Update OB/GYNs, 5*(5), 238–246.

7. Czelusta, A. J., Yen-Moore, A., Evans, T. Y., & Tyring, S. K. (1999). Periodic synopsis: Sexually transmitted diseases. *Journal of the American Academy of Dermatology, 41*(4), 614–623.

8. American Social Health Association (ASHA). (1999, Spring). HPV and JORRP. *HPV News, 9*(1), 1–12.

9. Cunningham, F. G., Gant, N. F., Leveno, K. J., Gilstrap, L. C., Hauth, J. C., & Wenstrom, K. D. (Eds.). (2001). *Williams obstetrics* (21st ed., pp. 1485–1513). New York: McGraw-Hill.

10. Östör, A. G. (1993). Natural history of cervical intraepithelial neoplasia: A critical review. *International Journal of Gynecological Pathology, 12*(2), 186–192.

11. American Social Health Association (ASHA). (2000, Winter). The vaccine marathon. *HPV News, 10*(4), 1–12.

12. National Cancer Institute. (2001). *Human papillomaviruses and cancer.* Fact Sheet 3.20. Available at: http://cis.nci.nih.gov/fact/3-20.htm.

Syphilis

Syphilis is a complex STD caused by the spirochete *Treponema pallidum*. Infectivity is high, with 60% of individuals acquiring the disease during the first exposure to a partner with a primary lesion.[1] Maternal infection may be transmitted to the fetus (congenital syphilis).

Epidemiology[1-4]

- Syphilis in the United States currently is characterized by geographic concentration, with southern states experiencing the highest rates. It disproportionately affects populations living near or below the poverty level, as well as those involved in high-risk activities such as prostitution, illicit drug use, and multiple sexual partners.
- Rates of primary and secondary syphilis are much higher among communities of color. In the year 1999, the reported rate in African Americans was 30 times the rate reported in Caucasians; rates increased 20% (from 1998 to 1999) among Hispanics and were 45% higher for men than for women.[2]
- Overall, both the number and rates for primary and secondary syphilis currently are decreasing.
- Maternal infection is primarily found in the young and unmarried and among those who receive inadequate or no prenatal care.[3]
- Racial/ethnic minority populations have the highest rates of congenital syphilis.[4]
- Failure of health care provider adherence to congenital syphilis screening recommendations may also result in congenital syphilis.[4]

Clinical Features[3,5-7]

- Stages of the disease are divided into primary, secondary, and latent phases.
- The incubation period for primary syphilis ranges from 10 to 90 days. A chancre usually develops 3 to 4 weeks after exposure.
- The chancre of *primary syphilis* occurs at the site of inoculation and appears as a red, painless ulcer with raised edges and a granulation base. Cervical chancres are common in exposed pregnant women, probably because of the friable cervix, which is easily infected. The chancre persists for 2 to 6 weeks and heals spontaneously. Often, nontender, enlarged inguinal lymph nodes can be palpated.
- *Secondary syphilis* occurs about 4 to 10 weeks after the primary chancre has healed. In approximately 15% of women, a chancre may still be present. This secondary stage involves more widespread dissemination of the *T. pallidum* and is therefore characterized by symptoms of systemic involvement: low-grade fever, sore throat, headache, malaise, adenopathy, and rashes on mucosal and skin surfaces. Alopecia, mild hepatitis, and kidney involvement may develop.
- The lesions of secondary syphilis may be mild and even go unnoticed. Some women will develop characteristic genital lesions of secondary syphilis called *condylomata lata*. They appear as white, raised, and moist lesions and are highly infectious. These lesions resolve in 3 to 12 weeks, and the disease enters the latent phase.
- *Latent syphilis* refers to infection in individuals who have reactive serologic tests but no clinical manifestations. *Latency* is divided into *early* (1 year or less from the beginning of infection) and *late* (more than 1 year from the beginning of infection). Infectiousness continues throughout these periods.
- *Tertiary syphilis* develops after years of untreated disease. The skeletal, nervous, and cardiovascular systems may be seriously affected.
- The clinical course of syphilis is not affected by pregnancy.
- Pregnancy outcomes are drastically affected by syphilis. Transmission of the disease largely depends on the duration of maternal disease.
- The most affected infants are those *conceived* in mothers with primary or secondary syphilis. The less affected are those infants *conceived* in mothers with early-late or late-stage disease.[7]

Perinatal Consequences[3,5-8]

- Syphilis causes infection in both the unborn and newborns.
- A twofold to fivefold increase in the risk of HIV transmission occurs in the presence of syphilis.[8] Direct contact with a syphilitic lesion (chancre) found on external genitalia, vagina, anus, rectum, and lips and in the mouth has a very high infection occurrence.
- The risk of prematurity, perinatal death, and congenital infection is directly related to the stage of maternal syphilis during pregnancy. Untreated early syphilis of 4 years' duration or less results in higher rates of dead or diseased infants and a significantly increased pos-

sibility of neonatal death. Adverse consequences of late latent syphilis of more than 4 years' duration are lessened, but stillbirth rates are high.[3]

- The infection can be transmitted to the fetus in utero, presumably by a transplacental route or during delivery by newborn contact with a genital lesion.
- It was formerly believed that fetal infection did not occur before the fourth month of pregnancy. This has been disproved through electron microscopy, silver staining, and immunofluorescent techniques. Infection can cause fetal morbidity during early gestation (e.g., spontaneous abortion at 9 and 10 weeks' gestation).
- Pregnancy outcomes in the presence of untreated syphilis are commonly spontaneous abortion during the second or third trimester, stillbirth, nonimmune hydrops, premature delivery, and perinatal death.
- *Most infants delivered to mothers with untreated syphilis, irrespective of disease stage or duration, do not have clinical or laboratory evidence of infection at birth. If left untreated, these infants may develop clinical signs and symptoms months or years later.[3]*
- The infection *is not* transmitted via breastfeeding *unless* an infectious lesion is present on the breast.[3]

Screening/Diagnosis[3,5-7,9-11]

Diagnostic workup and treatment of syphilis infection in the pregnant woman requires a thorough understanding of the natural history of the disease and how it relates to stages (primary, secondary, and latency), clinical progressions and relapse, and the proper evaluation of therapeutic results.[7] Laboratory techniques, their degrees of accuracy, and available applicability at given stages of the disease are essential. The following statements highlight some key points.

- Establishing the diagnosis in a pregnant woman is essentially the same as that for a nonpregnant woman.
- Dark-field microscopic examination to identify spirochetes is the most accurate method of diagnosing syphilis. However, serology is the most common method of confirming infection.
- Two basic types of serology are used: the nonspecific antibody test and the specific antitreponemal antibodies test.
- Diagnosis of syphilis in the pregnant woman is most often made by serologic screening at the first visit and repeated at 28 to 32 weeks' gestation. Testing is required by law in all 50 states.
- Nonspecific antibody tests include the rapid plasma regain (RPR) and the Venereal Disease Research Laboratory (VDRL). The tests are reported as reactive or nonreactive. A positive test is reported as reactive with a titer. These tests will be positive in the majority of women with primary syphilitic lesions and in all women with secondary syphilis. *However, it should be noted that most will be positive only after 4 to 6 weeks of initial infection.* These tests are not highly specific; therefore, a second confirmatory test is performed on anyone with an initial positive test.
- The confirmatory test is based on identification of treponemal antibodies: fluorescent treponemal antibody absorption test (FTA-ABS) or the microhemagglutination assay for antibodies to *T. pallidum* (MHA-TP). The MHA-TP has replaced the FTS-ABS in most clinical laboratories.[9] Newer, more sensitive and specific tests are evolving. The WHO's new recommendations suggest that treponemal antigen-based enzyme immunoassays (EIAs) are an appropriate alternative to the combined VDRL/RPR and MHA-TP screen. It is a single screening test and is being used in many laboratories, especially in Europe.[9]

NOTE: *Approximately 15% of individuals with primary syphilis will be seronegative at initial testing.[9] This is due to the prozone phenomenon, which is the result of an excess amount of anticardiolipin antibody present in a patient's serum, which interferes with the test chemically. Therefore, repeat testing should be performed on anyone at risk of recent infection.[3,9]*

- False-positive nontreponemal tests are relatively common and can be caused by recent febrile illness; intravenous drug use; autoimmune disease such as systemic lupus erythematosus; and viral (Epstein-Barr and hepatitis), protozoal, or mycoplasmal infection. A false-positive reaction may also be seen in elderly patients, those with malignancy or other chronic diseases, and even in pregnant women.[3]
- Treponemal antibody tests FTA-ABS and MHA-TP rarely give false-positive results. Once positive, these tests remain positive for life in most individuals.
- *When there is not a documented history of adequate treatment, a negative VDRL/RPR or EIA result does not mean that treatment is not needed. Inadequate treatment may lead to nonresolution of infection and relapses that can result in congenital infection.[9]*

Diagnosis of Fetal Syphilis
- Evidence of the disease in the fetus is usually not seen until about 18 weeks' gestation.[5]
- Prenatal diagnosis is possible using ultrasonography, which can identify fetal hydrops when maternal syphilis is documented.
- Most often, the diagnosis depends on testing after birth, at which time serology testing, physical examination, and laboratory testing are used.
- Detection of spirochetes in amniotic fluid and in fetal blood through cordocentesis can also be done.

Diagnosis of Congenital Syphilis
- Syphilis is confirmed by the demonstration of spirochetes in lesions, body fluids, or tissue using dark-field microscopy, immunofluorescence, or histologic examination.[3]
- PCR technique is highly specific for detecting *T. pallidum* in amniotic fluid and neonatal serum and spinal fluid.[6]
- The two most common clinical findings are hepatosplenomegaly and jaundice.[5,11]
- Comparison of the maternal nontreponemal serum titer with the newborn titer can be helpful. A newborn titer that is fourfold or greater supports a diagnosis of congenital syphilis.
- Newer tests that detect *anti–T. pallidum* IgM for maternal or fetal diagnosis have become available and may provide a major advancement in diagnosis.

Treatment[5,6,10]

Maternal Therapy

- Benzathine penicillin is the drug of choice for both acquired and congenital syphilis.
- There are no proven alternatives to penicillin treatment during pregnancy. Erythromycin may affect a maternal cure but not prevent congenital syphilis. Currently, it is not recommended for infected pregnant women.
- Penicillin desensitization is recommended for pregnant women with penicillin allergy. This requires hospitalization and careful monitoring but is usually successful. Desensitization produces a temporary tolerance of penicillin but will not prevent future allergic reactions.
- Recommended treatment according to CDC guidelines is as follows[10]:

Primary:	
Secondary:	Benzathine penicillin G 2.4 million units
Early latent (≤1 year):	
Late latent (>1 year):	IM as a single injection; some authorities recommend a second dose 1 week later
Unknown duration:	Benzathine penicillin G 2.4 million units IM weekly for three doses

- A treatment reaction occurring in up to 60% of patients treated for early syphilis in pregnancy is called the Jarisch-Herxheimer reaction. Manifestations include fever, chills, hypotension, tachycardia, and myalgia, which occur within a few hours of treatment and resolve by 24 to 36 hours. Pregnant women may experience frequent uterine contractions and even premature labor. Nonreassuring fetal heart rate patterns and decreased fetal activity can occur.[5,6]

Treatment of Congenital Syphilis

- The CDC recommends that every infant with suspected or proven congenital syphilis have a cerebrospinal examination before treatment.

Symptomatic infants:	Aqueous penicillin G
Infants with abnormal spinal fluid examination:	Administered as 50,000 U/kg IV every 12 hours for the first 7 days of life. This is followed by 50,000 U/kg for 10 days **OR** aqueous procaine penicillin G, 50,000 U/kg IM each day *so that a total of 10 days of treatment is completed*
Asymptomatic positive:	Benzathine penicillin G, 50,000 U/kg IM for a single dose

  Infants born to mothers treated with erythromycin for syphilis during pregnancy should be retreated as though they have congenital syphilis.[6]

REFERENCES

1. Bofill, J. A., & Rust, O. A. (1996). The diagnosis and treatment of syphilis in women. *Pregnancy Care Update for OB/GYNs, 3*(1), 13–19.
2. Centers for Disease Control and Prevention. (1998). Primary and secondary syphilis—United States, 1999. *MMWR Morbidity and Mortality Weekly Report, 50*(7), 113–117.
3. Sanchez, P. J., & Wendel, G. D. (1997) Syphilis in pregnancy. *Clinics in Perinatology, 22*(1), 71–90.
4. Centers for Disease Control and Prevention. (2000). Congenital syphilis, United States, 2000. *MMWR Morbidity and Mortality Weekly Report, 50*(27), 573–577.
5. Gilstrap, L. C., & Faro. S. (1997). *Syphilis in pregnancy. Infections in pregnancy* (2nd ed., pp. 135–149) New York: John Wiley & Sons.
6. Cunningham, F. G., Gant, N. F., Leveno, K. J., Gilstrap, L. C., Hauth, J. C., & Wenstrom, K. D. (Eds.). (2001) *Williams obstetrics* (21st ed., pp. 1485–1513). New York: McGraw-Hill.
7. Wicher, V., & Wicher, K. (2001). Pathogenesis of maternal-fetal syphilis revisited. *Clinical Infectious Diseases, 33*(3), 354–363.
8. Centers for Disease Control and Prevention, Division of Sexually Transmitted Diseases. (2001, May). *Syphilis elimination: History in the making.* Available at: http://www.cdc.gov/nchstp/dstd/ Fact_Sheets/Syphilis_Facts.htm.
9. Young, H. (2000). Guidelines for serological testing for syphilis. *Sexually Transmitted Infections, 76*(5), 403–405.
10. Centers for Disease Control and Prevention. (1998). 1998 guidelines for treatment of sexually transmitted diseases. *MMWR Morbidity and Mortality Weekly Report, 47*(RR-1): 74–75.
11. Hollier, L. M., Harstrad, T. W., Sanchez, P. J., Twickler, D. M., & Wendel, G. D. (2001). Fetal syphilis: Clinical and laboratory characteristics. *Obstetrics & Gynecology 97*(6), 947–953.

Trichomonas (Trichomoniasis)

Trichomonas vaginalis is a vaginal infection caused by a flagellated protozoan and is spread through sexual activity.

Epidemiology[1,2]

- The Vaginal Infections and Prematurity Study Group identified a 13% infection rate in 14,000 women who had cultures done at mid-pregnancy. The highest incidence was found in African American women, with a lower rate for Hispanic and Caucasian women.[1]
- Approximately 5 million new cases occur each year in men and women; it is especially prevalent in the 16- to 35-year-old age group.

Clinical Features[3,4]

- Women may be asymptomatic. Common symptoms include foul-smelling or frothy green (yellow/green) vaginal discharge, pruritus, and redness. Occasionally, abdominal pain, dysuria, and dyspareunia are experienced.
- In men the infection tends to be asymptomatic, but occasionally, urethritis epididymitis and prostatitis can occur.
- BV is a common coinfection in pregnant women diagnosed with trichomonas.[4]

Perinatal Consequences[5,6]

- Recent clinical studies point to an association between vaginal infections and preterm premature rupture of membranes, preterm delivery, and low birth weight. Common infections such as *Trichomonas,* chlamydia, and BV are being evaluated.

Screening/Diagnosis[3]

- The most accurate method of testing is by culture technique, but this is more costly. A DNA probe test is 90% sensitive and 99.8% specific.
- Wet mount preparation for microscope examination is the most common technique. This can be done immediately in an office setting, and sensitivity is considered approximately 85%. This allows for immediate treatment.

Treatment[2,3,7]

- Metronidazole (Flagyl) is the only drug available in the United States that is effective against the organism.
- Although a *vaginal* preparation of metronidazole exists, the CDC does not recommend its use in treating *Trichomonas; oral* administration is the effective treatment method.
- The dosage is 250 mg orally, three times a day for 7 days, **or** 2 g orally as a single dose **or** 500 mg orally twice daily for 7 days.
- The CDC cites that metronidazole may be used during pregnancy. Burtin et al., reporting on an analysis of 30 years' experience with metronidazole in pregnant women, conclude that the drug does not appear to be associated with an increased teratogenic risk.
- Alcohol consumption should be avoided while taking metronidazole and for a few days after the last dose because it may induce nausea/vomiting.
- Sexual partners should be treated, and sexual intercourse should be avoided until both partners have completed treatment.
- A test of cure is not recommended.

REFERENCES

1. Cotch, M. F., Pastorek, J. G., II, Nugent, R. P., Yerg, D. E., Martin D. H., & Eschenbach, E. A. (1991). (Vaginal infections and prematurity study group). Demographic and behavioral predictors of *Trichomonas vaginalis* infection among pregnant women. *Obstetrics & Gynecology, 78,* 1087.
2. Centers for Disease Control and Prevention. (1998). 1998 guidelines for treatment of sexually transmitted diseases. *MMWR Morbidity and Mortality Weekly Report, 47*(RR-1), 74–75.
3. Cunningham, F. G., Gant, N. F., Leveno, K. J., Gilstrap, L. C., Hauth, J. C., & Wenstrom, K. D. (Eds.). (2001). *Williams obstetrics* (21st ed., pp. 1485–1513). New York: McGraw-Hill.
4. Franklin, T. L., & Monif, G. R. G. (2000). *Trichomonas vaginalis* and bacterial vaginosis: Coexistence in vaginal wet mount preparations from pregnant women. *The Journal of Reproductive Medicine, 45*(2), 131–134.
5. Goldenberg, R. L. (1998). *Low birthweight in minority and high-risk women. Patient Outcomes Research Team Final Report* (Agency for Health Care Policy and Research. Contract Number 290-92-0055) (pp. 16–20, 64–65). Rockville, MD: Agency for Health Care Policy and Research.
6. Berkman, N. D., Thorp, J. M., Hartman, K. E., et al. (2000, December). Management of preterm labor. Evidence Report/Technology Assessment No. 18 (Prepared by Research Triangle Institute under Contract, No. 290-97-0011). AHRQ Publication No. 01-E021 (pp. 18–20). Rockville, MD: Agency for Healthcare Research and Quality.
7. Burtin, P., Taddio, A., Ariburnu, O., Einarson, T. R., & Koren, G. (1995). Safety of metronidazole in pregnancy: A meta-analysis. *American Journal of Obstetrics and Gynecology, 172*(2) 525–529.

A P P E N D I X   B

Treatment of Diabetes During Pregnancy

The three hallmarks in the treatment of diabetes during pregnancy are as follows:

1. Medical nutritional therapy
2. Exercise
3. Insulin therapy

Careful attention to each component is essential to optimizing glucose control.

Medical Nutritional Therapy

Medical nutritional therapy (MNT) is an essential component of successful diabetic management. Adherence to the plan is often challenging for pregnant women but is essential for successful management. To facilitate adherence, the MNT needs to be sensitive to culture, ethnicity, and financial considerations. Each patient needs an *individualized plan* appropriate to her lifestyle and diabetic management goals. Monitoring of blood glucose, HbA_{1c}, lipids, blood pressure, and renal status is included in the MNT plan.

Goals may differ depending on whether the patient has type 1, type 2, or gestational diabetes. The overall goal is to assist the woman in developing healthy nutrition and exercise habits that will lead to improved metabolic control.

The recommended amount of calories must be individualized. The appropriate recommended calorie intake depends on pregravid weight (Table B.1).

TABLE B.1	Recommendations for Caloric Intake During Pregnancy
BODY WEIGHT	**CALORIE REQUIREMENTS (kcal/kg)**
Less than 10% of ideal body weight	36–40
Ideal body weight	30
20%–50% above ideal body weight	24
Greater than 50% above ideal body weight	12–18

The recommended distribution of calories is 40% to 50% carbohydrates, 20% protein, and 30% to 40% fat.[1] **For obese women, carbohydrate restriction to 35% to 40% of calories has been shown to decrease maternal glucose values and improve maternal and fetal outcomes.**[2] Most plans consist of three meals and three snacks each day.

Many methods for teaching meal planning exist. The choice of method must be individualized for each woman. **The exchange list method and carbohydrate counting method are the most commonly used.**

The Exchange List Method
- This method was developed and published by the American Dietetic Association and the American Diabetes Association.
- Foods are listed based on calorie and macronutrient composition.
- Foods in each list can be exchanged for other foods in the same list.
- The meal plan specifies when and how many exchanges for each group can be eaten at each meal or snack.

The Carbohydrate Counting Method
- This method is endorsed by the American Diabetes Association.
- It offers greater flexibility in food and choices.
- More self-monitoring of blood glucose and decision making by the patient is required.
- Emphasis is on the total amount of carbohydrate in each food, not the type of carbohydrate.
- The patient must count the total amount of carbohydrate in each food item.

To calculate the required carbohydrates per day:

1. Calculate the amount of calories the patient requires each day.
2. Calculate the percentage of carbohydrates the patient needs based on the required calories per day.
3. Divide the number of calories by 4 because there are 4 calories per gram of carbohydrate.

Example:

1. Patient's weight is 66 kg $\times$ 30 kcal/kg/day = 1,980 kcal/day
2. If 50% of diet is carbohydrates, divide 1,980 by 2 = 990 kcal in carbohydrates
3. Divide 990 kcal by 4 (4 kcal per carbohydrate) = 247 g of carbohydrates per day

The many variations in carbohydrate counting include counting carbohydrate servings, counting carbohydrate exchanges, counting carbohydrate grams, counting carbohydrates plus proteins, and counting total available glucose (TAG), which includes carbohydrates, protein, and fat. Three levels of carbohydrate counting have been identified and are based on the increasing level of complexity and skills required for each level (Table B.2).[3]

TABLE B.2 Three Levels of Carbohydrate Counting

LEVEL OF CARBOHYDRATE COUNTING	REQUIREMENTS
Level 1 (basic)	Counting consistent amounts of carbohydrates at each meal and snack
Level 2 (intermediate)	Level 1 + learning the relationship between food, medication, activity, and blood glucose
Level 3 (advanced)	Level 1 + level 2 + learning to match insulin to carbohydrate intake using a carbohydrate:insulin ratio

Exercise

Because metabolism is affected by exercise, the pregnant woman with diabetes must be aware of the impact of exercise on her diabetes. Maternal fitness and sense of well-being may be enhanced by exercise.

Because of the physiologic changes that occur with pregnancy, diabetic women should be aware of the following:

- The impact of pregnancy on exercise
- The impact of exercise on diabetes

For women without obstetric or medical complications, cardiorespiratory and muscular fitness can be maintained during pregnancy with moderate levels of physical activity. Pregnancy causes physiologic changes in the cardiovascular, respiratory, mechanical, thermoregulatory, and metabolic systems.

During exercise in individuals *without diabetes, the plasma insulin normally decreases, along with an increase in plasma counterregulatory hormones* (Table B.3). This allows hepatic glucose production and lipolysis to match glucose utilization during exercise. However, in individuals *with type 1 diabetes, these hormonal adaptations are absent and the insulin is exogenous* (by injection). Therefore, too little insulin with an excess release of counterregulatory hormones during exercise may cause a rise in already elevated glucose levels. It can even precipitate diabetic ketoacidosis (DKA). On the other hand, excess exogenous insulin can prevent the increased mobilization of glucose and produce hypoglycemia (see Table B.3). With type 2 diabetic and gestational diabetic patients, exercise benefits include an improvement in carbohydrate metabolism and insulin sensitivity.

TABLE B.3 Effects of Exercise

TYPE OF PATIENT	INSULIN	COUNTERREGULATORY HORMONES	BLOOD GLUCOSE LEVEL
Type 1 diabetic (exogenous insulin)	Too little *or*	Excess release	Hyperglycemia (DKA is possible)
	Too much	Absent adaptation	Hypoglycemia
Nondiabetic (endogenous insulin)	Decreased	Increased	Normal blood glucose

General guidelines that should be followed during exercise include the following[4]:

- Obtain metabolic control before exercising. *Avoid exercising if fasting blood glucose is greater than 250 mg/dL and ketones are present.* Use caution if blood glucose is greater than 300 mg/dL and no ketones are present. Carbohydrates should be eaten if blood glucose is less than 100 mg/dL.
- Monitor blood glucose before and after exercise. Identify when changes in the insulin regimen or diet are necessary. Learn the way the body responds to different types of exercise.
- Monitor necessary food intake. Eat extra carbohydrates as needed to prevent hypoglycemia and always have carbohydrates available during and after exercise. Typical carbohydrate replacement includes 15 g of carbohydrates each hour for moderate-intensity exercise of 30 to 60 minutes in duration and 30 to 50 g of carbohydrates each hour for high-intensity exercise that last more than 1 hour.
- Include a warm-up an cool-down period with each exercise session.

Insulin and Treatment Regimens

Insulin is formed from a substance called proinsulin. It is a hormone produced by the beta cells of the islets of Langerhans in the pancreas. When the pancreas is stimulated by elevated blood glucose, the proinsulin molecule is broken apart into insulin and the connecting peptide referred to as C-peptide. These two molecules are then secreted into the bloodstream in equal amounts. Because insulin has a short half-life, the C-peptide level can be measured to monitor endogenous insulin production and to determine the type of diabetes an individual has. *Normal daily insulin secretion in a healthy, nonpregnant woman is 0.5 to 0.7 U/kg each day.*

The goal of insulin therapy is to mimic the physiologic profile of insulin secretion. In a person without diabetes, insulin is released gradually throughout the day to counteract ongoing hormonal influences. This is called the **basal rate.** When food is ingested, a quick release of insulin occurs. This is called the **bolus.** Insulin management involves developing a regimen to provide exogenous insulin when it is necessary.

Proper use of exogenous insulin must be formulated based on the type of insulin selected and the amount of insulin prescribed. The three sources of insulin are beef, pork, and human. *Human insulin is preferred during pregnancy because it is less antigenic than beef and slightly less antigenic than pork.* Insulin is usually classified based on the peak effect and on duration of action.

The most common types of insulin used during pregnancy are as follows:

- Regular: short-acting
- NPH: intermediate-acting
- Lispro (Humalog): rapid-acting
- Ultralente: long-acting

The major complication of insulin therapy is hypoglycemia.

The choice of insulin for each patient is individualized. For patients with a regular schedule and set mealtimes, usually regular and NPH insulin are used. This choice involves only two injections each day. For patients with a hectic schedule and irregular mealtimes, usually Humalog and Ultralente are used. This choice allows for flexibility because Humalog is given immediately before each meal; however, it involves three injections each day. See Table B.4 for characteristics of regular, NPH, Lispro, and Ultralente insulin.

TABLE B.4	Action of Insulin			
INSULIN	**ONSET OF ACTION (hr)**	**PEAK ACTION (hr)**	**THERAPEUTIC DURATION (hr)**	**APPEARANCE**
Lispro	10–15 min	$1/2$–$1^{1}/2$	3–4	Clear
Regular	$1/2$–1	2–4	6–8	Clear
NPH	1–2	6–14	10–16	Cloudy
Ultralente	4–6	8–24	24–36	Cloudy

The currently available concentrations of insulin in the United States are **U-100** and **U-500. U-100** is the most commonly used. The choice of insulin should be made based on the patient's individual needs. Fixed mixtures of NPH and regular insulin, such as 70/30 or 50/50, are available, but their use is not encouraged during pregnancy because the fixed combinations do not allow flexibility in adjustments for tight control.

The total dose of insulin is calculated based on the patient's weight, blood glucose values, and caloric intake. When insulin therapy is started in the first trimester, the initial total dose is usually calculated at approximately 0.7 U/kg per day. The insulin requirement increases throughout pregnancy as a result of the rising levels of human placental lactogen.

TABLE B.5	Insulin Requirements During Pregnancy	
GESTATIONAL PERIOD	**INSULIN REQUIREMENT (U/kg)**
Preconception	0.6
First trimester	0.7
18–26 weeks	0.8
26–36 weeks	0.9
36 weeks to term	1.0

Obese woman and type 2 diabetic patients may require up to 1.5 to 2.0 U/kg because of the high degree of insulin resistance.

Data from Jovanovic, L. (2000). Acute complications of diabetes: Medical emergencies in the patient with diabetes during pregnancy. *Endocrinology and Metabolism Clinics, 29*(4), 771–787.

Many insulin regimens can be used to obtain glycemic control. These include a single-dose injection, a two-injection regimen, a three-injection regimen, a four-injection regimen, or a continuous subcutaneous insulin infusion by an insulin pump.

The three most common insulin regimens are as follows:

1. Two-injection regimen with regular and NPH insulin
2. Three-injection regimen with Ultralente and Humalog
3. Insulin pump with Humalog

The two-injection regimen with Regular and NPH insulin consists of two thirds of the dose in the morning, with one third of the dose in the evening (Table B.6). Of the morning dose, one third is regular insulin and two thirds is NPH. Of the afternoon dose, half is regular insulin and half is NPH.

TABLE B.6	Calculation of Insulin for Two-Injection Regimen		
TIME OF DAY	**TOTAL DAILY DOSE**	**REGULAR INSULIN**	**NPH INSULIN**
Morning dose	$^2/_3$	$^1/_3$	$^2/_3$
Evening dose	$^1/_3$	$^1/_2$	$^1/_2$

With the **three-injection regimen involving Ultralente and Humalog,** half of the dose is Ultralente and half of the dose is Humalog. The Humalog dose is divided into three doses. One third is given as the breakfast dose, one third is given as the lunch dose, and one third is given as the supper dose. The Ultralente dose is divided into two doses. Half is given as the breakfast dose, and the other half is given as the supper dose (Table B.7).

TABLE B.7	Calculation of Insulin for Three-Injection Regimen	
TIME OF DAY	**HUMALOG** **($^1/_2$ Total Daily Dose)**	**ULTRALENTE** **($^1/_2$ Total Daily Dose)**
Breakfast	$^1/_3$	$^1/_2$
Lunch	$^1/_3$	0
Dinner	$^1/_3$	$^1/_2$

Last, with the **continuous subcutaneous infusion using the insulin pump,** a basal rate is programmed into the pump to deliver a set rate of insulin throughout the day; the rate may be altered depending on the time of day and the patient's activity. Most patients have three basal rates. The first is a low rate from midnight to approximately 4 AM to prevent nocturnal hypoglycemia. The second is an increased rate from 4 AM until approximately 10 AM to counteract the increased release of the cortisol and growth hormone that causes the dawn phenomenon. The third is an intermediate rate from 10 AM until midnight. The patient activates the pump to deliver a bolus of insulin with each meal to cover the glycemic response to food.[5]

Oral antidiabetic agents are not the drugs of choice to use during pregnancy. A recent study compared the use of glyburide, an oral second-generation sulfonylurea, to the use of insulin in women with gestational diabetes. Glyburide was a clinically effective alternative to insulin; however, it has not been approved for use during pregnancy.[6]

REFERENCES

1. Jovanovic, L. (2000). Acute complications of diabetes: Medical emergencies in the patient with diabetes during pregnancy. *Endocrinology and Metabolism Clinics, 29*(4), 771–787.
2. Major, C., Henry, M., De Veciana, M., & Morgan, M. (1998). The effects of carbohydrate restriction in patients with diet-controlled gestational diabetes. *Obstetrics and Gynecology, 91*(4), 600–604.
3. Franz, M., Kulkarni, K., Daly, A., & Gillespie, S. (1998). Therapies: Nutrition. In M. Funnell, C. Hunt, K. Kulkarni, R. Rubin, & P. Yarborough (Eds.), *A core curriculum for diabetes educators* (3rd ed., pp. 188–253). Chicago: American Association of Diabetes Educators.
4. American Diabetes Association. (2001). Position statement: Diabetes mellitus and exercise. *Diabetes Care, 24*(Suppl 1). Available at: http://journal.diabetes.org/FullText/Supplements/DiabetesCare/ Supplement101/S51.htm [Accessed February 5, 2001].
5. Fredrickson, L., & Graff, M. (Eds.). (1998). *MiniMed certified pump trainer manual for insulin pump therapy.* Sylmar, CA: MiniMed.
6. Langer, O., Conway, D., Berkus, M., Xenakis, E., & Gonzales, O. (2000). A comparison of glyburide and insulin in women with gestational diabetes. *New England Journal of Medicine, 343,* 1134–1138.

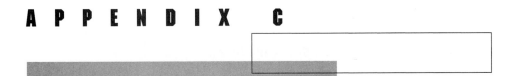

Comfort Care for the Dying Newborn

FRANCINE R. MARGOLIUS, EdD, MSN, RN, FAAN

To everything there is a season, . . .
A time to be born, and a time to die . . .
　　　(Book of Ecclesiastes)

Please take the following mini self-assessment quiz before reading this section.

MINI SELF-ASSESSMENT QUIZ	TRUE	FALSE
1. A newborn can feel pain as early as 20 weeks' gestation.[1]	☐	☐
2. Newborns increase their pain tolerance level during and after multiple heel sticks.	☐	☐
3. Newborns feel pain less then adults because of their immature neurologic and physiologic systems.[2]	☐	☐
4. Morphine is never the analgesic drug of choice for newborns because of the risk of respiratory depression.	☐	☐
5. Newborns are subjected to 50 to 132 procedures every 24 hours, many of which are painful.[3]	☐	☐

Answers can be found just before the References.

Now look at the correct answers. If you answered all the statements correctly, you are well on your way to providing excellent comfort care for the dying newborn.

What Is Comfort Care?

Comfort care, often called palliative care, ensures that each newborn experiences the highest quality of life possible until his or her life ends. This multifaceted concept is more encompassing than preventing and relieving unnecessary pain and suffering. Providing comfort is a holistic approach for compassionately meeting the individual and developmental needs of a newborn. Kolcaba[4] defines *comfort* as "the immediate experience of having met basic human needs for relief, ease, and transcendence." Because newborns are unable to verbally communicate, discomfort must be inferred through physiologic and behavioral indicators and basic developmental needs. Newborns are vulnerable and dependent on caregivers to interpret their every need. This unique circumstance challenges caregivers to know how to accurately assess, evaluate, and interpret their basic and individualized needs.

What Are Newborns' Basic Comfort Needs?

Newborns need consistent nurturing, nourishing, uninterrupted sleep, and a stable environment to promote trust, comfort, and growth. For the dying newborn, the ability to meet these needs is at risk. Promoting parental involvement should be encouraged when possible to provide bathing rituals, gentle rocking, non-nutritive sucking, and swaddling/containment. Parents should be provided support and taught that their involvement, touch, cuddle, voice, and love all contribute to meeting basic needs. Recording parents' voices to play when they are not present and providing appropriate sensory motor stimulus such as mobiles, soft music, and reduced environmental noises and lights help individualize attention to enhance a newborn's life experiences. In addition, nurses' efforts for organized care to allow maximum sleep and positive developmental stimulation greatly contribute to excellence in comfort care.

Are There Misconceptions About Newborn Comfort Needs?

For years it was thought that newborns did not experience discomfort and pain because their central nervous system was not fully developed, lacking myelinization nerve function.[5] Open-heart surgery and other painful procedures were routinely performed without analgesia or comfort relief. It is now known that unmyelinated (C-polymodal) nerve fibers are quite capable of carrying nociceptive impulses. In addition, the descending pathways from the central nervous system that inhibit the transmission of pain signals may not be well developed at birth, particularly in the premature newborn, thus raising the level of pain perception higher than that of adults.[5] Despite these facts, procedures known to be painful continue to be performed without adequate pain relief.

What Are Ways to Know When Newborns Are Uncomfortable or in Need of Comfort Measures?

Newborn Discomfort Relief Tips

Whatever would make an adult uncomfortable or hurt, assume a newborn would feel the same.

Circumcision involves amputating the foreskin, causing tissue damage and significant pain.[6] Adults undergoing circumcision are provided adequate analgesia, whereas neonates are often provided inadequate or no analgesia, resulting in "breath holding, apnea, cyanosis, gagging and vomiting."[6]

Expert assessment skills for normal newborns lead to expertise in identifying deviations from normal.

Learning effective assessments skills takes time and practice. Differentiating facial cues of healthy newborns from those of newborns in pain and discomfort requires repetitive observations based on known behavioral clues (see suggested exercise following).

Be aware of differences in pain and discomfort behaviors among newborns of varying gestational ages.

A term newborn in pain often cues discomfort by loud crying, compared with a premature newborn who may not have the energy to display outward cues and instead "shuts down" with pain.[7]

Term newborns are more likely to receive effective analgesia for painful procedures than are premature newborns.

Research demonstrates that newborns displaying robust pain behaviors receive analgesics and other comfort measures significantly more often than newborns displaying "shut-down" behaviors.[7]

Strong barriers to pain relief measures for newborns are beliefs, misconceptions, and lack of knowledge among health professionals.[8]

Relief of newborn discomfort and pain remains a low priority of health professionals. When opioids are ordered by physicians, nurses avoid administering effective doses approximately two thirds of the time needed. Fear of addiction is the most frequent reason physicians and nurses state for not relieving newborn pain.

Experiential Exercise for Improving Assessment Skills

From this day on, promise yourself that you will be more observant of newborns of varying gestational ages and health status. Current research shows that observing facial expressions of newborns is a useful measure of emotional status,[9,10] so begin your observations comparing newborn faces. Start by observing a healthy, term newborn's face for at least 1 hour. How does the skin appear? Note the color, consistency of color, and mucous membranes. What facial changes do you notice before, during, and after crying? How would you describe the newborn's skin and expression when he or she is relaxed versus when he or she is tense? What facial changes do you notice when the newborn is fussy? Organize and document the details you notice. Then compare your observations with another healthy newborn and then with another until you are confident you are able to identify pertinent observations. Are there similar facial expressions and cues? When do changes in facial expressions occur? What facial cues are given when newborns are hungry, tired, or wet? Challenge yourself to note the differences. Keep practicing these observations until you are able to discuss patterns, changes, similarities, and differences for a healthy newborn. Progress to healthy newborns of varying gestational ages and again compare differences. Developing expertise takes time, motivation, and commitment. The outcomes are well worth your time and affect the quality of comfort care you are able to provide. When you are ready, progress to comparing newborns of varying gestational ages with moderately ill newborns and lastly with a dying newborn. Again, notice similarities and differences. This exercise can be done alone, with a peer, or with a group of peers to compare results and enhance the experience.

This and other similar experiential activities not only will allow you to acquire a level of expertise for assessing newborn comfort levels but will support developing standards of care, policies, and teaching interventions for consistent, effective, and efficient comfort management for dying newborns (see CARE Model).

Are There Pharmacologic Guidelines for Relieving Pain in Newborns?

Even though interest in managing pain in children and infants has escalated over the last 10 years, newborns remain at high risk for poor pain assessment and treatment.[11] Nurses can and should play a major role in ensuring that comfort measures are initiated. Perhaps the strongest impetus so far is the pain management standards published by the Joint Commission on Accreditation of Health Care Organizations (JCAHO),[12] which mandate pain assessment on all newborns on admission and at regular intervals during their hospitalization; these standards went into effect in 2001. However, the most effective method for accomplishing this need has not yet been agreed upon.

A general rule for dosages for newborn infants to those 3 months of age is one half to one third an adult dose.[13] However, this must be individualized to the newborn's size, gestational age, and health status. Principles for using analgesics should be guided by the World Health Organization (WHO) three-step analgesic ladder using adjuvant drugs for mild pain, using non- opioids and adjuvant drugs for moderate pain, and including opioids for severe discomfort and pain.[14] For moderate to severe pain, Anand[15] recommends morphine sulfate 0.05 to 0.1 mg/kg intravenously (IV) with the infusion dose 0.01 to 0.3 mg/kg per hour, and fentanyl citrate 0.5 to 3 mg/kg IV with the infusion dose 0.5 to 2 mg/kg per hour. Other recommendations include lidocaine for local and topical needs, EMLA (lidocaine and prilocaine hydrochloride in an emulsion base), ketamine hydrochloride (systemic) 0.5 to 2 mg/kg IV, infusing 0.5 to 1 mg/kg per hour and for decreasing pain, and acetaminophen 10 to 15 mg/kg orally (20 to 30 mg/kg rectally). In addition, sucrose 12% to 24% solution can be given orally just before mild pain-producing procedures are performed.

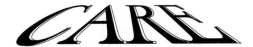

CARE

**(Children's Analgesia, Research and Education
Pain Management Team)**

Clinical Practice	Education	Clinical Research

Education, Clinical Research and Clinical Practice serve as CARE's framework for improving pain management practices for children.

1. Goals
    Clinical Practice: Prevent, relieve, and/or reduce pain and suffering experienced by children.
    Education: Promote current and ongoing evidence-based nursing related to pain management practices.
    Clinical Research: Develop & implement collaborative clinical research studies and performance improvement projects that support current practice and/or advance pain management practices for children.

2. Principles
    a. Prevention of pain is better than treatment. Pain that is established and severe is difficult to control.
    b. Accurate assessment and effective control of pain is partially dependent on a positive relationship between health care professionals and children and their families.
    c. Children who may have difficulty communicating their pain require particular attention; unexpected intense pain should be immediately evaluated.
    d. Unrelieved pain has negative physical and psychologic consequences.
    e. It may not be practical or desirable to eliminate all postoperative and procedure-related pain, but pain reduction to acceptable levels is usually a realistic goal.

    (Adapted from DHHS guidelines.)

3. Requirements:
    a. Pain intensity and pain relief must be assessed and reassessed at regular intervals.
    b. Children's and families' preferences must be respected when determining methods to be used for pain management.
    c. An organized program must be developed to evaluate the effectiveness of pain assessment and management of children.

    (Adapted from DHHS guidelines.)

Developed by Francine R. Margolius, EdD, MSN, RN, FAAN; and Karen A. Hudson, MN, RN, Co-Directors; Children's Analgesia, Education and Research (CARE) Interdisciplinary Pain Team at the Medical University of South Carolina, College of Nursing and Children's Hospital, Charleston, South Carolina.

Aside From Relieving Pain and Discomfort Through Effective Pain Management, What Other Effects Occur?

Effective pain and comfort management for newborns not only prevents and relieves unnecessary suffering but also potentiates other benefits, such as strengthening the immune system, reducing hyperglycemia, improving developmental and adaptive behaviors, helping in maintaining fat and carbohydrate storage, and lowering morbidity rates.[16]

Summary

There is much more to be learned about preventing and relieving unnecessary pain and discomfort in newborns. Closing the gap between currently known research-based evidence and clinical practice is an important goal. Nurses can promote this effort by ensuring their own knowledge and practice is current. Collaborating with peers in practice and clinical research will further promote effective ways to assess newborn comfort. The more nurses know and understand about providing comfort, the more likely the dying newborn will experience a dignified and peaceful life, without unnecessary suffering, until his or her death.

Answers to Mini Self-Assessment Quiz

T, F, F, F, T

REFERENCES

1. Fitzgerald, M., Anand, K., & McIntosh, N. (1989). Pain and analgesia in the newborn. *Archives of Disease in Childhood, 64,* 441–443.
2. Anand, K., & Carr, B. (1989). The neuroanatomy, neurophysiology and neurochemistry of pain, stress and analgesia in newborns and children. *Pediatric Clinics of North America, 36,* 795–822.
3. Lynam, L. (1995). Research utilization: Nonpharmacological management of pain in neonates. *Neonatal Network, 14*(5), 59–62.
4. Kolcaba, K. (1992). Holistic comfort: Operationalizing the construct as a nurse-sensitive outcome. *Advances in Nursing Science, 15,* 1–10.
5. Price, D., & Dubner, R. (1977). Neurons that subserve the sensory-discriminative aspects of pain. *Pain, 2,* 307–338.
6. ASPMN Position Statement. (2001). Neonatal circumcision pain relief. American Society of Pain Management Nurses. Available at: http://www.aspmn.org/html/PScircum.htm
7. Margolius, F. R., Bissinger, R., & Hulsey, T. (2002). Pain assessment in neonates [Unpublished manuscript].
8. Margolius, F. R., Hudson, K. A., & Michel, Y. (1995, March–April). Beliefs, misconceptions and perceptions about children in pain: A survey. *Pediatric Nursing, 21*(2), 111–115, 132–133.
9. Grunau, R., & Craig, K. (1987). Pain expression in neonates: Facial action and cry. *Pain, 28,* 395–410.
10. Grunau, R., Johnston, C., & Craig, K. (1990). Neonatal facial responses to invasive and non-invasive procedures. *Pain, 42,* 295–305.
11. McCaffery, M., & Pasero, C. (1999). *Pain: Clinical management* (2nd ed.). St. Louis: Mosby.
12. Joint Commission on Accreditation of Health Care Organizations. (2001). *Pain management standards for 2001.* Available at: http://www.jcaho.org/standards/pain_hap.html
13. Gaukroger, P., & van der Walt, J. (1995). The clinical aspect of pain control in neonates and children. *Pain Reviews, 2,* 92–110.
14. World Health Organization. (1990). Cancer pain relief and palliative care. *Technical report Series 804.* Geneva, Switzerland: Author.
15. Anand, K., DPhil, M., & The International Evidence-Based Group for Neonatal Pain. (2001). Consensus statement for the prevention and management of Pac's in the newborn. *Archives of Pediatric Medicine, 155,* 173–180.
16. Anand, K., Grunau, R., & Oberlander, T. (1997). Development character and long-term consequences of pain in infants and children. *Child and Adolescent Psychiatry Clinicals of North America, 6*(4), 703–724.

SUGGESTED READINGS

Anand, K., & Hickey, P. (1987). Pain and its effects in the human neonate and fetus. *New England Journal of Medicine, 317,* 1321–1329.

Anand, K., Schmitz, M., & Koh, J. (1998). Future directions for neonatal pain management. *Research Clinical Forums, 20,* 73–81

Anand, K., Stevens, B., & McGrath, P. (Eds.). (2000). *Pain in neonates: Pain research and clinical management* (Vol. 10). New York: Elsevier.

Porter, F. L., & Anand, K. J. S. (1998). Epidemiology of pain in neonates. *Research and Clinical Forums, 20,* 9–18.

Stevens, B. (1999). Pain in infants. In M. McCaffery & C. Pasera (Eds.), *Pain: Clinical manual for nursing practice* (2nd ed., pp. 626–673). St. Louis: Mosby.

RESOURCES

Agency for Healthcare Research and Quality: www.ahrq.gov

American Academy of Hospice and Palliative Care: www.aahpm.org

Department of Health and Human Resources (DHHS), Agency for Healthcare Research and Quality: Acute Pain Management in Infants, Children, and Adolescents: Operative and Medical Procedures, Number 1: 800-358-9295

ELNEC: End-of-Life Nursing Education Consortium; American Association of Colleges of Nursing: www.aacn.nche.edu/elnec

Hospice Foundation of America: www.hospicefoundation.org

Links to websites related to pain and end-of-life care: www.harcourthealth.com/Mosby/Wong/fyi_05.html

Mayday Pain Resource Center at the City of Hope e-mail: mayday_pain

National Hospice and Palliative Care Organization: www.npcho.org

National Library of Medicine (access to Medline and other sources of health information): www.nlm.nih.gov/hinfo.html

Project on Death in America: www.soros.org/death

A P P E N D I X   D

Guidelines for Implementing a Perinatal Education Program[a]

This text has been developed for use by the individual caregiver, an institution, or agency. Accordingly, it may be promoted as:

- An orientation guide for the new labor and delivery nurse
- A continuing education resource for the experienced caregiver, whether that be an advanced nurse practitioner, primary care provider, nurse, physician's assistant, or emergency medical technician (i.e., anyone whose professional responsibilities are involved with a laboring woman)
- A program of study for nurses involved in private obstetric practice settings or in prenatal clinics
- A perinatal outreach education program sponsored by a regional hospital or public health agency
- An adjunct text in nursing education programs, nurse-midwifery education programs, or advanced nurse practitioner programs

The following pages contain materials that are offered to assist an agency or regional center in implementing the text as a perinatal education program throughout a region that encompasses many community hospitals.

Protocol

The protocol gives a general outline of the time required for the regional center to implement the educational program. The time required may vary from center to center. Completion of the self-instructional materials by the community hospital should average approximately 10 weeks, but this too may vary among community hospitals and allowances can be made for individual hospital requirements.

0–1 week	Regional center sends contact letters to community hospitals (to hospital administrator, chief of staff, and director of nursing) to introduce the program.
2–3 weeks	Follow-up phone calls are made to those who receive the letter.
1–2 months	Community hospitals prepare for the program. Regional educators prepare for the workshop. (Educators may wish to visit participating hospitals at this time if they have not had previous contact with the hospital.)
2 months	Workshop is held for nurses designated as coordinators from their hospital (two for each hospital).
2½ months	Introductory meetings for hospital staff are held and modules distributed.
3–5 months	Community hospital staff work through education program.
5 months	Final meeting is held.

Repeat of the entire process with another group of hospitals may be started about halfway through the sequence of the first group.

Introductory Letter

The sample letter that follows on p. 670 is a draft of one that can be used for initial contact with your community hospitals. This letter should be sent to the hospital administrator, chief of staff, and director of nursing of each community hospital, along with a copy of the table of contents of the program.

[a]The implementation forms included in this section, such as the letter, checklist, and survey, were developed for the first edition by Donna M. Childs-Vincent, RN, BSN, MA.

Dear _____ :

We are writing to introduce you to *Intrapartum Management Modules: A Perinatal Education Program* and to explore the possibility of bringing it to your hospital. The program consists of a text and training workshop designed to enhance perinatal care in your institution. The goal of this program is to provide staff nurses in the intrapartum hospital setting with a self-paced, essentially self-instructional syllabus that addresses issues related to the care of the laboring woman and skills essential to nursing assessment and intervention. We have enclosed an outline of the program, which includes information and skill/practice modules.

If your hospital decides to participate, we request that two nurses from your hospital be selected as coordinators for the program. These nurses would then attend a 2-day workshop at [name of the regional center] to learn how to teach the skills included in the program and to become familiar with the administrative details required for the smooth functioning of the program within your hospital. This workshop is the only aspect of the program that does not take place within your hospital and will be held on [workshop dates].

We would appreciate your joining us in an effort to improve perinatal care in [your state], and we look forward to the opportunity of working with your hospital in this endeavor. We will be calling within the next few days to determine your hospital's interest in participating and to answer any questions you might have about the program.

Sincerely,

Regional Center Physician or Administrator
Regional Center Nurse Educator

Sample Workshop Agenda

The agenda outlines just one possible schedule for a 2-day coordinators' workshop at which two nurses from each community hospital are taught the skills that accompany the written material of the program. The nurses (or coordinators) then return to their community hospitals, prepare their staff for the educational program, and schedule a time for the regional center staff to conduct the introductory meeting. During this meeting, which takes place at the community hospital, *Intrapartum Management Modules: A Perinatal Education Program* will be distributed to each participant.

NOTE: The community hospital coordinators should receive their copy of the book before their attendance at the workshop to review and become familiar with its contents.

The workshop is intended to enhance the education program, but should institutions or agencies choose not to use the workshop component, program effectiveness need not be altered.

Day One

8:30 AM	Introduction to the *Perinatal Education Program*
	–Goals
	–Coordinator's role
	–Evaluation of program
10:00 AM	Physical Examination Discussion/Demonstration (Patient Demonstration)
	–General physical examination
	–Abdominal measurement of fundal height
	–Abdominal palpation, evaluation of fetal position and presentation
	–Auscultation of fetal heart tones
10:30 AM	Practice Session
10:45 AM	BREAK
11:00 AM	Assessing for Ruptured Membranes Discussion/Demonstration
	–Sterile speculum examination
	–Nitrazine paper test
	–Fern test
11:30 AM	Practice Session
12:30 PM	LUNCH
1:30 PM	Vaginal Examination Discussion/Demonstration
	–Evaluation of cervical effacement and dilatation
	–Evaluation of station and fetal presentation
2:00 PM	Practice Session
2:45 PM	Friedman Graph Plotting and Analysis Discussion/Demonstration
3:00 PM	Practice Session

Day Two

8:30 AM	Intrapartum Fetal Monitoring Discussion/Demonstration
	–Application of the external monitor
	–Application of the internal monitor
	–Assisting with application of the internal monitor
	–Strip graph interpretation
9:30 AM	Practice Session
10:30 AM	BREAK

10:45 AM	Oxytocin Administration Using an Infusion Pump Discussion/Demonstration
11:30 AM	Techniques for Breathing and Pushing Discussion/Demonstration
12:30 PM	LUNCH
1:30 PM	Managing an Unexpected Delivery Discussion/Demonstration
2:00 PM	Practice Session
2:45 PM	Apgar Scoring Discussion/Demonstration
3:00 PPm	Umbilical Cord Blood Sampling and Analysis Discussion/Demonstration
3:30 PM	Workshop Evaluation

Workshop Materials

Doll and pelvis
Ginny models (2)
Draw sheets (2)
K-Y Lubricating Jelly
Measuring tape
Speculums (variety of types and sizes)
Nitrazine paper
Lamp (gooseneck)
Gloves
Fetoscope and Doptone
Microscope and slides
Cotton-tipped applicators
Cotton balls and ring forceps
Delivery pack
Emesis basin
Bottle of water for pouring
Peribottle
Friedman graph paper (approximately five sheets per participant)
Fetal monitoring strips
Amniotic fluid (can use salt water solution—will give ferning effect when dried)

Consider employing a low-risk pregnant woman who is at 32 to 38 weeks' gestation to enable limited numbers of workshop participants to demonstrate fundal height measurement, Leopold's maneuvers, and fetal heart rate assessment.

Intrapartum Management Modules: A Perinatal Education Program Participant Checklist

To allow coordinators to maintain accurate records of participants' progress in the program, a checklist should be kept on each participant. Completion of module tests and successful skills demonstration should be dated and initialed by the coordinator or preceptor.

Name: _____   Hospital: _____
SS#: _____
License Number: _____
COMPLETED
_____   Module 1 Test: Date: _____
_____   Module 2 Test: Date: _____
_____   Module 3 Test: Date: _____
         Skills:
_____   Physical Examination of the Laboring Woman
         –Demonstrated skill correctly: Date: _____
_____   Testing for Ruptured Membranes Using Sterile Speculum
         Examination and Nitrazine Paper Test
         –Demonstrated skill correctly: Date: _____
_____   Fern Testing for Ruptured Membranes
         –Demonstrated skill correctly: Date: _____
_____   Vaginal Examination
         –Demonstrated skill correctly: Date: _____
         Preceptor Signature/Credentials: _____
_____   Module 4 Test: Date: _____
         Skills:
_____   Measuring Fundal Height
         –Demonstrated skill correctly: Date: _____
_____   Evaluating Fetal Lie, Presentation, and Position Using Leopold's Maneuvers
         –Demonstrated skill correctly: Date: _____
_____   Auscultation of Fetal Heart Tones
         –Demonstrated skill correctly: Date: _____

_____ Preceptor Signature/Credentials: _____

_____ Module 5 Test: Date: _____

Skills:

_____ Friedman Graph: Plotting and Analysis
        –Demonstrated skill correctly: Date: _____

_____ Techniques for Breathing and Relaxation
        –Demonstrated skill correctly: Date: _____

_____ Techniques for Second Stage and Birth
        –Demonstrated skill correctly: Date: _____

        Preceptor Signature/Credentials: _____

_____ Module 6 Test: Date: _____

_____ Module 7 Test: Date: _____

Skill:

_____ Oxytocin Labor Induction/Augmentation
        –Demonstrated skill correctly: Date: _____

        Preceptor Signature/Credentials: _____

_____ Module 8 Test: Date: _____

_____ Module 9 Test: Date: _____

_____ Module 10 Test: Date: _____

_____ Module 11 Test: Date: _____

_____ Module 12 Test: Date: _____

_____ Module 13 Test: Date: _____

_____ Module 14 Test: Date: _____

Skills:

_____ Managing an Unexpected Delivery
        –Demonstrated skill correctly: Date: _____

        Preceptor Signature/Credentials: _____

_____ Module 15 Test: Date: _____

Skills:

_____ Procedure for Obtaining Umbilical Cord Blood Sample
        –Demonstrated skill correctly: Date: _____

        Preceptor Signature/Credentials: _____

_____ Module 16 Test: Date: _____

_____ Module 17 Test: Date: _____

Intrapartum Management Modules: A Perinatal Education Program Evaluation

Having completed this module, you are in a good position to determine the relevancy of the content in enhancing your clinical knowledge and skills. Your answers will provide an important basis for evaluating the program's effectiveness. In addition, this survey offers regional centers or agencies a means of determining the degree of participant satisfaction with the program. A survey of each module studied should be completed by the participant, turned in to the coordinators, and returned to the regional center at the end of the program. You are encouraged to fill out the module survey as you complete the module. You may duplicate this form as needed.

NOTE: If you are applying for continuing education credits, you will need to include a copy of the module evaluation for each module studied.

Name: _____

SS#: _____

KEY

5   Strongly agree
4   Agree
3   Neither agree nor disagree
2   Disagree
1   Strongly disagree

Module Title: _____

Date: _____ Hours to Complete Module: _____

1.   I like this module.

      1   2   3   4   5

      Comments: _____
                _____
                _____

2. The information increased my understanding of topics in this module.

1   2   3   4   5

Comments: _____

_____

_____

3. I can use the information and/or skills learned in this module in my clinical practice.

1   2   3   4   5

Comments: _____

_____

_____

4. I believe that this module has an important place in this program.

1   2   3   4   5

Comments: _____

_____

_____

5. As a result of what I learned in this module, I will do some things differently in caring for the laboring woman.

1   2   3   4   5

Comments: _____

_____

_____

6. The material in this module was difficult to study and understand.

1   2   3   4   5

Comments: _____

_____

_____

7. The posttest helped me identify what I had learned from the module.

1   2   3   4   5

Comments: _____

_____

_____

8. The time it took to complete this module was reasonable.

1   2   3   4   5

Comments: _____

_____

_____

P O S T T E S T S

Posttest: Module 1. Overview of Labor

Answer the following questions without referring back to the information in the module. Select the ONE BEST answer for each question.

1. Which theory can explain the beginning of labor?
   A. Increase in gap junctions near term
   B. Fetal membrane production of arachidonic acid
   C. Efficient flow of calcium into myometrial cells
   D. All of these can play a part in the explanation

2. The first stage of labor is:
   A. Expulsion
   B. Dilatation
   C. Recovery
   D. Placental separation

3. Which tissue layer is responsible for the expulsion efforts during the birth process?
   A. Myometrium
   B. Perimetrium
   C. Endometrium

4. Which characteristic *best* describes the uterus during labor?
   A. Undergoes sporadic contractions
   B. Becomes thicker in all areas
   C. Never relaxes
   D. Differentiates into two separate areas

5. Effacement of the cervix takes place as a result of:
   A. Passive relaxation of the lower uterine segment
   B. Pressure of the presenting part of the baby
   C. Active contractions of the uterus
   D. All of these

6. Which characteristic of a uterine contraction best describes the *increment phase*?
   A. Occurs at the middle of the contraction
   B. Is approximately the same length as the decrement phase
   C. Is approximately the same length as the acme phase
   D. Is longer than either the acme or the decrement phase

7. The duration of a contraction is the time from the beginning of the:
   A. Increment to the end of the decrement
   B. Increment to the beginning of the decrement
   C. Acme to the beginning of the next acme
   D. Increment to the end of the acme

8. Which explanation is the *best* reason why the fingers are placed lightly on the fundus of the uterus when timing contractions?
   A. This is the least painful area for the mother.
   B. The fundus cannot be indented with light pressure.
   C. This is where the contraction usually begins.
   D. The mother is likely to feel the contraction here.

9. To time contractions efficiently, it is best to:
   A. Ask the mother to let you know when they begin and end
   B. Palpate the fundal area of the uterus
   C. Observe the mother's abdomen rise and fall with the contraction
   D. Use internal electronic fetal monitoring

10. The intensity of a contraction:
   A. Cannot be accurately measured
   B. Can be described as strong if the palpating fingers cannot indent the uterus at the peak of a contraction
   C. Cannot be accurately measured by an internal fetal monitor
   D. Can be accurately measured only by an external monitor

11. To make an accurate assessment of cervical dilatation, a vaginal examination should be performed:
   A. As the contraction is beginning
   B. Throughout the contraction
   C. Between contractions
   D. As the contraction is ending

12. Which situation can be characterized as *normal* labor?
   A. Intensity of contractions is 35 mm Hg with a frequency of every 10 minutes.
   B. Intensity of contractions is 12 mm Hg with a frequency of every 5 minutes.
   C. Intensity of contractions is 20 mm Hg with a frequency of every 8 minutes.
   D. Intensity of contractions approaches 50 mm Hg with a frequency of every 5 minutes.

13. The most effective support for the laboring woman includes:
   A. Reducing the number of decisions she is required to make by eliminating any choices she might make in her labor and birth
   B. Allowing a family member to visit at selected periods of time throughout labor
   C. Telling her that "it will make the pain easier to bear" as you administer a sedative
   D. Keeping her informed of her progress

14. Which action provides the most effective support for the laboring woman?
   A. Including her in conversations that you are having with others in her presence
   B. When leaving the room, informing her of the reason and when to expect your return
   C. Telling her in advance of examinations or special procedures
   D. All of these

15. Under the influence of labor contractions, the muscle fibers in the fundal portion of the uterus shorten as the fibers in the lower uterine segment lengthen.
   A. True
   B. False

16. *Effacement* refers to the process in which the cervix becomes shortened or thinned out.
   A. True
   B. False

17. The process of labor has been divided into four stages according to the changes in the mother's body brought about through the process of birthing.
   A. True
   B. False

18. The end of the first stage of labor is defined by:
   A. Rupture of membranes
   B. 5 cm of dilatation
   C. Complete effacement of the cervix
   D. Complete dilatation of the cervix

19. To determine the onset of true labor, it is necessary to identify:
   A. Onset of regular uterine contractions
   B. Complete cervical effacement
   C. Rupture of membranes
   D. Occurrence of bloody show

The patterns of contractions below was repeated over a 2- to 7-hour time segment. Answer questions 20–23 based on this pattern.

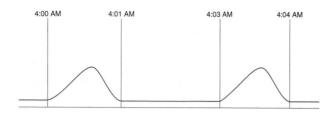

4:00 AM   4:01 AM   4:03 AM   4:04 AM

20. It is probably fair to conclude that the expectant woman is in labor.
    A. True
    B. False

21. Contractions are 60 seconds in duration.
    A. True
    B. False

22. The frequency of contractions is every 4 minutes.
    A. True
    B. False

23. The interval between contractions is 5 minutes.
    A. True
    B. False

24. Match the stage of labor in Column B with the appropriate description in Column A. Place the letter of your choice beside the appropriate number. You may use the choices more than once.

    Column A
    _____ 1. Is a 1-hour period of stabilizing
             of vital signs and body changes
    _____ 2. Ends with the expulsion
             of the placenta
    _____ 3. Includes a latent phase, which
             lasts several hours
    _____ 4. Begins with the onset
             of fairly regular contractions
    _____ 5. Begins with full dilatation of the cervix

    Column B
    A. Stage I
    B. Stage II
    C. Stage III
    D. Stage IV

25. Evidence-based findings show that the continuous presence of a supportive person for the laboring woman is associated with all of the following *except:*
    A. A reduction in the need for cesarean birth
    B. Less likelihood for an Apgar score below 7 at 5 minutes
    C. Avoidance of medication use
    D. Less likelihood of the need for operative vaginal delivery (e.g., forceps, vacuum extraction)

26. A culturally competent nurse will reflect all of the following characteristics *except:*
    A. Retains a sense of humor to keep a balanced perspective
    B. Moves beyond simply tolerating cultural differences to becoming comfortable with differences that exist between himself or herself and the patient
    C. Ignores his or her personal values and biases to interact effectively with a patient
    D. Becomes familiar with the unique needs of patients from different communities

Check your answers with the Module 1 Posttest Answer Key.

Answer the following questions without referring back to the information in the module. ONE OR MORE THAN ONE of the choices may be correct.

1. Which aspect of the fetal passenger is described by the statement, "The fetal head is entering the pelvis first"?
   A. Presentation
   B. Attitude
   C. Position
   D. Lie

2. During an abdominal examination, you determine that Mrs. Hall's baby is lying in a transverse position. What aspect of the fetal passenger are you describing, and is it normal or abnormal?
   A. Attitude; abnormal
   B. Lie; abnormal
   C. Position; normal
   D. Lie; normal

3. The female pelvis has a predominant shape called:
   A. Platypelloid
   B. Android
   C. Anthropoid
   D. Gynecoid

4. The true pelvis is located:
   A. Above the inlet and has narrow dimensions
   B. At the pelvic outlet and has ample room
   C. Below the false pelvis and has narrow dimensions
   D. Above the false pelvis and has narrow dimensions

5. The descent of the fetus is sometimes stopped by the narrowest diameter of the true pelvis, called the:
   A. Pelvic plane
   B. Inlet
   C. Plane of great dimensions
   D. Plane of least dimensions

6. An adaptation that permits the fetus to descend during birth is:
   A. Widening of the pelvic joints
   B. Change in size of the pelvic outlet
   C. Softening of the bony pelvis
   D. Molding of the fetal skull

7. During a vaginal examination, the posterior fontanelle is felt. Which part of the fetus is coming first?
   A. Breech
   B. Head
   C. Shoulder
   D. Foot

8. If you find that the fetal head is well flexed during a vaginal examination, you would expect to feel the:
   A. Sinciput
   B. Sagittal suture
   C. Mentum
   D. Vertex

9. While examining a laboring woman for admission, you discover that the fetus is in a transverse lie. You should know that (choose all answers that apply):
   A. This mother will not deliver vaginally
   B. This condition is associated with placenta previa
   C. There is something wrong with the baby
   D. The happens frequently and there is no reason for concern

10. Normally, the fetus assumes a flexed position because it:
    A. Is more comfortable
    B. Allows for better fetal circulation
    C. Permits the smallest fetal head measurements in relation to the pelvis
    D. Is easier for respirations to occur while labor is in progress

11. When the buttocks or feet enter the pelvis first, the denominator is the:
    A. Vertex
    B. Occiput
    C. Sacrum
    D. Mentum

12. If the occiput is in the left anterior portion of the mother's pelvis, which set of letters accurately describes the fetal position?
    A. ROA
    B. LOA
    C. ROP
    D. LOP

13. If the sacrum of the fetus is in the right posterior area of the mother's pelvis, which set of letters accurately describes the position?
    A. LSP
    B. LST
    C. LSA
    D. RSP

14. The fetal position of ROP describes the position of the fetus in which of the following diagrams?
    A. Diagram A
    B. Diagram B
    C. Diagram C

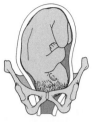
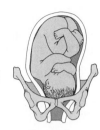

| Diagram A | Diagram B | Diagram C |

15. The fetal position of LSA describes the position of the fetus in which of the following diagrams?
    A. Diagram A
    B. Diagram B
    C. Diagram C

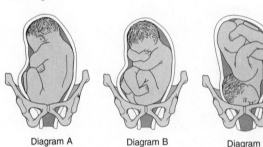

| Diagram A | Diagram B | Diagram C |

16. If the fetus is at a −1 station, it means that the presenting part is:
    A. At the pelvic outlet
    B. Engaged
    C. Above the ischial spines
    D. Below the ischial spines

17. The caput succedaneum is (more than one selection is possible):
    A. A result of the molding of the fetal skull
    B. A soft, swollen layer under the fetal scalp
    C. A cap of fetal hair
    D. Sometimes misleading to the examiner in evaluating fetal descent

18. An abdominal examination determines that the fetal head is "dipping," which means that the:
    A. Fetal head, although not easily moved, is not yet at station 0
    B. Fetal head is easily moved and is still not into the true pelvis
    C. Fetal presenting part is engaged
    D. Fetal presenting part is at station +2

19. Upon examining the newly admitted woman to labor and delivery, you find that the fetal position is LSA. This describes:
    A. Degree of fetal descent
    B. A malpresentation
    C. A fetal attitude
    D. A transverse lie

20. Which two clinical situations are associated with an abnormal lie?
    A. Hydramnios
    B. A fast labor
    C. A multiple pregnancy
    D. A gynecoid pelvis

21. A young primigravida with a fetus in a breech position is in early labor. You know that there is a better-than-average chance that (choose all answers that apply):
    A. The baby will turn
    B. The presenting part will descend quickly
    C. A prolapsed cord might occur
    D. The baby might be delivered by cesarean birth

22. Upon doing a vaginal examination, you determine that there is a prolapsed umbilical cord. Your first action should be to:
    A. Give the mother oxygen
    B. Help the mother into a knee–chest position
    C. Notify the primary care provider
    D. Cover the cord with a sterile pad soaked with saline solution

23. The most appropriate action to take when the membranes rupture in a laboring mother with an unengaged fetal presenting part is to:
    A. Take fetal heart tones
    B. Alert the primary care provider immediately
    C. Do a vaginal examination
    D. Give the mother some privacy

24. A previous difficult and unpleasant labor will have little influence on the progress of a woman's next labor.
    A. True
    B. False

25. The progress of labor usually depends on the adaptations between the fetus and the bony pelvis.
    A. True
    B. False

Check your answers with the Module 2 Posttest Answer Key.

Posttest: Module 3. Admission Assessment of the Laboring Woman (Includes Content from Appendix A)

Answer the following questions without referring back to the information in the module. ONE OR MORE THAN ONE of the choices may be correct.

1. Which statement is *not* an example of an open-ended question?
   A. "What is it that brings you into the hospital?"
   B. "Are you in labor?"
   C. "What did you eat last?"
   D. "How much weight have you gained during this pregnancy?"

2. All of the following questions are important to ask the laboring woman. What two questions should be asked before performing a vaginal examination?
   A. "How far apart are the contractions now?"
   B. "Have you had any problems during your pregnancy?"
   C. "Have you had any bleeding problems during your pregnancy?"
   D. "Has the bag of waters broken?"

3. Which of the following should *not* be done while taking a history on the woman being admitted for labor?
   A. Directing your questions to the person who comes with the laboring woman
   B. Following open-ended questions with more specific ones
   C. Maintaining good eye contact
   D. Avoiding asking questions during contractions

4. You admit a woman in advanced labor who cannot answer many questions. She is accompanied by her 16-year-old daughter. The method you select to obtain the *best* history on this mother before she delivers is to:
   A. Ask the daughter about her mother's pregnancy
   B. Quickly review the woman's prenatal record
   C. Have the medical records department find the delivery chart of the daughter from 16 years ago
   D. None of these methods

5. Which of the following women is *not* at risk for developing problems during labor? The woman who:
   A. Gained a total of 2 pounds with this pregnancy
   B. Has had no prenatal care
   C. Had preeclampsia with her last pregnancy
   D. Is 32 years old and having her first baby

6. A woman is expecting her fourth childbirth and is admitted in labor at 35 weeks' gestation. Compared with a term fetus at 40 weeks, this infant will:
   A. Weigh less and therefore be at risk for problems
   B. Be premature and therefore deliver more quickly
   C. Probably have little difficulty after birth
   D. Be preterm and therefore be at risk for problems

7. You are caring for four laboring women. As you plan your time, which woman will need continuous fetal monitoring?
   A. A 29-year-old woman expecting her fifth childbirth and who is in the early phase of labor
   B. A 21-year-old woman who is in premature labor with her first baby
   C. A 15-year-old who is in false labor
   D. A 34-year-old woman expecting her second childbirth who is progressing well

8. Which assessment indicates that true labor is in progress?
   A. Contractions are felt in the back and are regular; bloody show is present; walking causes the contractions to intensify.
   B. Bloody show occurred 3 days ago; contractions are irregular and disappear when the woman lies down.
   C. Fatigue is present; diarrhea and low backache have been present for the past 12 hours.
   D. Woman cleans house over a 2-day period; low backache and bloody show are present.

9. Characteristics of normal amniotic fluid are:
   A. Greenish color and composed of salts, fetal hair, and cells
   B. Highly alkaline and able to turn Nitrazine paper gray
   C. Clear or straw-colored with no foul odor
   D. Greenish brown color from fetal stool

10. Fresh meconium staining in any laboring woman requires careful assessment of the fetus through continuous fetal monitoring.
    A. True
    B. False

11. Match the terms in Column B with the appropriate amniotic fluid conditions in Column A.

Column A		Column B
1. _____	Greenish brown color	a. Oligohydramnios
2. _____	Less than 500 mL	b. Abruptio placentae
3. _____	Foul-smelling	c. Fresh meconium
4. _____	Yellow color	d. Old meconium
5. _____	More than 2,000 mL	e. Infection
6. _____	Port wine color	f. Hydramnios
		g. Eclampsia

12. Hydramnios is associated with:
    A. Problems in the mother
    B. Problems in the fetus
    C. Problems in both mother and fetus
    D. No problems in the mother or fetus

13. The infant born of a mother who had hydramnios during her pregnancy is best treated by:
    A. Immediate suctioning with a DeLee mucus trap
    B. Careful screening in the delivery room
    C. Routine newborn care
    D. Careful screening during the first 48 hours of life

14. A full bladder can make physical examination of the maternal abdomen:
    A. Inaccurate   C. Uncomfortable for the woman
    B. Difficult to do   D. More accurate

15. In conducting a physical examination on a woman who you are admitting to labor and delivery, you note that her blood pressure is elevated to 148/94 mm Hg. It is important to look for:
    A. An elevated temperature of greater than 99.6°F
    B. A glistening, rigid abdomen
    C. Bloody show
    D. Protein in the urine

16. To obtain an accurate blood pressure reading in a pregnant woman, which two positions are recommended?
    A. Lying supine   C. Sitting up
    B. Standing   D. On her left side

17. To determine whether a blood pressure of 138/88 mm Hg is elevated in a pregnant woman, you need to:
    A. Note whether she is extremely anxious
    B. Check her baseline blood pressure on her prenatal record
    C. Watch her carefully over the next 3 hours
    D. Determine whether she has a history of hypertension

18. A brisk reflex is characterized as:
    A. +1   C. +3
    B. +2   D. +4

19. Clonus in a laboring woman with brisk reflexes can be related to:
    A. Anxiety
    B. Central nervous system irritability
    C. The presence of preeclampsia
    D. All of these

20. The difference between the Graves and Pedersen speculum is that:
    A. The Graves speculum is used more often in women who are tense
    B. The Pedersen speculum is narrower and flatter than the Graves
    C. The Pedersen speculum is used for examining adult women
    D. There is no marked difference

21. To assist a woman in a vaginal examination, which action would *not* be helpful?
    A. Having her fold her arms across her abdomen
    B. Placing a pillow under her head
    C. Telling her to take slow deep breaths throughout the examination
    D. Using your hands to help her separate her legs

22. If the woman becomes upset during a speculum or vaginal examination, the first thing you should do is:
    A. Tell her to let herself relax like a rag doll
    B. Tell her what you are going to do next
    C. Stop what you are doing
    D. Remove the speculum or examining hand

23. To prevent discomfort to the sensitive bladder as the speculum is introduced into the vagina, you:
    A. Use a moderate downward pressure on the blades
    B. Warm the blades under the light
    C. Use a lubricant
    D. Tell the woman she might feel pressure

24. The *two* best methods of determining that the membranes have ruptured are:
    A. Viewing the leaking fluid as it escapes through the cervical opening
    B. Obtaining a blue-gray color using Nitrazine paper
    C. Obtaining a positive fern test
    D. Noting the smell of the amniotic fluid

25. In carrying out the fern test, how long must the slide be allowed to dry?
    A. 1 minute
    B. 15 minutes
    C. 5 to 7 minutes
    D. No drying period is necessary

26. An abdominal examination should always precede an *initial* vaginal examination.
    A. True
    B. False

27. When ruptured membranes are suspected, it is acceptable to use clean instead of sterile gloves in a vaginal examination.
    A. True
    B. False

28. A cervix that feels at least 1-inch thick is probably:
    A. 10% effaced   C. 100% effaced
    B. 50% effaced   D. Uneffaced

29. When the sagittal suture and posterior fontanelle are felt through the cervical opening during a vaginal examination, the fetal presentation is:
    A. Breech   C. Cephalic
    B. Face   D. Shoulder

30. Performing a vaginal examination between contractions will give you the most accurate assessment of cervical dilatation.
    A. True
    B. False

31. Which *two* statements reflect current knowledge about HSV type 1 and type 2?
    A. Asymptomatic infections can occur with either HSV type 1 or type 2.
    B. There is a high correlation between antepartum HSV infection and cervical shedding of the virus at the time of delivery.
    C. Cesarean birth is recommended for all pregnant women with recurrent HSV infection during early pregnancy.
    D. Cesarean birth is recommended only for women who have an active herpes virus lesion at time of delivery, regardless of whether membranes have ruptured.

32. A woman presenting for admission to the labor unit is having contractions every 6 to 8 minutes and is dilated 3 cm. Membranes ruptured 30 minutes ago. She tells you that she has a history of genital herpes infection and that she just noticed this morning that she is developing a painful blister on her right labia. You confirm by inspection that the blister is there. Your next step will depend on the fact that you anticipate:
    A. Admission with expected vaginal delivery
    B. Eventual admission after patient reaches 4 cm dilatation
    C. Admission with preparations begun for cesarean birth
    D. Admission with Pitocin augmentation of labor

33. A presenting fetal part felt at 1 cm below the ischial spines is described as at station:
    A. +1   C. +2
    B. 0   D. −1

34. You are evaluating a young primigravida who is at 35 weeks' gestation and presents with a complaint of "leaking fluid." She denies having any contractions. The initial step in determining her intrapartum risk status would be to:
    A. Perform a sterile speculum examination
    B. Perform a vaginal examination to rule out preterm labor
    C. Carry out 1 hour of electronic fetal monitoring
    D. Do a Nitrazine test

35. For which of the following women is it appropriate to perform a vaginal examination?
    A. A multiparous woman presenting at 30 weeks' gestation in early labor with ruptured membranes
    B. A primigravida at 38 weeks' gestation who has leaking membranes and is not in labor
    C. A multiparous woman with ruptured membranes presenting at 39 weeks' gestation, not in labor, but with a cervix dilated to approximately 3 cm as judged by sterile speculum examination
    D. A primigravida at 37 completed weeks' gestation with ruptured membranes, 90-second contractions every 2 minutes, and pronounced bloody show

36. Which of the women in question 35 has preterm premature rupture of membranes?
    A. A   C. C
    B. B   D. D

37. Fresh meconium staining in the absence of an abnormal fetal heart rate pattern:
    A. Indicates severe distress
    B. Can indicate that the fetus is not in distress
    C. Does not require continuous fetal heart rate auscultation
    D. Indicates fetal hypoxia

38. A mother who is at 43 weeks' gestation is admitted to the labor unit in advanced labor. Membranes are diagnosed as ruptured even though no amniotic fluid is seen. You anticipate that preparations for her delivery will include:
    A. Having a pediatrician or neonatal nurse practitioner present at delivery
    B. Setting up for a cesarean delivery
    C. No need for endotracheal suctioning because no meconium is visualized in the amniotic fluid
    D. The possible need for endotracheal suctioning

Check your answers with the Module 3 Posttest Answer Key.

Answer the following questions without referring back to the information in the module. ONE OR MORE THAN ONE of the choices may be correct.

1. Ms. T. tells you that her last normal menstrual period was October 1, 2002. According to Naegele's rule, the EDC would be:
   A. July 1, 2003
   B. August 8, 2003
   C. July 8, 2003
   D. August 1, 2002

2. To estimate an accurate gestational age you know that fetal heart tones are first heard during the:
   A. Tenth to twelfth week with a Doptone
   B. Thirteenth to fifteenth week with a fetoscope
   C. Eighteenth to twentieth week with a fetoscope

3. The correct order in the physical assessment of the fetus involves:
   A. Performing fundal height measurement after Leopold's maneuvers
   B. Obtaining fetal heart tones and rate before performing Leopold's maneuvers
   C. Obtaining fetal heart tones after fundal height assessment, fetal position, and fetal presentation are determined
   D. Determining fetal lie, position, and presentation before fundal height is measured

4. What steps are necessary to obtain an accurate fundal height measurement?
   A. Bring the measuring tape to the top of the fundus but not over the curve.
   B. Ask the woman to empty her bladder before the measurement is taken.
   C. Carefully identify the border of the symphysis pubis.
   D. Have the same person do the measuring each time.

5. At the twenty-fourth week of pregnancy, the fundal height is expected to range from 20 to 22 cm.
   A. True
   B. False

6. At 40 weeks, the fundal height usually approaches 38 cm.
   A. True
   B. False

7. You obtain a fundal height measurement of 34 cm in an actively laboring woman who is at term according to her EDC. Which of the following could be possibilities for the discrepancy in EDC and fundal height measurement?
   A. A multiple gestation
   B. A growth-restricted infant
   C. An inaccurate EDC
   D. A transverse lie

8. You obtain a fundal height measurement of 44 cm in a woman who is being admitted in early labor. Select the activity that could be omitted from your *immediate* care.
   A. Confirm the expected date of confinement.
   B. Palpate for the presence of twins or polyhydramnios.
   C. Review the mother's prenatal record for a history of diabetes.
   D. Begin an IV.

9. Referring to the situation in question 7, if the high fundal height is caused by hydramnios, which of the following situations is *not* usually associated with that condition?
   A. Tuberculosis
   B. Syphilis
   C. Twin gestation
   D. A blood incompatibility

10. It is determined that a fetus is severely growth restricted in a mother who is just admitted in advanced labor. If you are in a small community hospital, which of the following are priorities for your nursing interventions?
    A. Monitor the fetus electronically.
    B. Prepare for the delivery of a high-risk infant in the event delivery is imminent.
    C. Anticipate that the mother will be transferred to the nearest regional hospital if she is stable.
    D. Do a complete history and careful physical examination on the mother to determine the cause.

11. One of the reasons that Leopold's maneuvers are performed is to assess where to begin listening for fetal heart tones. If the baby's sacrum is pointing to the mother's lower right side and toward her back, what is the baby's position?
    A. LSP
    B. LSA
    C. RSP
    D. RSA

12. When the fetus is in an ROA position, the fetal heart tones are best heard in the:
    A. Right lower quadrant
    B. Right upper quadrant
    C. Left lower quadrant
    D. Left upper quadrant

13. During the examination of a woman who is approximately 39 weeks pregnant, you use Leopold's maneuvers to determine that the lowest level of the fetal head has moved deep into the pelvis. It is immovable. You *estimate* that the fetal head may be:
    A. Hyperextended
    B. Floating
    C. Dipping
    D. Engaged

14. Baseline FHR refers to the fetal heart rate when the woman is either not in labor or is between uterine contractions. It is established over at least a 10-minute interval.
    A. True
    B. False

15. The best time to begin taking a fetal heart rate is between contractions.
    A. True
    B. False

16. Fetal tachycardia is a baseline rate above 160 bpm sustained over at least a 10-minute interval.
    A. True
    B. False

17. Intermittent auscultation during labor has been found to be equivalent to EFM as a method of fetal surveillance in which of the following situations?
    A. In low-risk intrapartum situations
    B. When the laboring woman is at high risk
    C. When there is a 1:1 nurse:patient ratio
    D. When the nurse is experienced and skilled in the method and interpretation

18. In ensuring safe and sound clinical practice, decisions to use intermittent auscultation or EFM in laboring women will need to be guided by the:
    1. Degree of risk in each clinical situation
    2. Staffing on the unit
    3. Expertise of the staff
    4. Preference of the laboring woman and her provider
    A. 1, 2, 3
    B. 1, 3, 4
    C. 1, 2, 4
    D. 1, 2, 3, 4

19. Current research supports findings that the skilled and experienced nurse or provider can use intermittent auscultation to identify:
    A. FHR baseline, rhythm, and accelerations and decelerations from baseline
    B. Early and late decelerations
    C. Short-term variability
    D. Long-term variability

20. Select the one guideline given when using the EFM Doppler *for the purpose of fetal heart rate auscultation.*
    A. The paper recorder can be running, and the tracing must be interpreted.
    B. The paper recorder must not be running.
    C. The paper recorder can be running, but no interpretation of the tracing should be recorded.
    D. None of the above apply.

21. Electronic fetal monitoring for high-risk laboring women results in better neonatal outcomes than when the auscultation method is used.
    A. True
    B. False

22. In caring for a low-risk, actively laboring woman at 40 weeks' gestation, you auscultate fetal heart sounds for 2 full minutes on three separate occasions over a 10-minute period. The rate on each occasions is 100 bpm. Having assisted the mother to side-lying position, your next steps are to:
    A. Begin oxygen, and continue auscultation for at least 30 minutes to assess the true heart rate
    B. Request that another nurse validate the fetal heart rate by auscultation
    C. Change to electronic fetal monitoring
    D. Continue auscultation because 100 bpm is within an acceptable fetal heart rate range

23. Which of the following two choices explain the rationale for the step taken in question 22?
    A. Intermittent auscultation for fetal heart rate is not able to discriminate among types of fetal heart rate changes such as late decelerations or short-term variability.
    B. Continuous electronic fetal monitoring is effective in predicting the extent of fetal distress in utero.
    C. Auscultation by an experienced clinician can identify mild, as well as severe, fetal distress.
    D. Bradycardia accompanied by normal short- and long-term variability indicates that the fetus is tolerating a stressful event, but only electronic fetal monitoring will reveal these variability patterns.

24. Using the auscultation method to establish the baseline fetal heart rate in a woman, you would:
    A. Begin listening immediately after a contraction ends and count for a minimum of 30 seconds
    B. Listen and count throughout the contraction and for a minimum of 30 seconds after
    C. Begin listening as the contraction begins and listen for 30 seconds; then multiply by 2
    D. Listen at least every 60 minutes during early labor

25. A fetal alarm signal is identified as:
    A. The absence of fetal movement and fetal heart rate up to a 12-hour time period
    B. The presence of fetal heart rate accelerations
    C. The absence of fetal movement up to 12 hours while fetal heart tones are present
    D. The presence of fetal movement in the absence of fetal heart rate

26. A multiparous woman seen in the labor unit is reportedly at 38 weeks' gestation. As you review her prenatal record, which of the following is the most reliable criterion for confirming her gestational age?
    A. Reported LMP consisting of only 3 days of spotting
    B. Serum hCG levels less than 10,000 that decrease between 5 and 8 weeks
    C. An ultrasound that revealed a fetal crown-rump length correlating with 9 weeks' gestation
    D. Quickening reported at 20 weeks' gestation

27. Which of the following situations has the greatest risk for the fetus?
    A. A fundal height of 25 cm at 30 weeks' gestation
    B. A fetal heart rate of 170 bpm with fetal movements
    C. A breech lie
    D. A gestational age of 41 weeks

28. A young, expectant woman calls at 6 PM, stating that this is her first pregnancy and that she is due in 3 weeks. Having just completed an hour of "fetal kick counting," her concern is that only six movements were experienced. Further questioning confirms that she has had a normal pregnancy. You:
    A. Instruct her to come in immediately for further evaluation
    B. Tell her to drink two glasses of water or juice, continue counting for 1 more hour, and call back with the results
    C. Explain that this is normal and that she does not need to count anymore today
    D. Praise the mother and tell her to call her primary care provider in the morning for evaluation

29. Which of the following are examples of a fetal adaptive response?
    A. A significant reduction in breathing movements for a few hours in the presence of maternal ingestion of alcohol
    B. A significant reduction in gross body movements before the beginning of labor
    C. A decrease in fetal breathing movements during active labor
    D. Decreased activity in the presence of hypoxia

30. During an early morning admission to the labor unit for a scheduled induction for postdatism, the mother tells you that she has not felt any fetal movement since eating dinner last evening. An appropriate response to this would be to:
    A. Quickly finish the admission process and inform her primary care provider
    B. Auscultate for fetal heart tones as soon as the admission process is completed
    C. Alter your admission process and immediately place an external electronic fetal monitor on the mother
    D. Question the mother about her method of fetal movement assessment and about occurrences of contraction or bleeding activity

31. The rationale for your response to the situation in question 30 is:
    A. The primary care provider might alter the plan of management
    B. Completing the admission process will provide you with important information you need to complete a management plan
    C. Absence of fetal movement for more than 12 hours but with fetal heart tones present indicates a severely distressed fetus and a need for immediate intervention
    D. Maternal perceptions of fetal movement may not always correlate with actual fetal activity, so confirming the presence or absence of fetal heart tones is critical

32. Many expectant women do not seek care because they:
    A. Do not trust what they feel
    B. Have no prior experience on which to base a judgment
    C. Are fearful of advanced technology
    D. Fear being perceived as bothersome or overreacting

33. When an expectant woman in the third trimester of pregnancy calls to report decreased fetal movement, evaluation usually reveals:
    A. A normal fetal heart rate and activity pattern
    B. An overanxious expectant mother
    C. A fetal demise
    D. A fetus in some distress

Check your answers with the Module 4 Posttest Answer Key.

Posttest: Module 5. Caring for the Laboring Woman

Answer the following questions without referring back to the information in the module. ONE OR MORE THAN ONE of the choices may be correct.

1. Reducing a low-risk expectant mother's anxiety during labor can be accomplished by:
   A. Providing comfort measures, such as offering fluid and food choices throughout the first 12 hours of labor
   B. Giving her choices in resting in bed, ambulating, or using a rocking chair
   C. Looking at her and explaining in some detail what you are assessing during a vaginal examination
   D. Anticipating with her how long pushing might take to birth the baby

2. A supportive caregiver behavior(s) is (are):
   A. Nonverbal behaviors that enhance a woman's ability to cope
   B. Vital sign monitoring practices that adhere to standards for maternal and fetal assessments
   C. The provision of assistance with epidural administration
   D. Regulation of IV fluid administration to ensure adequate hydration

3. Maternal NPO (nothing by mouth) practices in labor and delivery units are associated with:
   A. Valid research to support its continuing practice
   B. Risk of fetal hyperglycemia
   C. High acidic gastric contents
   D. An assurance of little maternal stomach contents

4. Appropriate amnioinfusion fluid is:
   A. Sterile water
   B. Normal saline
   C. 5% dextrose and water
   D. Lactated Ringer's solution

5. Amnioinfusion hourly maintenance rates are recommended at:
   A. 100 mL per hour
   B. 150–200 mL per hour
   C. 300 mL per hour
   D. 400 mL per hour

6. Prophylactic amnioinfusion can be done in which of the following situations?
   A. Oligohydramnios
   B. Multiple gestation
   C. Persistent nonreassuring fetal heart rate patterns
   D. Impending delivery with late decelerations

7. Which of the following expectant women are candidates for amnioinfusion?
   A. 38 weeks' gestation, breech presentation with repetitive variable decelerations
   B. 40 weeks' gestation with moderate meconium-stained fluid and persistent late decelerations
   C. 34 weeks' gestation with chorioamnionitis and diminished fetal heart rate variability
   D. 37 weeks' gestation with thick meconium-stained amniotic fluid and reassuring fetal heart rate pattern

8. You are admitting a nulliparous patient who is 5 cm dilated with ruptured membranes and bloody show. She tells you that her contractions began today at approximately 8 AM. Which question is most likely to assist you in estimating the onset of true labor?
   A. When did the contractions begin to last more than 1 minute?
   B. When did the bag of waters rupture?
   C. When did you begin to have bloody show?
   D. When did the contractions begin to come fairly regularly?

9. A nulliparous woman who is having a normal pattern of labor will:
   A. Reach full dilatation in approximately 10 hours of labor
   B. Dilate at a rate of approximately 1 cm per hour in the active phase
   C. Have a pattern of descent at approximately 2 cm per hour in the active phase
   D. Not have a predictable pattern of labor

10. A woman laboring with her third birth remains at 2 cm of dilatation for the first 10 hours. This is:
    A. A normal latent phase
    B. A protracted active phase
    C. Best treated with oxytocin stimulation
    D. An indication that labor will be lengthy

11. Assuming that contractions became fairly regular at approximately 1 PM and using the data given, graph the following labor.

Time	Cervical Dilatation (cm)	Station
1:00 PM	2	−2
2:00 PM	1	−1
3:00 PM	3	−1
4:00 PM	5	0
5:00 PM	9	+1
6:00 PM	10	+3

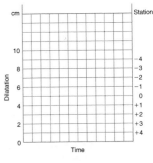

12. The labor in question 11 is most likely a multiparous labor.
    A. True
    B. False

13. The descent pattern in question 11 is protracted.
    A. True
    B. False

14. According to Friedman's recommendations, treatment at this time for the woman laboring in question 11 would include:
    A. Initiation of oxytocin stimulation
    B. A forceps delivery
    C. Continued observation
    D. A cesarean section

15. Which of the following steps ensures an effective but sensitive vaginal examination?
    A. Acknowledging the woman's pain if she indicates discomfort
    B. Performing the examination between contractions
    C. Waiting until the woman gives you consent to begin
    D. Because women will not usually give consent, beginning the examination gently without asking permission

16. A supportive companion (e.g., nurse, father, coach) can increase the laboring woman's chance to:
    A. Have a vaginal delivery
    B. Require less pain medication
    C. Deliver without the complication of meconium-stained amniotic fluid
    D. Experience a shorter labor than she might otherwise have had

The following two questions are about a nullipara who has been admitted to the labor and delivery unit. Her labor curve has been plotted on a Friedman graph and appears on the following figure.

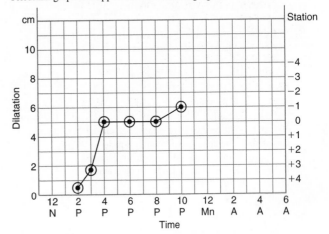

17. The endpoint (4 to 10 PM) of the curve shows:
    A. A prolonged latent phase
    B. Normal labor
    C. Arrested dilatation
    D. A protracted active phase

18. If cephalopelvic disproportion and malpresentation have been ruled out, which of the following treatments is *not likely* to improve the pattern, according to Friedman's recommendations?
    A. Sedation and rest
    C. Intravenous fluid
    B. Oxytocin stimulation
    D. Artificial rupture of membranes

19. A woman in active labor is dilating at an average rate of 1.5 cm per hour. Which of the following describes the woman's progress in labor?
    A. A protracted labor pattern for the multipara
    B. A precipitous labor pattern in the nullipara
    C. Normal rate of dilatation for the multipara
    D. A precipitous labor pattern in the multipara

20. A 28-year-old gravida, 10 para 9, is 8 cm dilated but remains at 12 station for 2 hours. She is having labor induction for preeclampsia. Which of the following is *not* effective in treating arrest of descent?
    A. Allowing excessive sedation to wear off
    B. Providing therapeutic rest
    C. Continuing the oxytocin stimulation
    D. Encouraging a family member to remain in the room for support

21. A protracted descent pattern might be caused by an occiput posterior position of the fetus.
    A. True
    B. False

22. A woman you are caring for is experiencing a protracted active phase. Select the statement or statements that identify appropriate treatment for this situation.
    A. Amniotomy
    B. Increasing the rate of IV fluid intake if it is running at a rate of less than 1,000 mL every 8 hours
    C. Oxytocin stimulation
    D. Offering constant support to reduce the need for added sedation

23. You are caring for M.J., a 22-year-old low-risk laboring woman who is 7 cm dilated. She does not have an electronic fetal monitor. Which of the following nursing actions are appropriate?
    A. Performing a vaginal examination every 15 minutes, as should be done on all laboring women who are dilated 7 cm or more
    B. When auscultating for fetal heart tones, counting the FHR throughout a contraction and for 30 seconds after the contraction
    C. Encouraging the mother to lie on either side during much of her remaining labor
    D. Discouraging any family members from remaining with M.J. during this difficult phase of labor

24. You auscultated M.J.'s fetal heart rate at 1:15 PM. The next time it should be evaluated is at:
    A. 1:20 PM
    C. 1:30 PM
    B. 1:25 PM
    D. 1:45 PM

25. M.J.'s blood pressure at 1:15 PM was 128/80 mm Hg. Her blood pressure has been fairly stable throughout labor. If her status remains basically stable, you will evaluate her blood pressure again at:
    A. 1:30 PM
    C. 2:00 PM
    B. 1:45 PM
    D. 2:15 PM

26. A young woman at 39 weeks' gestation is admitted to the hospital; she is having uterine contractions every 5 minutes, and they last for 40 seconds. The cervix is well effaced and dilated 2 cm. There is no change in the findings after 1 hour. This patient exhibits:
    A. Active labor
    C. Abruptio placentae
    B. False labor or latent-phase labor
    D. Precipitous labor

27. A woman presents with questionable ruptured membranes. The most accurate method for determining whether membranes have ruptured is:
    A. The Nitrazine test
    B. A careful history obtained from the mother
    C. An ultrasound examination
    D. A sterile speculum examination and fern test

28. Pressure, traction, and stretching of body tissues cause labor pain, making it impossible to reduce the mother's discomfort.
    A. True
    B. False

29. Pain experienced by the laboring woman can ultimately make the brain cells of the fetus more susceptible to damage during a hypoxic period.
    A. True
    B. False

30. Rapid breathing in the laboring mother can lead to a decreased blood supply to the uterus.
    A. True
    B. False

31. You have just come on duty and have not yet made rounds in the labor unit. An order for pain medication has been received for a young nullipara who is restless and calling out. Which of the following will you do before giving the pain medication?
    A. Quickly review her prenatal record.
    B. Take her blood pressure and FHR.
    C. Note the size and maturity of the fetus according to gestational age.
    D. Determine what progress she has made in labor.

32. Slow chest breathing:
    A. Involves taking deep breaths in through the nose and exhaling through the mouth or nose
    B. Is used during Stage II of labor
    C. Is done with the eyes closed
    D. Begins and ends with a cleansing breath

33. Effleurage is:
    A. A big deep sigh that begins and ends each contraction
    B. A massage technique that can be done by the mother, nurse, or support person
    C. Used between contractions
    D. Sometimes done by the coach

34. Which position for pushing does not make use of the effects of gravity or result in good circulation for the woman and fetus?
    A. Squatting
    B. Semi-Fowler's
    C. Sims
    D. Lithotomy

35. Select the statement that represents current recommendations for nursing assessment of maternal and fetal status during Stage II of labor.
    A. Fetal heart rate is checked before and during each contraction, and maternal blood pressure is taken every 5 minutes.
    B. Fetal heart rate is checked after each contraction, and maternal blood pressure is taken every 30 minutes.
    C. Fetal heart rate and maternal blood pressure are checked every 15 minutes.
    D. Fetal heart rate and maternal blood pressure are checked after each contraction.

36. When you begin your evening shift at 4 PM, you receive a report on an 18-year-old gravida 1 who is in active labor. At 2 PM, she was 5 cm dilated and 100% effaced, with the vertex at 0 station. Membranes ruptured at 11 AM. You evaluate her and note that she is on her back, restless, and requesting pain medication. Contractions are occurring every 3 minutes, are of 70 seconds' duration, and are strong on palpation. Her physician is performing an emergency cesarean section. Which sequence of steps will you take next?
    A. Take vital signs, including temperature; perform an abdominal palpation for fetal position; check fetal heart rate; perform a vaginal examination; inform the woman of progress made; assist her to a side-lying position.
    B. Perform a vaginal examination; perform an abdominal palpation for fetal position; check fetal heart rate; inform the woman of progress made; take vital signs, including temperature; assist her to a side-lying position.
    C. Assist the woman to the bathroom for voiding; take vital signs, including temperature; perform a vaginal examination; check fetal heart rate; assist her to a side-lying position.
    D. Perform an abdominal palpation for fetal position; check fetal heart rate; perform a vaginal examination; inform the woman of progress made; take vital signs, including temperature; assist her to a side-lying position.

37. When you administer IV pain medication to the laboring woman, you should:
    A. Use a filter needle when drawing the medication from glass ampules
    B. Always position the mother on her side
    C. Give the medication at the beginning of a contraction and over a period of a few minutes, if possible
    D. Give the medication at the end of a contraction and over a period of a few minutes, if possible

38. Which of the following situations is (are) more likely to result in a depressed infant?
    A. Protracted labor treated with Pitocin augmentation
    B. Secondary arrest of labor with subsequent vaginal delivery
    C. Secondary arrest of labor with subsequent cesarean delivery
    D. Arrest of descent treated with Pitocin augmentation and forceps delivery

39. Nursing measures carried out in preparation for and during the test dosing for epidural anesthesia include all of the following *except:*
    A. Noting maternal BP and pulse rate before and after administration of the test dose and at least every 5 minutes throughout the administration
    B. Ensuring that the woman's bladder is not full
    C. Explaining potential complications to the woman
    D. Confirming a reassuring fetal heart rate tracing prior to the procedure.

40. Select two statements that reflect what is currently appreciated about epidural anesthesia nursing care in the laboring woman.
    A. There are reliable, statistically significant data showing a cause-and-effect relationship between the use of epidural anesthesia and adverse effects.
    B. AWHONN guidelines for nursing care of women receiving epidural analgesia/anesthesia draw from considerable nursing research.
    C. While concern exists that epidural anesthesia may be associated with prolonged stages of labor, increased use of vacuum extractions and forceps, and higher rates of cesarean births, some clinicians believe the individual styles of obstetric management may play a significant role as well.
    D. Administration of bolus medications for an epidural anesthesia by the nurse is not supported in AWHONN guidelines.

Check your answers with the Module 5 Posttest Answer Key.

Posttest: Module 6. Intrapartum Fetal Monitoring

Answer the following questions without referring back to the information in the module. ONE OR MORE THAN ONE of the choices may be correct.

1. For each of the following statements, indicate whether the statement refers to external fetal monitoring (E), internal fetal monitoring (I), or both (B).
   a. _____ Procedure is noninvasive.
   b. _____ Decelerations can be detected in the fetal heart rate.
   c. _____ Intensity of the uterine contractions can be assessed.
   d. _____ Procedure is associated with no fetal or maternal morbidity.
   e. _____ Procedure requires partial dilatation of the cervix.
   f. _____ Frequency of the uterine contractions can be determined.
   g. _____ Short-term variability of the fetal heart rate can be assessed during labor.

2. The baseline fetal heart rate:
   A. Is between 110 and 160 bpm
   B. Is determined between contractions
   C. Can be influenced by maternal hyperthermia and hypoxia
   D. All of the above
   E. None of the above

3. Which of the following statements are *true* regarding baseline uterus tonus?
   A. Defined as the amount of tone in the uterus during a contraction
   B. Usually ranges between 5 and 15 mm Hg, but is not greater than 30 mm Hg
   C. Can be determined using an external or internal fetal monitor
   D. Can be increased with the use of Pitocin

4. Which of the following statements are *true* concerning fetal heart rate bradycardia?
   A. It is often defined as a decrease in the fetal heart rate to less than 110 bpm, lasting longer than 10 minutes.
   B. It can reflect prolonged fetal hypoxia.
   C. Oxygen therapy should be used in the treatment.
   D. All of the above are correct.

5. Uterine contractions can alter fetal heart rate via compression of the myometrial vessels, compression of the fetal head, and compression of the umbilical cord.
   A. True
   B. False

6. Indicate the appropriate type of periodic heart rate change using the following key. There may be more than one answer.
   Characteristics of Periodic Heart Rate Changes
   a. _____ Rarely falls below 110 bpm
   b. _____ Most common type of periodic change
   c. _____ Not a sign of fetal stress
   d. _____ Usually associated with good fetal outcome
   e. _____ Reflect(s) fetal hypoxia
   f. _____ Has (have) no consistent onset in relation to the contraction pattern
   g. _____ Uniform in shape and always last longer than the contraction
   h. _____ Often associated with poor variability
   i. _____ Usually associated with good variability
   j. _____ Should be treated with oxygen therapy
   k. _____ Caused by uteroplacental insufficiency
   l. _____ Caused by umbilical cord compression
   m. _____ Caused by fetal head compression

   Key
   A = accelerations
   ED = early decelerations
   VD = variable decelerations
   LD = late decelerations
   PD = prolonged decelerations

7. You are caring for a laboring patient who is being monitored. You notice several early decelerations. You should (more than one answer may be correct; list all):
   A. Continue to watch the monitor closely and perform a vaginal examination
   B. Begin oxygen therapy
   C. Notify the primary care provider immediately
   D. Change the patient's position

8. You are caring for a laboring patient who is being monitored. You notice a decrease in variability along with two subtle late decelerations in a 15-minute period. You should:
   A. Begin oxygen therapy
   B. Notify the primary care provider
   C. Change the patient's position to lateral
   D. Do the above *only* if the late decelerations begin to occur more frequently

9. Pitocin infusion should be stopped in the following situation(s):
   A. Occurrence of repetitive late decelerations with loss of variability
   B. Occurrence of severe and prolonged variable decelerations
   C. Occurrence of early decelerations
   D. All of the above

Questions 10 through 16 refer to the following strip graph. Use this strip to answer these questions. (This is an internal fetal monitor strip.)

10. What type of periodic heart rate change is present?
    A. Acceleration   C. Variable deceleration
    B. Early deceleration   D. Late deceleration

11. The fetal heart rate short-term variability is:
    A. Absent   C. Moderate
    B. Minimal   D. Marked

12. The baseline fetal heart rate is:
    A. 153 to 155 bpm   C. Increased
    B. 140 to 160 bpm   D. Decreased

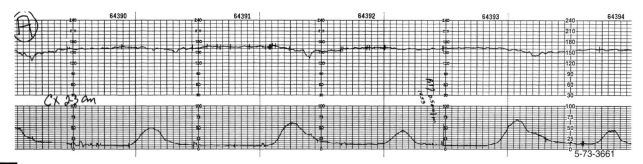

13. The cause of this periodic heart rate change is:
    A. Head compression
    B. Umbilical cord compression
    C. Uteroplacental insufficiency

14. The baseline uterine tone is:
    A. Within normal range
    B. Indeterminable with this type of monitoring
    C. Increased
    D. Decreased

15. The intensity of the uterine contractions is:
    A. 45 to 70 mm Hg
    B. 75 to 85 mm Hg
    C. Indeterminable with this type of monitoring
    D. Indicative of a moderate contraction

16. From the following list, determine the appropriate nursing action(s) for this type of periodic heart rate change. If the action is considered appropriate, write an "A" before the action. If the action is *not* considered appropriate, write an "N" before the action.
    a. _____ Turn the patient to her left side.
    b. _____ Continue watching the monitor closely.
    c. _____ Begin oxygen therapy.
    d. _____ Decrease the IV rate.
    e. _____ Place the patient on her back.
    f. _____ Turn off Pitocin (if infusing).
    g. _____ Notify the primary care provider immediately.

17. Mrs. S., a 35-year-old hypertensive patient at 38 weeks' gestation, is admitted in labor, and a fetal monitor is applied. Considering this patient's history, you must watch closely for:
    A. Early decelerations
    B. Late decelerations
    C. Variable decelerations

18. Hypoxia can be indicated by all of the following *except:*
    A. Late decelerations   C. Early decelerations
    B. Decreased variability   D. Fetal heart rate tachycardia

19. Complications of excessive oxytocin administration are:
    A. Uterine hypertonus   D. All of the above
    B. Uterine rupture   E. None of the above
    C. Fetal hypoxia

20. Variable decelerations:
    A. Start as a gradual drop from the baseline
    B. Must occur with contractions
    C. Are usually responsive to maternal position changes
    D. Rarely occur with shoulders

21. After administration of epidural anesthesia, late decelerations are observed. All of the following are appropriate interventions *except:*
    A. Increasing IV fluids
    B. Keeping the patient on her back
    C. Administering oxygen
    D. Discontinuing oxytocin infusion

22. Indications for internal FHR monitoring include all of the following *except:*
    A. Late decelerations with apparent good variability
    B. A fetus with an irregular heartbeat
    C. Accelerations of FHR
    D. An active fetus that is difficult to monitor externally

23. All of the following can cause prolonged FHR decelerations *except:*
    A. Cord prolapse
    B. Epidural anesthesia
    C. Hypertonic uterus
    D. Tetanic contractions
    E. Maternal fever

24. Which of the following is recommended *prior to* the initiation of electronic fetal monitoring?
    A. Auscultating the FHR
    B. Performing Leopold's maneuvers
    C. Starting IV fluids
    D. A and B
    E. B and C

25. In the presence of an intrauterine fetal death, the fetal electrode:
    A. Occasionally picks up the maternal ECG signal
    B. Always picks up the maternal ECG signal
    C. Will generate no signal
    D. Never picks up the maternal ECG signal

26. The spiral electrode permits accurate recording of:
    A. Variability   C. Accelerations
    B. Decelerations   D. All of the above

27. Ominous signs of fetal stress include all of the following *except:*
    A. Smooth baseline—absent FHR variability
    B. Accelerations of the FHR
    C. Late decelerations
    D. Sinusoidal pattern

28. Loss of *one shoulder* with variable decelerations probably indicates:
    A. Severe fetal distress
    B. The need for preparation for an aggressive resuscitation of the newborn
    C. Increasing placental dysfunction
    D. Respiratory acidosis
    E. A and D
    F. B and C

29. Absent short-term variability can be indicative of:
    A. Metabolic acidosis   E. A and B
    B. Fetal hypoxia   F. B and C
    C. Respiratory acidosis   G. C and D
    D. Mixed acidosis

30. Characteristic(s) of an abruptio placentae seen on the fetal monitor strip might include:
    A. A wavelike contraction pattern   E. B and C
    B. Increased baseline tone   F. A, B, and C
    C. Frequent contractions   G. All of the above
    D. Fetal tachycardia

Label the statements in questions 31 through 72 as:
    A. True
    B. False

31. _____ Variable decelerations indicate maternal hypotension.

32. _____ Early decelerations are uniform in shape.

33. _____ Some deceleration patterns may be corrected by giving terbutaline.

34. _____ The presence of short-term variability and periodic changes can usually be detected accurately with both internal and external monitoring.

35. _____ Fetal tachycardia, if untreated, can proceed to bradycardia and finally death.

36. _____ When fetal stress is suspected, it is appropriate to turn the patient on her side; discontinue the oxytocin, if it is infusing; administer a bolus of IV fluids; and perform a vaginal examination.

37. _____ Late decelerations are uniform in shape, last beyond the contraction, and often are associated with acidosis and hypoxia.

38. _____ The fetal heart rate baseline is determined in bpm during a contraction.

39. _____ Variable decelerations are believed to be a result of cord compression.

40. _____ Everything pertaining to the care of a patient should be on the tracing except the diagnosis or identification of periodic changes.

41. _____ Anything that affects maternal blood flow can affect the blood flow through the placenta.

42. _____ Chronic maternal diseases such as hypertension, diabetes mellitus, and collagen vascular disease can all compromise placental gas exchange.

43. _____ A persistent sinusoidal pattern can be associated with fetal asphyxia.

44. _____ Short-term variability is a sensitive indicator of adequate fetal oxygenation and reserve.

45. _____ A true sinusoidal pattern is uncommon.

46. _____ Early decelerations do not require intervention.

47. _____ Tachycardia usually proceeds bradycardia.

48. _____ The FSE can pick up the maternal heart rate if the fetus dies.

49. _____ Events such as blood pressure, VE, and medications should be accurately noted on the tracing. Therefore, tracings are replacements for conventional notes.

50. _____ Baroreceptors are stimulated by changes in the arterial blood pressure.

51. _____ Periodic changes should be marked and identified on all tracings.

52. _____ During cord compression, the arteries are the first vessels to be compressed.

53. _____ Late decelerations always begin at the peak of the contraction.

54. _____ Maturation of the parasympathetic nervous system is usually complete by week 28 to 32 of gestation.

55. _____ The fetal heart rate can stay within the normal range and still show signs of stress.

56. _____ A FHR baseline above 100 bpm with good variability is almost always benign.

57. _____ Variable decelerations can vary in shape and onset and are caused by placental dysfunction.

58. _____ Late decelerations usually remain within the normal FHR range.

59. _____ When determining whether the FHR pattern is reassuring or nonreassuring, one must assess variability.

60. _____ FHR accelerations can be a response to contractions, fetal movement, or abdominal palpation.

61. _____ Variable decelerations are thought to be caused by cord compression.

62. _____ The gradual decrease in FHR that occurs with increasing gestational age can be explained as increased maturation of the parasympathetic nervous system.

63. _____ In the presence of persistent late decelerations, there is nothing that the caregiver can do to improve the FHR pattern.

64. _____ FHR accelerations are almost always a sign of fetal well-being.

65. _____ When variability is absent, late decelerations, regardless of depth, should always be considered nonreassuring.

66. _____ Variables are uniform decelerations.

67. _____ Patients in labor should always lie on their backs so that the monitor can function properly.

68. _____ The fetal baseline heart rate is usually the best indicator of fetal oxygenation.

69. _____ FHR variability is determined exclusively by the sympathetic nervous system.

70. _____ The characteristic that distinguishes a variable deceleration from other kinds of deceleration is the abrupt drop from baseline.

71. _____ Periodic and nonperiodic changes (accelerations and decelerations) should be *marked* on all tracings.

72. _____ A sign on the monitor strip that might indicate *early* fetal hypoxia is bradycardia.

73. Select the appropriate interpretation of the following umbilical cord blood gas values. Choose from the following:
    1. Normal
    2. Normal with a shift toward metabolic acidosis
    3. Normal with a shift toward respiratory acidosis
    4. Metabolic acidosis
    5. Respiratory acidosis
    6. Metabolic and respiratory acidosis (mixed acidosis)
       a. _____   pH 7.12
                        Pco_2 69 mm Hg
                        Po_2 22 mm Hg
                        BD 4.4
       b. _____   pH 7.25
                        Pco_2 50 mm Hg
                        Po_2 24 mm Hg
                        BD 4.5
       c. _____   pH 7.16
                        Pco_2 36 mm Hg
                        Po_2 16 mm Hg
                        BD 12.0
       d. _____   pH 7.22
                        Pco_2 51 mm Hg
                        Po_2 17 mm Hg
                        BD 8.0

74. Given the following strip descriptions, state your expectations of the umbilical cord blood pH results (all baselines are within normal limits *unless otherwise stated*). Select from the choices given in question 73.
    a. _____ Absent variability, repetitive late decelerations, no accelerations
    b. _____ Repetitive variable decelerations, *no preshoulders,* postshoulders present, present STV
    c. _____ Present STV, moderate LTV, repetitive reassuring variable decelerations
    d. _____ Moderate LTV, present STV, occasional late decelerations
    e. _____ Absent STV, repetitive variable decelerations with loss of shoulders, overshoots present
    f. _____ Tachycardia 180 to 200 bpm, present STV, absent LTV.

Check your answers with the Module 6 Posttest Answer Key.

Answer the following questions without referring back to the information in the module. Select the ONE BEST answer for each question.

Mrs. Lea K. Waters is a 27-year-old woman admitted to the labor unit. She is at term with her second pregnancy. Her membranes ruptured 10 hours ago, and she has no palpable uterine contractions. Upon abdominal examination, you estimate fetal weight at 8 to 8.5 pounds and determine that the fetus is vertex presentation, ROA, and not engaged. Sterile vaginal examination reveals a roomy pelvis with presenting part at −2 station and cervix anterior soft, 80% effaced, and 3 cm dilated. The fluid is clear; vital signs and fetal heart rate are normal.

Mrs. Waters' first pregnancy was uneventful, and she delivered her 8-pound, 2-ounce son over an intact perineum. This pregnancy has been a good one for her. Family history; past medical, surgical, and gynecologic history; and current laboratory work are all normal. She and her husband plan to use their prepared childbirth techniques. Mrs. Waters will breastfeed this baby.

1. On the basis of this information, Mrs. Waters is a good candidate for oxytocin stimulation.
   A. True
   B. False

2. Her Bishop's score is:
   A. 6
   B. 8
   C. 10

You call Mrs. Waters' health care provider to give him your assessment. He informs you that he saw her several days ago in the office and that your vaginal examination findings are the same as his were at the time. He then directs you to start electronic fetal heart rate monitoring and to insert an intrauterine pressure catheter. After you have obtained a normal baseline evaluation, he wants you to start an oxytocin induction. He is readily available in his office next door and will be in to evaluate Mrs. Waters in an hour or two. You have his approved induction/augmentation protocols on file, and you are properly credentialed to initiate and conduct internal electronic monitoring, insert an intrauterine pressure catheter, and administer oxytocin per protocol.

3. The nurse should begin the oxytocin administration after a baseline evaluation to prevent delay and possible infection.
   A. True
   B. False

4. Before oxytocin is administered, the:
   A. Nurse must sedate the anxious woman if she refuses induction/augmentation
   B. Woman should be examined and a physician credentialed to perform a cesarean section must be readily available
   C. Woman's health care provider must write the order for the oxytocin administration rate that will dilate the woman's cervix most rapidly
   D. Nurse knows that if the woman is parous, her Bishop's score must be more than 5

5. Match the terms in Column B with the appropriate definition in Column A.

   Column A
   1. _____ Tetanic contractions
   2. _____ Fetal hypoxia
   3. _____ Water intoxication
   4. _____ Fetal bradycardia
   5. _____ Uterine dystocia
   6. _____ Pitocin
   7. _____ Secreted by the posterior pituitary
   8. _____ Augmentation of labor

   Column B
   a. Trade name for a synthetic hormone that makes the uterus contract
   b. Stimulating uterine contractions to become more powerful
   c. Retention of water, low serum levels of salt, and poor urinary output
   d. Powerful contractions without adequate rest periods
   e. Poor-quality contractions
   f. Slow heartbeat
   g. Decreased oxygen
   h. Oxytocin

6. For safe administration of oxytocin, the following is recommended.
   A. Piggyback setup, electronic fetal/uterine monitoring, and nasal oxygen
   B. Two-bottle IV administration setup, fluid administration setup, and fetal/uterine electronic monitoring
   C. IV fluid administration pump, piggyback setup, and electronic fetal/uterine monitoring
   D. Infusion control pump with filter needle attached, two-bottle setup, and fetal/uterine electronic monitoring

7. If sustained fetal bradycardia, tachycardia, or loss of variability is observed during the administration of an oxytocin infusion, the first thing the nurse must do is:
   A. Call the woman's health care provider
   B. Change the woman's position and reassure her
   C. Keep the rate of oxytocin administration at the same setting until the fetal heart rate improves
   D. Discontinue the administration of the oxytocin

8. When administering oxytocin for augmentation of labor, the nurse must be aware that it will:
   A. Usually cause tetanic contractions, which dilate the cervix quickly
   B. Cause a forceful and rapid birth of the baby
   C. Be safe when the woman is evaluated before the administration of the drug and the guidelines for administration are followed
   D. Be safe for any woman with a large pelvis who is at term

9. At least every 30 minutes, the nurse should take and record blood pressure, pulse, respiration, fetal heart tones, frequency and quality of contractions, and resting uterine tone.
   A. True
   B. False

10. Rate of fluid administration and dosage should be recorded every hour.
    A. True
    B. False

11. Noting maternal response to augmented labor contractions is more important than noting fetal response.
    A. True
    B. False

12. Elective induction/augmentation with oxytocin is not recommended.
    A. True
    B. False

13. Preinduction cervical ripening with Prepidil Gel (PGE₂) should be performed in the hospital. The Prepidil Gel:
    A. Should be carefully introduced into the extraamniotic space if the membranes have ruptured
    B. Should be warmed to 96.8°F before use and liberally applied to the cervix
    C. Should be inserted into the endocervical canal, below the level of the interval os
    D. Can be repeated every 4 hours until cervical changes occur or oxytocin induction is initiated

14. Cervidil Vaginal Insert dosing may be repeated as long as each insert is changed every 12 hours.
    A. True
    B. False

15. When misoprostol is used for safety and best outcomes, the 100-μg tablet should be cut by the pharmacist and placed in the posterior vaginal fornix with a small amount of lubricant.
    A. True
    B. False

16. All of the following are elements of active management of labor *except:*
    A. Is an attempt to reduce cesarean births resulting from dystocia
    B. Involves vigorous management of labor, often by using oxytocin induction and amniotomy
    C. Is carried out for nulliparas with a term single fetus in no distress who are in active labor, have ruptured membranes, and are progressing at less than 1 cm per hour
    D. Often uses higher starting dosages of oxytocin and increases at greater increments than does labor induction

Check your answers with the Module 7 Posttest Answer Key.

Posttest: Module 8. Caring for the Woman at Risk for Preterm Labor or With Premature Rupture of Membranes

Answer the following questions without referring back to the information in the module. Select the ONE BEST answer for each question.

1. When you admit a woman with ruptured membranes at 32 weeks' gestation, the greatest risk results from:
   A. Chorioamnionitis
   B. Spontaneous labor
   C. Immature fetus
   D. Impending cesarean birth

2. Mrs. A.M. is admitted to the labor unit at 38 weeks' gestation with leaking membranes. Labor has not begun. The plan of management probably will include:
   A. Beginning oxytocin induction of labor immediately
   B. Evaluating Mrs. A.M.'s white blood count to see if it is elevated
   C. Waiting until labor begins spontaneously unless signs of infection develop
   D. Beginning an oxytocin induction if labor does not start spontaneously within 24 to 48 hours

3. Treatment of premature ruptured membranes depends on:
   A. The gestational age of the fetus at the time of ruptured membranes
   B. The presence or absence of an infection
   C. Whether the fetus is assessed as mature or immature
   D. All of the above

4. A young primigravida comes to a small community hospital stating that her "bag of waters" has broken. She is at 29 weeks' gestation by dates and size. Labor has not begun. The nurse can anticipate that he or she will need to:
   A. Prepare the woman for transfer to a Level III regional center
   B. Prepare for a high-risk delivery
   C. Admit the woman to the labor unit and wait for labor to begin spontaneously
   D. Admit the woman to the labor unit for expectant management

5. A sterile speculum examination is recommended for the woman being seen at term for the first time after membranes have ruptured *prematurely* regardless of whether the woman is in labor. The main reason(s) for this is (are) to:
   A. Assess for infection
   B. Note whether a prolapsed cord is present
   C. Determine the extent of cervical dilatation
   D. Assess fetal maturity
   E. B and C

6. A *newly admitted* laboring woman with premature rupture of membranes at 37 weeks is 3 cm dilated. Select the *three* correct priorities for nursing intervention.
   1. Obtain a culture of the amniotic fluid.
   2. Attach the external fetal monitor.
   3. Take and record her temperature.
   4. Note the color and odor of the amniotic fluid.
   5. Time the contractions.
   6. Ensure that resuscitation equipment in the delivery room is in good working order.
   A. 2, 3, 4   C. 1, 4, 6
   B. 2, 5, 6   D. 3, 5, 6

7. The diagnosis of preterm labor can be made if:
   A. The cervix is 20% effaced and 2 cm dilated
   B. The cervix is dilated 4 cm on admission
   C. Contractions are lasting 45 seconds and are 18 minutes apart
   D. Contractions are 30 seconds long and are occurring 10 to 15 minutes apart

8. The primary action of ritodrine is to:
   A. Cause fetal lungs to mature
   B. Quiet the myometrium of the uterus and stop contractions
   C. Lower the possibility of convulsion
   D. Reduce fluid retention in the preeclamptic woman

9. Using the criteria given in each brief situation following, state whether the woman is a good candidate for terbutaline tocolysis.
   A. Melinda is at 18 weeks' gestation with her third child. Contractions are occurring every 3 minutes and lasting 60 seconds. _____
   B. Susan is at 25 weeks' gestation with contractions occurring every 6 minutes and lasting 45 seconds. _____
   C. Mary is an uncontrolled diabetic who is now 32 weeks pregnant. She has just started having 60-second contractions every 5 minutes. _____
   D. Yvonne is admitted to the labor unit at 37 weeks' gestation with heavy vaginal bleeding and 30-second contractions occurring every 4 minutes. _____
   E. Lou Ella is 32 weeks pregnant with ruptured membranes. Chorioamnionitis has just been diagnosed. Two hours ago she began having contractions of approximately 30 seconds' duration, 5 minutes apart. _____

10. Select the one most critical nursing action to be initiated during the administration of terbutaline.
    A. Allow the woman to assume any comfortable position.
    B. Using the fetoscope, listen for fetal heart tones at least every 15 minutes.
    C. Allow clear liquids for nourishment.
    D. Record intake and output every hour.

11. The standard initial dose of ritodrine *per minute* is:
    A. 0.1 mg   C. 1.1 mg
    B. 1 mg   D. 0.01 mg

12. The ritodrine infusion is increased by 0.05 mg per minute every:
    A. 5 minutes   C. 20 minutes
    B. 10 minutes   D. 30 minutes

13. When contractions have stopped under the influence of the ritodrine infusion, the nurse should:
    A. Stop the infusion
    B. Continue the infusion at its present rate for 1 hour
    C. Decrease the rate of the infusion by 0.05 mg per minute every 30 minutes
    D. Increase the rate of the infusion by 0.05 mg per minute every 30 minutes

14. A maintenance dose of ritodrine or terbutaline is that which:
    A. Does not cause side effects to occur
    B. Maintains a normal fetal heart rate
    C. Effectively inhibits contractions
    D. Effectively maintains vital signs within normal ranges

15. The major obstetric complication associated with perinatal mortality and morbidity is:
    A. Preeclampsia/eclampsia
    B. Premature delivery
    C. Maternal malnutrition
    D. Breech delivery

16. A pregnant woman presents to the delivery suite at 34 weeks' gestation. Her contractions are regular, occurring every 6 minutes, and are 50 seconds in duration. Progressive cervical changes occur with time. The diagnosis is:
    A. Braxton Hicks contractions
    B. Premature labor
    C. False labor
    D. Irritable uterus

17. Attempts to stop premature labor should be minimized if there is also associated:
    A. Placental separation
    B. Severe preeclampsia
    C. Dead fetus
    D. All of the above

18. In which situation will a pregnant uterus frequently become irritable?
    A. Enucleation of a fibroid   C. Pyelonephritis
    B. Appendectomy   D. All of the above

19. In which position is cardiac output and renal blood flow highest?
    A. Left lateral decubitus   C. Supine, horizontal
    B. Lithotomy   D. Trendelenburg

20. The number of vaginal examinations should be minimized in patients with premature labor because:
    A. The risk of infection is increased
    B. Plasma concentrations of oxytocin increase
    C. The risk of rupturing the membranes is increased
    D. Plasma concentrations of prostaglandins decrease

21. During the initial treatment of a patient in premature labor, the most important consideration is:
    A. Barbiturate sedation
    B. X-ray examination of the abdomen for fetal position
    C. Oral liquid diet
    D. Urine analysi

22. Signs and symptoms of premature labor that the patient can recognize include all of the following *except:*
    A. Backache   C. Constipation
    B. Change in vaginal   D. Pelvic pressure
       discharge

23. Which of the following actions is most likely to minimize the risk of pulmonary edema during tocolytic therapy?
    A. Avoidance of glucocorticoid therapy
    B. Meticulous monitoring of intake and output
    C. Bed rest
    D. Nothing by mouth

24. A woman who is 32 weeks pregnant with her first baby and who has no significant risk factors for preterm labor calls the office and states she has felt Braxton Hicks contractions all day long. A friend told her "she probably just overdid it." She has been lying down for an hour with no change in symptoms. An appropriate response would be to:
    A. Reassure her that what she is experiencing is normal
    B. Review signs and symptoms of labor
    C. Tell her to keep her appointment the next day
    D. Have her come in for immediate evaluation

25. Risk appraisal systems for identifying women at risk for preterm labor have been shown to be:
    A. More effective in identifying primigravidas at risk for preterm labor
    B. Effective in identifying most women at risk for preterm labor
    C. Ineffective in identifying 50% of women who enter preterm labor with no risk factors
    D. Ineffective in identifying any women at risk for preterm labor

26. Recent reports about care-seeking behaviors of pregnant women emphasize that:
    A. Pregnancy motivates women to seek help for discomforts quickly
    B. Having previous experience with contractions (a previous labor and delivery) ensures early recognition of preterm labor symptoms
    C. Most women are aware of the difference between symptoms of common discomforts of pregnancy and preterm labor
    D. Denial of significance of symptoms and seeking advice from family or friends often precedes obtaining medical assistance for preterm labor symptoms and results in delayed treatment

27. In the United States, the rate of preterm labor resulting in low-birth-weight infants:
    A. Contributes to the majority of all perinatal deaths
    B. Has improved significantly in the past 10 years because of widespread use of tocolysis
    C. Is a problem only in women of lower socioeconomic status
    D. Has been significantly lowered by risk assessment and preterm birth prevention programs

28. The NIH consensus statement on the antenatal use of corticosteroids concludes that:
    1. Antenatal corticosteroid therapy for fetal maturation reduces mortality, respiratory distress syndrome, and intraventricular hemorrhage in preterm infants
    2. All fetuses between 24 and 34 weeks' gestation at risk of preterm delivery should be considered candidates for antenatal treatment with corticosteroids
    3. The benefits of antenatal corticosteroids are additive to those derived from surfactant therapy
    4. There is no advantage in treating with antenatal corticosteroids if preterm delivery is anticipated in less than 24 hours
       A. 1
       B. 1, 2
       C. 1, 2, 3
       D. All of the above

29. Risk factors for preterm labor:
    1. Have been clearly defined in multiparas
    2. Can vary in different populations
    3. Include psychosocial and physical factors
    4. Are multifactorial and need further research
       A. 1, 2, 4
       B. 2, 3, 4
       C. 1, 2, 4
       D. All of the above

30. The American College of Obstetricians and Gynecologists recommends screening and treatment for bacterial vaginosis in which group of women?
    1. All women, whether symptomatic or asymptomatic
    2. Women at high risk for preterm delivery, whether symptomatic or asymptomatic
    3. All symptomatic pregnant women
    4. Low-risk asymptomatic women
       A. 1
       B. 2, 4
       C. 2, 3
       D. 2, 3, 4

Check your answers with the Module 8 Posttest Answer Key.

Answer the following questions without referring back to the information in the module. ONE OR MORE THAN ONE of the choices may be correct.

1. The primary goal of management in severe preeclampsia is to:
   A. Prevent nausea and vomiting
   B. Prevent convulsions and deliver the baby
   C. Ensure a mature fetus
   D. Prevent the premature onset of labor

2. Magnesium sulfate is a drug effective in treating preeclampsia. The drug:
   A. Causes blood vessels to constrict and therefore increases circulation to the placenta
   B. Aids in maturation of the fetus
   C. Lowers blood pressure
   D. Depresses central nervous system activity and reduces the chances of convulsions

3. Which of the following pregnant women are at increased risk for developing preeclampsia?
   A. A teenaged girl who is pregnant for the first time
   B. A 30-year-old woman who is pregnant for the first time and who has a twin gestation
   C. A multipara who is also a diabetic
   D. All of the above

4. A 35-year-old woman expecting her third child presents at the labor unit with a blood pressure of 160/100 mm Hg and 2+ proteinuria. You note in her prenatal record that she has had a history of elevated blood pressure (approximate range of 140/90 mm Hg) since age 30. According to the classification system given in Module 9, she has:
   A. Eclampsia
   B. Chronic hypertension with superimposed preeclampsia
   C. Superimposed eclampsia
   D. Gestational hypertension

5. According to the classification system used in Module 9, when pregnancy-related hypertension occurs with proteinuria after 20 weeks' gestation, it is called:
   A. Transient hypertension
   B. HELLP syndrome
   C. Preeclampsia
   D. Chronic hypertension

6. A 20-year-old gravida 1 had a blood pressure range of 90/60 to 98/64 mm Hg at 6 through 28 weeks' gestation. At 39 weeks' gestation, she presents on the labor unit with a complaint of headaches and a total weight gain of 50 pounds—8 pounds were gained in the previous 2 weeks. Her blood pressure today is 134/86 mm Hg with 2+ proteinuria. You determine that she is not in true labor. Your next step will be to:
   A. Call her primary care provider
   B. Discuss signs and symptoms of preeclampsia and send her home
   C. Ask her to walk for 2 hours and return for a blood pressure recheck
   D. Send her home with strict bed rest orders

7. Which of the following are acceptable screening procedures for predicting preeclampsia?
   A. The roll-over test
   B. Absence of a decline in blood pressure late in the second trimester
   C. Calculation of mean arterial pressure in the second trimester
   D. None of the above

8. A 27-year-old gravida 2 at 40 weeks' gestation experienced a normal labor and birth. During the third blood pressure check in the recovery room, you note that her blood pressure has risen from approximately 118/68 to 128/74 mm Hg (baseline pressure during pregnancy and labor) to 150/100 mm Hg. To determine whether this might be preeclampsia or late transient hypertension, you would:
   1. Review her prenatal record for any signs of preeclampsia
   2. Keep her in the recovery room for additional time to continue evaluation
   3. Evaluate her urine for proteinuria
   4. Question her regarding headaches or blurred vision

   A. 2, 3   C. 2, 4
   B. 1, 4   D. All of the above

9. You have been caring for a severely preeclamptic woman who is in labor. Laboratory tests indicate a hematocrit at 48 mg/dL, bilirubin at 2.1 mg/dL, ALT at 70 IU/L, LDH at 820 IU/L, and a platelet count of 70,000/mm³. This is suggestive of:
   A. Severe diabetes
   B. Late, transient hypertension
   C. HELLP syndrome
   D. Eclampsia

10. In which of the following situations is maternal transport from a Level I hospital to a high-risk regional center indicated?
    A. 21-year-old gravida 3 who is at 33 weeks' gestation with mild preeclampsia and in early labor
    B. 14-year-old gravida 1 at 39 weeks' gestation with severe preeclampsia and in advanced labor
    C. 42-year-old gravida 2 at 40 weeks' gestation with mild preeclampsia
    D. 30-year-old gravida 4, twin gestation, at 38 weeks with mild preeclampsia and not in labor

11. Match the clinical signs and symptoms with the pathophysiologic alteration that occurs in preeclampsia.

Clinical Signs and Symptoms	Pathophysiologic Alteration
a. Hyperreflexia/clonus	1. _____ Decreased blood supply to the placenta
b. Proteinuria	
c. Headaches	2. _____ Decreased intravascular volume with a shift of plasma to the tissues of the body
d. Fetal distress	
e. Rise in blood pressure	
f. Sudden weight gain and edema	3. _____ Hemoconcentration within the circulatory system
g. Blurred vision/scotomata	4. _____ Loss of renal integrity
h. Rising hematocrit	5. _____ Spasm of the blood vessels and edema in the optical bed of the eye
i. Rising blood glucose levels	
j. Epigastric pain	6. _____ Spasm of the blood vessels and edema in the brain
	7. _____ Irritation of the central nervous system
	8. _____ Spasm and hemorrhage in the liver capsule

12. To ensure that the woman receiving magnesium sulfate therapy is not at increasing risk for serum magnesium blood levels above the therapeutic range, the nurse should:
    A. Assess the hematocrit level every 4 hours
    B. Evaluate for proteinuria every hour
    C. Determine that urinary output is greater than 30 mL per hour
    D. Time the contractions

13. In which situations should the physician be consulted for possible magnesium toxicity during magnesium sulfate therapy?
    1. Serum magnesium level is 7 mg/dL (or 8.4 mEq/L).
    2. Maternal respirations are 10 per minute and shallow.
    3. The patellar reflex has disappeared.
    4. Proteinuria is 3+.
        A. 1, 4
        B. 2, 3
        C. 2, 4
        D. 3, 4

14. Select the appropriate set of calculations to administer $MgSO_4 \cdot 7H_2O$ intravenously at the rate of 2 g per hour by infusion pump. You have available ampules of 50% $MgSO_4 \cdot 7H_2O$ containing 5 g each.
    A. 1 ampule of $MgSO_4 \cdot 7H_2O$ added to 1,000 mL of 5% dextrose and water or lactated Ringer's and run at 125 mL per hour
    B. 2 ampules of $MgSO_4 \cdot 7H_2O$ added to 1,000 mL of 5% dextrose and water or lactated Ringer's and run at 200 mL per hour
    C. 8 mL from 1 ampule added to 1,000 mL of 5% dextrose and water or lactated Ringer's and run at 100 mL per hour
    D. 8 ampules of $MgSO_4 \cdot 7H_2O$ added to 1,000 mL of 5% dextrose and water or lactated Ringer's and run at 50 mL per hour

15. You are administering hydralazine (Apresoline) to a severely preeclamptic woman. The appropriate blood pressure evaluations should be done every:
    A. 2 to 5 minutes
    B. 10 minutes
    C. 15 minutes
    D. 20 minutes

16. The frequency of blood pressure evaluation by the nurse in a severely hypertensive woman who is receiving hydralazine (Apresoline) is critical because the:
    1. Peak effect of hydralazine is reached in 15 to 20 minutes
    2. Woman might have an increased intravascular blood volume and have a stroke
    3. Woman might have a decreased intravascular blood volume and become severely hypotensive
    4. Woman might experience a seizure
        A. 1, 3
        B. 2, 4
        C. 1, 2
        D. 3, 4

17. Pregnant women with moderate hypertension might need:
    1. More frequent prenatal visits
    2. Antihypertensive medication
    3. Moderate salt restriction
    4. Careful fetal growth surveillance
        A. 1, 3
        B. 1, 2, 3
        C. 1, 4
        D. All of the above

18. Sodium restriction in a moderately hypertensive woman during pregnancy:
    A. Reduces urinary output
    B. Can lead to lower plasma volume
    C. Promotes increased plasma volume
    D. Has been shown to benefit women with elevated diastolic blood pressure between 95 and 104 mm Hg

19. Select the best steps and correct order in which the following should be carried out when taking blood pressure readings on the laboring woman with a pregnancy complicated by hypertension.
    1. Use the same arm throughout.
    2. Either arm may be used provided that blood pressure is essentially the same in each arm on admission.
    3. If pressures differ in each arm by more than 10 mm Hg, use the arm with the lower pressure.
    4. If pressures differ in each arm by more than 10 mm Hg, use the arm with the higher pressure.
    5. Perform blood pressure readings with the woman in a supine position.
    6. Perform blood pressure readings with the woman in essentially the same position each time.
    7. Record the diastolic pressure at the point of disappearance.
    8. Record the diastolic pressure at the point of muffled pulse sound.
        A. 1, 4, 5, 8
        B. 2, 3, 4, 7
        C. 1, 4, 6, 7
        D. 2, 4, 5, 7

20. Select the appropriate set of calculations to prepare and administer a 4-g *loading dose* of magnesium sulfate from available ampules of 50% $MgSO_4 \cdot 7H_2O$ containing 5 g each.
    A. 2 ampules of the $MgSO_4 \cdot 7H_2O$ solution added to 1,000 mL of 5% dextrose and water and run at 125 mL per hour
    B. 8 ampules of the $MgSO_4 \cdot 7H_2O$ solution added to 1,000 mL of 5% dextrose and water and run at 100 mL over 25 minutes (4 mL per minute)
    C. 8 ampules of the $MgSO_4 \cdot 7H_2O$ solution added to 1,000 mL of 5% dextrose and water and run at 150 mL over 25 minutes (6 mL per minute)
    D. 8 ampules of the $MgSO_4 \cdot 7H_2O$ solution added to 1,000 mL of 5% dextrose and water and run at 50 mL per hour

21. A 28-year-old gravida 2 para 1 at 35 weeks' estimated gestational age presents complaining of a sharp pain just below her sternum. During the intake process, she also tells you she has had the "flu" for the past 3 days. In addition to the sharp pain below her sternum, her complaints include nausea and vomiting, diarrhea, and feeling "down" and tired all the time. Her blood pressure is 134/82 mm Hg, and she has 1+ proteinuria. She has gained 9 pounds since her last prenatal visit 5 days ago. You determine that she is not in true labor. After calling her primary care provider, the next steps you take are in anticipation of a differential diagnosis of:
    A. Gastroenteritis   C. HELLP syndrome
    B. Gallbladder disease   D. Eclampsia

22. You are caring for a woman at 35 weeks' estimated gestation who has HELLP syndrome. She is receiving magnesium sulfate therapy and undergoing induction of labor. While performing routine care, you notice that her IV site has begun oozing and that she has petechiae covering her extremities. Her urine is rose-colored, and she is complaining of pain in her right upper quadrant. Her last laboratory studies were taken 6 hours ago. Her blood has been typed and crossmatched. The physician is on the way to the hospital. You anticipate that a critical management step will be to:
    A. Draw a complete blood cell count with platelets and liver function tests
    B. Prepare for a cesarean delivery
    C. Keep the Pitocin infusion at its present rate
    D. Stop the magnesium sulfate therapy

23. The term *gestational hypertension* is applied to expectant women who:
    A. Have chronic hypertension before the twentieth week of pregnancy
    B. Will go on to develop preeclampsia
    C. Are at minimal risk from hypertension
    D. Have elevated blood pressure after 20 weeks' gestation but without proteinuria or edema

24. Which of the following reflect what is known about perinatal mortality/morbidity rates in pregnancies complicated by hypertension? (Select more than one choice.)
    A. HELLP syndrome, a form of preeclampsia, places both the mother and fetus at considerable risk related to cerebrovascular cranial hemorrhage accidents.
    B. As maternal blood pressure increases, so does the perinatal mortality rate.
    C. Perinatal morbidity rates are similar for both chronic hypertension and preeclampsia.
    D. Perinatal mortality is significantly higher in superimposed preeclampsia than in preeclampsia.

25. A 26-year-old gravida 1 at 38 weeks' gestation is seen in her primary care provider's office. She has gained 3 pounds over the past week, has a blood pressure of 130/80 mm Hg (first trimester blood pressure was 110/60 mm Hg), and on a clean-catch urine test, is noted to have 3+ proteinuria. Which of the following statements reflect an appreciation for this mother's status? (Select more than one choice.)
    A. A clean-catch urine dipstick is not sufficient to determine significant proteinuria.
    B. The 3+ proteinuria is considered "significant."
    C. The blood pressure elevation is not worrisome.
    D. In light of the proteinuria and the elevated diastole, the prognosis for perinatal risk increases.
    E. The 3-pound weight gain will be seen with the presence of edema.

26. Protein in urine (select more than one choice):
    A. Is difficult to quantify
    B. Can be the most ominous sign of preeclampsia
    C. Is normally seen in a 24-hour urine specimen in amounts less than 300 g
    D. Is normally seen in a 24-hour specimen in amounts of approximately 5 g

27. An elevated hematocrit level in a preeclamptic woman might be reflecting:
    A. An increase in intravascular blood volume
    B. A loss of intravascular blood volume
    C. Enhanced uteroplacental perfusion
    D. Hemodilution

28. A rising LDH can reflect (select more than one choice):
    A. Microangiopathic hemolytic anemia
    B. Thrombocytopenia
    C. Increased blood glucose
    D. Liver tissue damage

29. When personnel on a labor and delivery unit follow protocols for taking blood pressures by using the Korotkoff IV sound, they:
    A. Run the risk of underdiagnosing preeclampsia
    B. Will have abnormally low diastolic measurements
    C. Run the risk of overdiagnosing preeclampsia
    D. Will accurately diagnose preeclampsia if they use the criteria of a 30/15 mm Hg rise in blood pressure

30. A lateral recumbent position in an expectant woman receiving $MgSO_4 \cdot 7H_2O$ can (select more than one choice):
    A. Promote cardiac output
    B. Reduce the risk of magnesium toxicity
    C. Lower placental profusion
    D. Increase the likelihood of fetal hypoxia

31. Normal physiologic changes in renal blood flow and glomerular filtration during pregnancy are reflected in laboratory values that show a(n):
    A. Increase in both urine and blood creatinine levels
    B. Increase in urine creatinine levels and decrease in blood levels
    C. Decrease in urine creatinine levels and increase in blood levels
    D. Decrease in both urine and blood creatinine levels

32. A young mother with severe preeclampsia has been treated with magnesium sulfate throughout her labor induction and delivered a 5-pound, 12-ounce boy under epidural anesthesia. Besides a continued risk from hypertension immediately after delivery, what other serious maternal risks should be anticipated?
    A. Anemia   C. Uterine atony
    B. Liver dysfunction   D. Hypotension

33. In anticipation of delivery of a high-risk infant, the priority for preparation is to:
    A. Alert appropriate on-call neonatal resuscitation personnel
    B. Prepare the expectant parent
    C. Have crossmatched blood for the mother available on the labor and delivery unit
    D. Have appropriate neonatal resuscitation personnel in the delivery room

34. Which of the following statements reflects what is currently appreciated regarding the immediate postpartum period for the woman recovering from severe preeclampsia or HELLP syndrome?
    A. The signs and symptoms of her disease will resolve quickly.
    B. Pulmonary edema is a serious potential risk.
    C. Oliguria is unlikely to occur.
    D. Her abnormal laboratory values will steadily improve.

Check your answers with the Module 9 Posttest Answer Key.

Answer the following questions without referring back to the information in the module. ONE OR MORE THAN ONE of the choices may be correct.

1. The definition of intrauterine growth restriction is a fetus whose estimated weight is below which percentile for gestational age?
   A. 3rd
   B. 5th
   C. 10th
   D. 15th

2. Intrauterine growth-restricted babies and small-for-gestational-age babies are at increased risk of poor outcome.
   A. True
   B. False

3. It is possible to have a growth-restricted baby who weighs above the 10th percentile.
   A. True
   B. False

4. Which of the following factors does *not* influence fetal birth weight?
   A. Altitude
   B. Birth weight of siblings
   C. Maternal parity
   D. Paternal height

5. How is intrauterine growth restriction ranked as to leading causes of perinatal morbidity and mortality?
   A. First
   B. Second
   C. Third
   D. Fourth

6. Intrauterine fetal death can occur at any time during the pregnancy, but it is more common after which gestational week?
   A. Week 32
   B. Week 34
   C. Week 36
   D. Week 38

7. Select the appropriate terms to insert in the blanks from the following: Severe oligohydramnios represents a(n) _____ stress placed on the fetus and is considered _____ with respect to fetal well-being.
   A. Acute
   B. Chronic
   C. Reassuring
   D. Equivocal
   E. Ominous

8. Hypoxia during labor is evidenced by all of the following *except:*
   A. Late decelerations
   B. Early decelerations
   C. Bradycardia
   D. Absent variability

9. Meconium aspiration is a major cause of mortality and morbidity.
   A. True
   B. False

10. Which of the following blood glucose levels in the term infant is diagnosed as hypoglycemic?
    A. 25 mg/dL
    B. 30 mg/dL
    C. 35 mg/dL
    D. 40 mg/dL

11. Signs and symptoms of hypoglycemia include all of the following *except:*
    A. Jitteriness
    B. Tremors
    C. Strong cry
    D. Lethargy

12. IV hydration must be initiated immediately in the presence of a low blood sugar.
    A. True
    B. False

13. All of the following may be seen in a growth-restricted neonate *except:*
    A. Polycythemia
    B. Hypobilirubinemia
    C. Hypothermia
    D. Hypoglycemia

14. All of the following are physical characteristics of the growth-restricted newborn *except:*
    A. Loose, dry, and thin skin
    B. Meconium staining
    C. Large skull
    D. Alert appearance

15. The appearance of a growth-restricted baby and small-for-gestational-age baby is the same.
    A. True
    B. False

16. If an insult occurs early in the pregnancy (before 16 weeks' gestation), which phase of cellular growth will be affected?
    A. Hypertrophy
    B. Hypertrophy and hyperplasia
    C. Hyperplasia

17. The most important substrates a growing fetus needs are:
    A. Carbon dioxide, amino acids, and glucose
    B. Oxygen, amino acids, and calories
    C. Oxygen, amino acids, and glucose

18. What are the strongest indicators of birth weight?
    A. Maternal prepregnancy weight and paternal weight
    B. Paternal height and maternal height
    C. Maternal prepregnancy weight and maternal height
    D. Maternal prepregnancy weight and weight gain during the pregnancy

19. All of the following maternal factors contribute to IUGR *except:*
    A. Cigarette smoking
    B. Alcohol consumption
    C. Caffeine consumption
    D. Illicit drug use

20. All of the following fetal factors contribute to IUGR *except:*
    A. Multifetal gestation
    B. Chromosomal abnormalities
    C. Breech position
    D. Structural anomalies

21. The main prerequisite for determining IUGR is:
    A. Lagging fundal height
    B. Precise dating of the pregnancy
    C. Inadequate weight gain
    D. History of smoking two packs of cigarettes per day

22. Once IUGR is suspected, what is the first test ordered?
    A. Nonstress test
    B. Ultrasound
    C. Biophysical profile
    D. Doppler flow studies

23. The nonstress test should be reactive by which gestational week?
    A. 28
    B. 30
    C. 32
    D. 34

24. All of the following surveillance tests are ordered in a pregnancy complicated by growth restriction *except:*
    A. Daily fetal kick counts
    B. Weekly ultrasound for estimation of fetal weight
    C. Weekly or biweekly nonstress test
    D. Biophysical profile

25. How many contractions in 10 minutes are needed to perform a contraction stress test?
    A. 2
    B. 3
    C. 4
    D. 5

26. Which of the following parameters are included in a biophysical profile?
    A. Nonstress test, fetal movement, amniotic fluid volume, and placental grading
    B. Nonstress test, fetal breathing movements, fetal movement, and placental grading
    C. Fetal breathing movement, amniotic fluid volume, fetal tone, and placental grading
    D. Fetal breathing movements, fetal tone, nonstress test, and amniotic fluid volume

27. All of the following therapies are used in the treatment of IUGR *except:*
    A. Daily low-dose aspirin
    B. Corticosteroids
    C. Bed rest
    D. IV hydration

Questions 28 through 30 relate to the status of Mrs. Jones.

28. Mrs. Jones, a 30-year-old gravida 4 para 3003, is seen at the OB clinic for her first prenatal visit. She is unsure of the date of her last menstrual period, so an ultrasound is ordered. What is the best measurement for dating a pregnancy within the first trimester?
    A. Amniotic fluid volume
    B. Head circumference
    C. Crown-rump length
    D. Femur length

29. Mrs. Jones is underweight and wants to know the appropriate amount of weight she should gain this pregnancy. Your response will be:
    A. 15 to 25 pounds
    B. 25 to 35 pounds
    C. 28 to 40 pounds
    D. 35 to 45 pounds

30. At 18 weeks' gestation, Mrs. Jones has a low alpha-fetoprotein test result. Is she at risk for IUGR?
    A. No
    B. Yes

Questions 31 through 37 relate to the status of Mrs. Clancey.

31. Mrs. Clancey is a 38-year-old gravida 1 para 0 at 33 weeks' gestation with a fundal height of 32 cm. Is she at risk for having IUGR?
    A. No
    B. Yes

32. Mrs. Clancey is now 35 weeks' gestation with a fundal height of 32 cm. Is she at risk for having IUGR?
    A. No
    B. Yes

33. An ultrasound is performed on Mrs. Clancey and is compared against her previous ultrasound; IUGR is suspected. Mrs. Clancey is seen at the office to have a nonstress test. Which of the following would be an example of a *reactive* nonstress test?
    A. Baseline FHR of 120s with two 10-second accelerations to the 130s lasting 10 seconds
    B. Baseline 120s with two 10- to 15-second accelerations to the 140s lasting 10 to 15 seconds
    C. Baseline 120s with three 10- to 15-second accelerations to the 140s lasting 10 to 15 seconds
    D. Baseline 120s with two 15-second accelerations to the 140s lasting 15 seconds

34. Mrs. Clancey's nonstress test was similar to choice B from question 33. Based on her fetal monitor tracing, you anticipate that her care provider will:
    A. Send her home with instructions to perform daily fetal kick counts
    B. Order a biophysical profile
    C. Order Doppler studies
    D. Order an amniocentesis

35. Mrs. Clancey has a biophysical profile (BPP) with the following results: a nonreactive nonstress test, two episodes of fetal breathing, four discrete body movements, one episode of extension returning to flexion, and a 2.5-cm vertical pocket of amniotic fluid. What is Mrs. Clancey's BPP score?
    A. 4
    B. 6
    C. 8
    D. 10

36. Based on the score in question 35, you anticipate her care provider to:
    A. Send her home and order bed rest, with instructions to perform daily fetal kick counts
    B. Send her home and order bed rest, with instructions to perform weekly fetal kick counts
    C. Order an amniocentesis to assess fetal lung maturity
    D. Order Doppler flow studies

37. Mrs. Clancey has been very compliant and is now at 38 weeks' gestation. Her most recent nonstress test is reactive, with the most recent BPP score of 8. What do you anticipate her plan of care to be?
    A. Bed rest at home with instructions to perform fetal kick counts
    B. Induction of labor
    C. Scheduled cesarean section

Questions 38 through 42 relate to the status of Mrs. Hoffmann and her newborn.

38. Mrs. Hoffmann, a 24-year-old gravida 2 para 1001, is admitted for induction of labor at 39 weeks' gestation secondary to IUGR. Your plan of care includes all of the following *except:*
    A. Continuous fetal monitoring
    B. IV hydration
    C. Bed rest
    D. IV narcotics for pain management

39. Mrs. Hoffmann is 6 cm dilated, and her bag of waters just ruptured. Thick meconium is observed. What do you anticipate will be your next intervention?
    A. Increase the Pitocin dosage
    B. Begin continuous oxygen
    C. Start an amnioinfusion
    D. Empty her bladder

40. Mrs. Hoffmann progresses to 10 cm and delivers her baby without any problems. The pediatrician attended the delivery, and the baby did fine. Mrs. Hoffman is holding her baby and is concerned because he appears jittery. Your response should be to:
    A. Reassure her that all babies are jittery and that this is part of adjusting to extrauterine life
    B. Realize that this may be abnormal and order a complete blood count
    C. Realize that this may be abnormal and take his temperature
    D. Realize that this may abnormal and check his blood sugar

41. The result of his blood sugar is 35 mg/dL. Your next intervention should be to:
    A. Reassure her this is a normal value and promote bonding
    B. Explain to her that his blood sugar is low and because she plans to nurse, she could begin now
    C. Explain to her that his blood sugar is low and although she plans to nurse, he needs to be bottle-fed
    D. Explain to her that his blood sugar is low and IV hydration is needed immediately

42. Mrs. Hoffmann is concerned about her baby's long-term prognosis. Your response is based on your knowledge that most IUGR babies have a(n) _____ prognosis.
    A. Poor
    B. Fair
    C. Excellent
    D. The data are inconsistent; you are unable to answer this question

Check your answers with the Module 10 Posttest Answer Key.

Posttest: Module 11. Caring for the Laboring Woman With HIV Infection or AIDS

Answer the following questions without referring back to the information in the module. ONE OR MORE THAN ONE of the choices may be correct.

1. A 30-year-old newly delivered mother has been diagnosed as HIV positive. She has no symptoms of the infection as yet. Which activities do not carry the risk of transmitting the infection?
   A. Breastfeeding her newborn
   B. Resuming sexual activity with her husband 6 weeks after delivery
   C. Kissing her other two children
   D. Donating blood at the local Red Cross

2. A registered nurse works in a labor and delivery unit in a busy metropolitan area. Select the following activities that are most likely to put her at risk of contracting HIV infection.
   A. Using universal precautions only when caring for patients who are at high risk for HIV infection
   B. Recapping all needles carefully after use
   C. Wearing gloves only while bathing those babies whom have been born from intravenous drug users or from women who are partners of intravenous drug users
   D. Hugging an HIV-infected mother after the birth of her child

3. A patient is admitted to the labor unit and has had two positive (reactive) EIA tests and one unequivocal positive Western blot test. You can reasonably conclude that the patient:
   A. Does not have HIV infection
   B. Has HIV infection
   C. Is an intravenous drug abuser
   D. Has AIDS

4. In an HIV-infected woman who is not treated with antiretroviral medications, the rate of transmitting HIV infection to her newborn:
   A. Is estimated at 25.5%
   B. Is not a concern
   C. Is estimated at close to 100%
   D. Will depend on whether the mother has symptoms of AIDS

5. A pregnant nurse working on a labor and delivery, nursery, or postpartum unit should:
   A. Request a change to another hospital unit
   B. Be assigned to low-risk patients on those units
   C. Receive an HIV screen
   D. Use universal precautions

6. You are going to give a bath to an HIV-infected woman who has just delivered her baby. After the bath you need to begin an IV line. Which sequence of steps is recommended in universal precautions?
   A. No gloves are needed for the bath, but put gloves on when starting the IV line.
   B. Continue to use the same pair of gloves without interrupting for handwashing.
   C. Wash hands, put on gloves for the bath, remove gloves, wash hands, and put on the same pair of gloves if you see no tears.
   D. Remove gloves after the bath, wash hands immediately, and put on another pair of gloves before starting the IV line.

7. Measures that reduce the risk of HIV transmission to the newborn of an HIV-infected mother include:
   A. Using internal fetal monitoring for this high-risk infant
   B. Changing gloves after giving perineal care to the mother and before bathing the baby
   C. Bathing the baby before administering vitamin K
   D. Isolating the baby from the mother

8. What is seroconversion?
   A. When the patient has AIDS but blood tests are unable to isolate the virus
   B. The period of time before the patient developing full-blown AIDS
   C. The point when there are enough antibodies to HIV to make detection possible
   D. The period of time before there is enough antibodies to HIV to make detection possible

9. Which clinical situations place the mother with HIV infection and fetus at more risk than the non–HIV-infected woman?
   A. Premature rupture of membranes
   B. Multiparity
   C. Hypertension
   D. Anemia

10. Name the two mechanisms of transmission for HIV.
    A. Horizontal transmission
    B. Diagonal transmission
    C. Dominant transmission
    D. Vertical transmission

11. The drug currently recommended for pregnant women to prevent transmission of HIV to the newborn is:
    A. Zithromax
    B. Zovirax
    C. Zalcitabine
    D. Zidovudine

12. What is the current method of delivery recommended for the woman who is HIV positive with a viral load of 2150 copies/mL?
    A. Low forceps vaginal delivery
    B. Cesarean delivery
    C. Spontaneous vaginal delivery
    D. Vacuum extraction vaginal delivery

13. The highest percentage of perinatal transfer of HIV occurs in:
    A. The first trimester
    B. The third trimester
    C. Postpartum
    D. Intrapartum

14. When is antiretroviral treatment recommended for the pregnant woman?
    A. It is clinically indicated by her HIV status.
    B. If already initiated, it is continued (during the first trimester) throughout pregnancy, labor, and delivery.
    C. It is given only to women who have AIDS.
    D. It is not recommended for women who have full-blown AIDS.

15. What is the primary adverse effect of ZDV?
    A. Bone marrow suppression
    B. Nausea and vomiting
    C. Loss of hair and skin eruption
    D. Diarrhea

16. Name two educational topics that should be presented to the expectant woman during the intrapartum period.
    A. Risks and benefits of drug therapy
    B. Pain management options and their risks and benefits
    C. Contraceptive options after delivery
    D. Bathing the newborn

17. Which psychosocial considerations should be promoted in caring for the HIV-positive mother and her family during labor or immediately after delivery?
    A. Maternal–child bonding
    B. Family bonding
    C. Psychological adjustment
    D. None of the above

18. Name key ethical issues in the treatment of the HIV-positive patient.
    A. Confidentiality
    B. Advance directives
    C. Right to medical care
    D. Consent

19. What measures can be taken to help protect the fetus/newborn from HIV infection?
    A. Avoid internal monitoring if possible.
    B. Dry the infant immediately after delivery.
    C. Wait until 2 hours after delivery before bathing the baby.
    D. Avoid aspiration of gastric content.

20. The use of zidovudine therapy in HIV-infected pregnant women showed:
    A. No change in the risk of HIV vertical transmission
    B. A 8.3% increase in the risk of HIV vertical transmission
    C. A 25.5% decrease in the risk of HIV vertical transmission
    D. A 67.5% decrease in the risk of HIV vertical transmission

21. You are in an antepartum clinic providing care for an 18-year-old gravida 3 para 2 abortus 0 at 34 weeks' gestation. She was diagnosed as being HIV positive 1 year ago. She is presently receiving zidovudine therapy. Which of the following issues should be addressed in your education plans for this patient?
    A. The benefits and risks of zidovudine therapy during labor
    B. The benefits of breastfeeding
    C. The benefits and risks of zidovudine therapy for her newborn
    D. Pain management during labor

22. A 23-year-old gravida 4 para 1 abortus 2 at 38 4/7 weeks' gestation presents to the labor and delivery unit for evaluation of labor. She was diagnosed as being HIV positive 4 months ago when she began her prenatal care. Examination revealed that she was 5 cm, 75%, vertex −1 with intact membranes. Which of the following precautions should be taken to reduce her exposure to opportunistic organisms?
    A. Do not start an IV line.
    B. Insert a Foley catheter on admission.
    C. Limit vaginal examinations.
    D. Artificially rupture membranes and place helix and intrauterine pressure catheter to monitor her labor pattern.

Check your answers with the Module 11 Posttest Answer Key.

Posttest: Module 12. Hepatitis B Infection: Maternal–Newborn Management

Answer the following questions without referring back to the information in the module. Select the BEST answer for each question.

1. Which form of hepatitis can result in the *highest* rate of chronic infection among infected individuals?
   A. Hepatitis A
   B. Hepatitis B
   C. Hepatitis C
   D. Hepatitis E

2. When maternal infection exists, which of the following poses the *highest* risk of vertical transmission?
   A. HIV
   B. Hepatitis A
   C. Hepatitis B
   D. Hepatitis C

3. The *highest* risk of infection transmission from bloodborne exposures occurs from which one of the following diseases?
   A. HIV
   B. Hepatitis B
   C. Hepatitis C

4. All of the following statements reflect what is known about hepatitis A infection *except:*
   A. Infection with the hepatitis A virus results in subsequent immunity to the infection
   B. When the infection occurs during pregnancy, the disease is generally worse and teratogenic effects are possible
   C. No carrier state exists for this disease
   D. Hepatitis A vaccination may be given to pregnant women

5. All of the following statements regarding hepatitis A are accurate *except:*
   A. It is usually transmitted by blood
   B. It can be prevented by immunization
   C. It was previously known as "infectious hepatitis"
   D. It causes no serious problems in the well-nourished, healthy pregnant woman

6. Which type of hepatitis, not seen in the United States, is characterized by mild illness but also by a fulminant form of illness causing a high mortality rate?
   A. Hepatitis A
   B. Hepatitis C
   C. Hepatitis D
   D. Hepatitis E

7. Mr. Harvey Manfred contracted hepatitis C virus infection 1 year ago. Recent serologic testing reveals the presence of anti-HCV. This can be interpreted to indicate that he:
   A. Is immune
   B. Is infected
   C. Has cleared his system of the virus
   D. Is not infectious

8. Hepatitis B infection:
   A. Was formerly known as "infectious hepatitis"
   B. Is diagnosed by excluding other hepatitis types
   C. Can occur without the individual having symptoms of an acute infection
   D. Does not carry with it any long-term risks

9. Individuals with chronic hepatitis B infection:
   A. Have the potential for being a carrier
   B. Are never infectious
   C. Have few long-term risks
   D. Always have serious symptoms, which aid in the diagnosis

10. Which of the following hepatitis B serologic markers is done to screen pregnant women?
    A. HBsAg
    B. anti-HBs
    C. anti-HBc
    D. All of the above

11. A high possibility exists that a pregnant woman can transmit hepatitis B to her infant if her blood serum reveals the presence of HBsAg and:
    A. anti-HBc
    B. anti-HBe
    C. HBeAg
    D. HBcAg

12. Transmission of hepatitis B infection from an acutely infected or carrier mother to her infant:
    A. Occurs in a few infants transplacentally before birth
    B. Is unlikely if the mother has no symptoms of the infection throughout her pregnancy
    C. Is unlikely during labor and delivery in the mother who has no symptoms of the infection
    D. Rarely occurs from the infant's contact with infected blood or amniotic fluid at birth

13. In a hepatitis B virus–infected mother who is HBsAg and HBeAg positive, the rate of transmitting infection to her newborn:
    A. Is estimated at 30%
    B. Is estimated at 90%
    C. Is not a concern
    D. Will depend on whether the mother is symptomatic

14. A woman who has had two positive HBsAg tests 7 months apart is admitted to the labor unit. You can reasonably conclude that the woman:
    A. Does not have hepatitis B infection
    B. Has resolving hepatitis B infection
    C. Is a carrier
    D. Is susceptible to hepatitis B infection

15. Current recommendations for follow-up on a pregnant woman who tests positive for HBsAg include:
    A. Immediate immunization
    B. Liver function tests
    C. Hospitalization
    D. None of the above

16. Members in the household of a hepatitis B carrier are at risk for viral transmission through:
    A. Air contamination
    B. Water contamination
    C. Hugging and nonintimate kissing
    D. Shared toothbrushes and razor blades

17. The hepatitis B virus has been found in all body fluids of infected individuals. Which body fluid can be a source of transmission?
    A. Urine
    B. Tears
    C. Breast milk
    D. Vaginal secretions

18. Feces with gross contamination of blood is a source of hepatitis B virus transmission because:
    A. Hepatitis B virus is an enterically transmitted virus
    B. The blood contains concentrations of hepatitis B virus sufficient to cause disease
    C. Feces alone contains concentrations of hepatitis B virus sufficient to cause disease
    D. All of the above statements are correct

19. Pregnant women who contract hepatitis B usually experience:
    A. Severe jaundice, hepatitic tenderness, and weight loss
    B. Special dietary needs
    C. No symptoms
    D. An aggravated course of the disease because of pregnancy

20. If an infant is born to a mother who has not been screened for hepatitis B virus but who belongs to one of the risk groups, the recommendation for treating the infant is to:
    A. Obtain a blood specimen from the infant for a hepatitis screen
    B. Isolate the infant until discharge
    C. Immunize the mother
    D. Give the baby HBIG and hepatitis B vaccine within 12 hours of birth

21. To confer passive immunity quickly to the newborn whose mother is a hepatitis B carrier, administer 0.5 mL of:
    A. Engerix-B, Pediatric/Adolescent, IM within 2 to 12 hours of birth
    B. HBIG IM within 2 to 12 hours of birth
    C. Recombivax HB, Pediatric, IM within 12 hours of birth
    D. HBIG IM within 1 week of birth

22. The treatment regimen used to confer active immunity on the newborn is:
    A. An initial 0.5-mL dose of Recombivax HB, Pediatric, IM within 12 hours of birth, followed by two additional immunizations at 1 to 4 months after the first dose and 6 to 18 months after the second dose
    B. An initial 0.5-mL dose of HBIG IM within 12 hours of birth, followed by immunization with Recombivax HB, Pediatric, at 1 month of age and 5 months of age
    C. A single immunization with Engerix-B, Pediatric/Adolescent, or Recombivax HB, Pediatric, within 12 hours of birth
    D. An initial 0.5-mL dose of HBIG within 12 hours of birth, followed by immunization with HBIG at 2 months of age and 6 months of age

Case Studies (questions 23 and 24)

23. As a member of a health care team working in areas where exposure to body fluids, including blood, is common, you are tested for immune status to hepatitis B. The plan is to begin the three-part Recombivax HB vaccine if appropriate.
    Test Report 1: HBsAg = positive
    Test Report 2: anti-HBc = positive
    Test Report 3: anti-HBs = positive
    Test Report 4: HBsAg = positive; HBeAg = positive
    Test Report 5: HBsAg = positive; IgM anti-HBc = negative; IgG anti-HBc = positive
    Test Report 6: antigens = negative; antibodies = negative
    _____ A. Which of the laboratory reports above (1–6) is preferable?
    _____ B. Which laboratory report indicates that you are susceptible to hepatitis B infection?
    _____ C. Select the laboratory report that indicates a high degree of infectivity.
    _____ D. Select the laboratory report that documents a carrier state.

24. Alice Scottie, a 22-year-old gravida 1 who admits to intravenous drug abuse, received an initial physical examination and laboratory workup at 13 weeks' gestation. Her hepatitis B screen 1 week later revealed that she was HBsAg positive. Unfortunately, the health department personnel were unable to locate her and she never returned for further care. Approximately 6 months later she presents at the hospital emergency room in active labor. Her prenatal record reflects only information obtained at the initial visit. Select the statement(s) that accurately reflect what can be assessed about Alice's hepatitis B status from the information known to date.
    A. She might have cleared her system of HBsAg by now.
    B. A highly infectious state is present.
    C. An immune state exists.
    D. She is now a carrier.

25. In admitting a laboring woman who has been identified as a hepatitis B carrier, you will:
    A. Put her in isolation
    B. Label all soiled linens from her with "blood precautions"
    C. Send her blood specimens under separate cover and clearly label "hepatitis B precautions"
    D. Treat her laboratory specimens and linens as you would all other patients' blood and body fluids

26. Measures that reduce the risk of hepatitis B transmission to the fetus of an infected mother include:
    A. Using external fetal monitoring or intermittent auscultation of fetal heart tones
    B. Isolating the mother throughout labor
    C. Performing frequent vaginal examinations to assess progress
    D. Initiating early artificial rupture of membranes during labor

27. The blood of an infant of a drug-abusing 30-year-old mother showed the presence of hepatitis B surface antibodies. From this you can definitely conclude that the:
    A. Infant has hepatitis B virus infection
    B. Infant does not have hepatitis B virus infection
    C. Mother had hepatitis B virus infection at one time
    D. Mother is currently infected

28. What treatment is appropriate for the situation in question 27?
    A. Immunize the mother.
    B. Immunize the infant.
    C. Isolate the infant from the mother.
    D. No immunization is needed for the baby.

29. Carrier states:
    A. Are a key factor in the spread of hepatitis B worldwide
    B. Pose minimal problems for individual carriers themselves
    C. Are associated with high prevalence rates in most populations worldwide
    D. Are easily identified through symptoms of the disease

30. A hepatitis B carrier state never exists in an individual without the presence of _____ in his or her blood.
    A. HBsAg   C. HBcAg
    B. HBeAg   D. Anti-HBs

31. Gloves should be worn when:
    A. Giving a first bath to a newborn
    B. Changing the diaper of a newborn who received HBIG and the first hepatitis vaccine dose 2 days ago
    C. Bathing a 4-day-old infant who received HBIG only
    D. Changing diapers on all newborns

32. Postpartum education of the hepatitis B carrier mother includes all of the following except:
    A. The benefits of immunization for herself
    B. Handwashing procedures to reduce contamination
    C. The benefits of screening and immunization for members of her household
    D. Potential sources of contamination (e.g., saliva)

33. A mother diagnosed with acute infectious hepatitis B delivers and is discharged from the postpartum unit. The infant has received HBIG and his first vaccine dose. Plans regarding follow-up on the status of the mother's infection should include:
    A. Periodic breast milk testing for HBsAg
    B. Serologic testing for the continued presence of HBsAg or detection of anti-HBs
    C. Immunization with hepatitis B vaccine
    D. Serologic testing for HBcAg

34. What is the difference in the recommended schedule of immunoprophylaxis for an infant born to an HBsAg-positive mother and one who is known to be HBsAg negative and immune (select two answers)?
    A. The infant born to the HBsAg-negative mother need not receive HBIG at the time of birth.
    B. The infant born to the HBsAg-positive mother needs to have HBIG immediately and hepatitis B vaccine within the first 12 hours of life.
    C. There is no difference.
    D. The infant born to the HBsAg-negative mother needs no immunoprophylaxis.

35. Appropriate delivery plans for a laboring woman who has been identified as HBsAg positive include:
    A. Keeping the mother and baby separated until after the baby has been bathed
    B. Using an isolation room
    C. Obtaining consent for immunization of the newborn before delivery
    D. Assigning one nurse to attend to the baby after delivery

36. It is recommended that all newborns of hepatitis B carrier mothers have oropharyngeal and nasal suctioning because:
    A. All newborns of carrier mothers will have become infected with the hepatitis B virus
    B. Prompt removal of infectious fluids reduces the risk for newborns and caregivers for contracting the infection
    C. All newborns need suctioning regardless of the infection status of the mother
    D. This is an appropriate newborn stimulating intervention

37. Select the situation that typifies a nosocomial infection.
    A. A 26-year-old hepatitis B virus carrier mother was admitted and delivered at a community hospital.
    B. The infant of a hepatitis B virus carrier mother was diagnosed as HBsAg positive at 6 months of age.
    C. The HBsAg negative, anti-HBs negative nurse sustained a needlestick while caring for the hepatitis B carrier mother and her baby. She became acutely ill with hepatitis B 4 months later.

Case Studies (questions 38 through 41)

Read the following patient profiles and then answer questions 38 through 41 by matching the correct patient(s) with the statement.

Patient A: Mary is a 19-year-old who is expecting her second child in 7½ months. She contracted hepatitis B 8 months before becoming pregnant and now tests anti-HBs positive.

Patient B: Jane is a 21-year-old expecting her first child in approximately 4 weeks. A hepatitis B panel drawn last week reveals that she is HBsAg and HBeAg positive.

Patient C: Marla is 3 months pregnant. Her boyfriend has revealed that he is bisexual and a hepatitis carrier. Subsequently, Marla's hepatitis B workup indicates that she is HBsAg negative and possesses no antibodies for hepatitis B.

38. ____ Vertical transmission is a high risk.

39. ____ Vertical transmission is not a risk.

40. ____ Hepatitis B vaccine should be offered to this woman during her pregnancy.

41. ____ Hepatitis B immunization is not an appropriate intervention.

42. Which of the following newborns is *not* at risk for contracting hepatitis B virus infection?
    A. Baby A, born to a Vietnamese woman who has had no prenatal care
    B. Baby B, born to a mother whose hepatitis B panel has just been done because of late prenatal care
    C. Baby C, whose mother was immunized 6 months ago and now tests anti-HBs positive
    D. Baby D, whose mother cares for a father receiving renal dialysis and who tested anti-HBs negative 2 months ago

43. Indicate whether the following statements are true (T) or false (F).
    a. ____ The fetus of a hepatitis B virus carrier mother is presumed to be infected.
    b. ____ When caring for the fetus of a hepatitis B virus–infected mother, it is important to use fetal monitoring strategies that avoid inadvertent breaks in the skin barrier of the fetus.
    c. ____ Hepatitis B immunization is 100% effective.
    d. ____ A high rate of hepatitis B transmission occurs from infected health care personnel to newborns.
    e. ____ A high intrapartal morbidity rate is experienced by fetuses of hepatitis B virus carrier mothers.
    f. ____ The lowest risk of hepatitis B virus vertical transmission occurs during the second trimester.
    g. ____ Pregnant women in developing countries have a high fatality rate from fulminant hepatitis E.
    h. ____ Unvaccinated newborns have a higher likelihood of becoming chronically infected with hepatitis B than do exposed children.

44. The percentage of hepatitis B–infected health care workers who become chronically infected (i.e., a carrier state exists) is:
    A. 5% to 10%   C. 1%
    B. 3%   D. Rare

45. A nonvaccinated health care worker who experiences a needlestick injury has what chance of developing clinical hepatitis B if the source person is both HBsAg positive and HBeAg positive?
    A. 22% to 31%
    B. 10%
    C. 5%
    D. Little chance

46. When a health care worker experiences a blood exposure, OSHA's 1992 postexposure guidelines indicate that:
    A. Vaccination is mandatory
    B. Prescreening of the worker is not a requirement for receiving the vaccine
    C. Only a booster dose of the vaccine should be given
    D. It is not helpful to know the worker's serology status for hepatitis B

47. Postexposure prophylaxis for exposure to hepatitis B includes all of the following approaches *except:*
    A. Evaluating the nonresponder to determine whether he or she is HBsAg positive
    B. Giving one dose of HBIG and initiating revaccination if the nonresponder has not completed a second vaccine series
    C. Giving two doses of HBIG if the nonresponder has completed a second vaccine series but still fails to respond
    D. Giving a single booster injection

Check your answers with the Module 12 Posttest Answer Key.

Posttest: Module 13. Caring for the Pregnant Woman With Diabetes (Includes Content from Appendix B)

Answer the following questions without referring back to the information in the module. Select the ONE BEST answer for each question.

1. All the following metabolic changes occur during pregnancy *except:*
   A. Transplacental delivery of insulin to the fetus to promote growth
   B. Insulin resistance due to human placental lactogen, prolactin, and cortisol levels
   C. Increased blood volume
   D. Thermoregulatory changes, including an increase in basal metabolic rate and an increase in heat production

2. A vaginal delivery is contraindicated in a diabetic patient with:
   A. A macrosomic infant
   B. Neuropathy
   C. Elevated blood glucoses greater than 180 mg/dL
   D. Untreated proliferative retinopathy

3. Which of the following groups are at risk to have babies with congenital anomalies if their blood glucose is not in control?
   A. Gestational diabetic mothers
   B. Gestational diabetic and type 2 diabetic mothers
   C. Type 1 and type 2 diabetic mothers
   D. Gestational diabetic and type 1 diabetic mothers

4. Gestational diabetes can be diagnosed with which of the following tests?
   A. A fasting blood glucose and a 1-hour Glucola
   B. A 1-hour Glucola of 160 mg/dL and 1-hour glucose tolerance test
   C. A 1-hour Glucola of 146 mg/dL followed by a 3-hour glucose tolerance test with the following values: fasting, 101 mg/dL; 1-hour, 208 mg/dL; 2-hour, 155 mg/dL; and 3-hour, 150 mg/dL
   D. A 1-hour Glucola of 140 mg/dL followed by a 3-hour glucose tolerance test with the following values: fasting, 98 mg/dL; 1-hour, 185 mg/dL; 2-hour, 150 mg/dL; and 3-hour, 145 mg/dL

5. Pregestational diabetes can be diagnosed by all of the following tests if confirmed on a subsequent day *except:*
   A. Acute symptoms of diabetes plus a casual plasma glucose of 200 mg/dL or greater
   B. Fasting plasma glucose of 126 mg/dL or greater
   C. 2-hour plasma glucose of 200 mg/dL or greater during an oral glucose tolerance test
   D. Fasting plasma glucose of 105 mg/dL or greater plus a 2-hour glucose test of 195 mg/dL or greater

6. Pregnant women who need to be screened for gestational diabetes should be screened between:
   A. 20 and 24 weeks' gestation
   B. 24 and 28 weeks' gestation
   C. 28 and 32 weeks' gestation
   D. 32 and 36 weeks' gestation

7. Which type of diabetes is the most common?
   A. Type 1 diabetes
   B. Type 2 diabetes
   C. Gestational diabetes
   D. Secondary diabetes

8. The typical pattern of insulin requirements during pregnancy is:
   A. Decreased in first trimester, increased in second trimester, increased in third trimester, and increased during the postpartum period
   B. Decreased in first trimester, increased in second trimester, decreased in third trimester, and decreased during the postpartum period
   C. Increased in first trimester, increased in second trimester, increased in third trimester, and decreased during the postpartum period
   D. Decreased in first trimester, increased in second trimester, increased in third trimester, and decreased during the postpartum period

9. The American Diabetes Association recommends which of the following maternal glucose goals for type 1 and type 2 diabetic mothers?
   A. Fasting blood glucose between 60 and 90 mg/dL, premeal blood glucose between 60 and 105 mg/dL, 1-hour postprandial blood glucose between 100 and 120 mg/dL, and 2-hour postprandial blood glucose between 60 and 120 mg/dL
   B. Fasting blood glucose between 60 and 90 mg/dL, premeal blood glucose between 60 and 105 mg/dL, 1-hour postprandial blood glucose between 60 and 140 mg/dL, and 2-hour postprandial blood glucose between 60 and 120 mg/dL
   C. Fasting blood glucose between 60 and 90 mg/dL, premeal blood glucose between 60 and 105 mg/dL, 1-hour postprandial blood glucose between 60 and 140 mg/dL, and 2-hour postprandial blood glucose between 100 and 140 mg/dL
   D. Fasting blood glucose between 60 and 90 mg/dL, premeal blood glucose between 60 and 110 mg/dL, 1-hour postprandial blood glucose between 60 and 140 mg/dL, and 2-hour postprandial blood glucose between 60 and 120 mg/dL

10. Glucagon is:
    A. Intravenous glucose
    B. A hormone that can be given intramuscularly to stimulate hepatic glucose production from glycogen
    C. Glucose tablets that a patient can use during hypoglycemia
    D. The type of glucose produced by the liver

11. Which of the following methods of teaching for meal planning gives the patient the greatest flexibility?
    A. Carbohydrate counting
    B. Food pyramid
    C. Exchange list
    D. Calorie counting

12. Pregnancy causes which of the following physiologic changes?
    A. Cardiovascular, respiratory, mechanical, thermoregulatory, and metabolic
    B. Cardiovascular, respiratory, mechanical, thermoregulatory, and neurologic
    C. Cardiovascular, respiratory, immunologic, metabolic, and thermoregulatory
    D. Cardiovascular, immunologic, neurologic, thermoregulatory, and metabolic

13. A 37-year-old woman, gravida 3 para 2 abortus 0 with type 2 diabetes, presents at 6 weeks' gestation taking Glucophage. She is 5 feet, 6 inches tall and weighs 238 pounds. She has a hectic schedule and often misses lunch. Which is the best insulin regimen for her?
    A. Regular and NPH insulin
    B. Regular and Ultralente insulin
    C. Humalog and NPH insulin
    D. Humalog and Ultralente insulin

14. The prenatal patient in question 13, who is a type 2 diabetic and presents at 6 weeks' gestation with a weight of 238 pounds, would be started on which insulin dose?
    A. 12 units of Humalog at each meal with 19 units of Ultralente at breakfast and supper
    B. 8 units of Humalog at each meal with 14 units of Ultralente at breakfast and supper
    C. 16 units of regular insulin at breakfast, mixed with 32 units of NPH, and 12 units of regular insulin at supper, mixed with 12 units of NPH
    D. 16 units of regular insulin at breakfast, mixed with 32 units of NPH; 16 units of regular insulin at lunch; and 12 units of regular at supper, mixed with 12 units of NPH

15. The fetal pancreas begins to function at approximately:
    A. 13 weeks' gestation
    B. 20 weeks' gestation
    C. 28 weeks' gestation
    D. 35 weeks' gestation

16. The peak incidence of neonatal hypoglycemia is usually at:
    A. Immediate postpartum
    B. 2 to 6 hours postpartum
    C. 6 to 12 hours postpartum
    D. 24 hours postpartum

17. A type 1 diabetic mother presents for prenatal care at 14 weeks' gestation with a HbA_{1c} of 9.4%. What is her approximate risk of fetal congenital anomalies based on her HbA_{1c}?
    A. 3.4%
    B. 10.4%
    C. 22.4%
    D. 30.4%

18. The hallmarks in the treatment of diabetes are:
    A. MNT (medical nutritional therapy)
    B. SMBG (self-management of blood glucose)
    C. Exercise
    D. Medication if indicated
    E. All of the above

19. Preconception health care should be offered to which of the following women?
    A. All women of childbearing age
    B. All women with a poor obstetric history
    C. All women older than 35 years of age
    D. All diabetic women

20. The total number of daily carbohydrate grams required by a woman at her ideal body weight of 135 pounds is:
    A. 228 g each day
    B. 150 g each day
    C. 330 g each day
    D. 255 g each day

Check your answers with the Module 13 Posttest Answer Key.

Posttest: Module 14. Delivery in the Absence of a Primary Care Provider

Answer the following questions without referring back to the information in the module. Select the ONE BEST answer for each question.

1. Which of the following is a sign that the baby's birth is about to occur?
   A. The woman pushing at the peak of her contractions
   B. The woman's saying, "The baby is coming"
   C. An increasing fullness and pressure against the perineum
   D. A sudden gush of bright red blood

2. In the immediate care of the newborn, the nurse must *first:*
   A. Dry the baby thoroughly, especially the head
   B. Note and record the Apgar scores
   C. Weigh the baby and instill eye prophylaxis
   D. Maintain a clear airway

3. Excessive bright red bleeding from the vagina of a postpartum woman is a sign of:
   A. Uterine atony or retained placenta
   B. Lacerated cervix or retained placenta
   C. Lacerated cervix or lacerated vaginal wall
   D. Lacerated vaginal wall or uterine atony

4. When assisting the mother with the delivery of her baby, you must:
   A. Make sure a thorough skin prep is always done before delivering the head to prevent infection
   B. Wipe the baby's face, especially the nose and mouth, and check for a cord around the neck
   C. Suction the mouth and nose before pushing on the fundus to deliver the shoulders
   D. Wipe the baby's face and deeply suction the nose and mouth with the mucus trap

5. When the placenta is delivered:
   A. The cord should be pulled firmly in an upward direction to hasten its delivery
   B. The uterus should be vigorously rubbed to hasten its delivery
   C. Lengthening of the cord is a sign of placental separation
   D. A change in the shape of the uterus from globular to oval is a sign that the placenta has separated

6. Women at risk for excessive postpartum bleeding are those who have had:
   A. A gush of blood just before the delivery of the placenta
   B. Oxytocin administration and a long labor
   C. One or two babies previously
   D. Their placenta delivered in less than 5 minutes

7. Control of the delivering head is important to prevent damage to the head and the mother's tissues.
   A. True
   B. False

8. If the head is crowning and the primary care provider is on the way to the labor unit, the nurse should delay the birth by holding back the delivering head.
   A. True
   B. False

9. Pieces of the placenta can remain attached to the lining of the uterus or break off from the placenta.
   A. True
   B. False

10. If you know the mother's blood type, it is not necessary to obtain cord blood.
    A. True
    B. False

11. All umbilical cords should have two arteries and one vein.
    A. True
    B. False

12. By reviewing a woman's antepartum records, you will be able to eliminate shoulder dystocia as a concern.
    A. True
    B. False

13. Meconium-stained fluid may be associated with fetal hypoxia, uterine hyperstimulation, mature gastrointestinal tract, or biophysical profile of less than 6.
    A. True
    B. False

14. Match the phrase in Column B with the item in Column A.

Column A		Column B
a. _____	McRoberts maneuver	1. Aids in controlling the urge to push
b. _____	Bonding	2. Sign of impending birth
c. _____	Feather blow	3. A rapid labor
d. _____	Side-lying position	4. Use a mucus trap
e. _____	Umbilical cord	5. Cord around the neck
f. _____	Placenta	6. Maintaining infant's body heat
g. _____	Breech	7. Promotes good parenting
h. _____	Bulging of perineum	8. Less strain on the perineum
i. _____	Nuchal cord	9. Three vessels
j. _____	Meconium-stained amniotic fluid	10. Inspect for missing pieces
k. _____	Thermoregulation	11. Avoid excessive handling
l. _____	Possibility of postpartum hemorrhage	12. Exaggerated flexion of maternal knees and hips upon outward toward
		13. Apgar score

Check your answers with the Module 14 Posttest Answer Key.

Posttest: Module 15. Assessment of the Newborn and Newly Delivered Mother

Answer the following questions without referring back to the information in the module. Select the ONE BEST answer for each question.

1. What is the Apgar score of Baby Smith?

   Heart rate: 120 bpm
   Respiratory effort: Slow, irregular
   Muscle tone: Some extremity flexion
   Reflex irritability: Grimace
   Color: Blue extremities

   A. 4   C. 8
   B. 6   D. 3

2. Based on the score from question 1, Baby Smith needs:

   A. Immediate intubation   C. Assistance with resuscitation
   B. Routine newborn care   D. Further observation

3. Dr. Jones asks that umbilical cord gas samples be obtained on Baby Smith. The proper procedure includes:

   A. Collection of two specimens: one arterial and one venous
   B. Placement of needle through both vessels and specimen drawn
   C. Immediate analysis for accurate results
   D. Repetition of exam within 2 hours to ensure adequate treatment

4. The umbilical cord blood obtained on Baby Smith reveals the following arterial results:

   pH: 7.23 HCO_3:   24.3
   P_{CO_2}:   60.5 mm Hg   Base excess: 28.4
   P_{O_2}:   9.8 mm Hg

   The preceding values are:

   A. Normal
   B. Abnormal

5. Based on what is known about Baby Smith, it can be said that this baby's long-term outcome will be:

   A. Good, because all parameters are within normal limits
   B. Poor, because all parameters are abnormal
   C. Unknown, because not all variables have been examined
   D. Dependent on the care received before transport to the nursery

6. The most important factor to consider when evaluating the newborn at birth is:

   A. The baby's total clinical picture
   B. The baby's heart rate
   C. The Apgar score
   D. The baby's cord gases

7. Baby David has a 1-minute Apgar score of 3. Your first responsibility is to:

   A. Maintain an external heat source
   B. Conduct another Apgar assessment
   C. Initiate resuscitation
   D. Keep the parents informed of what is happening

8. The primary purpose of Apgar scoring is to:

   A. Clinically assess the newborn
   B. Predict long-term outcome
   C. Guide resuscitative efforts
   D. Determine the presence of hypoxia

9. Umbilical cord blood gas sampling allows identification of:

   A. Newborn response to oxygenation
   B. Intrapartum fetal distress
   C. Fetal maturity
   D. Undiagnosed congenital anomalies
   E. All of the above
   F. None of the above

10. Metabolic acidosis in the newborn is:

   A. Usually inconsequential and easily resolved
   B. Caused by the trauma of the vaginal birth process
   C. Potentially life threatening if uncorrected
   D. Readily diagnosed and easily responsive to treatment

11. For collection of the umbilical cord blood gas samples:

   A. Use at least a 10-mL syringe
   B. Flush the syringe with a heparinized solution
   C. Chill the syringe with ice before the sample is obtained
   D. Attach the syringe to an 18-gauge needle

12. The care of the newly delivered mother will be transferred from the nurse who followed the woman in labor to another nurse. What information will the new nurse need to care for this patient?

   A. Summary of antepartum events   D. Gender of the infant
   B. Plans for method of infant feeding   E. All of the above
   C. Time of delivery

13. During the immediate postpartum period, the fundus will be located:

   A. 2 fingerbreadths above the umbilicus, deviated to right of midline
   B. 3 fingerbreadths below the umbilicus
   C. At the level of the umbilicus or slightly below and in the midline

14. A 21-year-old woman delivers a 9-pound, 15-ounce infant after an 18-hour labor. The last 5 hours of labor required oxytocin augmentation and epidural anesthesia. During the immediate postpartum assessment, the single most critical element to be observant of is:

   A. A temperature elevation   C. Uterine atony
   B. Pregnancy-related hypertension   D. A full bladder

15. During the first hour postpartum, the newly delivered mother's temperature is 100.3°F. Which of the following may be the cause?

   A. Dehydration   C. Epidural anesthesia
   B. Infection   D. All of the above

16. Early signs of normal attachment to the newborn by the parent include:

   A. Asking the more experienced nurse to care for the infant
   B. Talking to the infant in a low-pitched voice
   C. Keeping the infant in a warmer to maintain temperature
   D. Calling the infant by name

17. A new mother plans to breastfeed. After a long labor, she asks that the infant be given a bottle for 24 hours so that she can rest. You:

   A. Respect the woman's wishes and bottle-feed the infant
   B. Tell the woman that she has to either bottle-feed or breastfeed and has to decide now
   C. Arrange for rest periods for the woman and wait to see if the lactation consultant can convince her to begin to nurse the baby
   D. Explain the advantages of early breastfeeding and plan with the woman ways to achieve adequate rest and initiate lactation

18. Normal findings after a cesarean delivery include:

   A. The woman is unable to move her legs after spinal anesthesia
   B. Bloody urine in the catheter bag
   C. A boggy uterus
   D. Elevated blood pressure

19. Before postpartum sterilization, a woman should:

   A. Be allowed to rest after a long labor
   B. Have documentation of informed consent
   C. Have a catheter inserted in her bladder
   D. Have at least two children

20. You have been assigned to care for a woman whose infant was stillborn. Which of the following behaviors are not supportive of this family's grief process?

   A. Allowing the family to see and hold the infant
   B. Asking the name of the infant
   C. Reminding the mother that she can have more children
   D. Offering to take pictures of the infant

21. Your patient will be discharged 8 hours after the birth of her infant. What information should she know before discharge?

   A. Who to call with questions or for help
   B. How to care for and feed her infant
   C. How to care for her episiotomy
   D. When to come for a postpartum examination
   E. All of the above

Check your answers with the Module 15 Posttest Answer Key.

Posttest: Module 16. Informed Consent and Documentation

Answer the following questions without referring back to the information in the module. Select the ONE BEST answer for each question.

1. As a nurse, you have been asked to obtain a patient's consent for a tubal ligation. Your response is to:
   A. Clearly explain the procedure to this woman
   B. Check the unit procedure/policy manual for the correct forms
   C. Refuse to obtain the consent
   D. Clearly explain the procedure and the risks to the woman

2. The difference between the professional and lay standards for the information part of a consent is:
   A. The language used to explain the procedure
   B. How the risk factors and outcomes are presented to the patient
   C. The length of the explanation about the procedure
   D. Only the professional standard requires a statement about the risks

3. Under what circumstances can a consent be invalid?
   A. When a 17-year-old gravida 2 para 1001 signs a consent for surgery
   B. When a patient's husband signs a consent for a cesarean birth
   C. When a procedure results in a negative outcome
   D. When the patient gives verbal consent for a nursing procedure

4. When you need to correct a charting error, the most appropriate action is to:
   A. Use correction fluid to cover the incorrect information and carefully write in the correct information
   B. Rewrite the whole page of notes
   C. With a single line, cross out the entry and write "error" above it with the date, time, and your initials
   D. Cross out the error and enter the correct information above it

5. Your initial assessment of the laboring patient should include all of the following *except:*
   A. Significant health problems
   B. The course of this pregnancy
   C. Facts about the onset of labor
   D. Your belief that the patient's husband is unsupportive of her plans for the birth

6. After instituting appropriate nursing interventions for a late deceleration in the fetal heart rate, you should document:
   A. The action taken
   B. Maternal and fetal response
   C. That the care provider was notified
   D. All of the above

7. According to current national standards of nursing practice, the person liable for an individual nurse's practice is the:
   A. Physician in charge of the case
   B. Individual professional nurse
   C. Hospital administration staff
   D. Nursing supervisor

8. When you are asked to chart a procedure for a co-worker, what should you do?
   A. Ask enough questions to be sure your notes are accurate.
   B. Have that person cosign your notes.
   C. Refuse to do the charting.
   D. Ask the person to dictate the information and both of you sign the entry.

9. When a patient refuses a medication, the most appropriate nursing action is to:
   A. Write a note documenting why the medication was not administered
   B. Try to talk the patient into accepting the medication
   C. Obtain assistance from a co-worker to administer the medication because it is in the best interest of the patient
   D. Write "withheld" on the medication record

10. A nurse can be held liable for malpractice in all of the following circumstances *except:*
    A. When it can be shown that the nurse did not meet a standard of care
    B. Whenever there is a poor outcome
    C. When in similar circumstances other nurses would have foreseen the possibility of a negative outcome for a particular action
    D. When the chart documents the patient's refusal of a nursing intervention that contributed to the negative outcome

11. You would expect a protocol delegating the responsibility for obtaining an informed consent for Pitocin augmentation to nursing personnel to include all of the following *except:*
    A. Criteria for patient selection
    B. Authorization for the protocol indicated by the medical director's signature
    C. Therapeutic goals for the augmentation
    D. Arguments to present if the patient refuses to sign the consent form

12. Documentation of a telephone triage contact should be determined by the:
    A. Patient's primary provider
    B. Seriousness of the problem
    C. Unit policy
    D. Person taking the call

13. You may discuss your preparation in a malpractice suit with:
    A. A nurse whose judgment you trust
    B. Counsel
    C. Other staff members present at the time of the incident
    D. Your spouse

Check your answers with the Module 16 Posttest Answer Key.

Posttest: Module 17. Maternal Transport

Answer the following questions without referring back to the information in the module. ONE OR MORE THAN ONE of the choices may be correct.

1. A primary advantage of maternal transport to a regional center is that:
   A. The community hospital experiences less strain on its limited resources
   B. The hospital stay of the mother and baby is increased to ensure complete stabilization
   C. Total cost of care and delivery is reduced
   D. A more accurate assessment of when and how to deliver the baby can be done

2. In preparing a high-risk mother for transport to a regional center, it is important that:
   A. Arrangements be made for a family member to accompany the mother
   B. The mother be in labor
   C. The mother be brought directly to the admitting office of the regional hospital
   D. A copy of the mother's records be sent with her

3. In initiating the referral of the mother to the regional center, it is recommended that:
   A. The nurse in the referring hospital call the physician in the regional center
   B. The physician in the referring hospital call the physician in the regional center
   C. The nurse in the referring hospital call the nurse in the regional center
   D. The physician in the referring hospital call the nurse in the regional center

4. The regional center has all of the following responsibilities in the maternal transport process *except:*
   A. A report by phone is given to the referring physician within 24 hours of an important change or outcome in the mother
   B. A discharge summary is sent to the referring hospital
   C. The consent for transport is obtained from the mother or a family member
   D. A physician sees the mother shortly after her arrival at the regional center

5. Which of the following conditions is characteristic of a high-risk transport situation?
   A. The mother's condition is stable.
   B. Time of delivery is not predictable.
   C. A skilled attendant may not need to accompany the mother.
   D. A transport incubator is unnecessary.

6. Which condition can require that a mother be transported from a small Level I community hospital to a regional center?
   A. A laboring woman with a breech baby
   B. A mother requiring a Pitocin induction
   C. A mother with poorly controlled diabetes mellitus
   D. A mother expecting her eighth child

7. A gravida 2 at 35 weeks' gestation is expecting twins. She is in early labor at a Level I hospital. The decision to transport her to a high-risk regional center is most likely because of the:
   A. Increased risk of the babies having birth weights below 2000 g
   B. Increased risk that preeclampsia can occur in multiple gestations
   C. Increased risk of a cesarean birth
   D. Desire to stop her labor by tocolysis

8. During a high-risk transport situation, when either the mother's condition is unstable or the time of delivery is unpredictable, the mother must be accompanied by a:
   A. Family member
   B. Certified registered nurse anesthetist
   C. Skilled medical attendant, such as an obstetrician
   D. Paramedic skilled in the delivery of the newborn

9. All of the following statements regarding maternal transport to a regional perinatal center are true *except:*
   A. Any woman whose membranes have ruptured prematurely should be referred to a regional center
   B. Transport of the undelivered woman to a regional center should be considered if it is anticipated that the infant might require intensive care not available at the referring hospital
   C. Transfer of high-risk women in early labor is recommended if time for transport will take less than 2 hours
   D. A woman with poorly controlled diabetes mellitus should be referred to a regional center

10. Select the nursing intervention most likely to assist the pregnant woman and her family in adjusting at the high-risk regional hospital.
    A. Delay orientation of the mother and family member to the unit until the mother has rested for a day or two.
    B. Limit the number of incoming and outgoing phone calls to and from family members to ensure adequate rest for the mother.
    C. To reduce the mother's anxiety about the pregnancy outcome, avoid paying too much attention to a fetus who might be greatly compromised.
    D. Assign one primary nurse to care for the mother for the first few days.

11. A nursing intervention critical to ensuring a safe maternal transport is to:
    A. Ensure the expectant woman's comfort in a supine position
    B. Make certain that the expectant woman knows what to expect during the transport
    C. Hang a new unit of IV solution just before transport
    D. Keep family members informed of the woman's status

12. All of the following statements reflect recommendations of the 1994 National Institutes of Health consensus conference on corticosteroid therapy for fetal maturation *except:*
    A. Corticosteroid therapy is strongly recommended for its effectiveness in decreasing RDS in infants born between 29 and 34 weeks' gestation
    B. Administration of a glucocorticoid to the mother is advised 24 to 48 hours before delivery
    C. Use of corticosteroids in infants born between 24 and 28 weeks' gestation will decrease the severity of the disease but not the incidence
    D. No strong recommendations were made because research data remain inconclusive

13. The National Institutes of Health recently released clinical recommendations on antenatal corticosteroid administration. Recommendations call for the administration of:
    A. Weekly doses   C. A single course
    B. Rescue therapy   D. Occasional doses

14. A single course of antenatal corticosteroid treatment using dexamethasone consists of:
    A. Two 12-mg doses given intramuscularly 6 hours apart
    B. Four 6-mg doses given intramuscularly 12 hours apart
    C. Four 12-mg doses given intramuscularly 24 hours apart
    D. Two 6-mg doses given intramuscularly 24 apart

15. Optimal benefits from antenatal corticosteroid treatment last:
    A. 1 day   C. 5 days
    B. 2 days   D. 7 days

16. Cyanosis from a cardiac abnormality rather than peripheral cyanosis should be suspected when it occurs in a:
    A. Term baby who has had a normal delivery with little respiratory distress
    B. Baby who has radiologic evidence of lung disease
    C. Baby experiencing premature rupture of membranes and passage of meconium in utero
    D. Premature baby who is in marked respiratory distress

17. A critical management step in caring for a woman with preterm premature rupture of membranes is to:
    A. Perform a sterile gloved vaginal examination
    B. Use a sterile cotton-tipped applicator to take a vaginal culture for group B streptococcus
    C. Keep the mother in a flat, supine position
    D. Insert an internal fetal monitor

18. Women presenting with premature rupture of membranes need to be observed for:
    A. Rising temperatures
    B. Ruptured uterus
    C. Any sign of abruptio placentae
    D. Eclampsia

19. At least two infusion lines should be established in any pregnant woman who is being transported.
    A. True
    B. False

20. Liability issues for health care personnel involved in transport are:
    A. Failure to stabilize before transport
    B. Failure or delay by the receiving hospital to diagnose a problem more significant than what was relayed by the referring hospital
    C. Delay in making a decision to transfer
    D. Failure to use treatment protocols

Check your answers with the Module 17 Posttest Answer Key.

POSTTEST ANSWER KEY

Module 1. Overview of Labor
1. D
2. B
3. A
4. D
5. D
6. D
7. A
8. C
9. B
10. B
11. B
12. D
13. D
14. D
15. A
16. A
17. A
18. D
19. A
20. A
21. A
22. B
23. B
24. 1. D
    2. C
    3. A
    4. A
    5. B
25. C
26. C

Module 2. Maternal and Fetal Response to Labor
1. A (D may also be selected)
2. B
3. D
4. C
5. D
6. D
7. B
8. D
9. A, B
10. C
11. C
12. B
13. D
14. C
15. A
16. C
17. B, D
18. A
19. B
20. A, C
21. C, D
22. B
23. C
24. B
25. A

Module 3. Admission Assessment of the Laboring Woman
1. B
2. C, D
3. A
4. B
5. D
6. D
7. B
8. A
9. C
10. A
11. 1. C
    2. A
    3. E
    4. D
    5. F
    6. B
12. C
13. D
14. C
15. D
16. C, D
17. B
18. C, D
19. D
20. B
21. D
22. C
23. A
24. A, C
25. C
26. A
27. B
28. D
29. C
30. B
31. A, D
32. C
33. A
34. A
35. D
36. A
37. B
38. A, D

Module 4. Admission Assessment of the Fetus
1. C
2. A, C
3. C
4. B, C, D
5. B
6. A
7. B, C, D
8. D
9. A
10. A, B
11. C

12. A
13. D
14. A
15. B
16. A
17. D
18. D
19. A
20. B
21. B
22. C
23. A, D
24. A
25. C
26. C
27. A
28. B
29. A, C, D
30. C
31. D
32. A, B, D
33. A

Module 5. Caring for the Laboring Woman
1. A, B, C, D
2. A
3. B, C
4. B, D
5. B
6. A
7. D
8. D
9. B
10. A
11.

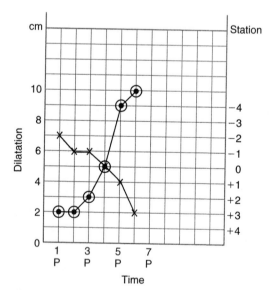

12. A (keep in mind that it could be a nullipara)
13. A (4 cm in 4 hours [active phase] = 1.0 cm/hr = protracted for a multiparous woman but a normal rate for a nullipara)
14. C
15. A, C
16. A, B, D
17. D
18. B, D
19. C
20. C
21. A
22. B, D
23. B, C
24. C
25. B
26. B
27. D
28. B
29. A
30. A
31. A, B, C, D
32. A, D
33. B, D
34. D
35. B
36. D
37. A, C
38. B, C, D
39. C
40. C, D

Module 6. Intrapartum Fetal Monitoring
1. a. E
    b. B
    c. I
    d. E
    e. I
    f. B
    g. I
2. D
3. B, D
4. D
5. A
6. a. ED, LD
    b. A
    c. A, ED
    d. A, ED, VD
    e. LD
    f. VD
    g. LD
    h. LD
    i. A, ED, VD
    j. VD, LD, PD
    k. LD
    l. VD
    m. ED
7. A
8. A, B, C
9. A, B

10. D
11. A
12. A
13. C
14. A
15. A
16. a. A
    b. A
    c. A
    d. N
    e. N
    f. A
    g. A
17. B
18. C
19. D
20. C
21. B
22. C
23. E
24. D
25. A
26. D
27. B
28. D
29. E
30. G
31. B
32. A
33. A
34. A
35. A
36. A
37. A
38. B
39. A
40. A
41. A
42. A
43. A
44. A
45. A
46. A
47. A
48. A
49. B
50. A
51. B
52. B
53. B
54. A
55. A
56. A
57. B
58. A
59. A
60. A
61. A
62. A
63. B

64. A
65. A
66. B
67. B
68. B
69. B
70. A
71. B
72. B
73. a. 5
    b. 1
    c. 4
    d. 2
74. a. 4
    b. 5
    c. 3
    d. 2
    e. 6
    f. 2

Module 7. Induction and Augmentation of Labor

1. A
2. C
3. A
4. B
5. 1. d
   2. g
   3. c
   4. f
   5. e
   6. a
   7 h
   8. b
6. C
7. D
8. C
9. A
10. B
11. B
12. A
13. C
14. B
15. A
16. B

Module 8. Caring for the Woman at Risk for Preterm Labor or With Premature Rupture of Membranes

1. C
2. D
3. D
4. A
5. E
6. A
7. B
8. B

9. A. No, tocolysis is not indicated at gestations less than 20 weeks.
    B. Yes.
    C. No, terbutaline tocolysis is not indicated with uncontrolled diabetes. MgSO$_4$ may be used along with insulin drip.
    D. No, tocolysis is not indicated with heavy vaginal bleeding or at-term gestation.
    E. No, tocolysis is not indicated in the presence of chorioamnionitis.
10. D
11. A
12. B
13. B
14. C
15. B
16. B
17. D
18. D
19. A
20. A
21. D
22. C
23. B
24. D
25. C
26. D
27. A
28. C
29. B
30. C

Module 9. Caring for the Laboring Woman With Hypertensive Disorders Complicating Pregnancy

1. B
2. D
3. D
4. B
5. C
6. A
7. D
8. D
9. C
10. A
11. 1. d, e
    2. f, h
    3. h
    4. b
    5. g
    6. c
    7. a
    8. j
12. C
13. B
14. D
15. A
16. A

17. C
18. B
19. C
20. B
21. C
22. A
23. D
24. A, B, D
25. B, D
26. B, C
27. B
28. A, D
29. C
30. A, B
31. B
32. C
33. D
34. B

Module 10: Intrauterine Growth Restriction: Perinatal Issues and Management

1. C
2. B
3. A
4. B
5. B
6. C
7. B, E
8. B
9. B
10. D
11. C
12. B
13. B
14. C
15. B
16. C
17. C
18. D
19. C
20. C
21. B
22. B
23. C
24. B
25. B
26. D
27. A
28. C
29. C
30. A
31. A
32. B
33. D
34. B
35. C
36. A
37. B
38. D
39. C

40. D
41. B
42. C

Module 11. Caring for the Laboring Woman With HIV Infection or AIDS

1. C
2. A, B, C
3. B
4. A
5. D
6. D (Initially, gloves are worn because of the presence of lochia.)
7. B, C
8. C
9. A
10. A, D
11. D
12. B
13. B
14. A, B
15. A
16. A, B
17. A, B, C
18. A, B, C, D
19. A, B
20. D
21. A, C, D
22. C

Module 12. Hepatitis B Infection: Maternal–Newborn Management

1. C
2. C
3. B
4. B
5. A
6. D
7. B
8. C
9. A
10. A
11. C
12. A
13. B
14. C
15. B
16. D
17. D
18. B
19. C
20. D
21. B
22. A
23. A. Test Report 3—this means you are immune
    B. Test Report 6—no immunity developed that can be documented
    C. Test Report 4—due to the presence of HBeAg
    D. Test Report 5—when IgM anti-HBc is negative, an acute infection is not present, hence the carrier state
24. A
25. D
26. A
27. C
28. B
29. A
30. A
31. A
32. A
33. B
34. A, B
35. C, D
36. B
37. C
38. Patients B and C
39. Patient A
40. Patient C
41. Patients A and B
42. C
43. a. F
    b. T
    c. F
    d. F
    e. F
    f. F
    g. T
    h. T
44. A
45. A
46. B
47. D

Module 13. Caring for the Pregnant Woman With Diabetes

1. A
2. D
3. C
4. C
5. D
6. B
7. B
8. D
9. A
10. B
11. A
12. A
13. D
14. A
15. A
16. C
17. C
18. E
19. A
20. A

Module 14. Delivery in the Absence of a Primary Care Provider

1. C
2. D
3. C
4. B
5. C
6. B
7. A
8. B
9. A
10. B
11. A
12. B
13. A
14. a. 12
   b. 7
   c. 1
   d. 8
   e. 9
   f. 10
   g. 11
   h. 2
   i. 5
   j. 4
   k. 6
   l. 3

Module 15. Assessment of the Newborn and Newly Delivered Mother

1. B
2. C
3. A
4. A
5. C
6. A
7. C
8. C
9. F
10. C
11. B
12. E
13. C
14. C
15. D
16. D
17. D
18. A
19. B
20. C
21. E

Module 16. Informed Consent and Documentation

1. C
2. B
3. B
4. C
5. D
6. D
7. B
8. C
9. A
10. B
11. D
12. C
13. B (When opposition counsel learns that you have discussed the case with an individual, the person can be called as a witness for the opposition. The only exception is your counsel.)

Module 17. Maternal Transport

1. D
2. A, D
3. B
4. C
5. B
6. C
7. A
8. C
9. A
10. D
11. C
12. D
13. C
14. B
15. D
16. A
17. B
18. A
19. A
20. A, B, C, D

Page numbers in *italics* denote figures; those followed by "t" denote tables.

INTRAPARTUM MANAGEMENT MODULES
MODULE 1
OVERVIEW OF LABOR

General Purpose: To provide registered professional nurses and other providers of women's health care with an overview of labor and interventions for supporting the laboring woman.

Objectives

After reading this module and taking this test you will be able to:

1. Describe the physiologic processes involved in initiating labor
2. Outline the stages of labor and the characteristics of uterine contractions
3. Discuss principles or factors helpful in planning interventions for the laboring woman

Directions

To earn continuing education credit, follow these instructions:

1. Read Module 1.
2. Complete the following posttest. Each question has only one answer. Choose the one that is best in each case and darken the corresponding box on the Enrollment Form (Section B).
3. Complete Section A and record your answers to the Evaluation Questions (Section C) on the Enrollment Form.
4. The passing score for this CE activity posttest is 7 correct answers (70%).
5. Registration deadline is April 30, 2004. After this date, please contact Lippincott Williams & Wilkins Continuing Education Department at 212-886-1330.
6. Send the completed Enrollment Form with the appropriate fee (U.S. checks only) to:

Lippincott Williams & Wilkins
Continuing Education Department
345 Hudson Street, 16th Floor
New York, NY 10014

1. The chemical substances that trigger smooth muscle contractions and help prepare the cervix for dilatation are synthesized by:
   A. Macrophages
   B. Calcium
   C. Cytokines
   D. Progesterone

2. In late pregnancy, muscle fibers in the uterine myometrium communicate with each other via:
   A. The decidua
   B. Calcium channels
   C. Gap junctions
   D. Cytokines

3. During which stage of labor does the cervix reach full dilatation?
   A. The latent phase of Stage I
   B. The active phase of Stage I
   C. Stage II
   D. Stage III

4. During labor, the upper portion of the uterus:
   A. Softens
   B. Recedes passively
   C. Becomes thicker
   D. Undergoes a lengthening of its muscle fibers

5. The strongest portion of a uterine contraction is represented on a waveform as the:
   A. Acme
   B. Increment
   C. Base
   D. Decrement

6. Prolonged labor is characterized by contractions:
   A. Less than 35 mm Hg in intensity and less frequently than five in 10 minutes
   B. Less than 25 mm Hg in intensity and less frequently than four in 10 minutes
   C. Less than 35 mm Hg in intensity and less frequently than two in 10 minutes
   D. Less than 25 mm Hg in intensity and less frequently than two in 10 minutes

7. The duration of a uterine contraction is the time that elapses from:
   A. One acme to the next
   B. The beginning of the increment to the end of the decrement
   C. The acme to the end of the decrement
   D. The beginning of one wave to the beginning of the next wave

8. While assessing a uterine contraction by the palpation method, you can indent the uterus only with firm fingertip pressure at the peak of a contraction. You would consider this contraction:
   A. Ineffective
   B. Mild
   C. Moderate
   D. Strong

9. Propagation of a uterine contraction begins at the:
   A. Cervix
   B. Pacemaker
   C. Decidua
   D. Pelvis

10. An appropriate intervention for the laboring woman is:
    A. Keeping her room darkened at all times to promote a soothing atmosphere
    B. Directing all progress reports to her and not to her coach because she is the focus of your care
    C. Avoiding the use of drapes and other coverings because they can create unnecessary pressure and inconvenience
    D. Encouraging a family member to remain with her because family can also provide comfort and reassurance

Intrapartum Management Modules
3rd Edition

A Perinatal Education Program

Module 1—Overview of Labor
Nursing CE contact hours: 2
Fee: $13.75 (If submitting two or more tests together, deduct $1.00 from each test fee.)
Registration Deadline: April 30, 2004

A. Name (Last) _____ (First) _____ (MI) _____

Address _____

City _____ State _____ Zip _____

Telephone _____ Social Security Number _____

State of Licensure #1 _____ License #1 Number _____

RN ☐   APN ☐   Other _____

State of Licensure #2 _____ License #2 Number _____

RN ☐   APN ☐   Other _____

State of Licensure #3 _____ License #3 Number _____

RN ☐   APN ☐   Other _____

B. There may be more response boxes than there are questions. Please indicate your answers in the appropriate boxes and disregard the extra boxes.

1. a ☐	b ☐	c ☐	d ☐	6. a ☐	b ☐	c ☐	d ☐
2. a ☐	b ☐	c ☐	d ☐	7. a ☐	b ☐	c ☐	d ☐
3. a ☐	b ☐	c ☐	d ☐	8. a ☐	b ☐	c ☐	d ☐
4. a ☐	b ☐	c ☐	d ☐	9. a ☐	b ☐	c ☐	d ☐
5. a ☐	b ☐	c ☐	d ☐	10. a ☐	b ☐	c ☐	d ☐

C. EVALUATION QUESTIONS

1. Did this educational activity's learning objectives relate to its general purpose? Yes ☐ No ☐
2. Was this format an effective way to present the material? Yes ☐ No ☐
3. Was the content current to your practice? Yes ☐ No ☐
4. How long did it take you to complete this educational activity? _____ hrs.
5. Suggestions for future topics.

Continuing Education Posttests

■ ■ ■ ■

INTRAPARTUM MANAGEMENT MODULES
MODULE 2
MATERNAL AND FETAL RESPONSE TO LABOR

General Purpose: To present registered professional nurses and other providers of women's health care with a description of both the fetal and the maternal responses to labor and techniques for assessing fetal descent and fetal malpresentation.

Objectives

After reading this module and taking this test, you will be able to:

1. Outline the dimensional and relational parameters that help predict the course of labor and delivery
2. Discuss assessment techniques used to help monitor the progress of labor
3. Plan interventions for evaluating and managing the laboring woman

Directions

To earn continuing education credit, follow these instructions:

1. Read Module 2.
2. Complete the following posttest. Each question has only one answer. Choose the one that is best in each case and darken the corresponding box on the Enrollment Form (Section B).
3. Complete Section A and record your answers to the Evaluation Questions (Section C) on the Enrollment Form.
4. The passing score for this CE activity posttest is 7 correct answers (70%).
5. Registration deadline is April 30, 2004. After this date, please contact Lippincott Williams & Wilkins Continuing Education Department at 212-886-1330.
6. Send the completed Enrollment Form with the appropriate fee (U.S. checks only) to:

Lippincott Williams & Wilkins
Continuing Education Department
345 Hudson Street, 16th Floor
New York, NY 10014

1. The relationship of the long axis of the fetus to the long axis of the mother is called the fetal:
   A. Position
   B. Lie
   C. Attitude
   D. Presentation

2. The pelvic cavity:
   A. Includes the true and the false pelvis
   B. Includes only one of the pelvic planes
   C. Extends from the pelvic inlet to the pelvic outlet
   D. Is another name for the false pelvis

3. Hyperextension of the fetal head results in which of the following presentations?
   A. Transverse
   B. Cephalic
   C. Shoulder
   D. Breech

4. The denominator in a vertex presentation is the:
   A. Occiput
   B. Mentum
   C. Sacrum
   D. Acromial process

5. When the level of the fetal presenting part is one-third the distance between the mother's ischial spines and the pelvic outlet, its station is:
   A. −1
   B. 0
   C. +1
   D. +3

6. When the fetal presenting part has entered the false pelvis but has yet to pass the pelvic inlet, the fetus is:
   A. Presenting
   B. Floating
   C. Molding
   D. Dipping

7. When it is possible to move the presenting part just above the symphysis pubis via abdominal examination, the fetus is:
   A. Presenting
   B. Floating
   C. Molding
   D. Dipping

8. When the station is high at the onset of labor:
   A. Labor tends to be short
   B. The cervix is likely to be considerably effaced
   C. Disproportion is a significant possibility
   D. Nonprogressive labor is unlikely

9. When you detect a prolapsed umbilical cord, you should:
   A. Reposition the mother
   B. Exert upward internal pressure on the cord
   C. Reposition the cord externally
   D. Exert downward external pressure on the presenting part

10. When a prolapsed cord extends outside the mother's vagina, you should:
    A. Clamp the cord
    B. Reposition the cord
    C. Cover the cord with saline-soaked gauze
    D. Reinsert the cord

Intrapartum Management Modules
3rd Edition

A Perinatal Education Program

Module 2—Maternal and Fetal Response to Labor
Nursing CE contact hours: 4
Fee: $25.00 (If submitting two or more tests together, deduct $1.00 from each test fee.)
Registration Deadline: April 30, 2004

A. Name (Last) _____ (First) _____ (MI) _____

    Address _____

    City _____ State _____ Zip _____

    Telephone _____ Social Security Number _____

    State of Licensure #1 _____ License #1 Number _____

    RN ☐   APN ☐   Other _____

    State of Licensure #2 _____ License #2 Number _____

    RN ☐   APN ☐   Other _____

    State of Licensure #3 _____ License #3 Number _____

    RN ☐   APN ☐   Other _____

B. There may be more response boxes than there are questions. Please indicate your answers in the appropriate boxes and disregard the extra boxes.

    1. a ☐ b ☐ c ☐ d ☐   6. a ☐ b ☐ c ☐ d ☐
    2. a ☐ b ☐ c ☐ d ☐   7. a ☐ b ☐ c ☐ d ☐
    3. a ☐ b ☐ c ☐ d ☐   8. a ☐ b ☐ c ☐ d ☐
    4. a ☐ b ☐ c ☐ d ☐   9. a ☐ b ☐ c ☐ d ☐
    5. a ☐ b ☐ c ☐ d ☐   10. a ☐ b ☐ c ☐ d ☐

C. EVALUATION QUESTIONS
    1. Did this educational activity's learning objectives relate to its general purpose? Yes ☐ No ☐
    2. Was this format an effective way to present the material? Yes ☐ No ☐
    3. Was the content current to your practice? Yes ☐ No ☐
    4. How long did it take you to complete this educational activity? _____ hrs.
    5. Suggestions for future topics.

Continuing Education Posttests

INTRAPARTUM MANAGEMENT MODULES
MODULE 3
ADMISSION ASSESSMENT OF THE LABORING WOMAN

General Purpose: To present registered professional nurses and other providers of women's health care with a detailed admission assessment procedure for the laboring woman, including the physical examination, testing for ruptured membranes, and the vaginal examination.

Objectives
After reading this module and taking this test, you will be able to:
1. List reasons why collecting an adequate admission history from a pregnant woman is vital for optimal perinatal outcomes
2. Discuss warning signs indicating perinatal compromise
3. Outline the essential actions and observations necessary for a thorough and appropriate vaginal examination of the laboring woman

Directions
To earn continuing education credit, follow these instructions:
1. Read Module 3.
2. Complete the following posttest. Each question has only one answer. Choose the one that is best in each case and darken the corresponding box on the Enrollment Form (Section B).
3. Complete Section A and record your answers to the Evaluation Questions (Section C) on the Enrollment Form.
4. The passing score for this CE activity posttest is 7 correct answers (70%).
5. Registration deadline is April 30, 2004. After this date, please contact Lippincott Williams & Wilkins Continuing Education Department at 212-886-1330.
6. Send the completed Enrollment Form with the appropriate fee (U.S. checks only) to:

Lippincott Williams & Wilkins
Continuing Education Department
345 Hudson Street, 16th Floor
New York, NY 10014

1. How many infants born to mothers who have experienced a primary genital herpesvirus infection during the pregnancy acquire the virus?
   A. 1 in 2
   B. 1 in 3
   C. 1 in 50
   D. 1 in 100

2. Which of the following is a sign of false labor?
   A. Contractions that start at the back and spread to the front
   B. Loose bowel movements
   C. Contractions that intensify with walking
   D. A brownish "bloody show"

3. Which of the following is a sign of true labor?
   A. Brief increases in fetal movement
   B. No change in contractions after sedation is administered
   C. Contractions that diminish temporarily with increased maternal activity
   D. Moderate contractions felt only in the back

4. Meconium-stained amniotic fluid is a dangerous sign because:
   A. Of its high bacterial content
   B. It always indicates fetal distress
   C. It is easily aspirated
   D. It is a sure marker of prematurity

5. Which of the following findings requires immediate surgical intervention?
   A. Too little amniotic fluid
   B. Too much amniotic fluid
   C. Meconium-stained amniotic fluid
   D. Port wine–colored amniotic fluid

6. You should forego the initial vaginal examination when admitting a pregnant woman who is:
   A. In labor and whose membranes have not yet ruptured
   B. Not in labor and whose membranes have ruptured
   C. In labor and whose membranes have ruptured
   D. Not in labor and whose membranes have not yet ruptured

7. When performing a vaginal examination on a woman in labor, you should:
   A. Have her empty her bladder before the examination
   B. Position her hands above her head for the examination
   C. Maintain a moderate upward pressure on the blades as you insert the speculum
   D. Apply a water-based lubricant to the speculum

8. Which of the following is a definitive sign of ruptured membranes?
   A. A glistening perineum
   B. A color change indicating alkalinity on Nitrazine paper
   C. Positive arborization
   D. Leakage of straw-colored fluid with a neutral odor

9. A cervix that is ¼-inch thick is:
   A. 25% effaced
   B. 50% effaced
   C. 75% effaced
   D. 100% effaced

10. During the vaginal examination of a laboring woman, you can fit the tips of three of your fingers inside the cervical opening. The cervix is approximately:
    A. 3 cm dilated
    B. 5 to 6 cm dilated
    C. 8 to 9 cm dilated
    D. Fully dilated

LIPPINCOTT WILLIAMS & WILKINS
CONTINUING EDUCATION ENROLLMENT FORM

Intrapartum Management Modules
3rd Edition

A Perinatal Education Program

Module 3—Admissions Assessment of the Laboring Woman
Nursing CE contact hours: 4
Fee: $25.00 (If submitting two or more tests together, deduct $1.00 from each test fee.)
Registration Deadline: April 30, 2004

A. Name (Last) _____ (First) _____ (MI) _____

Address _____

City _____ State _____ Zip _____

Telephone _____ Social Security Number _____

State of Licensure #1 _____ License #1 Number _____

RN ☐   APN ☐   Other _____

State of Licensure #2 _____ License #2 Number _____

RN ☐   APN ☐   Other _____

State of Licensure #3 _____ License #3 Number _____

RN ☐   APN ☐   Other _____

B. There may be more response boxes than there are questions. Please indicate your answers in the appropriate boxes and disregard the extra boxes.

1. a☐   b☐   c☐   d☐   6. a☐   b☐   c☐   d☐
2. a☐   b☐   c☐   d☐   7. a☐   b☐   c☐   d☐
3. a☐   b☐   c☐   d☐   8. a☐   b☐   c☐   d☐
4. a☐   b☐   c☐   d☐   9. a☐   b☐   c☐   d☐
5. a☐   b☐   c☐   d☐   10. a☐   b☐   c☐   d☐

C. EVALUATION QUESTIONS
1. Did this educational activity's learning objectives relate to its general purpose? Yes ☐ No ☐
2. Was this format an effective way to present the material? Yes ☐ No ☐
3. Was the content current to your practice? Yes ☐ No ☐
4. How long did it take you to complete this educational activity? _____ hrs.
5. Suggestions for future topics.

■ ■ ■ ■

INTRAPARTUM MANAGEMENT MODULES
MODULE 4
ADMISSION ASSESSMENT OF THE FETUS

General Purpose: To present registered professional nurses and other providers of women's health care with information on the components of a thorough fetal assessment.

Objectives
After reading this module and taking this test, you will be able to:
1. Discuss the assessment techniques used to approximate gestation
2. Outline principles essential for evaluating fetal position and movement
3. Describe actions that will yield information about fetal heart tones

Directions
To earn continuing education credit, follow these instructions:
1. Read Module 4.
2. Complete the following posttest. Each question has only one answer. Choose the one that is best in each case and darken the box on the Enrollment Form (Section B).
3. Complete Section A and record your answers to the Evaluation Questions (Section C) on the Enrollment Form.
4. The passing score for this CE activity posttest is 7 correct answers (70%).
5. Registration deadline is April 30, 2004. After this date, please contact Lippincott Williams & Wilkins Continuing Education Department at 212-886-1330.
6. Send the completed Enrollment Form with the appropriate fee (U.S. checks only) to:

Lippincott Williams & Wilkins
Continuing Education Department
345 Hudson Street, 16th Floor
New York, NY 10014

1. Using Naegele's rule, a pregnant woman whose last normal menstrual period began on November 13 would have an estimated date of confinement of:
   A. August 6
   B. August 10
   C. August 13
   D. August 20

2. With a Doppler ultrasound, the earliest that fetal heart tones can typically be heard is between:
   A. 6 and 8 weeks
   B. 10 and 12 weeks
   C. 14 and 16 weeks
   D. 18 and 20 weeks

3. Which of the following is a true statement about the effects of maternal behavior on fetal breathing movements (FBMs)?
   A. Smoking increases FBMs.
   B. Drinking alcohol stops FBMs for at least 6 hours.
   C. Eating decreases FBMs for 2 to 3 hours.
   D. FBMs increase during active labor.

4. When evaluating fetal movement, it is important to remember that:
   A. Most women feel at least 10 distinct fetal movements in 2 hours
   B. Fetal movement has been known to cease completely for as long as 20 hours before fetal death
   C. Any woman who does not feel the appropriate number of movements in 2 hours should count them for another 2 hours
   D. Hiccups should be counted as fetal movements

5. When measuring fundal height, the zero point of the tape measure should be positioned at the:
   A. Midline of the umbilicus
   B. Top of the fundus
   C. Anterior border of the symphysis pubis
   D. Lowermost edge of the curved fundus

6. Approximately where should the fundus be at 28 weeks' gestation?
   A. Approximately 3 fingerbreadths below the xiphoid
   B. Approximately 3 fingerbreadths above the umbilicus
   C. Approximately 1 to 2 fingerbreadths above the umbilicus
   D. Approximately 1 to 2 fingerbreadths below the umbilicus

7. Using one hand to stabilize the gravid uterus on one side of the abdomen and the other hand to feel along the side of the abdomen, you are attempting to palpate the fetal:
   A. Head
   B. Chest
   C. Back
   D. Cephalic prominence

8. While facing the mother's feet and moving your hands down the sides of her abdomen toward the symphysis pubis, you are attempting to palpate the fetal:
   A. Head
   B. Chest
   C. Back
   D. Cephalic prominence

9. With a breech position, the best place to auscultate fetal heart tones is:
   A. Below the umbilicus on the right side
   B. Below the umbilicus on the left side
   C. Above the umbilicus on the right side
   D. Above the umbilicus on the left side

10. The best place to begin listening for fetal heart tones when the fetus is at 20 weeks' gestation is:
    A. In the right lower quadrant
    B. 1 fingerbreadth above the umbilicus
    C. 2 fingerbreadths above the pubic hairline at the midline of the abdomen
    D. In the left lower quadrant at the upper border of the pubic hair

LIPPINCOTT WILLIAMS & WILKINS
CONTINUING EDUCATION ENROLLMENT FORM

Intrapartum Management Modules
3rd Edition

A Perinatal Education Program

Module 4—Admission Assessment of the Fetus
Nursing CE contact hours: 3.5
Fee: $22.75 (If submitting two or more tests together, deduct $1.00 from each test fee.)
Registration Deadline: April 30, 2004

A. Name (Last) _____ (First) _____ (MI) _____

   Address _____

   City _____ State _____ Zip _____

   Telephone _____ Social Security Number _____

   State of Licensure #1 _____ License #1 Number _____

   RN ☐   APN ☐   Other _____

   State of Licensure #2 _____ License #2 Number _____

   RN ☐   APN ☐   Other _____

   State of Licensure #3 _____ License #3 Number _____

   RN ☐   APN ☐   Other _____

B. There may be more response boxes than there are questions. Please indicate your answers in the appropriate boxes and disregard the extra boxes.

   1. a ☐ b ☐ c ☐ d ☐   6. a ☐ b ☐ c ☐ d ☐
   2. a ☐ b ☐ c ☐ d ☐   7. a ☐ b ☐ c ☐ d ☐
   3. a ☐ b ☐ c ☐ d ☐   8. a ☐ b ☐ c ☐ d ☐
   4. a ☐ b ☐ c ☐ d ☐   9. a ☐ b ☐ c ☐ d ☐
   5. a ☐ b ☐ c ☐ d ☐   10. a ☐ b ☐ c ☐ d ☐

C. EVALUATION QUESTIONS
   1. Did this educational activity's learning objectives relate to its general purpose? Yes ☐ No ☐
   2. Was this format an effective way to present the material? Yes ☐ No ☐
   3. Was the content current to your practice? Yes ☐ No ☐
   4. How long did it take you to complete this educational activity? _____ hrs.
   5. Suggestions for future topics.

■ ■ ■ ■

INTRAPARTUM MANAGEMENT MODULES
MODULE 5
CARING FOR THE LABORING WOMAN

General Purpose: To present registered professional nurses and other providers of women's health care with detailed guidelines for intrapartum care, including maternal and fetal assessment, hydration, and pain management strategies.

Objectives

After reading this module and taking this test, you will be able to:

1. Outline assessment parameters or techniques for monitoring the laboring woman and her fetus
2. Discuss the indications, rationale, and guidelines for appropriate maternal and fetal hydration
3. Plan pain control strategies for the laboring woman

Directions

To earn continuing education credit, follow these instructions:

1. Read Module 5.
2. Complete the following posttest. Each question has only one answer. Choose the one that is best in each case and darken the box on the Enrollment Form (Section B).
3. Complete Section A and record your answers to the Evaluation Questions (Section C) on the Enrollment Form.
4. The passing score for this CE activity posttest is 7 correct answers (70%).
5. Registration deadline is April 30, 2004. After this date, please contact Lippincott Williams & Wilkins Continuing Education Department at 212-886-1330.
6. Send the completed Enrollment Form with the appropriate fee (U.S. checks only) to:

Lippincott Williams & Wilkins
Continuing Education Department
345 Hudson Street, 16th Floor
New York, NY 10014

1. For a fetus in a normal position of flexion, the optimal location for auscultating the fetal heart tones is over the fetus':
   A. Chest
   B. Back
   C. Vertex
   D. Buttocks

2. For a high-risk woman in active labor, fetal heart sounds should be evaluated every:
   A. 5 minutes
   B. 10 minutes
   C. 15 minutes
   D. 30 minutes

3. Which of the following is an indication for amnioinfusion?
   A. A nuchal cord
   B. A nonvertex presentation
   C. Multiple gestation
   D. Absent fetal heart rate variability

4. During amnioinfusion, the laboring woman:
   A. Receives about 1,800 mL of fluid
   B. Is given normal saline or lactated Ringer's warmed in a microwave oven
   C. Is positioned on her back
   D. Is given infusate at the maintenance rate of about 150 to 180 mL per hour

5. Immediate delivery is indicated when fetal oxygenation, as monitored by pulse oximetry, drops below:
   A. 90%
   B. 70%
   C. 50%
   D. 30%

6. A laboring woman:
   A. Who is kept NPO will have reduced gastric acidity
   B. Needs routine IV hydration to reduce the risk of hypoglycemia in her newborn
   C. Should be encouraged to empty her bladder every 2 hours
   D. Must have routine IV hydration during the first 12 hours of labor

7. Pain experienced by the laboring woman can:
   A. Cause hyperventilation and subsequent increased blood flow to the uterus
   B. Trigger the release of epinephrine, which ultimately reduces blood flow to the placenta
   C. Reduce both her cardiac output and blood pressure
   D. Trigger the release of epinephrine, which ultimately causes fetal hypoglycemia

8. Intravenous medications should be administered to a laboring woman:
   A. At the beginning of a contraction and over a few minutes
   B. At the end of a contraction and over a few minutes
   C. At the beginning of a contraction and over a few seconds
   D. At the peak of a contraction and over a few minutes

9. Treatment for a postepidural spinal headache includes:
   A. Maintaining the patient in a semiupright position
   B. Using a blood patch to seal the puncture site
   C. Restricting fluid intake
   D. Withholding analgesia to prevent masking the symptoms

10. Effleurage is:
    A. Light abdominal massage recommended between contractions
    B. Gentle abdominal massage performed with the palm of the hand
    C. Firm abdominal massage performed with the fingertips
    D. Light abdominal massage recommended during contractions

LIPPINCOTT WILLIAMS & WILKINS
CONTINUING EDUCATION ENROLLMENT FORM

Intrapartum Management Modules
3rd Edition

A Perinatal Education Program

Module 5—Caring for the Laboring Woman
Nursing CE contact hours: 6.5
Fee: $29.25 (If submitting two or more tests together, deduct $1.00 from each test fee.)
Registration Deadline: April 30, 2004

A. Name (Last) _____ (First) _____ (MI) _____

    Address _____

    City _____ State _____ Zip _____

    Telephone _____ Social Security Number _____

    State of Licensure #1 _____ License #1 Number _____

    RN ☐   APN ☐   Other _____

    State of Licensure #2 _____ License #2 Number _____

    RN ☐   APN ☐   Other _____

    State of Licensure #3 _____ License #3 Number _____

    RN ☐   APN ☐   Other _____

B. There may be more response boxes than there are questions. Please indicate your answers in the appropriate boxes and disregard the extra boxes.

    1. a ☐ b ☐ c ☐ d ☐   6. a ☐ b ☐ c ☐ d ☐
    2. a ☐ b ☐ c ☐ d ☐   7. a ☐ b ☐ c ☐ d ☐
    3. a ☐ b ☐ c ☐ d ☐   8. a ☐ b ☐ c ☐ d ☐
    4. a ☐ b ☐ c ☐ d ☐   9. a ☐ b ☐ c ☐ d ☐
    5. a ☐ b ☐ c ☐ d ☐   10. a ☐ b ☐ c ☐ d ☐

C. EVALUATION QUESTIONS

    1. Did this educational activity's learning objectives relate to its general purpose? Yes ☐ No ☐
    2. Was this format an effective way to present the material? Yes ☐ No ☐
    3. Was the content current to your practice? Yes ☐ No ☐
    4. How long did it take you to complete this educational activity? _____ hrs.
    5. Suggestions for future topics.

Continuing Education Posttests

■ ■ ■ ■

INTRAPARTUM MANAGEMENT MODULES
MODULE 6
INTRAPARTUM FETAL MONITORING

General Purpose: To present registered professional nurses and other providers of women's health care with detailed guidelines for fetal monitoring.

Objectives
After reading this module and taking this test, you will be able to:
1. Compare and contrast the capabilities of and techniques and equipment involved with intermittent auscultation and electronic fetal monitoring
2. Discuss the physiologic basis for at least three parameters used to monitor fetal status
3. Plan interventions for the laboring woman based on interpretation of fetal monitoring parameters

Directions
To earn continuing education credit, follow these instructions:
1. Read Module 6.
2. Complete the following posttest. Each question has only one answer. Choose the one that is best in each case and darken the corresponding box on the Enrollment Form (Section B).
3. Complete Section A and record your answers to the Evaluation Questions (Section C) on the Enrollment Form.
4. The passing score for this CE activity posttest is 7 correct answers (70%).
5. Registration deadline is April 30, 2004. After this date, please contact Lippincott Williams & Wilkins Continuing Education Department at 212-886-1330.
6. Send the completed Enrollment Form with the appropriate fee (U.S. checks only) to:

Lippincott Williams & Wilkins
Continuing Education Department
345 Hudson Street, 16th Floor
New York, NY 10014

1. Using intermittent auscultation alone, an experienced clinician cannot necessarily:
   A. Determine baseline variations such as bradycardia
   B. Identify the baseline rhythm
   C. Approximate the baseline rate
   D. Distinguish the different kinds of decelerations accurately

2. Which of the following devices detects changes in the shape of the laboring woman's abdomen as a result of uterine contractions?
   A. An ultrasonic transducer
   B. A tocodynamometer
   C. A fetoscope
   D. An intrauterine pressure catheter

3. Essential to reading a fetal monitor strip is understanding that:
   A. The space between each light vertical line represents 10 seconds, while the space between each light horizontal line represents 10 beats per minute
   B. The space between each light vertical line represents 1 minute, while the space between each light horizontal line represents 30 beats per minute

C. The space between each light vertical line represents 10 seconds, while the space between each light horizontal line represents 30 beats per minute
D. The space between each light vertical line represents 1 minute, while the space between each light horizontal line represents 10 beats per minute

4. Blood flow to the placenta is completely blocked when uterine tone:
   A. Drops below 10 mm Hg
   B. Drops below 15 mm Hg
   C. Rises above 25 mm Hg
   D. Rises above 40 mm Hg

5. During a 10-minute period, a laboring woman has five contractions. The first two are 45 mm Hg in intensity, the third is 50 mm Hg, and the last two are 60 mm Hg. Resting uterine tone between each contraction is 10 mm Hg. Using the Montevideo units standard, what is the status of labor progression?
   A. The contraction pattern is inadequate.
   B. Labor is likely to progress normally.
   C. The contraction pattern indicates hyperstimulation.
   D. There is insufficient information to determine the labor progression.

6. A drop in the pH of fetal blood is recognized by:
   A. Baroreceptors, which trigger a decrease in fetal heart rate
   B. Baroreceptors, which trigger an increase in fetal heart rate
   C. Chemoreceptors, which trigger an initial decrease in fetal heart rate
   D. Chemoreceptors, which trigger an initial increase in fetal heart rate

7. Which of the following interventions is recommended for decreased long-term variability?
   A. Positioning the patient on her back
   B. Discontinuing oxygen therapy
   C. Turning the patient to the side
   D. Avoiding any actions that might stimulate the fetus

8. A drop in fetal heart rate that typically lasts less than 2 minutes and is usually associated with umbilical cord compression is called:
   A. An early deceleration
   B. A late deceleration
   C. A variable deceleration
   D. A prolonged deceleration

9. The fetal heart rate pattern most likely to indicate fetal metabolic acidosis is:
   A. Absent variability
   B. Early decelerations
   C. Variable decelerations with loss of one shoulder
   D. Overshoots

10. Which of the following fetal dysrhythmias requires immediate intervention?
    A. Premature atrial contractions
    B. Severe heart block
    C. Premature ventricular contractions
    D. Vagal cardiac arrest

LIPPINCOTT WILLIAMS & WILKINS
CONTINUING EDUCATION ENROLLMENT FORM

Intrapartum Management Modules
3rd Edition

A Perinatal Education Program

Module 6—Intrapartum Fetal Monitoring
Nursing CE contact hours: 10.5
Fee: $36.75 (If submitting two or more tests together, deduct $1.00 from each test fee.)
Registration Deadline: April 30, 2004

A. Name (Last) _____ (First) _____ (MI) _____

Address _____

City _____ State _____ Zip _____

Telephone _____ Social Security Number _____

State of Licensure #1 _____ License #1 Number _____

RN ☐   APN ☐   Other _____

State of Licensure #2 _____ License #2 Number _____

RN ☐   APN ☐   Other _____

State of Licensure #3 _____ License #3 Number _____

RN ☐   APN ☐   Other _____

B. There may be more response boxes than there are questions. Please indicate your answers in the appropriate boxes and disregard the extra boxes.

1. a ☐	b ☐	c ☐	d ☐	6. a ☐	b ☐	c ☐	d ☐
2. a ☐	b ☐	c ☐	d ☐	7. a ☐	b ☐	c ☐	d ☐
3. a ☐	b ☐	c ☐	d ☐	8. a ☐	b ☐	c ☐	d ☐
4. a ☐	b ☐	c ☐	d ☐	9. a ☐	b ☐	c ☐	d ☐
5. a ☐	b ☐	c ☐	d ☐	10. a ☐	b ☐	c ☐	d ☐

C. EVALUATION QUESTIONS
1. Did this educational activity's learning objectives relate to its general purpose? Yes ☐ No ☐
2. Was this format an effective way to present the material? Yes ☐ No ☐
3. Was the content current to your practice? Yes ☐ No ☐
4. How long did it take you to complete this educational activity? _____ hrs.
5. Suggestions for future topics.

Continuing Education Posttests

■ ■ ■ ■

INTRAPARTUM MANAGEMENT MODULES
MODULE 7
INDUCTION AND AUGMENTATION OF LABOR

General Purpose: To present registered professional nurses and other providers of women's health care with detailed guidelines for inducing and augmenting labor, including procedures for implementing various mechanical and pharmacologic interventions.

Objectives

After reading this module and taking this test, you will be able to:

1. Discuss the indications, contraindications, and precautions for implementing the various methods of labor induction and/or augmentation
2. Discuss at least two assessment parameters useful for monitoring pregnancy and labor progression
3. Plan interventions for the laboring woman undergoing labor induction and/or augmentation

Directions

To earn continuing education credit, follow these instructions:

1. Read Module 7.
2. Complete the following posttest. Each question has only one answer. Choose the one that is best in each case and darken the corresponding box on the Enrollment Form (Section B).
3. Complete Section A and record your answers to the Evaluation Questions (Section C) on the Enrollment Form.
4. The passing score for this CE activity posttest is 7 correct answers (70%).
5. Registration deadline is April 30, 2004. After this date, please contact Lippincott Williams & Wilkins Continuing Education Department at 212-886-1330.
6. Send the completed Enrollment Form with the appropriate fee (U.S. checks only) to:

Lippincott Williams & Wilkins
Continuing Education Department
345 Hudson Street, 16th Floor
New York, NY 10014

1. Of the following, which is an absolute contraindication for induction and for augmentation of labor?
   A. Multiple gestation
   B. Hydramnios
   C. Breech presentation
   D. Total placenta previa

2. At what gestational point can most multiparous women perceive quickening?
   A. 16 weeks
   B. 17 weeks
   C. 18 weeks
   D. 19 weeks

3. A Bishop's score includes evaluation of all of the following except:
   A. Station
   B. Cervical consistency
   C. Presentation
   D. Cervical effacement

4. Of the following, which is a contraindication for preinduction cervical ripening with prostaglandin E_2 vaginal inserts?
   A. Active genital herpes
   B. Ruptured membranes
   C. Vertex presentation
   D. Early decelerations in fetal heart rate

5. After endocervical instillation of prostaglandin E_2 gel, the patient should be positioned:
   A. On her side for 30 minutes
   B. On her back for 1 hour
   C. On her side for 1 to 2 hours
   D. Supine for 2 hours

6. If fetal bradycardia develops after prostaglandin E_2 is instilled, the patient should be placed:
   A. On her left side
   B. On her right side
   C. In semi-Fowler's position
   D. In Trendelenburg's position

7. Optimal safety for the mother and the fetus during misoprostol administration is most likely when:
   A. The woman is having 12 or more contractions per hour
   B. The Bishop's score is greater than 6
   C. The woman has had plenty of fluids by mouth in the previous 3 hours
   D. The fetus has had a reactive stress test before drug placement

8. During oxytocin administration:
   A. Flow rate should be adjusted initially every 10 minutes as needed
   B. Contractions should not exceed 60 to 70 mm Hg in strength
   C. Contractions should not occur more frequently than three in 10 minutes
   D. Contractions should not exceed 30 seconds in duration

9. A desirable pattern during oxytocin administration includes:
   A. A fetal heart rate of 150 to 180 beats per minute
   B. A resting uterine tone of 15 to 25 mm Hg
   C. Good variability in the fetal heart baseline
   D. Five contractions in 10 minutes

10. When oxytocin is used to augment labor, the infusion should be:
    A. Started at 0.5 to 1 mU per minute
    B. Increased 1 mU per minute every 15 minutes
    C. Started at 1 to 2 mU per minute
    D. Increased 1 mU per minute every 30 minutes

Intrapartum Management Modules
3rd Edition

A Perinatal Education Program

Module 7—Induction and Augmentation of Labor
Nursing CE contact hours: 3
Fee: $19.75 (If submitting two or more tests together, deduct $1.00 from each test fee.)
Registration Deadline: April 30, 2004

A. Name (Last) _____ (First) _____ (MI) _____

    Address _____

    City _____ State _____ Zip _____

    Telephone _____ Social Security Number _____

    State of Licensure #1 _____ License #1 Number _____

    RN ☐   APN ☐   Other _____

    State of Licensure #2 _____ License #2 Number _____

    RN ☐   APN ☐   Other _____

    State of Licensure #3 _____ License #3 Number _____

    RN ☐   APN ☐   Other _____

B. There may be more response boxes than there are questions. Please indicate your answers in the appropriate boxes and disregard the extra boxes.

    1. a ☐ b ☐ c ☐ d ☐   6. a ☐ b ☐ c ☐ d ☐
    2. a ☐ b ☐ c ☐ d ☐   7. a ☐ b ☐ c ☐ d ☐
    3. a ☐ b ☐ c ☐ d ☐   8. a ☐ b ☐ c ☐ d ☐
    4. a ☐ b ☐ c ☐ d ☐   9. a ☐ b ☐ c ☐ d ☐
    5. a ☐ b ☐ c ☐ d ☐   10. a ☐ b ☐ c ☐ d ☐

C. EVALUATION QUESTIONS
    1. Did this educational activity's learning objectives relate to its general purpose? Yes ☐ No ☐
    2. Was this format an effective way to present the material? Yes ☐ No ☐
    3. Was the content current to your practice? Yes ☐ No ☐
    4. How long did it take you to complete this educational activity? _____ hrs.
    5. Suggestions for future topics.

Continuing Education Posttests

■ ■ ■ ■

INTRAPARTUM MANAGEMENT MODULES
MODULE 8
CARING FOR THE WOMAN AT RISK FOR PRETERM LABOR
OR WITH PREMATURE RUPTURE OF MEMBRANES

General Purpose: To present registered professional nurses and other providers of women's health care with detailed guidelines for evaluating and managing preterm labor and premature rupture of membranes.

Objectives

After reading this module and taking this test, you will be able to:

1. Discuss the risk factors associated with preterm level and key assessment parameters
2. Outline the indications, contraindications, mechanisms of action, and side effects of various tocolytic agents
3. Plan interventions for the woman with premature rupture of membranes and/or undergoing preterm labor

Directions

To earn continuing education credit, follow these instructions:

1. Read Module 8.
2. Complete the following posttest. Each question has only one answer. Choose the one that is best in each case and darken the corresponding box on the Enrollment Form (Section B).
3. Complete Section A and record your answers to the Evaluation Questions (Section C) on the Enrollment Form.
4. The passing score for this CE activity posttest is 7 correct answers (70%).
5. Registration deadline is April 30, 2004. After this date, please contact Lippincott Williams & Wilkins Continuing Education Department at 212-886-1330.
6. Send the completed Enrollment Form with the appropriate fee (U.S. checks only) to:

Lippincott Williams & Wilkins
Continuing Education Department
345 Hudson Street, 16th Floor
New York, NY 10014

1. Which of the following is a key finding in preterm labor?
   A. Cervical effacement of at least 60%
   B. At least 16 weeks' gestation
   C. Cervical dilation of at least 2 cm
   D. Five to six contractions per 20 minutes

2. Which of the following factors is associated with an increased risk of preterm labor?
   A. Funneling
   B. A lengthy interpregnancy interval
   C. Previous first trimester abortion
   D. A cervix that is 4 cm or longer

3. Which of the following biochemical markers of preterm labor can be detected in cervicovaginal secretions?
   A. Estriol
   B. Fetal fibronectin
   C. Alpha-fetoprotein
   D. Corticotropin-releasing hormone

4. At the onset of symptoms of preterm labor, it is recommended that the woman:
   A. Restrict fluids
   B. Lie on her back
   C. Resume her usual activities
   D. Empty her bladder

5. Common side effects of tocolytic therapy include:
   A. Bradycardia
   B. Hypercalcemia
   C. Palpitations
   D. Diarrhea

6. Which of the following tocolytic agents works by reducing the production of prostaglandin?
   A. Calcium channel blockers
   B. Nonsteroidal anti-inflammatory drugs
   C. β-Mimetics
   D. Magnesium sulfate

7. Which of the following tocolytic agents specifically reduces the risk of uncontrolled hyperglycemia?
   A. Calcium channel blockers
   B. Nonsteroidal anti-inflammatory drugs
   C. β-Mimetics
   D. Magnesium sulfate

8. β-Mimetics are specifically contraindicated for women in preterm labor who have:
   A. Heart disease
   B. Myasthenia gravis
   C. Oligohydramnios
   D. Renal failure

9. Most women with premature rupture of membranes:
   A. Go on to deliver at term
   B. Deliver within a week of membrane rupture
   C. Can postpone delivery for 2 to 3 weeks with tocolytic therapy
   D. Deliver within 24 hours of membrane rupture

10. Antenatal corticosteroid therapy:
    A. Is most effective within the first 24 hours of administration
    B. Produces benefits that last up to 2 weeks
    C. Is especially effective before 24 weeks' gestation
    D. Reduces the risk of neonatal intraventricular hemorrhage

LIPPINCOTT WILLIAMS & WILKINS
CONTINUING EDUCATION ENROLLMENT FORM

Intrapartum Management Modules
3rd Edition

A Perinatal Education Program

Module 8—Caring for the Woman at Risk for Preterm Labor or With Premature Rupture of Membranes
Nursing CE contact hours: 3
Fee: $19.75 (If submitting two or more tests together, deduct $1.00 from each test fee.)
Registration Deadline: April 30, 2004

A. Name (Last) _____ (First) _____ (MI) _____

   Address _____

   City _____ State _____ Zip _____

   Telephone _____ Social Security Number _____

   State of Licensure #1 _____ License #1 Number _____

   RN ☐   APN ☐   Other _____

   State of Licensure #2 _____ License #2 Number _____

   RN ☐   APN ☐   Other _____

   State of Licensure #3 _____ License #3 Number _____

   RN ☐   APN ☐   Other _____

B. There may be more response boxes than there are questions. Please indicate your answers in the appropriate boxes and disregard the extra boxes.

1. a ☐	b ☐	c ☐	d ☐	6. a ☐	b ☐	c ☐	d ☐
2. a ☐	b ☐	c ☐	d ☐	7. a ☐	b ☐	c ☐	d ☐
3. a ☐	b ☐	c ☐	d ☐	8. a ☐	b ☐	c ☐	d ☐
4. a ☐	b ☐	c ☐	d ☐	9. a ☐	b ☐	c ☐	d ☐
5. a ☐	b ☐	c ☐	d ☐	10. a ☐	b ☐	c ☐	d ☐

C. EVALUATION QUESTIONS

   1. Did this educational activity's learning objectives relate to its general purpose? Yes ☐ No ☐

   2. Was this format an effective way to present the material? Yes ☐ No ☐

   3. Was the content current to your practice? Yes ☐ No ☐

   4. How long did it take you to complete this educational activity? _____ hrs.

   5. Suggestions for future topics.

■ ■ ■ ■

INTRAPARTUM MANAGEMENT MODULES
MODULE 9
CARING FOR THE LABORING WOMAN WITH HYPERTENSIVE DISORDERS COMPLICATING PREGNANCY

General Purpose: To present registered professional nurses and other providers of women's health care with comprehensive guidelines for understanding, evaluating, and managing the hypertensive disorders that complicate pregnancy.

Objectives

After reading this module and taking this test, you will be able to:

1. Discuss principles or factors helpful for understanding hypertension during pregnancy
2. List guidelines essential for evaluating hypertension during pregnancy
3. Describe interventions for the pregnant woman with a hypertensive disorder

Directions

To earn continuing education credit, follow these instructions:

1. Read Module 9.
2. Complete the following posttest. Each question has only one answer. Choose the one that is best in each case and darken the box on the Enrollment Form (Section B).
3. Complete Section A and record your answers to the Evaluation Questions (Section C) on the Enrollment Form.
4. The passing score for this CE activity posttest is 7 correct answers (70%).
5. Registration deadline is April 30, 2004. After this date, please contact Lippincott Williams & Wilkins Continuing Education Department at 212-886-1330.
6. Send the completed Enrollment Form with the appropriate fee (U.S. checks only) to:

Lippincott Williams & Wilkins
Continuing Education Department
345 Hudson Street, 16th Floor
New York, NY 10014

1. A woman whose blood pressure rises to 140/90 mm Hg after 20 weeks' gestation with no protein detected in her urine and whose blood pressure returns to baseline by the time she is 12 weeks' postpartum would probably be diagnosed as having:
   A. Gestational hypertension
   B. Chronic hypertension
   C. Preeclampsia
   D. Eclampsia

2. Mild preeclampsia is characterized by:
   A. More than 500 mg of protein in a 24-hour urine sample
   B. Weight gain of more than 2 pounds per week during the third trimester
   C. Infrequent seizures
   D. Two rises in blood pressure to 160/110 mm Hg or higher in a 4-hour period

3. Hemolysis, elevated liver enzymes, and low platelets (HELLP) syndrome is most common:
   A. In primigravid women
   B. In African American women
   C. Late in the first and early in the second trimester
   D. With cesarean delivery

4. Women with preeclampsia have a shift in the usual balances of vasoactive substances, with especially high levels of:
   A. Prostacyclin
   B. Angiotensin II
   C. Thromboxane
   D. Endothelin

5. When evaluating a pregnant woman's blood pressure, it is important to use which of the following guidelines?
   A. An elevated blood pressure reading on two occasions at least a week apart confirms gestational hypertension.
   B. A blood pressure of 140/90 mm Hg or higher constitutes an abnormally high blood pressure with diagnostic significance during pregnancy.
   C. Common preference is to use an electronic device to measure blood pressure because of its increased accuracy even in various positions.
   D. An elevation of 30 mm Hg systolic or 15 mm Hg diastolic over baseline constitutes an abnormally high blood pressure with diagnostic significance during pregnancy.

6. When checking for proteinuria, a false-positive value is likely when:
   A. Urine specific gravity is 1.030 or higher
   B. Urine pH is 8.0 or higher
   C. Urine specific gravity is less than 1.010
   D. Diluted urine is used

7. Management of preeclampsia includes all of the following except:
   A. Bed rest
   B. Magnesium sulfate to prevent seizures
   C. Evaluation by a clinician as often as twice per week
   D. Sodium restriction

8. The optimal resting position for a woman with severe preeclampsia is:
   A. Semirecumbent
   B. High Fowler's
   C. Supine
   D. Lateral Trendelenburg

9. Which of the following represents an appropriate guideline for administering magnesium sulfate?
   A. Mixing the drug in isotonic saline solution
   B. Giving a loading dose of 1 to 2 g
   C. Infusing the loading dose over 30 minutes
   D. Giving the drug at the rate of 1 g per minute to stop a seizure

10. The drug of choice for treating seriously elevated maternal blood pressure near term is:
    A. Labetalol
    B. Calcium gluconate
    C. Hydralazine
    D. Nifedipine

LIPPINCOTT WILLIAMS & WILKINS
CONTINUING EDUCATION ENROLLMENT FORM

Intrapartum Management Modules
3rd Edition

A Perinatal Education Program

Module 9—Caring for the Laboring Woman With Hypertensive Disorders Complicating Pregnancy
Nursing CE contact hours: 4
Fee: $25.00 (If submitting two or more tests together, deduct $1.00 from each test fee.)
Registration Deadline: April 30, 2004

A. Name (Last) _____ (First) _____ (MI) _____

   Address _____

   City _____ State _____ Zip _____

   Telephone _____ Social Security Number _____

   State of Licensure #1 _____ License #1 Number _____

   RN ☐   APN ☐   Other _____

   State of Licensure #2 _____ License #2 Number _____

   RN ☐   APN ☐   Other _____

   State of Licensure #3 _____ License #3 Number _____

   RN ☐   APN ☐   Other _____

B. There may be more response boxes than there are questions. Please indicate your answers in the appropriate boxes and disregard the extra boxes.

   1. a☐ b☐ c☐ d☐   6. a☐ b☐ c☐ d☐
   2. a☐ b☐ c☐ d☐   7. a☐ b☐ c☐ d☐
   3. a☐ b☐ c☐ d☐   8. a☐ b☐ c☐ d☐
   4. a☐ b☐ c☐ d☐   9. a☐ b☐ c☐ d☐
   5. a☐ b☐ c☐ d☐   10. a☐ b☐ c☐ d☐

C. EVALUATION QUESTIONS
   1. Did this educational activity's learning objectives relate to its general purpose? Yes ☐ No ☐
   2. Was this format an effective way to present the material? Yes ☐ No ☐
   3. Was the content current to your practice? Yes ☐ No ☐
   4. How long did it take you to complete this educational activity? _____ hrs.
   5. Suggestions for future topics.

Continuing Education Posttests

■ ■ ■ ■

INTRAPARTUM MANAGEMENT MODULES
MODULE 10
INTRAUTERINE GROWTH RESTRICTION: PERINATAL ISSUES AND MANAGEMENT

General Purpose: To present registered professional nurses and other providers of women's health care with comprehensive instructions for understanding, evaluating, and managing intrauterine growth restriction (IUGR).

Objectives

After reading this module and taking this test, you will be able to:

1. Discuss factors helpful for identifying IUGR and distinguishing it from nonpathologic states
2. Outline the common causes and characteristics of IUGR
3. Describe techniques for evaluating fetal health, growth, and development

Directions

To earn continuing education credit, follow these instructions:

1. Read Module 10.
2. Complete the following posttest. Each question has only one answer. Choose the one that is best in each case and darken the corresponding box on the Enrollment Form (Section B).
3. Complete Section A and record your answers to the Evaluation Questions (Section C) on the Enrollment Form.
4. The passing score for this CE activity posttest is 7 correct answers (70%).
5. Registration deadline is April 30, 2004. After this date, please contact Lippincott Williams & Wilkins Continuing Education Department at 212-886-1330.
6. Send the completed Enrollment Form with the appropriate fee (U.S. checks only) to:

Lippincott Williams & Wilkins
Continuing Education Department
345 Hudson Street, 16th Floor
New York, NY 10014

1. Small for gestational age babies:
   A. Have reached their growth potential
   B. Are small as a result of intrauterine stress
   C. Are at considerable risk for poor outcomes
   D. Have a birth weight below the 15th percentile for gestational age

2. With IUGR, fetal death is most common:
   A. After 36 weeks' gestation and after the onset of labor
   B. Before 32 weeks' gestation and after the onset of labor
   C. After 36 weeks' gestation and before the onset of labor
   D. Before 32 weeks' gestation and before the onset of labor

3. Neonatal hypoglycemia is defined as blood glucose levels lower than:
   A. 40 mg/dL both in term and in preterm infants
   B. 40 mg/dL in term infants and lower than 25 mg/dL in preterm infants
   C. 90 mg/dL in term infants and lower than 25 mg/dL in preterm infants
   D. 90 mg/dL in term infants and lower than 40 mg/dL in preterm infants

4. Which of the following is often observed in IUGR newborns?
   A. A larger than usual skull
   B. A limp umbilical cord
   C. Taut, moist skin
   D. Abundant scalp hair

5. The phase of cell growth during which cells increase rapidly in size takes place:
   A. From conception through 16 weeks' gestation
   B. From 16 to 32 weeks' gestation
   C. After 32 weeks' gestation
   D. Consistently throughout gestation

6. Which of the following is a true statement about substance abuse in pregnancy?
   A. Cocaine use reduces blood pressure to dangerous levels.
   B. Alcohol abuse in the second trimester causes fetal alcohol syndrome.
   C. Alcohol abuse in the first trimester causes IUGR.
   D. Alcohol collapses umbilical vessels.

7. Symmetric IUGR is:
   A. Sometimes the result of an infection early in the pregnancy
   B. "Brain sparing" because it redirects nutrients from other organs
   C. About four times more common than asymmetric IUGR
   D. Usually the result of a problem that alters cellular hypertrophy

8. Which of the following ultrasonic parameters, once considered the gold standard for evaluating fetal growth, is now known to be unreliable because of normal variability?
   A. Abdominal circumference
   B. Crown to rump length
   C. Biparietal diameter
   D. Femur length

9. Using the amniotic fluid index (AFI) to screen for oligohydramnios, you note that the largest pocket of fluid found in each of two uterine quadrants measures approximately 2.5 cm. In the third, a 1.5-cm pocket is found, and in the fourth, a 0.5-cm pocket is found. You would conclude that the AFI of:
   A. 3.5 indicates a severe degree of oligohydramnios
   B. 7 indicates a decreased amount of amniotic fluid
   C. 8.5 indicates a decreased amount of amniotic fluid
   D. 10 indicates adequate amniotic fluid

10. A nonstress test is considered reactive when:
    A. Two fetal heart rate accelerations are noted in a 20-minute period
    B. Three uterine contractions are noted in a 10-minute period
    C. Two fetal heart rate accelerations are noted in a 10-minute period
    D. Late decelerations follow at least 50% of all uterine contractions

LIPPINCOTT WILLIAMS & WILKINS
CONTINUING EDUCATION ENROLLMENT FORM

Intrapartum Management Modules
3rd Edition

A Perinatal Education Program

Module 10—Intrauterine Growth Restriction: Perinatal Issues and Management
Nursing CE contact hours: 3.5
Fee: $22.75 (If submitting two or more tests together, deduct $1.00 from each test fee.)
Registration Deadline: April 30, 2004

A. Name (Last) _____ (First) _____ (MI) _____

Address _____

City _____ State _____ Zip _____

Telephone _____ Social Security Number _____

State of Licensure #1 _____ License #1 Number _____

RN ☐   APN ☐   Other _____

State of Licensure #2 _____ License #2 Number _____

RN ☐   APN ☐   Other _____

State of Licensure #3 _____ License #3 Number _____

RN ☐   APN ☐   Other _____

B. There may be more response boxes than there are questions. Please indicate your answers in the appropriate boxes and disregard the extra boxes.

1. a☐   b☐   c☐   d☐   6. a☐   b☐   c☐   d☐
2. a☐   b☐   c☐   d☐   7. a☐   b☐   c☐   d☐
3. a☐   b☐   c☐   d☐   8. a☐   b☐   c☐   d☐
4. a☐   b☐   c☐   d☐   9. a☐   b☐   c☐   d☐
5. a☐   b☐   c☐   d☐   10. a☐   b☐   c☐   d☐

C. EVALUATION QUESTIONS

1. Did this educational activity's learning objectives relate to its general purpose? Yes ☐ No ☐
2. Was this format an effective way to present the material? Yes ☐ No ☐
3. Was the content current to your practice? Yes ☐ No ☐
4. How long did it take you to complete this educational activity? _____ hrs.
5. Suggestions for future topics.

■ ■ ■ ■

INTRAPARTUM MANAGEMENT MODULES
MODULE 11
CARING FOR THE LABORING WOMAN WITH HIV INFECTION OR AIDS

General Purpose: To present registered professional nurses and other providers of women's health care with a detailed overview of HIV infection, with specific guidelines for testing and managing HIV infection and preventing mother-to-baby transmission.

Objectives

After reading this module and taking this test, you will be able to:
1. Discuss factors helpful for understanding HIV infection
2. Outline the criteria for identifying HIV infection
3. Describe interventions for an HIV-infected mother and her baby

Directions

To earn continuing education credit, follow these instructions:
1. Read Module 11.
2. Complete the following posttest. Each question has only one answer. Choose the one that is best in each case and darken the corresponding box on the Enrollment Form (Section B).
3. Complete Section A and record your answers to the Evaluation Questions (Section C) on the Enrollment Form.
4. The passing score for this CE activity posttest is 7 correct answers (70%).
5. Registration deadline is April 30, 2004. After this date, please contact Lippincott Williams & Wilkins Continuing Education Department at 212-886-1330.
6. Send the completed Enrollment Form with the appropriate fee (U.S. checks only) to:

Lippincott Williams & Wilkins
Continuing Education Department
345 Hudson Street, 16th Floor
New York, NY 10014

1. Replication of HIV includes which of the following steps?
   A. Viral DNA is released from the host lymphocyte surface.
   B. Transcription of viral RNA generates multiple copies of viral DNA.
   C. The virus' RNA is converted to DNA via reverse transcription.
   D. Viral RNA is incorporated into host RNA.

2. False-positive enzyme immunosorbent assay (EIA) results are common in people who:
   A. Have hemophilia
   B. Are in the first trimester of pregnancy
   C. Have diabetes
   D. Have never been pregnant

3. An acceptable sequence of confirming HIV infection is:
   A. A positive Western blot confirmed with a reactive EIA
   B. Two reactive EIAs followed by an indeterminate Western blot followed by a positive immunofluorescent antibody test
   C. A positive single-use diagnostic system (SUDS)
   D. A reactive EIA followed by a positive SUDS

4. HIV is transmitted via:
   A. Vaginal secretions
   B. Amniotic fluid
   C. Urine
   D. Cerebrospinal fluid

5. To reduce the risk of vertical transmission of HIV, which of the following is advised?
   A. Giving eye prophylaxis immediately as the infant is delivered
   B. Performing an episiotomy to prevent unexpected blood flow from a perineal tear
   C. Conducting internal fetal monitoring throughout labor
   D. Bathing the infant with soap and water before blood sampling

6. An HIV-infected pregnant woman with a high viral load can reduce her risk of vertical transmission from 25% to 2% with:
   A. Zidovudine (ZDV) therapy
   B. ZDV therapy and vaginal delivery without forceps and without an episiotomy
   C. ZDV therapy and cesarean section as soon as labor begins
   D. ZDV therapy and cesarean section before labor and with amniotic membranes intact

7. All of the following vaccines are considered safe for an HIV-infected pregnant woman except:
   A. The hepatitis B series
   B. The pneumococcal vaccine
   C. Measles/mumps/rubella (MMR)
   D. *Haemophilus influenzae* type B (Hib)

8. Which of the following is recommended for infants of HIV-infected women?
   A. *Pneumocystis carinii* prophylaxis at birth and before initiation of ZDV therapy
   B. A baseline complete blood count with differential just after initiation of ZDV therapy
   C. *Pneumocystis carinii* prophylaxis at 12 weeks of age
   D. Hemoglobin measurements at the completion of ZDV therapy and again at 12 weeks of age

9. Which of the following is used to confirm HIV infection in the baby of an HIV-infected mother?
   A. Western blot
   B. Serial EIAs
   C. DNA polymerase chain reaction
   D. Maternal HIV antibodies in the baby's blood

10. When caring for an HIV-infected woman during delivery and the postpartum period, you would:
    A. Promote maternal–infant contact as soon as possible after delivery
    B. Encourage the mother to breastfeed to foster maternal–infant bonding
    C. Discourage family participation in the birth to reduce the risk of opportunistic infection
    D. Plan your interventions carefully to minimize contact with the mother to reduce your risk of occupational exposure

LIPPINCOTT WILLIAMS & WILKINS
CONTINUING EDUCATION ENROLLMENT FORM

Intrapartum Management Modules
3rd Edition

A Perinatal Education Program

Module 11—Caring for the Laboring Woman With HIV Infection or AIDS
Nursing CE contact hours: 4
Fee: $25.00 (If submitting two or more tests together, deduct $1.00 from each test fee.)
Registration Deadline: April 30, 2004

A. Name (Last) _____ (First) _____ (MI) _____

   Address _____

   City _____ State _____ Zip _____

   Telephone _____ Social Security Number _____

   State of Licensure #1 _____ License #1 Number _____

   RN ☐   APN ☐   Other _____

   State of Licensure #2 _____ License #2 Number _____

   RN ☐   APN ☐   Other _____

   State of Licensure #3 _____ License #3 Number _____

   RN ☐   APN ☐   Other _____

B. There may be more response boxes than there are questions. Please indicate your answers in the appropriate boxes and disregard the extra boxes.

  1. a ☐   b ☐   c ☐   d ☐   6. a ☐   b ☐   c ☐   d ☐
  2. a ☐   b ☐   c ☐   d ☐   7. a ☐   b ☐   c ☐   d ☐
  3. a ☐   b ☐   c ☐   d ☐   8. a ☐   b ☐   c ☐   d ☐
  4. a ☐   b ☐   c ☐   d ☐   9. a ☐   b ☐   c ☐   d ☐
  5. a ☐   b ☐   c ☐   d ☐   10. a ☐   b ☐   c ☐   d ☐

C. EVALUATION QUESTIONS

  1. Did this educational activity's learning objectives relate to its general purpose? Yes ☐ No ☐
  2. Was this format an effective way to present the material? Yes ☐ No ☐
  3. Was the content current to your practice? Yes ☐ No ☐
  4. How long did it take you to complete this educational activity? _____ hrs.
  5. Suggestions for future topics.

Continuing Education Posttests

■ ■ ■ ■

INTRAPARTUM MANAGEMENT MODULES
MODULE 12
HEPATITIS B INFECTION: MATERNAL–NEWBORN MANAGEMENT

General Purpose: To present registered professional nurses and other providers of women's health care with a detailed overview of viral hepatitis and specific guidelines for testing, managing hepatitis infection, and preventing mother-to-baby transmission.

Objectives

After reading this module and taking this test, you will be able to:

1. Discuss factors helpful for understanding viral hepatitis and distinguishing the five types
2. Outline the criteria for identifying hepatitis infection status
3. Discuss interventions for a hepatitis-infected mother and her baby

Directions

To earn continuing education credit, follow these instructions:

1. Read Module 12.
2. Complete the following posttest. Each question has only one answer. Choose the one that is best in each case and darken the box on the Enrollment Form (Section B).
3. Complete Section A and record your answers to the Evaluation Questions (Section C) on the Enrollment Form.
4. The passing score for this CE activity posttest is 7 correct answers (70%).
5. Registration deadline is April 30, 2004. After this date, please contact Lippincott Williams & Wilkins Continuing Education Department at 212-886-1330.
6. Send the completed Enrollment Form with the appropriate fee (U.S. checks only) to:

Lippincott Williams & Wilkins
Continuing Education Department
345 Hudson Street, 16th Floor
New York, NY 10014

1. Which of the following is a true statement about the danger of hepatitis infection during pregnancy and postpartum?
   A. Hepatitis B cannot be transmitted via breast milk.
   B. Hepatitis A is usually much more severe in pregnant women than it is in other individuals.
   C. Maternal antibodies to the hepatitis C virus protect the infant from transmission.
   D. Neonatal mortality is greater with hepatitis E than with any other type of viral hepatitis.

2. Hepatitis B e antigen (HBeAg):
   A. Is found only when the hepatitis B core antigen (HBcAg) is also found
   B. Reflects a high level of hepatitis B infectivity
   C. Seems to be derived from the hepatitis B surface antigen (HBsAg)
   D. Can be detected only through liver biopsy

3. Immunity to hepatitis B is indicated by the presence of:
   A. The antibody to the hepatitis B surface antigen (anti-HBs)
   B. The antibody to the hepatitis B core antigen (anti-HBc)
   C. The antibody to the hepatitis B e antigen (anti-HBe)
   D. The hepatitis B surface antigen (HBsAg)

4. Hepatitis B carriers:
   A. Represent about 25% of adults who acquired acute hepatitis B infection
   B. Always have symptoms intermittently
   C. Show evidence of viral infection on liver biopsy
   D. Can clear HBsAg from their blood despite high levels of anti-HBs

5. The risk of vertical transmission of hepatitis B during pregnancy is greatest when the mother becomes infected:
   A. During the first trimester
   B. During the second trimester
   C. During the third trimester
   D. At any time during the pregnancy because no single trimester increases the infant's risk

6. Maternal hepatitis B infection during pregnancy:
   A. Often goes unrecognized
   B. Results in jaundice and liver tenderness in most women
   C. Usually requires hospitalization and careful dietary restrictions
   D. Causes symptoms within 2 to 3 weeks of exposure

7. Hepatitis B vaccination tends to be less effective in pregnant women who are:
   A. In the third trimester
   B. Smokers
   C. Undernourished
   D. Younger than the age of 18 years

8. The best choice for conferring immediate passive immunity to someone who has had a significant exposure to the hepatitis B virus is:
   A. Recombivax HB
   B. Engerix-B
   C. Hepatitis B immune globulin (HBIG)
   D. A plasma-derived hepatitis B vaccine

9. After a hepatitis B series, boosters are recommended:
   A. After 10 years in all individuals
   B. For immunosuppressed individuals with low antibody titers
   C. For those who have responded adequately to the primary course
   D. For anyone who has since contracted another sexually transmitted disease

10. An infant born to a woman whose hepatitis B status cannot be immediately identified must be:
    A. Given HBIG and hepatitis B vaccine within 24 hours of delivery
    B. Breastfed to receive protection from maternal antibodies
    C. Given HBIG immediately and the hepatitis B vaccine within the first 3 months of life
    D. Considered a carrier

LIPPINCOTT WILLIAMS & WILKINS
CONTINUING EDUCATION ENROLLMENT FORM

Intrapartum Management Modules
3rd Edition

A Perinatal Education Program

Module 12—Hepatitis B Infection: Maternal–Newborn Management
Nursing CE contact hours: 5.5
Fee: $27.50 (If submitting two or more tests together, deduct $1.00 from each test fee.)
Registration Deadline: April 30, 2004

A. Name (Last) _____ (First) _____ (MI) _____

   Address _____

   City _____ State _____ Zip _____

   Telephone _____ Social Security Number _____

   State of Licensure #1 _____ License #1 Number _____

   RN ☐   APN ☐   Other _____

   State of Licensure #2 _____ License #2 Number _____

   RN ☐   APN ☐   Other _____

   State of Licensure #3 _____ License #3 Number _____

   RN ☐   APN ☐   Other _____

B. There may be more response boxes than there are questions. Please indicate your answers in the appropriate boxes and disregard the extra boxes.

   1. a ☐   b ☐   c ☐   d ☐   6. a ☐   b ☐   c ☐   d ☐
   2. a ☐   b ☐   c ☐   d ☐   7. a ☐   b ☐   c ☐   d ☐
   3. a ☐   b ☐   c ☐   d ☐   8. a ☐   b ☐   c ☐   d ☐
   4. a ☐   b ☐   c ☐   d ☐   9. a ☐   b ☐   c ☐   d ☐
   5. a ☐   b ☐   c ☐   d ☐   10. a ☐   b ☐   c ☐   d ☐

C. EVALUATION QUESTIONS

   1. Did this educational activity's learning objectives relate to its general purpose? Yes ☐ No ☐
   2. Was this format an effective way to present the material? Yes ☐ No ☐
   3. Was the content current to your practice? Yes ☐ No ☐
   4. How long did it take you to complete this educational activity? _____ hrs.
   5. Suggestions for future topics.

■ ■ ■ ■

INTRAPARTUM MANAGEMENT MODULES
MODULE 13
CARING FOR THE PREGNANT WOMAN WITH DIABETES

General Purpose: To provide registered professional nurses and other providers of women's health care with information on diabetes during pregnancy, including the physiology, implications, screening guidelines, and management of mother and baby.

Objectives
After reading this module and taking this test, you will be able to:
1. Discuss factors helpful for understanding diabetes during pregnancy
2. Outline the risks to mother and baby, as well as screening recommendations for diabetes during pregnancy
3. Discuss interventions for the pregnant woman with diabetes and her baby

Directions
To earn continuing education credit, follow these instructions:
1. Read Module 13.
2. Complete the following posttest. Each question has only one answer. Choose the one that is best in each case and darken the box on the Enrollment Form (Section B).
3. Complete Section A and record your answers to the Evaluation Questions (Section C) on the Enrollment Form.
4. The passing score for this CE activity posttest is 7 correct answers (70%).
5. Registration deadline is April 30, 2004. After this date, please contact Lippincott Williams & Wilkins Continuing Education Department at 212-886-1330.
6. Send the completed Enrollment Form with the appropriate fee (U.S. checks only) to:

Lippincott Williams & Wilkins
Continuing Education Department
345 Hudson Street, 16th Floor
New York, NY 10014

1. Gestational diabetes is a result of:
   A. Increased insulin secretion
   B. Overeating during pregnancy
   C. Increased insulin resistance
   D. Decreasing levels of human placental lactogen

2. Diabetic women who become pregnant are most likely to have an increased need for insulin:
   A. At the beginning of the first trimester
   B. At the end of the first trimester
   C. During the second and third trimesters
   D. In the postpartum period

3. Which of the following is a true statement about diabetic nephropathy during pregnancy?
   A. Nephropathy with hypertension can lead to intrauterine growth restriction.
   B. Preeclampsia develops in about 50% of women whose urinary protein levels are between 190 and 499 mg/day.
   C. Progression toward renal failure accelerates with pregnancy.
   D. Even without hypertension, nephropathy usually has a profound adverse effect on the fetus.

4. The most common cause of diabetic ketoacidosis in pregnancy is:
   A. Preeclampsia
   B. Infection
   C. Multiparity
   D. Polyhydramnios

5. Maternal hyperglycemia results in fetal:
   A. Distress
   B. Hypotension
   C. Hypoglycemia
   D. Hyperinsulinism

6. A neonate born to a diabetic mother is at risk for:
   A. Hypoglycemia, typically 6 to 12 hours after birth
   B. Hypoglycemia, typically 24 to 48 hours after birth
   C. Hyperglycemia, typically 6 to 12 hours after birth
   D. Hyperglycemia, typically 24 to 48 hours after birth

7. To control maternal blood glucose levels during delivery, which of the following is recommended?
   A. Increasing the woman's morning dose of insulin
   B. Infusing regular insulin to maintain a maternal glucose level between 80 and 120 mg/dL
   C. Infusing only isotonic saline or lactated Ringer's throughout delivery
   D. Adding a long-acting insulin to the usual morning insulin regimen

8. When breastfeeding her infant, a mother with diabetes is likely to experience:
   A. A sudden steady increase in blood glucose over time
   B. An increased need for insulin
   C. Good glycemic control with oral hypoglycemic agents
   D. A 50- to 100-mg/dL decrease in blood sugar during a typical nursing session

9. Which of the following statements about screening for gestational diabetes is true?
   A. Screening is routinely recommended for all pregnant women.
   B. Screening with a 1-hour glucose challenge test is recommended between 24 and 28 weeks' gestation.
   C. Screening with a 3-hour glucose tolerance test is recommended between 18 and 28 weeks' gestation.
   D. Screening is routinely recommended for all underweight pregnant women older than the age of 30 years.

10. Infants of diabetic mothers are especially at risk for shoulder dystocia when:
    A. The first stage of labor is prolonged
    B. It is a preterm delivery
    C. The mother is a primigravida
    D. The baby is macrosomic

LIPPINCOTT WILLIAMS & WILKINS
CONTINUING EDUCATION ENROLLMENT FORM

Intrapartum Management Modules
3rd Edition

A Perinatal Education Program

Module 13—Caring for the Pregnant Woman With Diabetes
Nursing CE contact hours: 3
Fee: $19.75 (If submitting two or more tests together, deduct $1.00 from each test fee.)
Registration Deadline: April 30, 2004

A. Name (Last) _____ (First) _____ (MI) _____

   Address _____

   City _____ State _____ Zip _____

   Telephone _____ Social Security Number _____

   State of Licensure #1 _____ License #1 Number _____

   RN ☐   APN ☐   Other _____

   State of Licensure #2 _____ License #2 Number _____

   RN ☐   APN ☐   Other _____

   State of Licensure #3 _____ License #3 Number _____

   RN ☐   APN ☐   Other _____

B. There may be more response boxes than there are questions. Please indicate your answers in the appropriate boxes and disregard the extra boxes.

   1. a ☐   b ☐   c ☐   d ☐   6. a ☐   b ☐   c ☐   d ☐
   2. a ☐   b ☐   c ☐   d ☐   7. a ☐   b ☐   c ☐   d ☐
   3. a ☐   b ☐   c ☐   d ☐   8. a ☐   b ☐   c ☐   d ☐
   4. a ☐   b ☐   c ☐   d ☐   9. a ☐   b ☐   c ☐   d ☐
   5. a ☐   b ☐   c ☐   d ☐   10. a ☐   b ☐   c ☐   d ☐

C. EVALUATION QUESTIONS

   1. Did this educational activity's learning objectives relate to its general purpose? Yes ☐ No ☐
   2. Was this format an effective way to present the material? Yes ☐ No ☐
   3. Was the content current to your practice? Yes ☐ No ☐
   4. How long did it take you to complete this educational activity? _____ hrs.
   5. Suggestions for future topics.

Continuing Education Posttests

■ ■ ■ ■

INTRAPARTUM MANAGEMENT MODULES
MODULE 14
DELIVERY IN THE ABSENCE OF A PRIMARY CARE PROVIDER

General Purpose: To present registered professional nurses and other providers of women's health care with detailed guidelines for managing an unexpected delivery in the absence of a primary care provider.

Objectives

After reading this module and taking this test, you will be able to:

1. List the signs of imminent delivery and plan appropriate interventions for safe delivery
2. Describe the appropriate actions for handling at least two potential problems during delivery

Directions

To earn continuing education credit, follow these instructions:

1. Read Module 14.
2. Complete the following posttest. Each question has only one answer. Choose the one that is best in each case and darken the box on the Enrollment Form (Section B).
3. Complete Section A and record your answers to the Evaluation Questions (Section C) on the Enrollment Form.
4. The passing score for this CE activity posttest is 7 correct answers (70%).
5. Registration deadline is April 30, 2004. After this date, please contact Lippincott Williams & Wilkins Continuing Education Department at 212-886-1330.
6. Send the completed Enrollment Form with the appropriate fee (U.S. checks only) to:

Lippincott Williams & Wilkins
Continuing Education Department
345 Hudson Street, 16th Floor
New York, NY 10014

1. A sign of impending delivery is:
   A. Spontaneous amniotic membrane rupture
   B. Anal bulging
   C. Strong, regular contractions
   D. Panting respirations

2. You would instruct a woman about to deliver to "feather blow" to help:
   A. Increase intraabdominal pressure
   B. Her control her urge to push
   C. Enhance her uterine contractions
   D. Improve her oxygenation

3. After the baby's head is delivered and before the shoulders are delivered, you would first:
   A. Suction the baby's oropharynx
   B. Stimulate respirations
   C. Suction the baby's nasopharynx
   D. Have the mother push

4. You would manage shoulder dystocia by:
   A. Placing the mother in an upright position
   B. Applying suprapubic pressure from the side opposite the fetal back
   C. Having two attendants pull back on the mother's legs to sharply flex her knees and hips
   D. Trying to manipulate the baby so that the shoulders are in an anteroposterior position

5. If you suspect a hematoma in the perineal area, you would:
   A. Apply firm pressure to the area
   B. Reduce the infusion rate to just enough to keep the vein "open"
   C. Massage the fundus
   D. Take and record the patient's blood pressure and pulse

6. For an unexpected delivery of an infant with a breech presentation, you would:
   A. Maintain a firm hold on the infant's abdomen until the head is delivered
   B. Use a towel to lift the body after the shoulders are delivered
   C. Keep the baby's head flexed using suprapubic pressure
   D. Lower the baby's body to deliver the shoulders

7. If the amniotic membranes do not rupture spontaneously, you would:
   A. Rupture them when the head crowns
   B. Attempt delivery with the membranes intact
   C. Rupture them as the head is delivered
   D. Rupture them before active labor begins

8. If the umbilical cord is tightly wrapped around the baby's neck, you would:
   A. Try to force a loop of cord down over the head
   B. Leave it alone until the baby is delivered and remove it then
   C. Clamp the cord and deliver the baby, then cut the cord
   D. Apply two clamps 1 inch apart, cut the cord between them, and loosen the cord

9. Between delivery of the anterior and the posterior shoulder, you would:
   A. Apply upward, outward traction to the head
   B. Apply upward, inward traction to the head
   C. Apply downward, outward traction to the head
   D. Apply downward, inward traction to the head

10. As you deliver the placenta, you would:
    A. Massage the fundus vigorously
    B. Exert gentle downward traction on the cord
    C. Tug firmly on the cord once you see a gush of blood
    D. Instruct the mother to avoid bearing down

LIPPINCOTT WILLIAMS & WILKINS
CONTINUING EDUCATION ENROLLMENT FORM

Intrapartum Management Modules
3rd Edition

A Perinatal Education Program

Module 14—Delivery in the Absence of a Primary Care Provider
Nursing CE contact hours: 2.5
Fee: $16.75 (If submitting two or more tests together, deduct $1.00 from each test fee.)
Registration Deadline: April 30, 2004

A. Name (Last) _____ (First) _____ (MI) _____

   Address _____

   City _____ State _____ Zip _____

   Telephone _____ Social Security Number _____

   State of Licensure #1 _____ License #1 Number _____

   RN ☐   APN ☐   Other _____

   State of Licensure #2 _____ License #2 Number _____

   RN ☐   APN ☐   Other _____

   State of Licensure #3 _____ License #3 Number _____

   RN ☐   APN ☐   Other _____

B. There may be more response boxes than there are questions. Please indicate your answers in the appropriate boxes and disregard the extra boxes.

1. a ☐	b ☐	c ☐	d ☐	6. a ☐	b ☐	c ☐	d ☐
2. a ☐	b ☐	c ☐	d ☐	7. a ☐	b ☐	c ☐	d ☐
3. a ☐	b ☐	c ☐	d ☐	8. a ☐	b ☐	c ☐	d ☐
4. a ☐	b ☐	c ☐	d ☐	9. a ☐	b ☐	c ☐	d ☐
5. a ☐	b ☐	c ☐	d ☐	10. a ☐	b ☐	c ☐	d ☐

C. EVALUATION QUESTIONS
1. Did this educational activity's learning objectives relate to its general purpose? Yes ☐ No ☐
2. Was this format an effective way to present the material? Yes ☐ No ☐
3. Was the content current to your practice? Yes ☐ No ☐
4. How long did it take you to complete this educational activity? _____ hrs.
5. Suggestions for future topics.

INTRAPARTUM MANAGEMENT MODULES
MODULE 15
ASSESSMENT OF THE NEWBORN AND NEWLY DELIVERED MOTHER

General Purpose: To present registered professional nurses and other providers of women's health care with detailed guidelines for assessing the mother and her baby immediately after delivery.

Objectives

After reading this module and taking this test, you will be able to:

1. Describe assessment parameters for the infant immediately after delivery and plan appropriate interventions
2. Describe assessment parameters for the mother immediately after delivery and plan appropriate interventions
3. Discuss key aspects of infant and mother care after delivery

Directions

To earn continuing education credit, follow these instructions:

1. Read Module 15.
2. Complete the following posttest. Each question has only one answer. Choose the one that is best in each case and darken the corresponding box on the Enrollment Form (Section B).
3. Complete Section A and record your answers to the Evaluation Questions (Section C) on the Enrollment Form.
4. The passing score for this CE activity posttest is 7 correct answers (70%).
5. Registration deadline is April 30, 2004. After this date, please contact Lippincott Williams & Wilkins Continuing Education Department at 212-886-1330.
6. Send the completed Enrollment Form with the appropriate fee (U.S. checks only) to:

Lippincott Williams & Wilkins
Continuing Education Department
345 Hudson Street, 16th Floor
New York, NY 10014

1. A recommended stimulus for evaluating a newborn's reflexes for Apgar scoring is:
   A. Tapping the sole of the infant's foot
   B. Slapping the infant on the buttocks
   C. Pricking the heel for a capillary blood specimen
   D. Taking a rectal temperature

2. The 1-minute Apgar score of an infant with a heart rate of 120 bpm, a sporadic respiratory effort, a grimace response to a catheter placed in the nares, some extremity flexion, and who is mostly pinkish with blue extremities is:
   A. 4
   B. 5
   C. 6
   D. 7

3. Some degree of resuscitation is usually indicated when an infant's Apgar score is below:
   A. 10
   B. 9
   C. 8
   D. 7

4. Cord compression just before delivery is most likely to cause which of the following in the infant?
   A. Respiratory acidosis
   B. Metabolic acidosis
   C. Respiratory alkalosis
   D. Mixed acidosis

5. The appropriate procedure for assessing the fundus after delivery includes:
   A. Cupping your hand and applying pressure just above the symphysis pubis
   B. Starting palpation at midline well above the umbilicus
   C. Calculating fundal height in fingerbreadths above or below the symphysis pubis
   D. Starting palpation at midline just below the umbilicus

6. Normal lochia immediately after delivery should be:
   A. Brown and scant
   B. Red and flowing lightly
   C. Red and flowing moderately
   D. Red and flowing heavily

7. When evaluating fundal height, it is helpful to understand that the fundus:
   A. Might be displaced to one side if the baby was unusually large
   B. Should be at the level of the umbilicus on the second postpartum day
   C. Should be at the level of the symphysis pubis about 5 days after delivery
   D. Might be higher than usual if the uterus contains multiple blood clots

8. Guidelines for assisting with breastfeeding include:
   A. Not initiating breastfeeding until several hours after delivery to be sure the infant is able to suck and to swallow water
   B. Positioning the mother so that she is semireclining
   C. Making sure the mother always begins with the same breast
   D. Encouraging the mother to breastfeed her infant as often as every 2 to 3 hours initially

9. Breastfeeding is contraindicated for women who:
   A. Are recovering from spinal anesthesia
   B. Have preeclampsia
   C. Are HIV positive
   D. Have a boggy uterus

10. When assisting parents whose infant has died, it is helpful to:
    A. Save any declined mementos of the infant in case the parents request them weeks or months later
    B. Dissuade them from holding the child's body for more than a few minutes
    C. Spend as little time as possible with the family, even if asked to stay, so that they can better share their grief with each other privately
    D. Repress one's own feelings about perinatal loss to better focus on the situation at hand

Intrapartum Management Modules
3rd Edition

A Perinatal Education Program

Module 15—Assessment of the Newborn and Newly Delivered Mother
Nursing CE contact hours: 3.5
Fee: $22.75 (If submitting two or more tests together, deduct $1.00 from each test fee.)
Registration Deadline: April 30, 2004

A. Name (Last) _____ (First) _____ (MI) _____

   Address _____

   City _____ State _____ Zip _____

   Telephone _____ Social Security Number _____

   State of Licensure #1 _____ License #1 Number _____

   RN ☐   APN ☐   Other _____

   State of Licensure #2 _____ License #2 Number _____

   RN ☐   APN ☐   Other _____

   State of Licensure #3 _____ License #3 Number _____

   RN ☐   APN ☐   Other _____

B. There may be more response boxes than there are questions. Please indicate your answers in the appropriate boxes and disregard the extra boxes.

1. a ☐	b ☐	c ☐	d ☐	6. a ☐	b ☐	c ☐	d ☐
2. a ☐	b ☐	c ☐	d ☐	7. a ☐	b ☐	c ☐	d ☐
3. a ☐	b ☐	c ☐	d ☐	8. a ☐	b ☐	c ☐	d ☐
4. a ☐	b ☐	c ☐	d ☐	9. a ☐	b ☐	c ☐	d ☐
5. a ☐	b ☐	c ☐	d ☐	10. a ☐	b ☐	c ☐	d ☐

C. EVALUATION QUESTIONS
1. Did this educational activity's learning objectives relate to its general purpose? Yes ☐ No ☐
2. Was this format an effective way to present the material? Yes ☐ No ☐
3. Was the content current to your practice? Yes ☐ No ☐
4. How long did it take you to complete this educational activity? _____ hrs.
5. Suggestions for future topics.

Continuing Education Posttests

■ ■ ■ ■

INTRAPARTUM MANAGEMENT MODULES
MODULE 16
INFORMED CONSENT AND DOCUMENTATION

General Purpose: To present registered professional nurses and other providers of women's health care with an overview of informed consent and nursing documentation as it applies to perinatal care.

Objectives

After reading this module and taking this test, you will be able to:
1. Discuss principles relating to the process of obtaining informed consent
2. Define the standards that apply to counseling a patient about the risks and outcomes of treatment
3. Outline legal requirements for medical documentation

Directions

To earn continuing education credit, follow these instructions:
1. Read Module 16.
2. Complete the following posttest. Each question has only one answer. Choose the one that is best in each case and darken the box on the Enrollment Form (Section B).
3. Complete Section A and record your answers to the Evaluation Questions (Section C) on the Enrollment Form.
4. The passing score for this CE activity posttest is 7 correct answers (70%).
5. Registration deadline is April 30, 2004. After this date, please contact Lippincott Williams & Wilkins Continuing Education Department at 212-886-1330.
6. Send the completed Enrollment Form with the appropriate fee (U.S. checks only) to:

> Lippincott Williams & Wilkins
> Continuing Education Department
> 345 Hudson Street, 16th Floor
> New York, NY 10014

1. The essential components of informed consent are:
   A. Condition, information, and voluntariness
   B. Capacity, information, and permission
   C. Emancipation, information, and permission
   D. Capacity, information, and voluntariness

2. In most states, all of the following qualify a person for emancipated status except:
   A. Getting married
   B. Becoming orphaned
   C. Becoming a parent
   D. Becoming financially independent

3. A patient's need for information about risks specifically related to that particular individual's lifestyle is considered the:
   A. Subjective patient standard
   B. Professional standard
   C. Objective patient standard
   D. Reasonable patient standard

4. A patient's need for information about risks and expected outcomes for that patient is considered the:
   A. Subjective patient standard
   B. Professional standard
   C. Objective patient standard
   D. Reasonable patient standard

5. The informed refusal is:
   A. A patient's decision not to receive treatment
   B. Information given to the patient about that patient's risk when declining to receive treatment or testing
   C. A health care provider's decision not to offer a patient a specific treatment or test
   D. A family's decision to override a patient's wish for a specific treatment

6. Which of the following is a true statement about informed consent?
   A. Written consent must be obtained for every patient contact.
   B. Consent is necessary only for major procedures, such as surgery.
   C. The components of informed consent must be integral to every patient contact.
   D. Written consent is especially necessary when the patient's health is rapidly deteriorating.

7. When an adult patient is comatose:
   A. Informed consent is not needed
   B. Family members may give consent
   C. A cohabitating significant other may give consent
   D. The patient's attorney may give consent

8. When a patient questions the advisability of having a surgical procedure done, the person responsible for answering the patient's questions is:
   A. The nurse
   B. The nurse practitioner
   C. The physician
   D. Any licensed health care professional

9. The correct procedure for correcting an error in a medical chart is:
   A. Erasing the error or obscuring it with liquid correction fluid, writing in the correct information over the error, and writing in the date and time and initialing it
   B. Drawing a line through the error, writing in the correct information just above the crossed-out information, and writing in the date and time and initialing it
   C. Erasing the error or obscuring it with liquid correction fluid, writing in the date and time and initialing it, and entering the new material as an addendum in the next available space
   D. Drawing a line through the error, writing in the date and time and initialing it, and entering the new material as an addendum in the next available space

10. Countersigning another person's charting means that you:
    A. Also provided the documented care to that patient
    B. Approved the care that person gave
    C. Are passing no judgment on that person's care or documentation but are just following your institution's policies
    D. Carry no legal responsibility for that person's actions

LIPPINCOTT WILLIAMS & WILKINS
CONTINUING EDUCATION ENROLLMENT FORM

Intrapartum Management Modules
3rd Edition

A Perinatal Education Program

Module 16—Informed Consent and Documentation
Nursing CE contact hours: 1.5
Fee: $11.75 (If submitting two or more tests together, deduct $1.00 from each test fee.)
Registration Deadline: April 30, 2004

A. Name (Last) _____ (First) _____ (MI) _____

Address _____

City _____ State _____ Zip _____

Telephone _____ Social Security Number _____

State of Licensure #1 _____ License #1 Number _____

RN ☐   APN ☐   Other _____

State of Licensure #2 _____ License #2 Number _____

RN ☐   APN ☐   Other _____

State of Licensure #3 _____ License #3 Number _____

RN ☐   APN ☐   Other _____

B. There may be more response boxes than there are questions. Please indicate your answers in the appropriate boxes and disregard the extra boxes.

1. a☐ b☐ c☐ d☐   6. a☐ b☐ c☐ d☐
2. a☐ b☐ c☐ d☐   7. a☐ b☐ c☐ d☐
3. a☐ b☐ c☐ d☐   8. a☐ b☐ c☐ d☐
4. a☐ b☐ c☐ d☐   9. a☐ b☐ c☐ d☐
5. a☐ b☐ c☐ d☐   10. a☐ b☐ c☐ d☐

C. EVALUATION QUESTIONS
1. Did this educational activity's learning objectives relate to its general purpose? Yes ☐ No ☐
2. Was this format an effective way to present the material? Yes ☐ No ☐
3. Was the content current to your practice? Yes ☐ No ☐
4. How long did it take you to complete this educational activity? _____ hrs.
5. Suggestions for future topics.

Continuing Education Posttests

■ ■ ■ ■

INTRAPARTUM MANAGEMENT MODULES
MODULE 17
MATERNAL TRANSPORT

General Purpose: To present registered professional nurses and other providers of women's health care with detailed guidelines for maternal transport to a regional perinatal center.

Objectives

After reading this module and taking this test, you will be able to:

1. Outline the indications and contraindications for maternal transport to a regional center
2. Describe three interventions for the high-risk mother and her infant

Directions

To earn continuing education credit, follow these instructions:

1. Read Module 17.
2. Complete the following posttest. Each question has only one answer. Choose the one that is best in each case and darken the corresponding box on the Enrollment Form (Section B).
3. Complete Section A and record your answers to the Evaluation Questions (Section C) on the Enrollment Form.
4. The passing score for this CE activity posttest is 7 correct answers (70%).
5. Registration deadline is April 30, 2004. After this date, please contact Lippincott Williams & Wilkins Continuing Education Department at 212-886-1330.
6. Send the completed Enrollment Form with the appropriate fee (U.S. checks only) to:

Lippincott Williams & Wilkins
Continuing Education Department
345 Hudson Street, 16th Floor
New York, NY 10014

1. Transferring a potentially ill infant to a Level III regional center is best:
   A. When delivery is not expected for the next 24 hours
   B. When delivery is expected within the next 12 hours
   C. When delivery is expected within the next 8 hours
   D. Immediately after stabilization postdelivery

2. Transferring a mother who is in early labor and is expected to deliver a compromised neonate is best when:
   A. Delivery is anticipated within 3 hours
   B. Transport time is estimated to be 4 hours or less
   C. The family can transport the mother in a private vehicle
   D. Transport time is estimated to be 2 hours or less

3. Transport to a regional center should be deferred for a mother who:
   A. Has reached term and is 3 cm dilated
   B. Has mild preeclampsia
   C. Is in preterm labor and is 6 cm dilated
   D. Has placenta previa but is not bleeding

4. Which of the following circumstances is least likely to require maternal transport to a regional center?
   A. Preterm labor at 35 weeks' gestation with a fetus likely to weigh more than 2,000 g
   B. Preterm labor at 34 weeks' gestation with a fetus likely to weigh between 1,500 and 2,000 g
   C. Preterm labor at 33 weeks' gestation in a mother with poorly controlled diabetes mellitus
   D. Ruptured amniotic membranes at 33 weeks' gestation

5. A cyanotic neonate is most likely to have a cardiac abnormality when he or she:
   A. Has only peripheral cyanosis
   B. Also has significant respiratory distress
   C. Is term
   D. Experiences a rise in Po_2 while on 100% oxygen

6. A consensus panel sponsored by the National Institutes of Health concluded that corticosteroid therapy:
   A. Decreased the incidence of respiratory distress syndrome (RDS) in infants born between 24 and 28 weeks' gestation
   B. Decreased the severity of RDS in infants born between 24 and 28 weeks' gestation
   C. Decreased both the severity and the incidence of RDS in infants born between 24 and 28 weeks' gestation
   D. Decreased the severity of RDS only in infants born after 29 weeks' gestation

7. Current recommendations for corticosteroid therapy include:
   A. Giving repeat courses of betamethasone or dexamethasone over the entire month before delivery is anticipated
   B. Giving four doses of betamethasone intramuscularly 24 hours apart within 7 days of the anticipated delivery
   C. Giving two doses of dexamethasone intramuscularly 24 hours apart within 14 days of the anticipated delivery
   D. Giving two doses of betamethasone intramuscularly 24 hours apart within 7 days of the anticipated delivery

8. The most appropriate way to transport most women expected to deliver a compromised neonate is by:
   A. Ambulance
   B. Helicopter
   C. Private vehicle
   D. Fixed-wing aircraft

9. When the infant is in the neonatal intensive care unit, it is appropriate to:
   A. Restrict parental visits until the infant is stable
   B. Stay with the parents throughout all visits
   C. Have the attending neonatologist make all decisions about the infant's care
   D. Make sure the parents participate, even if minimally, in the infant's care during visits

10. During maternal transport, the patient should be positioned:
    A. Supine
    B. In high semi-Fowler's
    C. In Trendelenburg
    D. Lying on her right side

LIPPINCOTT WILLIAMS & WILKINS
CONTINUING EDUCATION ENROLLMENT FORM

Intrapartum Management Modules
3rd Edition

A Perinatal Education Program

Module 17—Maternal Transport
Nursing CE contact hours: 1.5
Fee: $11.75 (If submitting two or more tests together, deduct $1.00 from each test fee.)
Registration Deadline: April 30, 2004

A. Name (Last) _____ (First) _____ (MI) _____

Address _____

City _____ State _____ Zip _____

Telephone _____ Social Security Number _____

State of Licensure #1 _____ License #1 Number _____

RN ☐　　APN ☐　　Other _____

State of Licensure #2 _____ License #2 Number _____

RN ☐　　APN ☐　　Other _____

State of Licensure #3 _____ License #3 Number _____

RN ☐　　APN ☐　　Other _____

B. There may be more response boxes than there are questions. Please indicate your answers in the appropriate boxes and disregard the extra boxes.

1. a ☐　b ☐　c ☐　d ☐　　　6. a ☐　b ☐　c ☐　d ☐
2. a ☐　b ☐　c ☐　d ☐　　　7. a ☐　b ☐　c ☐　d ☐
3. a ☐　b ☐　c ☐　d ☐　　　8. a ☐　b ☐　c ☐　d ☐
4. a ☐　b ☐　c ☐　d ☐　　　9. a ☐　b ☐　c ☐　d ☐
5. a ☐　b ☐　c ☐　d ☐　　10. a ☐　b ☐　c ☐　d ☐

C. EVALUATION QUESTIONS
1. Did this educational activity's learning objectives relate to its general purpose? Yes ☐ No ☐
2. Was this format an effective way to present the material? Yes ☐ No ☐
3. Was the content current to your practice? Yes ☐ No ☐
4. How long did it take you to complete this educational activity? _____ hrs.
5. Suggestions for future topics.

■ ■ ■ ■

Self Study Modules
8/12 1 Abnormal Pt Results Not available
2 Aseptic tecnique
3 Basic Chemo precautions
4 CHF
5 Critical test Result
6 Critical thinking
7 Emergency detention
8 How Aging Influences Drug therapy
9 Insulin
10 Issue, transport + verification of
Blood

Housewide
X 1 2006 Blood Comp.
X 2 Administration
Housewide
X 3 Moderate/Deep
+ 4 Restraints Sed
+ 5 waived lab test
X 6 AHA BLS Guideline
7 Self Study Mod